Recent Advances in Immunology

Recent Advances in Immunology

Edited by Avery Steele

hayle
medical

New York

Hayle Medical,
750 Third Avenue, 9th Floor,
New York, NY 10017, USA

Visit us on the World Wide Web at:
www.haylemedical.com

ISBN: 978-1-63241-644-5

Cataloging-in-Publication Data

Recent advances in immunology / edited by Avery Steele.
    p. cm.
Includes bibliographical references and index.
ISBN 978-1-63241-644-5
1. Immunology. 2. Clinical immunology. 3. Immunologic diseases.
4. Serology. I. Steele, Avery.
QR181 .R43 2019
616.079--dc23

Table of Contents

Preface

The main aim of this book is to educate learners and enhance their research focus by presenting diverse topics covering this vast field. This is an advanced book which compiles significant studies by distinguished experts in the area of analysis. This book addresses successive solutions to the challenges arising in the area of application, along with it; the book provides scope for future developments.

Immunology is involved with the study of the immune system and related conditions. Research in immunology is making it increasingly clearer that the development of many disorders, whether metabolic, neurodegenerative or cardiovascular has an immunological contribution. Besides these, infectious diseases such as hepatitis, dysentery, tuberculosis, pneumonia, etc. have a direct correlation with the immune system. The immune conditions affecting the human body can be classified as autoimmune diseases, hypersensitivity and immunodeficiencies. Hypersensitive responses or allergies can be diagnosed with a patch test, allergy blood test, skin test, etc. The treatment of immunological conditions depends on the severity and type of condition. Immunosuppressants, anti-inflammatory drugs and NSAIDs are used for the management of autoimmune diseases. Treatment strategies for boosting the immune system are employed for immune deficiency states. This book contains some path-breaking studies in the field of immunology. It outlines the principles and applications of immunology in detail. Those in search of information to further their knowledge will be greatly assisted by this book.

It was a great honour to edit this book, though there were challenges, as it involved a lot of communication and networking between me and the editorial team. However, the end result was this all-inclusive book covering diverse themes in the field.

Finally, it is important to acknowledge the efforts of the contributors for their excellent chapters, through which a wide variety of issues have been addressed. I would also like to thank my colleagues for their valuable feedback during the making of this book.

Editor

Antigen presenting capacity of murine splenic myeloid cells

Ying-Ying Hey[1,2], Benjamin Quah[3] and Helen C. O'Neill[2*]

Abstract

Background: The spleen is an important site for hematopoiesis. It supports development of myeloid cells from bone marrow-derived precursors entering from blood. Myeloid subsets in spleen are not well characterised although dendritic cell (DC) subsets are clearly defined in terms of phenotype, development and functional role. Recently a novel dendritic-like cell type in spleen named 'L-DC' was distinguished from other known dendritic and myeloid cells by its distinct phenotype and developmental origin. That study also redefined splenic eosinophils as well as resident and inflammatory monocytes in spleen.

Results: L-DC are shown to be distinct from known splenic macrophages and monocyte subsets. Using a new flow cytometric procedure, it has been possible to identify and isolate L-DC in order to assess their functional competence and ability to activate T cells both in vivo and in vitro. L-DC are readily accessible to antigen given intravenously through receptor-mediated endocytosis. They are also capable of $CD8^+$ T cell activation through antigen cross presentation, with subsequent induction of cytotoxic effector T cells. L-DC are $MHCII^-$ cells and unable to activate $CD4^+$ T cells, a property which clearly distinguishes them from conventional DC. The myeloid subsets of resident monocytes, inflammatory monocytes, neutrophils and eosinophils, were found to have varying capacities to take up antigen, but were uniformly unable to activate either $CD4^+$ T cells or $CD8^+$ T cells.

Conclusion: The results presented here demonstrate that L-DC in spleen are distinct from other myeloid cells in that they can process antigen for $CD8^+$ T cell activation and induction of cytotoxic effector function, while both L-DC and myeloid subsets remain unable to activate $CD4^+$ T cells. The L-DC subset in spleen is therefore distinct as an antigen presenting cell.

Keywords: Myeloid cells, Dendritic cells, Antigen presentation/processing, Spleen

Background

Spleen is a secondary lymphoid organ that specialises in filtering blood-borne antigen and recycling the heme group from damaged erythrocytes. The spleen is also important for myelopoiesis, and myeloid cells are primarily located within the red pulp region. The white pulp contains the periarteriolar lymphoid sheath in the T-cell zone, B cell follicles and the marginal zone, located at the interface of the red pulp and the periarteriolar lymphoid sheath for screening blood-borne antigens and pathogens [1, 2]. Multiple subsets of dendritic cells (DC) have been described in spleen, located mainly within the white pulp where immune responses against blood-borne antigens and pathogens are initiated.

The "myeloid" subset in spleen includes granulocytes, monocytes and macrophages. Granulocytes like neutrophils, eosinophils, basophils and mast cells are $Ly6G^+$ cells mainly localised in the red pulp region, with some cells in transition through the marginal zone into red pulp [3]. Monocytes develop in bone marrow from a common myeloid/dendritic cell progenitor [4, 5], and continuously migrate into blood and spleen as mature cells [6]. When monocytes enter tissues they terminally differentiate to give macrophages, although recent evidence suggests that blood precursors may not be the only source of tissue macrophages, with evidence that they can derive from endogenous progenitors of yolk sac and embryonic origin [7–9].

* Correspondence: honeill@bond.edu.au
[2]Clem Jones Research Centre for Regenerative Medicine, Bond University, Gold Coast, Queensland, Australia
Full list of author information is available at the end of the article

Two clear subsets of monocytes were originally identified in blood as the $CX_3CR1^{lo}Ly6C^{hi}$ inflammatory monocytes, and the $CX_3CR1^{hi}Ly6C^-$ resident monocytes [5, 6]. However, the characterization of monocyte subsets in tissues is still in its infancy, and our own recent investigations suggest that these early phenotypic descriptors do not exactly mirror the phenotype of similar subsets in spleen [10]. Current thinking is that inflammatory monocytes, now sometimes referred to as "classical monocytes" [11], home to sites of infection where they induce an inflammatory response, and may also differentiate to give TNF/iNOS-producing dendritic cells [12]. Resident monocytes are sometimes referred to as "non-classical monocytes" and migrate under steady-state conditions as precursors of tissue-resident macrophages, for example in liver, spleen, lung and skin [11, 13]. However, there are still gaps in our knowledge of the relationship between resident macrophages and resident or non-classical monocytes. Some studies now indicate a multitude of pathways for development, influenced by environmental and infectious states, with a recent evidence for the wound healing capacity of some monocytes. A reservoir of undifferentiated monocytes resident in spleen was found to be similar to blood monocytes in terms of phenotype and gene expression [14]. Monocytes were shown to mobilise from spleen into sites of inflammation in heart, with inflammatory monocytes clearing damaged tissues, and resident monocytes promoting wound healing [14].

Spleen also contains several subsets of resident macrophages. Marginal zone metallophilic macrophages stain with the MOMA-1 antibody and are localised near the PALS and B cell follicles [15]. These macrophages are thought to function in induction of cytotoxic T cell responses against blood-borne and self antigens [15, 16]. Marginal zone macrophages are located closer to red pulp and express a number of Toll-like receptors (TLR), the MARCO scavenger receptor and the C-type lectin, SIGNR1, for clearance of microorganisms [15, 17]. Tangible body macrophages in the white pulp of spleen are involved in phagocytosis of apoptotic B cells during germinal center reactions and can be distinguished as $CD11b^-F4/80^-CD68^+$ cells [18]. Red pulp macrophages which clear old or damaged red blood cells and recycle of heme groups, are distinct by F4/80 expression ($CD11b^+F4/80^+CD68^+$) [2]. In addition, macrophages can be further classified as pro-inflammatory (classical) or anti-inflammatory (non-classical) subsets of M1 and M2 macrophages on the basis of functions, adding further functional diversification to the myeloid lineage [19].

Extensive studies on the lineage origin and immune function of splenic DC subsets has led to definition of conventional (c) DC and plasmacytoid (p) DC derived from a common dendritic progenitor in bone marrow [20, 21]. Plasmacytoid-preDC and pre-cDC can then be found in blood [22], and precursors enter and mature in spleen to form three main subsets which activate both $CD4^+$ and $CD8^+$ T cells [22]. The $CD8^+$ and $CD8^-$ subsets of cDC are distinct in production pf interleukin-12 and ability to cross -present antigen to $CD8^+$ T cells [23], while pDC are strong producers of interferon-α in response to viral infection [24, 25]. However, monocyte-derived DC can also form in spleen in response to inflammatory stimuli [26], and these are distinguishable both marker phenotypically and functionally from cDC [6, 27, 28].

A novel subset of dendritic-like cells, namely L-DC, has also been identified in both murine and human spleen [10, 29, 30]. These cells were discovered on the basis of their resemblance to cells produced in splenic long term cultures [31, 32]. An equivalent L-DC subset in spleen has been identified following comprehensive flow cytometric analysis of many splenic myeloid and dendritic subsets [10]. That study distinguished L-DC from cDC subsets, and served to better define the splenic subsets of inflammatory monocytes, resident monocytes and eosinophils in mice [10]. L-DC are now identifiable by their phenotype as $CD11b^{hi}CD11c^{lo}CD43^{lo}CX_3CR1^{lo}$ cells, also lacking expression of MHCII, Ly6C, Ly6G, and Siglec-F. They are clearly distinct from inflammatory monocytes, neutrophils and eosinophils on the basis of phenotype and morphology. Inflammatory monocytes were found to be phenotypically and morphologically distinct from resident monocytes, Resident monocytes were found to be more closely related in phenotype to L-DC than to inflammatory monocytes, although all three subsets were morpologically distinct. In order to assess the functional role of L-DC in relation to resident monocytes and other myeloid subsets, pure populations of cells have been sorted for comparison of their antigen presenting capacity.

Methods

Animal

C57BL/6J, C57BL/6.Tg(TcraTcrb)1100Mjb (OT-I TCR-transgenic (TCR-tg) (anti-H-2K^b/OVA$_{257-264}$), C56BL/6. SJL/J.OT-II.CD45.1 (OT-II TCR-tg (anti-IA^b/OVA$_{323-339}$) mice) and C57BL/6-Tg(CAG-OVA)916Jen:WehiAnu (Act-mOVA) mice were obtained from the John Curtin School of Medical Research at the Australian National University (Canberra, ACT, Australia). Mice were housed and handled according to the guidelines of the Animal Experimentation Ethics Committee at the Australian National University. Mice were euthenased through carbon dioxide asphyxiation.

Fractionation of cells

Dendritic and myeloid cells were separated from splenocytes via negative depletion of T, B and red blood cells using MACS® magnetic bead technology (Miltenyi: Bergisch Gladbach, Germany). Splenocytes were incubated with red blood cell lysis buffer for 5 minutes and washed with fluorescence activated cell sorting (FACS) buffer (1% FSC, 0.1% sodium azide in Dulbecco's Modified Eagle Medium). Cells were then stained with 0.25 µg biotinylated anti-Thy1.2 antibody/10^8 cells (T cells), 0.25 µg biotinylated anti-CD19 antibody/10^8 cells (B cells) and 0.25 µg biotinylated anti-Ter119 antibody/10^8 cells (red blood cells) in 1 mL FACS buffer for 20 min on ice. Cells were washed and supernatant aspirated. They were then resuspended in MACS labelling buffer (2 mM EDTA/0.5% bovine serum albumin in PBS) at 10^8 cells/mL and 20 µl of anti-biotin microbeads/10^8 cells on ice for 25 min. Cells were washed twice in MACS buffer and resuspended in 500 µl of buffer prior to running cells through LS columns (Miltenyi) in a SuperMACS II Separation Unit (Miltenyi). T, B and red blood cells were removed via binding to microbeads in the LS columns. The column was washed thrice with MACS buffer and unbounded cells collected as flow-through.

CD8$^+$ T cells were isolated from OT-I TCR-tg mice specific for ovalbumin (OVA)$_{257-264}$/H-2K^b and CD4$^+$ T cells were isolated from OT-II TCR-tg mice specific for IA^b/OVA$_{323-339}$, using MACS magnetic microbead separation technology as described above. CD8$^+$ T cells were enriched from splenocytes via negative depletion of myeloid cells, granulocytes, DC, B cells and CD4$^+$ T cells using specific antibodies: 0.25 µg biotinylated anti-CD19 antibody/10^8 cells (B cells), 0.25 µg biotinylated anti-MHCII antibody/10^8 cells (DC), 0.25 µg biotinylated anti-Gr1 antibody/10^8 cells (granulocytes and myeloid cells) and 0.25 µg biotinylated anti-CD4 antibody/10^8 cells. Similarly, CD4$^+$ T cells were enriched by substituting antibody to deplete CD8$^+$ T cells in the above cocktail: 0.25 µg biotinylated anti-CD8 antibody/10^8 cells.

Flow cytometry

Methods used for antibody staining and flow cytometry for analysis of cell surface marker expression have been described previously [10, 33, 34]. Prior to antibody staining, non-specific antibody binding to cells was inhibited by absorption of anti-CD16/32 (FcBlock: Biolegend: San Diego, CA, USA) used at 5 µg/10^6 cells in 1 mL of FACS buffer. Fluorochrome- or biotin-conjugated antibodies specific for CD11c (N418), CD11b (M1/70), CD8 (53–6.7), CD19 (1D3), CD43 (IBII), F4/80 (CI:A3-1), Ter119 (Ter119), Thy1.2 (30-H12), Siglec-F (E50-2440), Ly6C (HK1.4), Ly6G (1A8) and I-A/I-E (M5/114.15.2) were purchased from Biolegend. Antibodies specific for CD68 (FA-11) and SIGN-R1 (ER-TR9) were purchased from AbD Serotec. Lastly, antibody specific for MOMA-1 (MOMA-1) was purchased from AbCam. Propidium iodide (PI) staining prior to flow

cytometry was used to distinguish live and dead cells. Flow cytometry was performed on a BD LSRII flow cytometer (Becton Dickinson: Franklin Lakes, NJ, USA). Data were collected in terms of forward scatter, side scatter and multiple fluorescence channels. BD FACSDiva Software (Becton Dickinson) was used to acquire data and analysis post-acquisition employed FlowJo software (Tree Star: Ashland, OR, USA).

For sorting, cells were stained with fluorochrome-labelled antibodies and subsets identified as described in Hey et al. [10] and summarised in Table 1. All incubation and washing steps were performed in sodium azide-free FACS buffer. Sorted populations were collected in complete medium for use in functional assays.

Endocytosis assay

The capacity of cells to take up antigen in vivo was assessed by measuring uptake of labelled antigen using flow cytometry. Ovalbumin conjugated to FITC (OVA-FITC) was delivered intravenously to mice at 1 mg/mouse at different time points, as described previously [30], with spleens collected at the same time (Fig. 2a). Mannan conjugated to FITC (mannan-FITC) was a new compound and so an initial time course study was conducted using 1 mg of mannan-FITC per mouse. A dose response was then conducted using 3 h as the time for maximum uptake (Fig. 2b). Splenocytes were prepared by red blood cell lysis and enrichment of T and B cells by depletion as described above. Cells were then stained with specific antibodies to identify subsets and determine uptake of labelled antigen via flow cytometry.

Cell culture

Cells were cultured in Dulbecco's Modified Eagle Medium supplemented with 22.2 mM D-glucose, 13 µM folic acid, 27 µM L-asparagine, 5.5 mM L-arganine HCL,

Table 1 Phenotypic identification of myeloid and dendritic subsets in spleen

Subsets	Phenotype[a]
CD8$^+$ cDC	CD11b$^-$CD11c^{hi}CD8$^+$CD43$^-$Ly6C$^-$Ly6G$^-$MHCII$^+$
CD8$^-$ cDC	CD11b$^+$CD11c^{hi}CD8$^-$CD43$^-$Ly6C$^-$Ly6G$^-$MHCII$^+$
L-DC	CD11b^{hi}CD11c^{lo}CD8$^-$CD43$^+$Ly6C$^-$Ly6G$^-$MHCII$^-$Siglec-F$^-$
Resident monocytes	CD11b^{hi}CD11c^{lo}CD8$^-$CD43^{hi}Ly6C$^+$Ly6G$^-$MHCII$^-$Siglec-F$^-$
Inflammatory monocytes	CD11b^{hi}CD11c$^-$CD8$^-$CD43$^+$Ly6C^{hi}Ly6G$^-$MHCII$^-$Siglec-F$^-$
Eosinophils	CD11b^{hi}CD11c$^-$CD8$^-$CD43$^+$Ly6C$^+$Ly6G$^-$MHCII$^-$Siglec-F$^+$
Neutrophil	CD11b^{hi}CD11c$^-$CD8$^-$CD43$^+$Ly6C$^+$Ly6G$^+$MHCII$^-$Siglec-F$^-$

[a] Splenocytes were prepared by removal of red blood cells and T and B lymphocytes, and then cells stained with cocktails of antibodies for separation of subsets and sorting using flow cytometry. The phenotype of myeloid subsets was delineated previously in Hey et al. [10]. The phenotype of cDC subsets was taken from Merad et al. [56]

10% heat inactivated fetal calf serum (JRH Biosciences: Lenexa, Kansas, USA), 10 mM Hepes (JRH Biosciences), 2 mM L-glutamine (JRH Biosciences), 17.1 µM streptomycin, 100U penicillin and 50 µM 2-mercaptoethanol (BDH Ltd.: Poole, England) per litre of medium. For culture, cells were maintained in 5% CO_2 in air with 97% humidity at 37 °C.

T cell activation

The ability of sorted dendritic and myeloid cells to activate T cells was measured by their capacity to induce antigen-specific activation and proliferation of anti-OVA $CD4^+$ T cells isolated from OT-II TCR-tg mice, or anti-OVA $CD8^+$ T cells isolated from OT-I TCR-tg mice. Dendritic and myeloid subsets were sorted from splenocytes prepared from transgenic Act-mOVA mice. Sorted cells express OVA peptides on MHCI and MHCII molecules after in vivo uptake and clearance of dead cells in mice. Thus, cDC isolated from Act-mOVA mice can cross-present antigen to $CD8^+$ T cells. Antigen presenting cells (APC) were sorted as described in Hey et al. [10] and summarised in Table 1. Cells were plated in diluting numbers in the presence or absence of lipopolysaccharide (LPS: 10 µg/mL), prior to addition of T cells. In order to measure proliferation, T cells were labelled with 5-(and 6-) carboxyfluorescein diacetate succinimidyl ester (CFSE: Molecular Probes: Eugene, Oregon, USA) as described previously [33]. T cells were labelled at a final concentration of 2.5 µM CFSE per 10^7cells/mL in CFSE labelling buffer (PBS/0.1%BSA). T cells were cocultured with APC and collected after 72 h to determine T cell proliferation flow cytometrically by quantitation of CFSE staining. Proliferation was assessed in terms of dilution of fluorescent stain with each cell division.

Measuring a cytotoxic T cell response in vivo

The ability of APC to induce a cytotoxic T lymphocyte response was investigated via lysis of target cells. Targeted cell lysis was measured using a fluorescent target array developed by Quah et al. [35]. The experimental protocol is summarised in Fig. 4a. On Day 0, $CD8^+$ T cells were isolated from OT-I TCR-Tg mice. Equal numbers of $CD8^+$ T cells were delivered into individual host mice (C57BL/6 J) via intravenous injection (3.5×10^6 cells/mouse). At one hour after delivery of T cells, APC subsets sorted from Act-mOVA mice were also delivered into host mice. Three concentrations of APC were used: 90,000, 9000 and 900 cells. The effector function of activated $CD8^+$ T cells was measured on Day 7 via lysis of peptide-pulsed target cells adoptively transferred intravenously on Day 6. Target cells were isolated from B6. SJL spleen and labelled with CFSE, Cell Trace Violet (Molecular Probes, Invitrogen) and Cell Proliferation

Dye (eBioscience). Splenocytes were resuspended at 0.5-2×10^8 cells/mL in 20 °C in medium and labelled with a final concentration of 0, 400, 2250 and 12,500nM of each dye. Labelled splenocytes were pulsed with SIIN (SIIN-FEKL), N6 (SIINFNKL), G4 (SIIGFEKL) and E1 (EIIN-FEKL), respectively, for an hour at 37 °C. All peptides were synthesised at the Biomolecular Research Facility (Australian National University). Pulsed target cells (2.5×10^7) were delivered intravenously into host mice one day prior to harvesting host splenocytes for flow cytometric analysis of target cells. Flow cytometry was used to estimate the total number of target cells left in spleen. Specific killing of target cells was determined by the following formula which has been described previously [35].

$$\% \text{ specific lysis} = \left[1 - \left(\frac{\text{Targets}_{\text{primed}}^{+\text{peptide}} \Big/ \text{Targets}_{\text{primed}}^{+\text{nil}}}{\text{Targets}_{\text{naive}}^{+\text{peptide}} \Big/ \text{Targets}_{\text{naive}}^{+\text{nil}}} \right) \right] \times 100$$

Statistical analysis

Data have been presented as mean ± standard error for sample size n. Where a normal distribution could be assumed, Students' t-test was used to determine significance ($p \leq 0.05$). For sample size $n \leq 5$, where normal distribution cannot be assumed, the Wilcoxon Rank Sum test was used to test significant ($p \leq 0.05$).

Results

Phenotypic identification of dendritic and myeloid subsets in spleen

A combination of cell surface markers was used to identify DC and myeloid subsets in spleen following a recent published procedure [10]. Conventional DC were gated as $CD11c^{hi}MHCII^+$ cells, then further delineated to give $CD8^+$ cDC and $CD8^-$ cDC on the basis of CD8 and CD11b expression (Table 1). Myeloid cells were initially gated as $CD11b^{hi}CD11c^-$ cells, then further delineated to give neutrophils, inflammatory monocytes and eosinophils on the basis of Ly6C, Ly6G and Siglec-F expression (Table 1). While L-DC and resident monocytes share a common $CD11b^{hi}CD11c^{lo}$ profile, they can be distinguished on the basis of Ly6C, Ly6G, CD43 and CX_3CR1 expression (Table 1) [10].

L-DC are distinct from splenic macrophages

Macrophages have been historically characterised in spleen by immunohistological analysis. While some macrophage-specific markers have been identified, macrophage subsets are not well defined. Expression of markers like MOMA-1, SIGNR1, CD68 and F4/80 was therefore investigated on splenocytes. For each of the four macrophage markers, marker positive cells were initially gated and found to display a majority phenotype (40–50%) as CD11b$^+$CD11c$^-$Ly6C$^{+/-}$Ly6G$^-$ macrophages (data not shown). Subsequently, myeloid subsets and L-DC were gated as described in Table 1 and Hey et al. [10], and assessed for expression of specific macrophage markers (Fig. 1). Gated inflammatory monocytes, eosinophils and neutrophils did not stain for any of the macrophage markers, except F4/80. However, all gated myeloid and DC subsets stained for F4/80, and this is consistent with multiple studies which have demonstrated that F4/80 staining is not restricted to red pulp macrophages

[36–38]. Neither resident monocytes, cDC nor L-DC showed expression of macrophage specific markers (Fig. 1).

Antigen uptake capacity of L-DC compared with myeloid subsets

A primary function of spleen is to filter and trap blood-borne antigens, and this involves uptake and processing of antigen by dendritic and myeloid cells. Antigen presenting cells express a combination of receptors for uptake of antigen of different type via different pathways for endocytosis. In this study, pinocytosis and receptor-

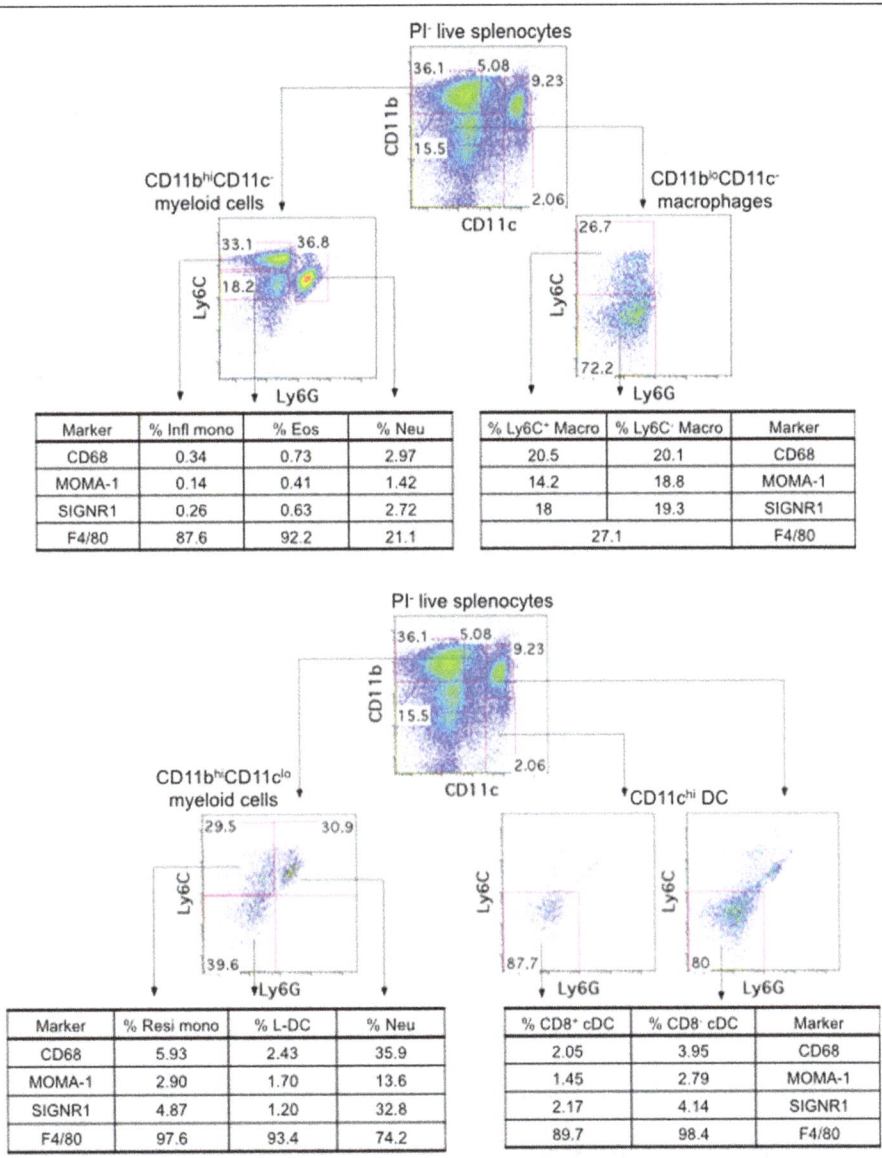

a

Marker	% Infl mono	% Eos	% Neu
CD68	0.34	0.73	2.97
MOMA-1	0.14	0.41	1.42
SIGNR1	0.26	0.63	2.72
F4/80	87.6	92.2	21.1

% Ly6C$^+$ Macro	% Ly6C$^-$ Macro	Marker
20.5	20.1	CD68
14.2	18.8	MOMA-1
18	19.3	SIGNR1
27.1		F4/80

b

Marker	% Resi mono	% L-DC	% Neu
CD68	5.93	2.43	35.9
MOMA-1	2.90	1.70	13.6
SIGNR1	4.87	1.20	32.8
F4/80	97.6	93.4	74.2

% CD8$^+$ cDC	% CD8$^-$ cDC	Marker
2.05	3.95	CD68
1.45	2.79	MOMA-1
2.17	4.14	SIGNR1
89.7	98.4	F4/80

Fig. 1 Expression of macrophage specific markers. Splenocytes were clear of red blood cells by lysis and enriched for myeloid and DC subsets via T and B cell depletion. Cells were then stained with fluorochrome-conjugated antibodies specific for CD11b (PE-Cy7), CD11c (APC), Ly6C (FITC), Ly6G (PE), along with biotinylated antibodies to CD68, MOMA-1, SIGNR1 and F4/80. APC-Cy7-streptavidin was used as a secondary conjugate. L-DC, dendritic and myeloid subsets were gated as described in Table 1 and Hey et al., (2016) [10]. **a** Expression of CD68, MOMA-1, SIGNR1 and F4/80 on inflammatory monocytes (Infl mono), eosinophils (Eos), neutrophils (Neu) and macrophages (Macro). **b** Expression of CD68, MOMA-1, SIGNR1 and F4/80 on resident monocytes (Resi mono), L-DC and cDC subsets. Data are reflective of three independent analyses

mediated endocytosis of antigen were investigated for the splenic myeloid subsets described in Table 1. FITC-labelled antigens were delivered intravenously into mice with subsequent isolation of subsets to compare uptake over time. Pinocytosis was studied by uptake of OVA-FITC as a soluble antigen under conditions described previously [30]. Amongst the splenic myeloid subsets, both resident and inflammatory monocytes showed ability to endocytose and retain OVA, with resident monocytes the most potent (Fig. 2a). Only ~10% of neutrophils and eosinophils took up and retained OVA (Fig. 2a). Their endocytic capacity was relatively weak compared with monocytes (Fig. 2a). L-DC displayed some uptake of OVA, but the level was relatively low compared with monocytes (Fig. 2a).

Mannose receptor-mediated uptake of antigen in DC has been found to contribute to cross-presentation of antigen to CD8[+] T cells [39, 40]. Cross-presentation is a defining property of DC, and is clearly a property of splenic CD8[+] cDC [23]. In order to determine if L-DC and other myeloid subsets can endocytose antigen via mannose receptors, mannan-FITC was prepared and delivered intravenously to mice and cell uptake monitored in a pilot study to determine optimal time for uptake. A further experiment using a 3 h time for uptake, then determined the minimum saturating dose of FITC-mannan as 0.1 mg per mouse. In the time course study, both resident and

inflammatory monocytes demonstrated the strongest ability to take up mannan, with >75% uptake after 1 h, and >50% of resident monocytes retaining mannan after 6 h (Fig. 2b). In contrast, inflammatory monocytes displayed peak uptake of 88% at 3 h, with retention of antigen for 6 h by ~50% of cells (Fig. 2b). Delayed uptake by inflammatory monocytes, could reflect lower accessibility to antigen in comparison with resident monocytes. About 35% of eosinophils took up mannan by 3 h after delivery, but this diminished by 6 h (Fig. 2b). Neutrophils showed no endocytosis of mannan-FITC. Notably, L-DC showed high ability to take up and retain mannan although at lower levels than monocytes (~50%) (Fig. 2b). In the dose response experiment, both L-DC and resident monocytes gave strong early uptake, while inflammatory monocytes required infusion of more FITC-mannan to reach the same level of uptake (Fig. 2b). In an in vivo assay of this type, the level of mannan in cells is indicative of both the accessibility of cells to blood-borne antigen and the endocytic ability of cells. Resident monocytes took up and retained the highest level of mannan, followed by inflammatory monocytes, then L-DC (Fig. 2b).

Ability of splenic myeloid and DC subsets to activate CD4[+] T cells

A known property of antigen presenting DC and some macrophages is their ability to process exogenous

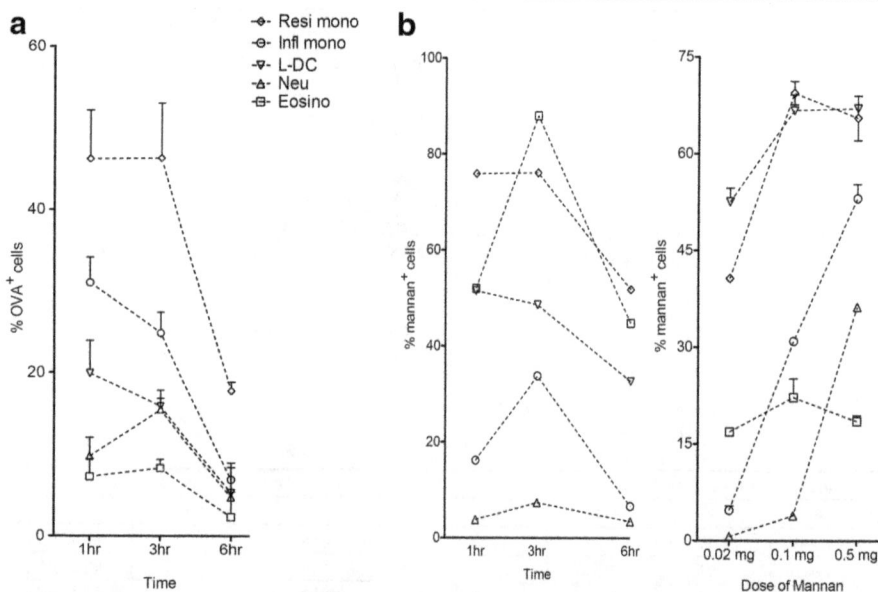

Fig. 2 Comparison of endocytic ability of myeloid and dendritic subsets. The ability of cells to endocytose antigen was measured by uptake of OVA-FITC and mannan-FITC. Spleens were collected for analysis at the same time, and splenocytes prepared by lysis of red blood cells with enrichment for dendritic and myeloid cells via T and B cell depletion. Cells were stained with antibodies to identify L-DC and myeloid subsets as shown in Table 1. Uptake of antigen was assessed in terms of % FITC staining cells. C57BL/6 J mice were given: **a** OVA-FITC at 1, 3, and 6 h prior to euthanasia for spleen collection (intravenously; 1 mg per mouse). Data reflect mean ± SE (n = 4); **b** mannan-FITC (intravenously; 0.5 mg per mouse) at 1, 3 and 6 h prior to euthanasia for spleen collection. Single mice only were analysed tin a pilot study to determibe optimal time of 3 h used in a subsequent dose response experiment. Data reflect mean ± SE (n = 2). Control mice were given PBS

antigen and present it as peptides on MHC-II molecules for CD4[+] T cell activation. Previously it was shown that L-DC generated in vitro in long-term splenic cultures, or in stromal co-cultures, lack ability to activate CD4[+] T cells, consistent with their absence of cell surface MHC-II expression [30, 33, 41]. Improved methodology for distinguishing dendritic and myeloid subsets in spleen now allows the question of the antigen presenting capacity of different subsets to be addressed with more certainty. The Act-mOVA mouse model was employed as a source of OVA antigen-expressing APC. Splenic myeloid and DC subsets were therefore sorted from Act-mOVA mice according to the criteria shown in Table 1, and compared for capacity to induce proliferation of CD4[+] T cells isolated from OT-II TCR-tg anti-OVA mice.

Consistent with the literature [42], CD8[−] cDC were found to be very strong inducers of CD4[+] T cell proliferation (Fig. 3). Neutrophils, inflammatory monocytes and eosinophils induced no CD4[+] T cell proliferation. L-DC and resident monocytes induced no or very low levels of CD4[+] T cell proliferation, equivalent to the control population of only T cells (Fig. 3). The addition of lipopolysaccharide (LPS) as a stimulator of APC did not improve the activation of CD4[+] T cells, except in the case of CD8[−] cDC where there was a minor increase at the highest T cell: APC ratio (Fig. 3). L-DC and monocyte

subsets lacked ability to activate CD4[+] T cells, despite their ability to endocytose and process mannan as an antigen, or OVA as a soluble antigen in the case of resident monocytes. Inability to activate CD4[+] T cells is also consistent with lack of MHC-II expression by L-DC and the two monocyte subsets. These data serve to distinguish L-DC from professional APC like cDC.

Can L-DC cross present antigen for CD8[+] T cell activation?
Cross presentation appears to be a property of DC, and has been clearly demonstrated for the CD8α[+] subset of cDC [42–44]. Early studies suggested that cross presentation was restricted to DC [45], although some macrophage and neutrophil subsets were found to have cross presenting ability under specific conditions [45–50]. The techniques used to isolate pure subsets of cells in those earlier studies were not as specific as those used here. The cross presenting ability of L-DC and the myeloid subsets listed in Table 1 has been assessed in relation to CD8[+] cDC. Subsets were isolated from Act-mOVA mice and used to activate purified OTI (TCR-tg; anti-OVA) CD8[+] T cells. T cells and APC were co-cultured for 72 h at ratios of 33, 100, 300 and 900:1 T cells:APC. The % proliferation of T cells was measured, and the ratio of T cell/APC required to induce 50% proliferation of CD8[+] T cells used to compare data across replicate experiments (Table 2). The

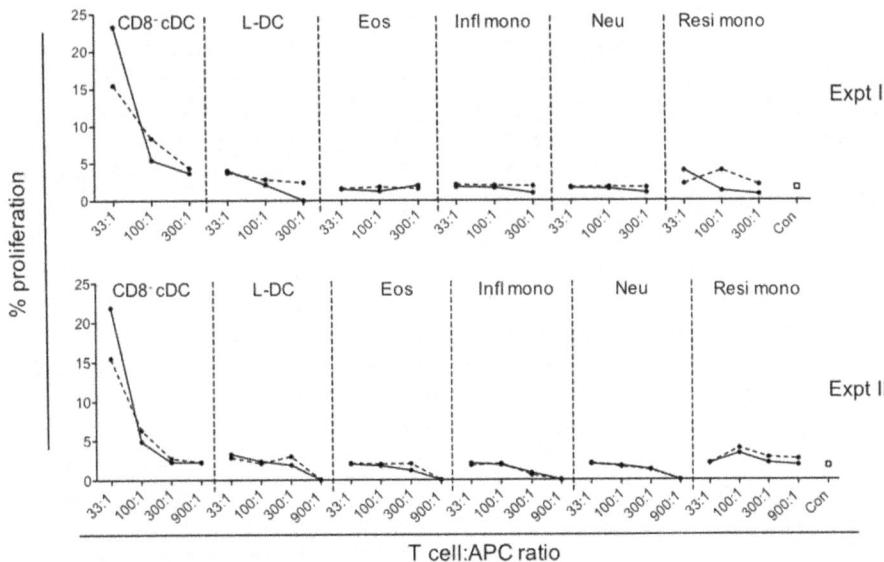

Fig. 3 Activation of CD4[+] T cells by splenic dendritic and myeloid subsets. Antigen presenting ability of myeloid subsets purified from spleens of Act-mOVA mice was assessed. L-DC, eosinophils (Eos), inflammatory monocytes (Infl mono), neutrophils (Neu), resident monocytes (Resi mono) and CD8[−] cDC (as a control), were sorted as described in Table 1 following enrichment of splenocytes by depletion of red blood cells and T and B lymphocytes using magnetic bead technology. Diluting numbers of APC were plated following treatment with LPS (10 μg/ml) (solid line) and without LPS (dotted line) for 2 h. This was followed by addition of 10[5] CFSE-labelled OT-II (TCR-tg) CD4[+] T cells purified from mouse spleen through depletion of B cells, CD8[+] T cells, DC and myeloid cells using magnetic bead protocols. Cells were cultured at T cell:APC ratios of 33:1, 100:1, 300:1 and 900:1 for 72 h. CD4[+] OT-II T cells were then gated as PI[−]Thy1.2[+]Vα2[+]CD8[−] cells, and assessed flow cytometrically for CFSE dilution as an indicator of T cell proliferation. OT-II T cells cultured alone served as controls (con). Graphs show % proliferating OT-II cells. Two independent replicate experiments were conducted

Table 2 Cross priming capability of L-DC compared with myeloid cells

Expt	Condition	T cell: APC ratio giving 50% maximum proliferation of OT-I T cells[ab]				
		L-DC	Resi Mono	Infl mono	Neu	cDC
I	+ LPS	33	-	-	33	300
	- LPS	33	-	-	<33	300
II	+ LPS	33	33	-	-	300
	- LPS	33	<33	-	-	300
III	+ LPS	100	42	-	-	300
	- LPS	100	42	-	-	141
IV	+ LPS	100	42	<33	-	300
	- LPS	100	33	<33	-	300
V	- LPS	100	33	0	<33	-
VI	+ LPS	141	0	-	<33	-
	- LPS	100	0	-	<33	-

[a]For preparation of APC, splenocytes were harvested from Act-mOVA mice and prepared by red blood cell lysis followed by T and B cell depletion. L-DC, cDC, resident monocytes (Resi mono), inflammatory monocytes (Infl mono), neutrophils (Neu) were sorted as described in Table 1
[b] APC, with and without LPS (10ug/ml), were cocultured with 10^5 CFSE-labelled OT-I (TCR-tg) CD8$^+$ T cells, sorted as PI$^-$Thy1.2$^+$Va2$^+$CD4$^-$ cells, at T cell:APC ratios of 33, 100, 300 and 900:1. After 72 h, CD8$^+$ OT-I T cells were gated as PI$^-$CD11b$^-$Thy1.2$^+$Va2$^+$ cells, and CFSE dilution assessed flow cytometrically to estimate % proliferating T cells. OT-I T cells alone served as a control (Con)

assay was performed in the presence and absence of LPS which can act as a potent inflammatory stimulus for some APC [51]. Consistent with previous reports in the literature, CD8$^+$ cDC were superior in their ability to cross present antigen for CD8$^+$ T cell activation and proliferation (Table 2), and this was shown over 6 independent experiments. In these experiments, neutrophils and inflammatory monocytes did not induce T cell proliferation through cross presentation of antigen. L-DC were up to 3-fold better activators of T cell proliferation than resident monocytes, but also 3-fold less effective than cDC in cross presentation of antigen for CD8$^+$ T cell activation. In most experiments, the proliferation of T cells was not increased in the presence of LPS, suggesting it is not an activator of most of the APC subsets tested here. While outcomes from different experiments varied slightly, there was an overall trend showing that L-DC were better APC than resident monocytes, but were less effective than cDC. Inflammatory monocytes and neutrophils did not activate T cells.

Induction of cytotoxic T cells by L-DC
The ability of APC to induce cytotoxic effector function along with proliferation of CD8$^+$ T cells was tested by adoptive transfer in vivo. Experiments compared the ability of L-DC, resident monocytes and CD8$^+$ cDC to induce cytotoxic effector function in CD8$^+$ T cells using an in vivo cytotoxic killing assay developed by Quah et al. [35]. Sorted CD8$^+$ OT-I (TCR-tg; anti-OVA) T cells

were delivered intravenously into mice one hour ahead of APC sorted from ACTm-OVA mice as described in Table 1. Three doses of sorted APC were given to mice: 90,000, 9,000 and 900 cells. Six days later, labelled peptide-pulsed splenocytes were delivered intravenously to act as target cells for cytotoxic effectors primed by the sorted APC (Fig. 4a). At 1-day after delivery of target cells, host splenocytes were harvested to quantitate number of viable target cells in spleen to estimate % target cell lysis (Fig. 4). Ahead of adoptive transfer, target splenocytes were labelled with three different dyes used at four different concentrations. These were then pulsed with four different OVA peptides, either (SIIN) SIIN-FEKL, N6 (SIINFNKL), G4 (SIIGFEKL) or E1 (EII-FEKL), used at six different concentrations, so creating a multiplex assay. OT-I T cells can recognise the SIIN peptide but not the G4 and E1 peptides included as negative controls. The N6 peptide is a variant of SIIN peptide with phenylalanine and glutamic acid removed, which is also recognised by OT-I T cells. The response to N6 peptide determined in this in vivo response was of similar magnitude to that induced by the specific SIIN peptide. This could be a feature of this highly sensitive in vivo cytotoxic T cell assay [35].

The APC subsets of L-DC, resident monocytes and CD8$^+$ cDC each induced cytotoxic T lymphocytes which then lysed target cells pulsed with SIIN and N6 peptides, but not target cells pulsed with the G4 or E1 peptides (Fig. 4b). In addition, the level of lysis of target cells reduced with decreasing concentration of peptides used to pulse APC, and the number of APC used to prime host mice (Fig. 4b). In order to directly compare APC subsets, the concentration of peptide required to prime cytotoxic T cells for 50% lysis of target cells was determined for each APC. With the N6 peptide, cytotoxic T cells generated by priming with 9,000 resident monocytes required 100 times more peptide to induce 50% lysis of target cells in comparison with L-DC and CD8$^+$ cDC (Table 3). After priming with 90,000 APC, cytotoxic T lymphocytes generated using CD8$^+$ cDC as APC, required 10 times more SIIN peptide to give 50% lysis of target cells in comparison with L-DC and resident monocytes (Table 3). When the number of priming APC was reduced to 9,000, cytotoxic T cells generated by resident monocytes required a higher concentration of SIIN to induce 50% lysis of target cells when compared with L-DC and CD8$^+$ cDC (Table 3). Overall, resident monocytes were weaker inducers of a cytotoxic T lymphocyte response in comparison with L-DC and CD8$^+$ cDC, which appear to induce similar cytotoxic effector responses.

Discussion
Spleen plays a central role in immunity to blood-borne pathogens and cancer antigens. Ineffective immunity to

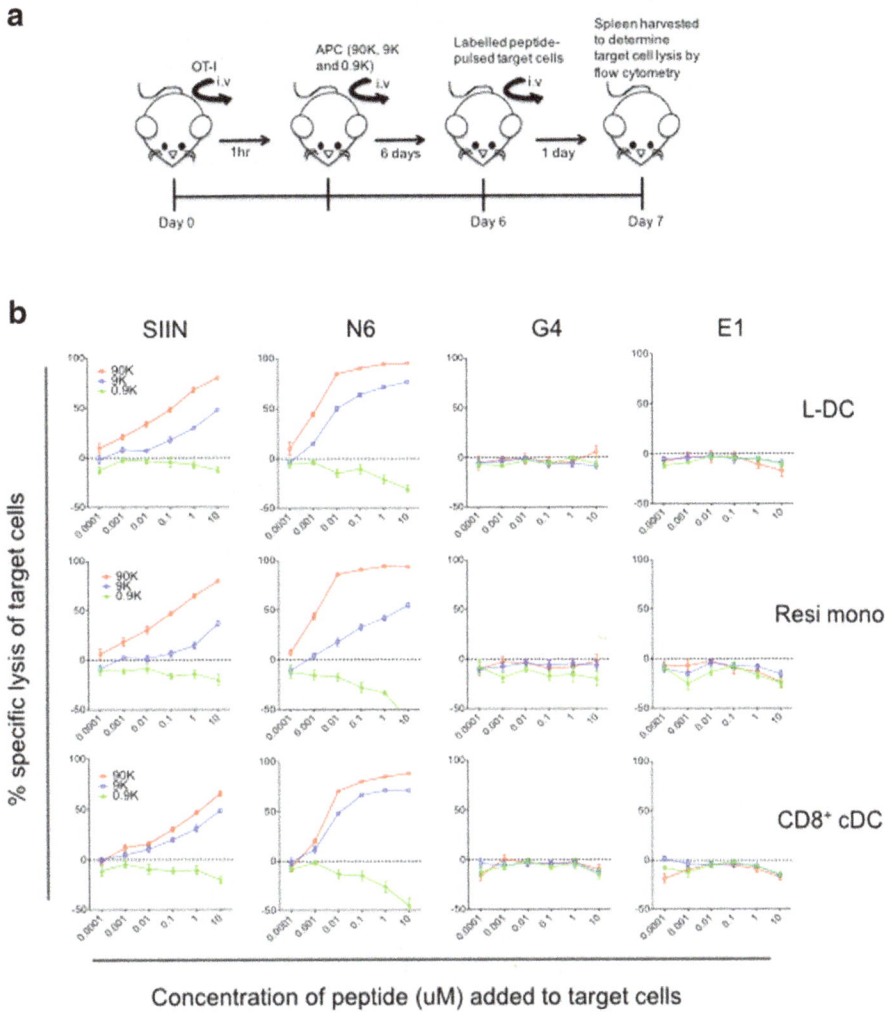

Fig. 4 Ability of splenic APC to induce a cytotoxic T cell response. The ability of APC subsets to induce cytotoxic effector function in CD8+ T cells was assessed by measuring lysis of OVA peptide-pulsed target cells in a fluorescent target assay (FTA). **a** The experimental procedure is shown as a timeline. On Day 0, CD8+ T cells from OT-I TCR-Tg mice were prepared by red blood cell lysis of splenocytes and sorting for PI-Thy1.2+Vα2+CD4- cells. OT-I T cells (3.5 × 10^6) were delivered intravenously into host mice (C57BL/6). An hour later, several APC subsets sorted from Act-mOVA mice were also delivered into host mice. These were sorted as described in Table 1 and three cell doses (90 K, 9 K or 0.9 K) given intravenously. In order to measure the effector function of activated CD8+ T cells after 7 days, B6. SJL splenocytes were prepared as targets and adoptively transferred intravenously on Day 6. Target cells were labelled with several concentrations of CFSE, CTV and CPD for later identification. Overall, labelled target cells were then pulsed with 6 different concentrations of 4 distinct OVA peptides: SIINFEKL (SIIN), GLEQLESIINFEKL (N6), SIIGFEKL (G4) and EIINFEKL (E1). Specific killing of the distinctly labelled, antigen-pulsed target cells was determined by flow cytometric analysis to determine the number of target cells remaining in the test mouse compared with the control mouse given OT-I T cells only. Calculation of target lysis involved the formula described in Materials and Methods. **b** Data shows % specific lysis of target cells pulsed with different concentrations of peptides by OT-I T cells primed with three different APC types. Data is expressed as mean ± SE (n = 6)

bacteria at the level of spleen results in sepsis which can be both lethal and a costly complication of surgery and emergency medicine. Perisinusoidal niches housing hematopoietic stem cells were recently described in spleen red pulp [52], and this finding now opens fresh debate about the specific contribution of spleen to myelopoiesis and immunity. While the DC subsets in spleen have been well defined, other myeloid cells have not been systematically identified, with subset characterisation based only on the phenotype of similar cells in blood. With recent systematic identification of dendritic and myeloid subsets in spleen, and redefinition of monocytes and eosinophils [10], it is now possible to compare these subsets in terms of their capacity to uptake antigen, to activate CD4+ T cells, and to cross prime CD8+ T cells.

Several distinct dendritic and myeloid subsets were compared initially for capacity to endocytose antigen in vivo. While L-DC and resident monocytes have a similar CD11c^lo CD11b^hiMHCII- phenotype, differing in expression of

Table 3 Capacity of splenic subset to induce a cytotoxic T cell response

Peptide	No. APC from Actm-OVA mice used for priming[a] Targets:	Concentration of peptide (uM) required to activate CTL for 50% lysis of targets		
		L-DC	Resi Mono	CD8+cDC
SIIN	90 K	0.1	0.1	1.0
	9 K	10.0	>> 10	10.0
	0.9 K	0	0	0
N6	90 K	0.001	0.001	0.001
	9 K	0.01	1.0	0.01
	0.9 K	0	0	0
G4	90 K	0	0	0
	9 K	0	0	0
	0.9 K	0	0	0
E1	90 K	0	0	0
	9 K	0	0	0
	0.9 K	0	0	0

[a] The table summarises data obtained from the fluorescent target experiment described in Fig. 3. Mice were given sorted OT-I CD8+ T cells ahead of APC sorted from Act-mOVA mice. These included L-DC, Resident monocytes (Resi mono) and CD8+ cDC. Target cells were added after 6 days, and their lysis measured in terms of % cell recovery at 24 h

Ly6C, CD43 and CX$_3$CR1 (Table 1), they have very distinct antigen uptake abilities. Resident monocytes demonstrated superior ability to pinocytose soluble antigen in vivo, while L-DC were very weak, like eosinophils and neutrophils. However, L-DC and resident monocytes both showed high capacity for uptake of antigen by receptor-mediated endocytosis. Despite this similarity, only L-DC and not resident monocytes, could activate CD8+ T cells and induce cytotoxic effector cells. L-DC were also distinct from neutrophils which did not undergo receptor-mediated endocytosis or cross presentation. As shown previously by others, CD8+ cDC were highly endocytic of both soluble and particulate antigen, although resident and inflammatory monocytes demonstrated stronger receptor-mediated uptake. Previously, antigen uptake via mannose receptors was correlated with cross priming ability in DC [39, 40], although that study did not investigate the comparative ability of other myeloid subsets. Here we have been able to demonstrate that both resident and inflammatory monocyte subsets cannot cross prime CD8+ T cells, despite strong ability to take up antigen via mannose receptors. This suggests that cross presentation of antigen is unlinked to that antigen uptake pathway, and may require specific uptake or processing mechanisms.

One main aim of this project has been to compare L-DC with resident monocytes and cDC subsets in terms of capacity for T cell activation. A major limitation for in vitro studies of antigen presentation has been the low number of dendritic and myeloid cells present in spleen, and the difficulty of their isolation. Both CD8+ cDC and L-DC are very rare cell types, representing <1% of splenic leukocytes, and resident monocytes represent a 3-4-fold smaller population [10]. In order to overcome the limitation of low cell numbers, the Act-mOVA mouse model was used as a source of APC. These mice constitutively express high levels of cell-associated OVA under the actin promotor, and isolated APC express OVA peptides in association with MHCI and MHCII, without the need for antigen pulsing and washing of cells. In the animal, APC acquire OVA as an exogenous antigen through uptake of dead and dying cells then presented on MHCI and MHCII. However, when OVA is transcribed and expressed within the cell, there is also the possibility that OVA enters the endogenous antigen processing pathway whereby defective OVA is ubiquitin tagged for destruction in the cytoplasm. Since this type of processing could occur in all cells including APC, it has been necessary to use a control cell population as an indicator of endogenous cross presentation. In experiments described here, neutrophils which do not cross present antigen in the steady-state have served as an adequate control. In all experiments they induced little or no response in either CD8+ or CD4+ T cells.

Activation of CD4+ T cells is essential for induction of T helper cells, which then activate B cells and macrophages. Both CD8+ and CD8− cDC induce activation of CD4+ T cells, although CD8− cDC have been described as the strongest inducers [53]. Consistent with those findings, CD8− cDC were shown to be strong activators of CD4+ T cells, while L-DC which lack MHCII expression show no capacity common to other MHCII− myeloid cell types like eosinophils, neutrophils, inflammatory monocytes and resident monocytes. This is consistent with previous findings on L-DC produced in longterm spleen co-cultures, and in spleen stromal co-cultures [30, 33, 41].

While cross presentation is recognised as a characteristic property of DC, questions still remain as to the cross presenting capability of monocytes/macrophages and other myeloid subsets. Interpretation of published data is limited by the purity and certainty of subsets isolated for analysis, and of the conditions under which cells have been assessed. Indeed, a number of studies have described macrophages and neutrophils as able to cross present antigens to CD8+ T cells under inflammatory conditions. For example, it was recently shown that neutrophils from inflammatory peritoneal exudates could cross-prime CD8+ T cells both in vivo and in vitro [46, 54], While those studies demonstrated cross-priming by neutrophils, the described response occurred only under inflammation and so would not be reflective of neutrophils in steady-state spleen. Here two distinct assays have been used to analyse cross presenting ability, involving both in vitro and in vivo analyses, and measurement of a response in terms of both T cell proliferation and induction of T cell cytotoxicity. Both of these approaches have demonstrated the capacity of both cDC and L-DC to cross present antigen. Resident monocytes were quite distinctly different, at least 10-fold weaker then cDC, and 3- or 10-fold weaker than L-DC across two assays. Inflammatory monocytes and neutrophils were also incapable of cross presentation, and at least 10-fold weaker than cDC in inducing T cell proliferation. The treatment of all APC subsets with LPS did not improve activation of CD8[+] T cells. Since L-DC were insensitive to LPS activation, it is unlikely that L-DC are monocyte-derived DC.

Cross priming for activation of CD8[+] T cells is essential in the generation of cytotoxic T lymphocytes [55]. Cytotoxic T lymphocytes play an important dual functional role in maintaining self-tolerance by lysing self-targets and infected or cancerous cells. The ability of APC to cross present antigen and to induce cytotoxic T lymphocytes was investigated using a fluorescent target array which assesses cytotoxic T cell formation within the animal, where lytic activity against target cells is directly measured [35]. Cytotoxic T lymphocytes generated by OVA-expressing L-DC, lysed target cells pulsed with the SIIN and N6 peptides of OVA, but not with the G4 and E1 peptides. The cytotoxic T cell response induced was antigen-specific, since OT-I CD8[+] T cells can only recognise SIIN and N6 peptides in the context of MHCI. Similarly, both CD8[+] cDC and resident monocytes generated cytotoxic T lymphocytes which gave antigen-specific lysis of target cells when 9,000 APC were used, although at 90,000 APC, the activation capacity of CD8[+] cDC was 10-fold lower. We attribute this to a saturation response in the presence of too many cells and too much peptide antigen. However, resident monocytes required a much higher concentration of peptide on target cells to give a similar level of lysis. Thus, resident monocytes are weaker inducers of cytotoxic T lymphocytes than both L-DC and CD8[+] cDC, consistent with their lack of cross-presenting ability. These data serve to functionally distinguish the L-DC and resident monocyte subsets despite their similar but distinct phenotypes.

Conclusion

This study identifies the distinct functional capacity of L-DC in terms of antigen presenting ability for CD4[+] and CD8[+] T cells. L-DC have been shown to be both phenotypically and functionally distinct from cDC subsets, resident and inflammatory monocytes, as well as neutrophils and eosinophils. They are not macrophages since they do not express markers which identify macrophage subsets unique to spleen. L-DC reflect a unique subset of cells resembling myeloid cells by phenotype, but a dendritic-like cell in terms of morphology, function in cross presentation, and ability to induce a cytotoxic T cell response.

Abbreviations
APC: Antigen presenting cell; cDC: Conventional DC; CFSE: Carboxyfluorescein diacetate succinimidyl ester; DC: Dendritic cell; LPS: Lipopolysaccharide; OVA: Ovalbumin; pDC: Plasmacytoid DC; PI: Propidium iodide; TCR-tg: TCR transgenic

Acknowledgements
Mannan-FITC used in the endocytosis assays was kindly donated by Dr. Craig Freeman (John Curtin School of Medical Research, Australian National University, Canberra, Australia).

Funding
This work was supported by funding from the National Health and Medical Research Council of Australia to HO (Project grant #585443). YH was supported by an Australian National University Graduate School scholarship.

Authors' contributions
This study was designed by YH, BQ and HO. Data collection and analysis was performed by YH and BQ. YH wrote the first draft. YH and HO prepared the final manuscript which was approved by all authors.

Competing interests
The authors declare that they have no competing interests.

Author details
[1]Research School of Biology, Australian National University, Canberra, ACT, Australia. [2]Clem Jones Research Centre for Regenerative Medicine, Bond University, Gold Coast, Queensland, Australia. [3]John Curtin School of Medical Research, Australian National University, Canberra, Australia.

References
1. Cesta MF. Normal structure, function, and histology of the spleen. Toxicol Pathol. 2006;34(5):455–65.
2. Kurotaki D, Uede T, Tamura T. Functions and development of red pulp macrophages. Microbiol Immunol. 2015;59(2):55–62.
3. Nolte MA, Hoen ENM T, Van Stijn A, Kraal G, Mebius RE. Isolation of the intact white pulp. Quantitative and qualitative analysis of the cellular composition of the splenic compartments. Eur J Immunol. 2000;30(2): 626–34.
4. Akashi K, Traver D, Miyamoto T, Weissman IL. A clonogenic common myeloid progenitor that gives rise to all myeloid lineages. Nature. 2000; 404(6774):193–7.
5. Yona S, Kim KW, Wolf Y, Mildner A, Varol D, Breker M, Strauss-Ayali D, Viukov S, Guilliams M, Misharin A, et al. Fate mapping reveals origins and dynamics of monocytes and tissue macrophages under homeostasis. Immunity. 2013; 38:79–91.
6. Geissmann F, Auffray C, Palframan R, Wirrig C, Ciocca A, Campisi L, Narni-Mancinelli E, Lauvau G. Blood monocytes: distinct subsets, how they relate to dendritic cells, and their possible roles in the regulation of T-cell responses. Immunol Cell Biol. 2008;86(5):398–408.

7. Hashimoto D, Chow A, Noizat C, Teo P, Beasley MB, Leboeuf M, Becker CD, See P, Price J, Lucas D, et al. Tissue-resident macrophages self-maintain locally throughout adult life with minimal contribution from circulating monocytes. Immunity. 2013;38(4):792–804.

8. Schulz C, Perdiguero EG, Chorro L, Szabo-Rogers H, Cagnard N, Kierdorf K, Prinz M, Wu B, Jacobsen SEW, Pollard JW, et al. A lineage of myeloid cells independent of myb and hematopoietic stem cells. Science. 2012;335(6077): 86–90.

9. van de Laar L, Saelens W, De Prijck S, Martens L, Scott CL, Van Isterdael G, Hoffmann E, Beyaert R, Saeys Y, Lambrecht BN, et al. Yolk sac macrophages, fetal liver, and adult monocytes can colonize an empty niche and develop into functional tissue-resident macrophages. Immunity. 2016;44(4):755–68.

10. Hey YY, Tan JKH, O'Neill HC. Redefining myeloid cell subsets in murine spleen. Front Immunol. 2016. https://doi.org/10.3389/fimmu.2015.00652.

11. Geissmann F, Gordon S, Hume DA, Mowat AM, Randolph GJ. Unravelling mononuclear phagocyte heterogeneity. Nat Rev Immunol. 2010;10(6):453–60.

12. Serbina NV, Salazar-Mather TP, Biron CA, Kuziel WA, Pamer EG. TNF/iNOS-producing dendritic cells mediate innate immune defense against bacterial infection. Immunity. 2003;19(1):59–70.

13. Geissmann F, Jung S, Littman DR. Blood monocytes consist of two principal subsets with distinct migratory properties. Immunity. 2003;19(1):71–82.

14. Swirski FK, Nahrendorf M, Etzrodt M, Wildgruber M, Cortez-Retamozo V, Panizzi P, Figueiredo JL, Kohler RH, Chudnovskiy A, Waterman P, et al. Identification of splenic reservoir monocytes and their deployment to inflammatory sites. Science. 2009;325(5940):612–6.

15. Mebius RE, Kraal G. Structure and function of the spleen. Nat Rev Immunol. 2005;5(8):606–16.

16. Backer R, Schwandt T, Greuter M, Oosting M, Jüngerkes F, Tüting T, Boon L, O'Toole T, Kraal G, Limmer A, et al. Effective collaboration between marginal metallophilic macrophages and CD8+ dendritic cells in the generation of cytotoxic T cells. Proc Natl Acad Sci U S A. 2010;107(1):216–21.

17. Kang YS, Yamazaki S, Iyoda T, Pack M, Bruening SA, Kim JY, Takahara K, Inaba K, Steinman RM, Park CG. SIGN-R1, a novel C-type lectin expressed by marginal zone macrophages in spleen, mediates uptake of the polysaccharide dextran. Int Immunol. 2003;15(2):177–86.

18. Noel G, Guo X, Wang Q, Schwemberger S, Byrum D, Ogle C. Postburn monocytes are the major producers of TNF-alpha in the heterogeneous splenic macrophage population. Shock. 2007;27(3):312–9.

19. Italiani P, Boraschi D. From monocytes to M1/M2 macrophages: phenotypical vs. functional differentiation. Front Immunol. 2014;5:514.

20. Naik SH, Sathe P, Park HY, Metcalf D, Proietto AI, Dakic A, Carotta S, O'Keeffe M, Bahlo M, Papenfuss A, et al. Development of plasmacytoid and conventional dendritic cell subtypes from single precursor cells derived in vitro and in vivo. Nat Immunol. 2007;8(11):1217–26.

21. Onai N, Obata-Onai A, Schmid MA, Ohteki T, Jarrossay D, Manz MG. Identification of clonogenic common Flt3 + M-CSFR+ plasmacytoid and conventional dendritic cell progenitors in mouse bone marrow. Nat Immunol. 2007;8(11):1207–16.

22. Naik SH, Metcalf D, van Nieuwenhuijze A, Wicks I, Wu L, O'Keeffe M, Shortman K. Intrasplenic steady-state dendritic cell precursors that are distinct from monocytes. Nat Immunol. 2006;7:663–71.

23. Heath WR, Belz GT, Behrens GMN, Smith CM, Forehan SP, Parish IA, Davey GM, Wilson NS, Carbone FR, Villadangos JA. Cross-presentation, dendritic cell subsets, and the generation of immunity to cellular antigens. Immunol Rev. 2004;199:9–26.

24. Cella M, Jarrossay D, Faccheth F, Alebardi O, Nakajima H, Lanzavecchia A, Colonna M. Plasmacytoid monocytes migrate to inflamed lymph nodes and produce large amounts of type I interferon. Nat Med. 1999;5(8):919–23.

25. Kadowaki N, Antonenko S, Lau JYN, Liu YJ. Natural interferon α/β-producing cells link innate and adaptive immunity. J Exp Med. 2000;192(2):219–25.

26. Randolph GJ, Beaulieu S, Lebecque S, Steinman RM, Muller WA. Differentiation of monocytes into dendritic cells in a model of transendothelial trafficking. Science. 1998;282(5388):480–3.

27. León B, López-Bravo M, Ardavín C. Monocyte-derived dendritic cells. Semin Immunol. 2005;17(4):313–8.

28. León B, López-Bravo M, Ardavín C. Monocyte-derived dendritic cells formed at the infection site control the induction of protective T helper 1 responses against leishmania. Immunity. 2007;26(4):519–31.

29. Petvises S, Talaulikar D, O/'Neill HC. Delineation of a novel dendritic-like subset in human spleen. Cell Mol Immunol. 2015;13:443–50.

30. Tan JKH, Quah BJC, Griffiths KL, Periasamy P, Hey YY, O'Neill HC. Identification of a novel antigen cross-presenting cell type in spleen. J Cell Mol Med. 2011;15(5):1189–99.

31. Quah B, Ni K, O'Neill HC. In vitro hematopoiesis produces a distinct class of immature dendritic cells from spleen progenitors with limited T cell stimulation capacity. Int Immunol. 2004;16:567–77.

32. Wilson HL, Ni K, O'Neill HC. Identification of progenitor cells in long-term spleen stromal cultures that produce immature dendritic cells. Proc Natl Acad Sci U S A. 2000;97(9):4784–9.

33. Periasamy P, O'Neill HC. Stroma-dependent development of two dendritic-like cell types with distinct antigen presenting capability. Exp Hematol. 2013;41(3):281–92.

34. Petvises S, O'Neill HC. Distinct progenitor origin distinguishes a lineage of dendritic-like cells in spleen. Front Immunol. 2014;4:501.

35. Quah BJC, Wijesundara DK, Ranasinghe C, Parish CR. Fluorescent target array killing assay: a multiplex cytotoxic T-cell assay to measure detailed T-cell antigen specificity and avidity in vivo. Cytometry A. 2012;81 A(8): 679–90.

36. McGarry MP, Stewart CC. Murine eosinophil granulocyte bind the murine macrophage-monocyte specific monoclonal antibody F4/80. J Leukoc Biol. 1991;50(5):471–8.

37. Murray PJ, Wynn TA. Protective and pathogenic functions of macrophage subsets. Nat Rev Immunol. 2011;11(11):723–37.

38. Rose S, Misharin A, Perlman H. A novel Ly6C/Ly6G-based strategy to analyze the mouse splenic myeloid compartment. Cytometry A. 2012;81 A(4):343–50.

39. Burgdorf S, Kautz A, Böhnert V, Knolle PA, Kurts C. Distinct pathways of antigen uptake and intracellular routing in CD4 and CD8 T cell activation. Science. 2007;316(5824):612–6.

40. Burgdorf S, Lukacs-Kornek V, Kurts C. The mannose receptor mediates uptake of soluble but not of cell-associated antigen for cross-presentation. J Immunol. 2006;176(11):6770–6.

41. Periasamy P, Tan JKH, Griffiths KL, O'Neill HC. Splenic stromal niches support hematopoiesis of dendritic-like cells from precursors in bone marrow and spleen. Exp Hematol. 2009;37(9):1060–71.

42. Pooley JL, Heath WR, Shortman K. Cutting edge: Intravenous soluble antigen is presented to CD4 T cells by CD8- dendritic cells, but cross-presented to CD8 T cells by CD8+ dendritic cells. J Immunol. 2001;166(9): 5327–30.

43. del Hoyo GM, Martín P, Arias CF, Marín AR, Ardavín C. CD8α + dendritic cells originate from the CD8α – dendritic cell subset by a maturation process involving CD8α, DEC-205, and CD24 up-regulation, vol. 99. 2002.

44. Schulz O, Reis E, Sousa C. Cross-presentation of cell-associated antigens by CD8+ dendritic cells is attributable to their ability to internalize dead cells. Immunology. 2002;107(2):183–9.

45. Shortman K, Heath WR. The CD8+ dendritic cell subset. Immunol Rev. 2010; 234(1):18–31.

46. Beauvillain C, Delneste Y, Scotet M, Peres A, Gascan H, Guermonprez P, Barnaba V, Jeannin P. Neutrophils efficiently cross-prime naive T cells in vivo. Blood. 2007;110(8):2965–73.

47. Harding CV, Song R. Phagocytic processing of exogenous particulate antigens by macrophages for presentation by class I MHC molecules. J Immunol. 1994;153(11):4925–33.

48. Kovacsovics-Bankowski M, Clark K, Benacerraf B, Rock KL. Efficient major histocompatibility complex class I presentation of exogenous antigen upon phagocytosis by macrophages. Proc Natl Acad Sci U S A. 1993; 90(11):4942–6.

49. Norbury CC, Hewlett LJ, Prescott AR, Shastri N, Watts C. Class I MHC presentation of exogenous soluble antigen via macropinocytosis in bone marrow macrophages. Immunity. 1995;3(6):783–91.

50. Pfeifer JD, Wick MJ, Roberts RL, Findlay K, Normark SJ, Harding CV. Phagocytic processing of bacterial antigens for class I MHC presentation to T cells. Nature. 1993;361(6410):359–62.

51. Akira S, Takeda K. Toll-like receptor signalling. Nat Rev Immunol. 2004;4(7): 499–511.

52. Inra CN, Zhou BO, Acar M, Murphy MM, Richardson J, Zhao Z, Morrison SJ. A perisinusoidal niche for extramedullary haematopoiesis in the spleen. Nature. 2015;527(7579):466–71.

53. Behrens G, Li M, Smith CM, Belz GT, Mintern J, Carbone FR, Heath WR. Helper T cells, dendritic cells and CTL Immunity. Immunol Cell Biol. 2004; 82(1):84–90.

54. Tvinnereim AR, Hamilton SE, Harty JT. Neutrophil involvement in cross-priming CD8+ T cell responses to bacterial antigens. J Immunol. 2004; 173(3):1994–2002.
55. Barry M, Bleackley RC. Cytotoxic T lymphocytes: All roads lead to death. Nat Rev Immunol. 2002;2(6):401–9.
56. Merad M, Sathe P, Helft J, Miller J, Mortha A. The dendritic cell lineage: ontogeny and function of dendritic cells and their subsets in the steady state and the inflamed setting. Annu Rev Immunol. 2013;31:563–604.

2

Altered endotoxin responsiveness in healthy children with Down syndrome

Dean Huggard[1,2,3,8,9]* (iD), Fiona McGrane[1,3], Niamh Lagan[1,3], Edna Roche[1,3], Joanne Balfe[1,3], Timothy Ronan Leahy[1,6], Orla Franklin[1,7], Ana Moreno[1,2], Ashanty M. Melo[1,2], Derek G. Doherty[1,2] and Eleanor J. Molloy[1,2,3,4,5,8]

Abstract

Background: Down syndrome (DS) is the most common syndromic immunodeficiency with an increased risk of infection, mortality from sepsis, and autoinflammation. Innate immune function is altered in DS and therefore we examined responses in CD11b and Toll like receptor 4 (TLR-4), which are important immune cell surface markers upregulated in response to Lipopolysaccharide (LPS) endotoxin, and the immunomodulator melatonin. Neutrophil and monocyte responses to LPS and melatonin in children with Down syndrome (DS) who were clinically stable were compared to age-matched controls. Whole blood was incubated with LPS and melatonin and the relative expression of CD11b and TLR-4 evaluated by flow cytometry.

Results: Children with DS had an increased response to LPS in neutrophils and intermediate monocytes, while also having elevated TLR-4 expression on non-classical monocytes compared to controls at baseline. Melatonin reduced CD11b expression on neutrophils, total monocytes, both classical and intermediate sub-types, in children with DS and controls.

Conclusion: Melatonin could represent a useful clinical adjunct in the treatment of sepsis as an immunomodulator. Children with DS had increased LPS responses which may contribute to the more adverse outcomes seen in sepsis.

Keywords: Down syndrome, Inflammation, Endotoxin, Innate immunity, Immunomodulation

Background

Down syndrome (DS) is caused by an extra copy of genetic material from chromosome 21, and is the most prevalent chromosomal abnormality, affecting approximately 1 in 550 births in Ireland [1], and 1 in 700 births in the USA [2]. Co-morbidities associated with DS include developmental disability, congenital heart disease (CHD), gastrointestinal tract anomalies, and an increased risk of haematological malignancy [3]. In addition, it is the most common genetic syndrome associated with abnormal immune function and immune defects [4]. There is significant evidence of immune dysregulation in Down syndrome including T-cell and B-cell lymphopenia due to impaired expansion of these cell lines in infancy [5], a smaller thymus gland with reduced naïve Tcell and regulatory T-cell numbers [6], suboptimal antibody responses to vaccination [7–10], and abnormal levels of serum cytokines [11–13].

Children with Down syndrome are, therefore, at increased risk of infection, especially in early childhood, particularly respiratory tract infections [14]. Hilton et al. [15] reported a higher risk of admission to hospital and intensive care with respiratory tract infections (RTIs) in children with DS. Mortality from sepsis is 30% greater in patients with DS in comparison to children without DS who also had sepsis [16].

It is challenging to attribute causation to a specific deficit of the immune system with the increased incidence of infections and sepsis seen in this cohort. A normal innate immune system is crucial in providing first line defence against infection. Neutrophils and monocytes are crucial cellular components of the innate immune system. Defective phagocytic activity and neutrophil chemotaxis have previously been reported in DS [17, 18]. Monocyte function in DS is poorly described. Increased numbers of the non-classical (CD14dim/CD16+) monocyte pro-inflammatory sub-type have been described in DS in comparison to controls [19].

* Correspondence: dean.huggard@gmail.com
[1]Paediatrics, Trinity College, the University of Dublin, Dublin, Ireland
[2]Trinity Translational Medicine Institute (TTMI), Trinity College Dublin, Dublin, Ireland
Full list of author information is available at the end of the article

This monocyte population has previously been implicated in sepsis and chronic disease [20].

CD11b is a cell surface marker involved in mediating neutrophil and monocyte adhesion and diapedesis [21] and is an indicator of activation. Dysfunction in neutrophil adherence and migration has been shown to increase the risk of infection in adults and neonates [22]. Toll-like receptor 4 (TLR-4) is the key receptor involved in lipopolysaccharide (LPS) endotoxin recognition and activation of the innate immune system [23], and has also been implicated in the pathogenesis of autoimmune conditions such as systemic lupus erythematosus (SLE) and rheumatoid arthritis [24].

Immunomodulators can alter responses to infection, alleviate autoimmunity and ultimately improve patient care. Melatonin is an endogenous hormone which mediates its anti-inflammatory effects by modulating pro-inflammatory cytokines and inflammasome de-activation, thereby ameliorating results in endotoxaemia [25, 26]. Melatonin has a very good safety profile and is used in paediatrics in sleep management [27]. Clinical trials in adults and neonates with sepsis have demonstrated improved clinical outcomes [28, 29].

We hypothesized that children with DS have altered neutrophil and monocyte function which contributes to their increased susceptibility to infection and increased mortality from sepsis. We aimed to evaluate the in vitro effect of LPS endotoxin, and the anti-inflammatory melatonin on CD11b and TLR4 expression on neutrophils and monocytes in children with DS.

Methods

Study population

This study was approved by the ethics committees in the National Children's Hospital, Tallaght and Our Lady's Children's Hospital, Crumlin (OLCHC), Dublin, Ireland. All parents and participants received verbal and written information on the study and written consent was obtained in advance of recruitment. There were two patient groups studied: a) Healthy children with Down syndrome < 16 years old attending the dedicated Down syndrome clinic. All children were clinically well with no recent fever or evidence infection and were undergoing annual routine health surveillance and b) Age-matched Controls: healthy controls attending phlebotomy or for day case procedures. Blood sampling occurred at induction of general anaesthetic and controls had no recent fever or evidence of infection.

Experimental design

All blood samples (1-3 mL) for in vitro experiments were collected in a sodium citrate anti-coagulated blood tube and analysed within 2 h of sample acquisition.

Blood sampling coincided with routine phlebotomy or at induction of anaesthesia for day case procedures. Whole blood was incubated at 37 °C for 1 h with the pro-inflammatory stimulant Lipopolysaccharide (LPS; *E.coli* 0111:B4: SIGMA Life Science, Wicklow, Ireland) 10 ng/mL, the anti-inflammatory agent Melatonin (SIGMA Life Science, Wicklow, Ireland) at 42 μM and both combined.

Blood samples were incubated with a dead cell stain (100 μL; (Fixable Viability Dye eFlour 506, Invitrogen, California USA), diluted to working concentration in phosphate buffered saline (PBS). The following fluorochrome-labelled monoclonal antibodies (mAb) were added to each sample (2.5 μL per tube): CD14-PerCP, CD15-PECy7, CD16-FITC, CD66b-Pacific Blue and TLR4-APC (BioLegend®, California, USA) and PE labelled CD11b (BD Biosciences, Oxford, UK; 10 μL per tube. PBA buffer (PBS containing 1% bovine serum albumin and 0.02% sodium azide) was used to make up the antibody cocktail. Samples were incubated in the dark for 15 min. Next 1 mL of FACS lysing solution (BD Biosciences, Oxford, UK) was added to each tube, the samples were then incubated for 15 min in the dark. Cells were pelleted by centrifugation at 450 g for 7 min at room temperature, washed twice with PBA buffer and fixed in 300 μL of 1% paraformaldehyde. The final cell pellet was resuspended in 100 μL PBA buffer and analysed on a BD FACS Canto II flow cytometer.

Quantification of cell surface antigen expression

The expression of CD11b and TLR-4 antigens on the surface of neutrophils and monocytes was evaluated by flow cytometry on the BD FACS Canto II cytometer. Neutrophils were delineated based on SSC-A and CD66b + positivity as previously described [30], monocytes were defined based on SSC-A, CD66b- and subsets based on relative CD14+ CD16 + populations; classical (CD14+/CD16-), intermediate (CD14+/CD16+), non-classical (CD14dim/CD16+), Fig. 1. A minimum of 10,000 events were collated and relative expression of CD11b and TLR-4 was expressed as mean channel fluorescence (MFI), and analysed using FloJo software (Oregon, USA). Every sample was processed and analysed by the same researcher (DH) thereby reducing variability in results.

Statistics

Statistical analysis was done using paired and un-paired *t* tests to compare mean results between two independent cohorts. Significance was defined as $p < 0.05$. Results shown are expressed as mean +/- standard error of the mean (SEM) unless otherwise stated. Data was analysed with FloJo software (Oregon, USA) and GraphPad Prism.

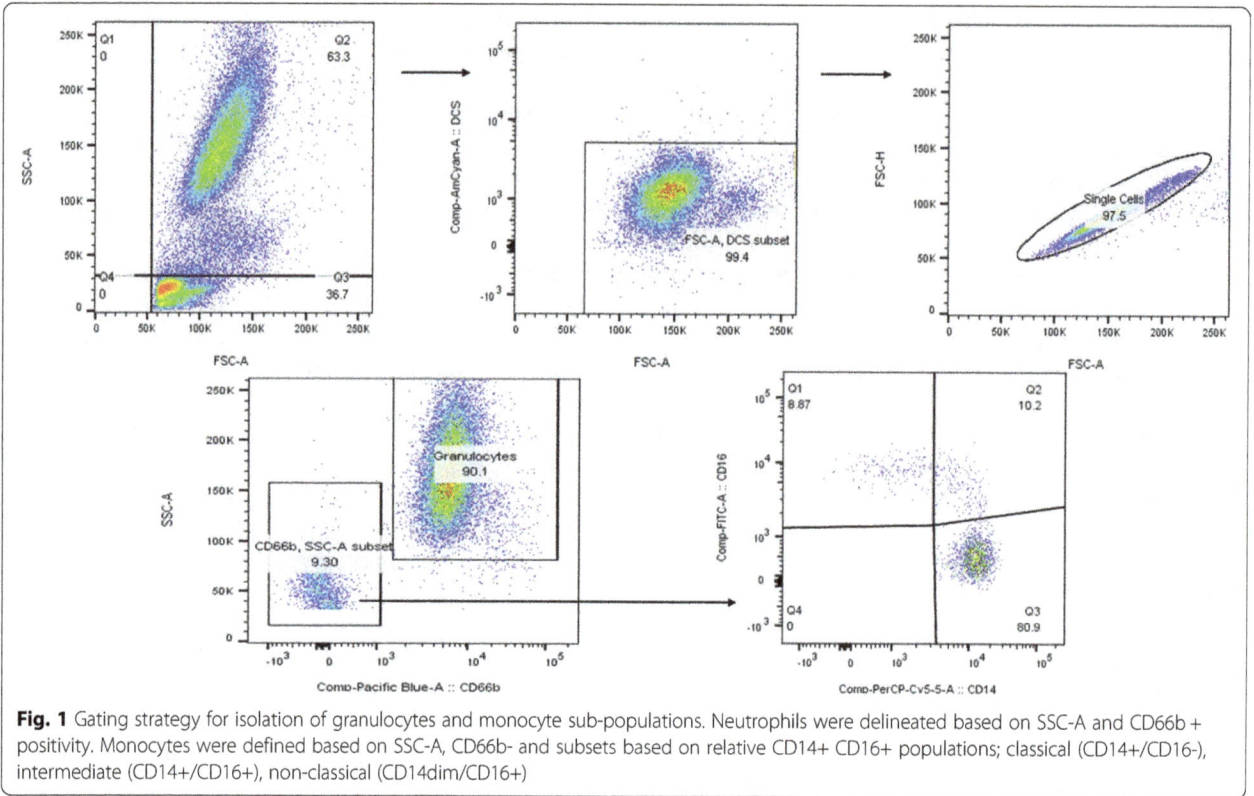

Fig. 1 Gating strategy for isolation of granulocytes and monocyte sub-populations. Neutrophils were delineated based on SSC-A and CD66b + positivity. Monocytes were defined based on SSC-A, CD66b- and subsets based on relative CD14+ CD16+ populations; classical (CD14+/CD16-), intermediate (CD14+/CD16+), non-classical (CD14dim/CD16+)

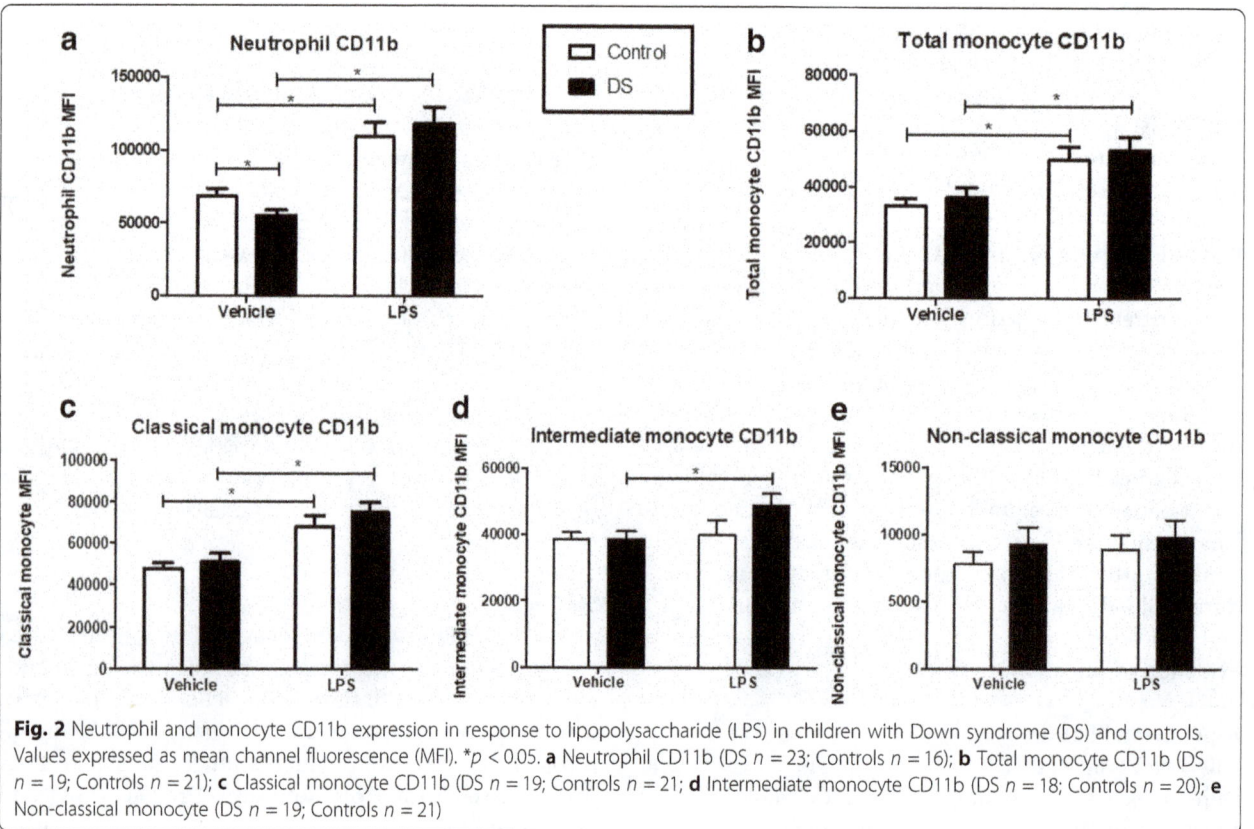

Fig. 2 Neutrophil and monocyte CD11b expression in response to lipopolysaccharide (LPS) in children with Down syndrome (DS) and controls. Values expressed as mean channel fluorescence (MFI). *$p < 0.05$. **a** Neutrophil CD11b (DS $n = 23$; Controls $n = 16$); **b** Total monocyte CD11b (DS $n = 19$; Controls $n = 21$); **c** Classical monocyte CD11b (DS $n = 19$; Controls $n = 21$; **d** Intermediate monocyte CD11b (DS $n = 18$; Controls $n = 20$); **e** Non-classical monocyte (DS $n = 19$; Controls $n = 21$)

Results

Patient characteristics

There were 23 healthy children with Down syndrome (DS) with a mean ±SD age of 8.67 ± 4 years(y) of which 13 were female (57%), and 21 healthy controls with a mean age of 7.4 ± 4.60 y, of which 10 were female (48%). In the DS cohort, children with a history of significant congenital heart disease requiring surgery in infancy ($n = 7$) were all clinically stable with no further cardiology intervention. All control participants had no significant medical history. Both groups were well at the time of blood sampling with no recent history of infection.

Effects of LPS endotoxin on CD11b expression

Neutrophil baseline CD11b expression in children with DS was significantly lower compared with controls ($p = 0.045$). Following incubation with LPS, CD11b significantly increased in both groups (Fig. 1a: DS $p < 0.0001$; Control $p = 0.0001$). When comparing the fold increase in CD11b expression from baseline, children with DS had a significantly higher rise after LPS stimulation (DS: Controls: 116% versus 62.4%; $p = 0.03$; Fig. 3a).

CD11b expression on total monocytes showed no difference at baseline or after LPS stimulation between both groups (Fig. 2b $p = 0.48$). The percentage rise of CD11b expression after LPS was similar in both groups also (DS versus Control: 53 v 55%; $p = 0.92$ Fig. 4b). Monocyte subset CD11b expression analysis revealed no significant differences at baseline or after LPS stimulation in classical (CD14 +/CD16-) ($p = 0.74$), and non-classical (CD14dim/CD16+) ($p = 0.21$) sub-populations in children with DS versus controls (Figs. 2c, e and 4c ($p = 0.55$), e ($p = 0.56$)). Intermediate monocytes (CD14+/CD16+) demonstrated no difference in CD11b expression at baseline in children with DS and controls ($p = 0.87$). After LPS stimulation there was a significant increase in CD11b in children with DS ($p = 0.004$) but not in controls ($p = 0.78$; Fig. 2d). The mean percentage rise in CD11b expression in children with DS was not significantly increased compared to controls (DS vs controls: 31.8 v 5.8%; $p = 0.088$; Fig. 4d).

Classical monocytes (CD14+/CD16-) exhibited the highest CD11b expression at baseline compared with the other sub-populations in both cohorts (DS vs Control -classical vs intermediate: $p = 0.009$ v 0.01). This sub-population also demonstrated the largest mean percentage rise in CD11b after LPS treatment in both children with DS and controls. (DS – classical % rise vs intermediate vs nonclassical = 52.1 vs 31.8 vs 15.3%; Controls - 44 vs 5.8 vs 24%). Non-classical monocytes (CD14dim/CD16+) demonstrated the lowest mean CD11b expression at baseline of any sub-population, in both children with DS and controls. This was significantly lower compared to both intermediate and classical monocyte CD11b in both cohorts.

Effects of LPS endotoxin on TLR4 expression

Neutrophil TLR-4 expression at baseline was not significantly different between children with DS compared to controls ($p = 0.57$). After LPS incubation there was no significant response in TLR4 expression in either cohort (DS $p = 0.15$ v Control $p = 0.057$; Fig. 3a). On comparing the mean percentage rise in TLR-4 expression after LPS, there was a 9.4% rise in children with DS versus 28.7% in the control group (Fig. 5a ($p = 0.23$)).

TLR-4 expression on total monocytes did not show any difference at baseline between children with DS and controls ($p = 0.24$). TLR-4 expression post LPS treatment increased significantly in controls ($p = 0.016$) but did not reach significance in the children with DS ($p = 0.07$; Fig. 3b). The mean percentage rise after LPS stimulation was 8.4% in children with DS versus 17.2% in controls (($p = 0.2$)) Fig. 5b. Monocyte subset TLR-4 expression analysis revealed no significant differences at baseline or after LPS treatment in classical (CD14+/CD16-) or intermediate (CD14+/CD16+) subpopulations between children with DS and controls (Fig. 3c ($p = 0.51$), d ($p = 0.4$) and Fig. 5c ($p = 0.75$), d ($p = 0.84$)). Non-classical monocyte (CD14dim/CD16+) TLR-4 expression was found to be significantly higher at baseline in children with DS compared to controls ($p = 0.02$; Fig. 3e). There were no significant differences in TLR-4 expression after LPS stimulation in either cases or controls (Fig. 5e ($p = 0.96$)).

The classical monocytes in both cohorts exhibited the largest mean percentage rise in TLR-4 expression after LPS treatment (DS – classical vs intermediate vs non-classical = 15.2 vs 3.6 vs 9.9%; Control - 17.9 vs 1.2 vs 10.7%). Intermediate monocytes had the largest mean TLR-4 MFI at baseline of any monocyte subpopulation in both children with DS and the control group (DS v control: intermediate vs classical $p = 0.003$ versus 0.005). Non-classical monocytes displayed the lowest mean TLR-4 at baseline of the three monocyte subsets and was significantly lower than intermediate monocyte TLR-4 in both cohorts.

Effects of melatonin on CD11b expression

Neutrophil CD11b expression decreased significantly after melatonin treatment in both cohorts (DS $p = < 0.0001$; Controls $p = < 0.0001$), compared with baseline the mean percentage fall in CD11b expression was 25.8% in children with DS versus 23.1% in controls ($p = 0.63$)). There were no differences in mean percentage fall in CD11b expression when comparing LPS treated samples and those treated with LPS and melatonin in both cohorts (Fig. 4a($p = 0.64$)).

Total monocyte CD11b expression reduced significantly after melatonin incubation in children with DS ($n = 12$; $p = 0.02$), but not in the control group ($n = 17$; $p = 0.12$). The mean percentage fall in CD11b MFI was

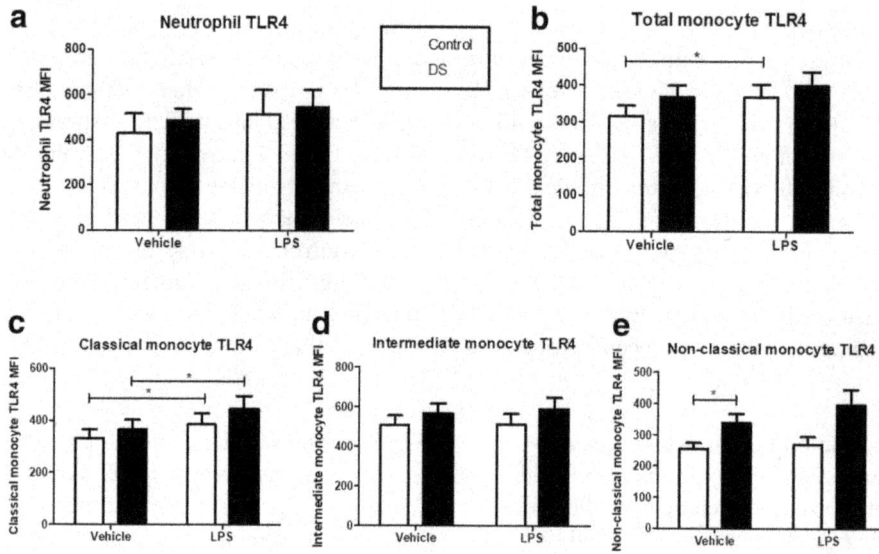

Fig. 3 Neutrophil and monocyte Toll-like receptor (TLR-4) expression in response to lipopolysaccharide (LPS) in children with Down syndrome (DS) and controls. Values expressed as mean channel fluorescence (MFI). *$p < 0.05$. **a** Neutrophil TLR4 (DS $n = 19$; Controls $n = 10$); **b** Total monocyte TLR-4 (DS $n = 22$; Controls $n = 15$); **c** Classical monocyte TLR4 (DS $n = 16$; Controls $n = 15$); **d** Intermediate monocyte TLR4 (DS $n = 15$; Controls $n = 14$); **e** Non-classical monocyte TLR-4 (DS $n = 16$; Controls $n = 20$)

19% in children with DS versus 3.4% in controls (Fig. 4b($p = 0.24$)). In classical and intermediate monocytes there were significant decreases in CD11b expression from baseline after melatonin in both cohorts) DS ($p = 0.001$); Control ($p = 0.05$); (d) DS ($p = 0.02$); Control ($p = 0.03$)]. Non-classical monocytes (CD14dim/CD16-)

showed a significant increase in CD11b expression after melatonin in children with DS ($p = 0.03$), and in controls but not to a significant level in the latter ($p = 0.1$). The mean percentage rise in CD11b expression after melatonin was 45% in children with DS versus 15.3% in controls (Fig. 4e ($p = 0.12$)).

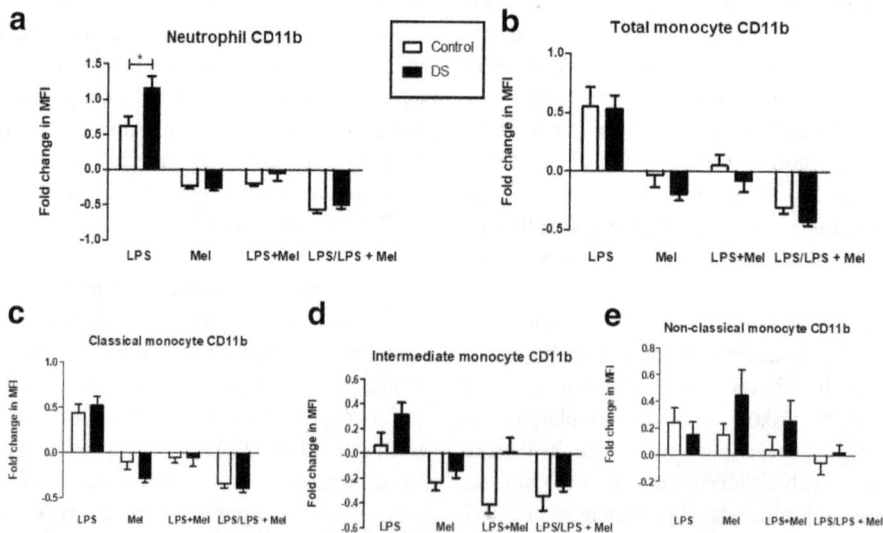

Fig. 4 Neutrophil and monocyte CD11b expression in response to LPS and melatonin in children with DS versus controls: Samples were treated with Lipopolysaccharide (LPS), Melatonin (Mel), Lipopolysaccharide and melatonin (LPS + Mel) and Lipopolysaccharide (LPS) versus Lipopolysaccharide and melatonin (LPS/ LPS + Mel) and expressed as fold changes in mean channel fluorescence (MFI). p* < 0.05. **a** Neutrophil CD11b (DS $n = 23$; Controls $n = 16$); **b** Total monocyte CD11b (DS $n = 19$; Controls $n = 21$); **c** Classical monocyte CD11b (DS $n = 19$; Controls $n = 21$); **d** Intermediate CD11b (DS $n = 18$; Controls $n = 20$); **e** Non-classical monocyte CD11b (DS $n = 19$; Controls $n = 21$)

Effects of melatonin on TLR-4 expression

Neutrophil TLR-4 expression showed no significant change after melatonin treatment in either group. The mean percentage fall in TLR-4 expression was 4.4% in children with DS and 1.3% in controls ($p = 0.82$). Comparing LPS and LPS + melatonin treated samples there was a 17.5% mean reduction in TLR-4 expression on neutrophils of children with DS compared to a fall of 4.8% in controls ($p = 0.48$), Fig. 5a.

Total monocyte TLR-4 was significantly reduced after melatonin incubation in both groups (DS $p = 0.03$; Controls $p = 0.05$). The average percentage fall in TLR-4 expression after melatonin treatment was 13% in children with DS versus 11.4% in controls (Fig. 5b ($p = 0.81$)). Monocyte subset analysis of melatonin on TLR-4 expression showed no significant reduction in either group (Fig. 5c ($p = 0.74$), d ($p = 0.23$), e ($p = 0.52$)).

Discussion

Neutrophil CD11b expression at baseline was significantly lower in children with DS compared with controls. Following LPS treatment children with DS upregulated CD11b, and this was significantly greater than controls. Novo et al. [18] reported that, at baseline, CD11b expression on neutrophils was not significantly different between children with DS ($n = 12$) and controls, although the smaller numbers and older population in this study may contribute to these findings. Our research suggests that although the level of CD11b may be lower under normal conditions, after contact with endotoxin there is an increased ability to activate and mobilise neutrophils in

response to this stimulus. Neutrophils in children with DS may be hyper-responsive to endotoxin, which may have detrimental effects in the setting of sepsis. Adults with sepsis and renal injury in the absence of hypotension, have been shown to have increased activation of neutrophils with upregulation of CD11b [31], worsening prognosis. Furthermore, neutrophil mediated lung injury in sepsis, and multi-organ dysfunction (MODS) have been associated with increased CD11b expression on these cells [32, 33]. A blockade of this receptor could have potential benefits in these clinical contexts [34]. In paediatric studies LPS hyper-responsiveness has been demonstrated through increased CD11b expression on neutrophils and monocytes of neonates with encephalopathy [35, 36], these infants having developed significant immune dysregulation. Zhou et al. [37] examined TLR4 signalling and the CD11b response on polymorphonuclear cells in mice. The authors concluded that TLR4 mediates CD11b upregulation and is key for PMN activation in response to LPS. Further correlation between CD11b and TLR4 has been described by Guang et al. [38] who reported that CD11b mediates TLR4 signalling and trafficking in a cell specific manner in dendritic cells and macrophages, having a crucial role in balancing the innate and adaptive response to LPS. It appears that the two receptors are inter-linked and have important regulatory roles on one another in initiating the innate immune response.

Zhang et al. [39] demonstrated that mice deficient in CD11b exposed to *Mycobacterium tuberculosis* developed more severe granulomas, higher leucocyte recruitment and elevated pro-inflammatory cytokines. This

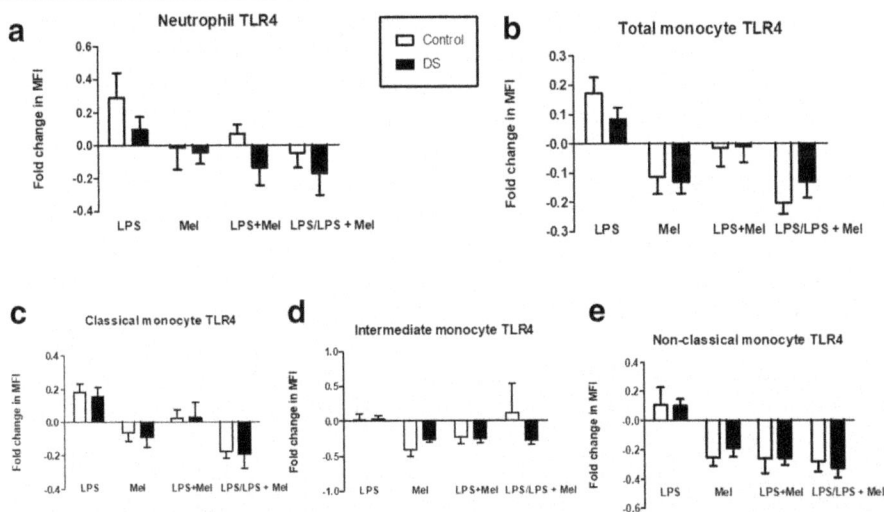

Fig. 5 Neutrophil and monocyte TLR-4 expression in response to LPS and melatonin in children with DS versus controls: Samples were treated with Lipopolysaccharide (LPS), Melatonin (Mel), Lipopolysaccharide and melatonin (LPS + Mel) and Lipopolysaccharide (LPS) versus Lipopolysaccharide and melatonin (LPS/ LPS + Mel) and expressed as fold changes in mean channel fluorescence (MFI). **a** Neutrophil TLR-4 (DS $n = 19$; Controls $n = 10$); **b** Total monocyte TLR-4 (DS $n = 22$; Controls $n = 15$); **c** Classical monocyte TLR-4 (DS $n = 16$; Controls $n = 15$); **d** Intermediate monocyte TLR-4 (DS $n = 15$; Controls $n = 14$); **e** Non-classical monocyte TLR-4 (DS $n = 16$; Controls $n = 20$)

demonstrates the immunomodulatory effect neutrophil CD11b expression exerts on the host response to infection. A persistent inflammatory response can be seen in autoimmunity and there is a higher prevalence in DS, recent studies suggest that reduced CD11b is associated with chronic inflammation in SLE and lupus nephritis [40, 41]. Neutrophil CD11b is also decreased in septic shock and correlated with poorer outcomes [42, 43]. In this context, the increased incidence of both autoimmunity and sepsis in DS is particularly noteworthy [16, 44]. We demonstrated that melatonin caused a predominant decrease in CD11b expression in both cohorts; Fig. 4. We also showed that children with DS exhibited a hyper-responsive CD11b response to LPS in neutrophils Fig. 4a. In the acute setting of sepsis/SIRS an upregulation of CD11b may be associated with deleterious effects [45], furthermore, a positive correlation between CD11b expression and the degree of systemic inflammation has been described [46], making melatonin a potential adjunct in acute sepsis/SIRS.

The classical monocyte (CD14+/CD16-) accounts for the largest proportion of monocytes (80–85%) and its main functions include antigen presentation and phagocytosis [47]. We found classical monocytes exhibited significantly higher CD11b expression at baseline, and greater fold increases in CD11b after LPS than other monocyte sub-populations in both groups. This sub-group also displayed the largest rise in TLR-4 after LPS compared with other monocyte subpopulations in both cohorts. This suggests that classical monocytes are significantly pro-inflammatory with the largest CD11b and TLR4 response to LPS than any other sub-population. Regarding differential CD11b expression on monocyte subsets Tak et al. [48] reported no significant differences, whereas another study examining differential in vivo activation of monocyte subsets reported the most significant rise in CD11b on the intermediate monocyte [49]. However, these studies [48, 49] characterised CD11b expression after lower doses of LPS with longer incubations in an adult in vivo setting as compared to our study which was undertaken in a paediatric cohort. Monocyte CD11b was highest on classical and intermediate monocytes [50].

Intermediate monocytes (CD14+/CD16+) are elevated in the setting of acute illness such as sepsis in children [51]. In our study, there was a significant rise in CD11b expression after LPS stimulation in children with DS but not in controls on intermediate monocytes. This adds to the evidence that there are hyper-responsive elements to the innate immune system in children with DS. Indeed, intermediate monocytes produce significant quantities of TNF-α once activated [50]. Previous studies have demonstrated elevated levels of TNF-α in patients with DS

compared with healthy controls [13] at baseline. Intermediate monocytes demonstrated the greatest TLR-4 at baseline compared with other monocytes in both groups which has also been demonstrated in adults [20].

Non-classical monocytes (CD14dim/16+) have been implicated in both acute and chronic disease and have a pro-inflammatory phenotype with increased production of IL-1β and TNF-α [47]. This monocyte sub-group had significantly lower CD11b and TLR-4 expression in both groups at baseline. Furthermore, non-classical monocytes demonstrated a relative hypo-responsiveness to LPS versus the other sub-populations. Boyette et al. [50] assessed the phenotype, function, and differentiation monocyte subsets, and reported that non-classical monocytes had the lowest CD11b MFI and that there was the smallest response in this subset following TLR-4 stimulation. We found baseline TLR-4 expression was significantly raised in children with DS versus controls. The TLR-4 response plays a significant role in fighting infection but may also be responsible for the dysregulated inflammation seen in septic shock [52]. Williams et al. noted an increased mortality in mice with polymicrobial sepsis who exhibited early up-regulation of TLR-4, and improved survival in those with suppressed TLR gene expression [53]. Suppression of TLR-4 activation, pro-inflammatory cytokine release, and developing endotoxin tolerance is important in limiting the adverse effects of sepsis. Furthermore, a failure of this protective negative feedback process may contribute to increased mortality in sepsis [54].

We demonstrated that melatonin has an anti-inflammatory influence on innate immune function by reducing CD11b expression on neutrophils and total monocytes in children with DS and controls, thereby inhibiting neutrophil and monocyte activation and migration. Although there is a paucity of literature on the effect of melatonin on CD11b, Alvarez-Sanchez et al. reported a reduction in CD11b in melatonin-treated mice [55]. A significant reduction in TLR-4 expression only occurred in total monocyte populations. Melatonin may act as a TLR-4 antagonist and may be modulated via TLR-4 mediated inflammatory genes through molecule myeloid differentiation factor 88 (MyD88)-dependent and TRIF-dependent signalling pathways [56], thereby attenuating inflammation.

Melatonin has beneficial immunomodulatory effects in the setting of sepsis by inhibiting mitochondrial dysfunction and inflammation, reducing nitrosative and oxidative stress [29]. Melatonin has a robust antioxidant or free radical scavenging activity of [57, 58] and melatonin administration also impairs NF-κB transcriptional activity, reducing pro-inflammatory cytokine (IL-1β, TNF-α, IFN-γ) release and inhibiting activation of the NLRP3 inflammasome [59]. Melatonin improved survival and clinical outcomes in neonates versus controls in sepsis [28, 60, 61]. We have demonstrated that the immuno-modulatory effects of melatonin in sepsis can also be broadened to include reducing neutrophil and monocyte activation.

Melatonin increased CD11b expression on non-classical monocytes and to a significant level in the children with DS. However, it has been shown that melatonin can have pro-inflammatory actions in response to endotoxaemia. Effenberger et al. [62] reported that melatonin enhanced the general immune response following LPS treatment. Melatonin may have differing actions on distinct cell lines, with the pro-inflammatory non-classical monocyte being preferentially activated. Further evaluation of the immuno-modulatory properties of melatonin in children with DS will allow assessment of its potential as a therapeutic agent.

Conclusion

This research highlights important differences in the innate immunity of children with DS versus age-matched controls. To our knowledge this has not been studied previously in this population. Children with DS have an increased response to LPS in neutrophils and intermediate monocytes, while also having elevated TLR-4 expression on non-classical monocytes compared to controls. These variations may be a contributory factor in a heightened/dysregulated innate immune response, which may have deleterious effects, leading to the worse outcomes seen in sepsis in these children. Lastly, melatonin could represent a useful clinical adjunct in the treatment of sepsis as an immunomodulator and our study suggests its anti-inflammatory effects also influence neutrophil and monocyte function.

Abbreviations

CHD: Congenital heart disease; DS: Down syndrome; LPS: Lipopolysaccharide; MFI: Mean channel fluorescence; MODS: Multi organ dysfunction syndrome; MyD88: Myeloid differentiation factor 88; NS: Not significant; OLCHC: Our lady's children's hospital Crumlin; PBA: PBS containing 1% bovine serum albumin and 0.02% sodium azide; PBS: Phosphate buffered solution; RTIs: Respiratory tract infections; SD: Standard deviation; SEM: Standard error of the mean; SLE: Systemic lupus erythematosus; TLR-4: Toll like receptor 4

Acknowledgements
N/A

Funding
This study was funded by the National Children's Research Centre (NCRC), Crumlin, Dublin 12 and the National Children's Hospital Fund, Tallaght, Dublin, Ireland.

Authors' contributions
The manuscript is being submitted on behalf of all the authors and is the original work of all authors. DH was responsible for recruitment, sample acquistion, lab experiments, analysis and was responsible for writing the main draft of the manuscript. FM, NL, ER, JB, OF were responsible for patient recruitment, sample acquisition, reviewing and editing the manuscript. AM, and AMM provided expertise in sample analysis on the flow cytometer, review of those results and of the manuscript. TRL, DD and EM were instrumental in study design, supervising the research and its outcomes and providing key editorial assistance. All authors had editorial license to review and re-draft the manuscript, and all contributors had to approve the final edit. All authors are accountable for the accuracy and scientific integrity of this work.

Competing interests
The authors declare that they have no competing interests.

Author details
[1]Paediatrics, Trinity College, the University of Dublin, Dublin, Ireland. [2]Trinity Translational Medicine Institute (TTMI), Trinity College Dublin, Dublin, Ireland. [3]Paediatrics, Tallaght Hospital, Dublin, Ireland. [4]Coombe Women and Infants University Hospital, Dublin, Ireland. [5]Neonatology, Our Lady's Children's Hospital, Crumlin, Dublin, Ireland. [6]Immunology, Our Lady's Children's Hospital, Crumlin, Dublin, Ireland. [7]Cardiology, Our Lady's Children's Hospital, Crumlin, Dublin, Ireland. [8]National Children's Research Centre, Our Lady's Children's Hospital, Crumlin, Dublin, Ireland. [9]Department of Paediatrics, Trinity Centre for Health Sciences, Tallaght Hospital, Dublin 24, Ireland.

References

1. Down's Syndrome Medical Interest Group (DSMIG) (UK & Ireland), Department of Paediatrics University of Dublin TCTNCsH, Tallaght Hospital. Medical management of children & adolescents with Down syndrome in Ireland 2015.
2. Parker SE, Mai CT, Canfield MA, Rickard R, Wang Y, Meyer RE, et al. Updated National Birth Prevalence estimates for selected birth defects in the United States, 2004-2006. Birth defects research part A, clinical and molecular. Teratology. 2010;88(12):1008–16.
3. van Trotsenburg AS, Heymans HS, Tijssen JG, de Vijlder JJ, Vulsma T. Comorbidity, hospitalization, and medication use and their influence on mental and motor development of young infants with Down syndrome. Pediatrics. 2006;118(4):1633–9.
4. Cruz NV, Mahmoud SA, Chen H, Lowery-Nordberg M, Berlin K, Bahna SL. Follow-up study of immune defects in patients with dysmorphic disorders. Ann Allergy Asthma Immunol. 2009;102(5):426–31.
5. de Hingh YC, van der Vossen PW, Gemen EF, Mulder AB, Hop WC, Brus F, et al. Intrinsic abnormalities of lymphocyte counts in children with Down syndrome. J Pediatr. 2005;147(6):744–7.
6. Murphy M, Epstein LB. Down syndrome (trisomy 21) thymuses have a decreased proportion of cells expressing high levels of TCR alpha, beta and CD3. A possible mechanism for diminished T cell function in Down syndrome. Clin Immunol Immunopathol. 1990;55(3):453–67.
7. Kusters MA, Bok VL, Bolz WE, Huijskens EG, Peeters MF, de Vries E. Influenza A/H1N1 vaccination response is inadequate in Down syndrome children when the latest cut-off values are used. Pediatr Infect Dis J. 2012;31(12):1284–5.
8. Kusters MA, Jol-Van Der Zijde EC, Gijsbers RH, de Vries E. Decreased response after conjugated meningococcal serogroup C vaccination in children with Down syndrome. Pediatr Infect Dis J. 2011;30(9):818–9.

9. Kusters MA, Jol-van der Zijde CM, van Tol MJ, Bolz WE, Bok LA, Visser M, et al. Impaired avidity maturation after tetanus toxoid booster in children with Down syndrome. Pediatr Infect Dis J. 2011;30(4):357–9.

10. Valentini D, Marcellini V, Bianchi S, Villani A, Facchini M, Donatelli I, et al. Generation of switched memory B cells in response to vaccination in Down syndrome children and their siblings. Vaccine. 2015;33(48):6689–96.

11. Cetiner S, Demirhan O, Inal TC, Tastemir D, Sertdemir Y. Analysis of peripheral blood T-cell subsets, natural killer cells and serum levels of cytokines in children with Down syndrome. Int J Immunogenet. 2010;37(4):233–7.

12. Nateghi Rostami M, Douraghi M, Miramin Mohammadi A, Nikmanesh B. Altered serum pro-inflammatory cytokines in children with Down's syndrome. Eur Cytokine Netw. 2012;23(2):64–7.

13. Zhang Y, Che M, Yuan J, Yu Y, Cao C, Qin XY, et al. Aberrations in circulating inflammatory cytokine levels in patients with Down syndrome: a meta-analysis. Oncotarget. 2017;8(48):84489–96.

14. Ram G, Chinen J. Infections and immunodeficiency in Down syndrome. Clin Exp Immunol. 2011;164(1):9–16.

15. Hilton JM, Fitzgerald DA, Cooper DM. Respiratory morbidity of hospitalized children with trisomy 21. J Paediatr Child Health. 1999;35(4):383–6.

16. Garrison MM, Jeffries H, Christakis DA. Risk of death for children with Down syndrome and sepsis. J Pediatr. 2005;147(6):748–52.

17. Licastro F, Melotti C, Parente R, Davis LJ, Chiricolo M, Zannotti M, et al. Derangement of non-specific immunity in Down syndrome subjects: low leukocyte chemiluminescence activity after phagocytic activation. Am J Med Genet Suppl. 1990;7:242–6.

18. Novo E, Garcia MI, Lavergne J. Nonspecific immunity in Down syndrome: a study of chemotaxis, phagocytosis, oxidative metabolism, and cell surface marker expression of polymorphonuclear cells. Am J Med Genet. 1993;46(4):384–91.

19. Bloemers BL, van Bleek GM, Kimpen JL, Bont L. Distinct abnormalities in the innate immune system of children with Down syndrome. J Pediatr. 2010; 156(5):804–9 9.e1–9.e5.

20. Mukherjee R, Kanti Barman P, Kumar Thatoi P, Tripathy R, Kumar Das B, Ravindran B. Non-classical monocytes display inflammatory features: validation in sepsis and systemic lupus erythematous. Sci Rep. 2015;5:13886.

21. Carr R. Neutrophil production and function in newborn infants. Br J Haematol. 2000;110(1):18–28.

22. Romero R, Chaiworapongsa T, Espinoza J. Micronutrients and intrauterine infection, preterm birth and the fetal inflammatory response syndrome. J Nutr. 2003;133(5 Suppl 2):1668s–73s.

23. O'Hare FM, Watson W, O'Neill A, Grant T, Onwuneme C, Donoghue V, et al. Neutrophil and monocyte toll-like receptor 4, CD11b and reactive oxygen intermediates, and neuroimaging outcomes in preterm infants. Pediatr Res. 2015;78(1):82–90.

24. Liu Y, Yin H, Zhao M, Lu Q. TLR2 and TLR4 in autoimmune diseases: a comprehensive review. Clin Rev Allergy Immunol. 2014;47(2):136–47.

25. Escames G, Leon J, Macias M, Khaldy H, Acuna-Castroviejo D. Melatonin counteracts lipopolysaccharide-induced expression and activity of mitochondrial nitric oxide synthase in rats. FASEB J. 2003;17(8):932–4.

26. Favero G, Franceschetti L, Bonomini F, Rodella LF, Rezzani R. Melatonin as an anti-inflammatory agent modulating Inflammasome activation. Int J Endocrinol. 2017;2017:1835195.

27. Abdelgadir IS, Gordon MA, Akobeng AK. Melatonin for the management of sleep problems in children with neurodevelopmental disorders: a systematic review and meta-analysis. Arch Dis Child. 2018. https://doi.org/10.1136/archdischild-2017-314181. [Epub ahead of print]

28. El Frargy M, El-Sharkawy HM, Attia GF. Use of melatonin as an adjuvant therapy in neonatal sepsis. J Neonatal-Perinatal Med. 2015;8(3):227–32.

29. Hu W, Deng C, Ma Z, Wang D, Fan C, Li T, et al. Utilizing melatonin to combat bacterial infections and septic injury. Br J Pharmacol. 2017;174(9):754–68.

30. Prabhu SB, Rathore DK, Nair D, Chaudhary A, Raza S, Kanodia P, et al. Comparison of human neonatal and adult blood leukocyte subset composition phenotypes. PLoS One. 2016;11(9):e0162242.

31. Rinder CS, Fontes M, Mathew JP, Rinder HM, Smith BR. Neutrophil CD11b upregulation during cardiopulmonary bypass is associated with postoperative renal injury. Ann Thorac Surg. 2003;75(3):899–905.

32. Asaduzzaman M, Zhang S, Lavasani S, Wang Y, Thorlacius H. LFA-1 and MAC-1 mediate pulmonary recruitment of neutrophils and tissue damage in abdominal sepsis. Shock. 2008;30(3):254–9.

33. Maekawa K, Futami S, Nishida M, Terada T, Inagawa H, Suzuki S, et al. Effects of trauma and sepsis on soluble L-selectin and cell surface expression of L-selectin and CD11b. J Trauma. 1998;44(3):460–8.

34. Maiguel D, Faridi MH, Wei C, Kuwano Y, Balla KM, Hernandez D, et al. Small molecule-mediated activation of the integrin CD11b/CD18 reduces inflammatory disease. Sci Signal. 2011;4(189):ra57.

35. O'Hare FM, Watson RW, O'Neill A, Blanco A, Donoghue V, Molloy EJ. Persistent systemic monocyte and neutrophil activation in neonatal encephalopathy. J Matern Fetal Neonatal Med. 2016;29(4):582–9.

36. Eliwan HO, Watson RWG, Aslam S, Regan I, Philbin B, O'Hare FM, et al. Neonatal brain injury and systemic inflammation: modulation by activated protein C ex vivo. Clin Exp Immunol. 2015;179(3):477–84.

37. Zhou X, Gao XP, Fan J, Liu Q, Anwar KN, Frey RS, et al. LPS activation of toll-like receptor 4 signals CD11b/CD18 expression in neutrophils. Am J Phys Lung Cell Mol Phys. 2005;288(4):L655–62.

38. Ling GS, Bennett J, Woollard KJ, Szajna M, Fossati-Jimack L, Taylor PR, et al. Integrin CD11b positively regulates TLR4-induced signalling pathways in dendritic cells but not in macrophages. Nat Commun. 2014;5:3039.

39. Zhang Q, Lee W-B, Kang J-S, Kim LK, Kim Y-J. Integrin CD11b negatively regulates Mincle-induced signaling via the Lyn–SIRPα–SHP1 complex. Exp Mol Med. 2018;50(2):e439.

40. Faridi MH, Khan SQ, Zhao W, Lee HW, Altintas MM, Zhang K, et al. CD11b activation suppresses TLR-dependent inflammation and autoimmunity in systemic lupus erythematosus. J Clin Invest. 2017;127(4):1271–83.

41. Khan SQ, Khan I, Gupta V. CD11b activity modulates pathogenesis of lupus nephritis. Front Med. 2018;5:52.

42. Muller Kobold AC, Tulleken JE, Zijlstra JG, Sluiter W, Hermans J, Kallenberg CG, et al. Leukocyte activation in sepsis; correlations with disease state and mortality. Intensive Care Med. 2000;26(7):883–92.

43. Chishti AD, Shenton BK, Kirby JA, Baudouin SV. Neutrophil chemotaxis and receptor expression in clinical septic shock. Intensive Care Med. 2004;30(4):605–11.

44. Pellegrini FP, Marinoni M, Frangione V, Tedeschi A, Gandini V, Ciglia F, et al. Down syndrome, autoimmunity and T regulatory cells. Clin Exp Immunol. 2012;169(3):238–43.

45. Rosenbloom AJ, Pinsky MR, Napolitano C, Nguyen TS, Levann D, Pencosky N, et al. Suppression of cytokine-mediated beta2-integrin activation on circulating neutrophils in critically ill patients. J Leukoc Biol. 1999;66(1):83–9.

46. Delanghe JR, Speeckaert MM. Translational research and biomarkers in neonatal sepsis. Clin Chim Acta. 2015;451(Pt A):46–64.

47. Wong KL, Yeap WH, Tai JJ, Ong SM, Dang TM, Wong SC. The three human monocyte subsets: implications for health and disease. Immunol Res. 2012; 53(1–3):41–57.

48. Tak T, van Groenendael R, Pickkers P, Koenderman L. Monocyte subsets are differentially lost from the circulation during acute inflammation induced by human experimental endotoxemia. J Innate Immun. 2017;9(5):464–74.

49. Thaler B, Hohensinner PJ, Krychtiuk KA, Matzneller P, Koller L, Brekalo M, et al. Differential in vivo activation of monocyte subsets during low-grade inflammation through experimental endotoxemia in humans. Sci Rep. 2016;6:30162.

50. Boyette LB, Macedo C, Hadi K, Elinoff BD, Walters JT, Ramaswami B, et al. Phenotype, function, and differentiation potential of human monocyte subsets. PLoS One. 2017;12(4):e0176460.

51. Skrzeczynska J, Kobylarz K, Hartwich Z, Zembala M, Pryjma J. CD14+CD16+ monocytes in the course of sepsis in neonates and small children: monitoring and functional studies. Scand J Immunol. 2002;55(6):629–38.

52. Rosadini CV, Kagan JC. Early innate immune responses to bacterial LPS. Curr Opin Immunol. 2017;44:14–9.

53. Williams DL, Ha T, Li C, Kalbfleisch JH, Schweitzer J, Vogt W, et al. Modulation of tissue toll-like receptor 2 and 4 during the early phases of polymicrobial sepsis correlates with mortality. Crit Care Med. 2003;31(6):1808–18.

54. Skinner NA, MacIsaac CM, Hamilton JA, Visvanathan K. Regulation of toll-like receptor (TLR)2 and TLR4 on CD14dimCD16+ monocytes in response to sepsis-related antigens. Clin Exp Immunol. 2005;141(2):270–8.

55. Alvarez-Sanchez N, Cruz-Chamorro I, Lopez-Gonzalez A, Utrilla JC, Fernandez-Santos JM, Martinez-Lopez A, et al. Melatonin controls experimental autoimmune encephalomyelitis by altering the T effector/regulatory balance. Brain Behav Immun. 2015;50:101–14.

56. Xia MZ, Liang YL, Wang H, Chen X, Huang YY, Zhang ZH, et al. Melatonin modulates TLR4-mediated inflammatory genes through MyD88- and TRIF-dependent signaling pathways in lipopolysaccharide-stimulated RAW264.7 cells. J Pineal Res. 2012;53(4):325–34.

57. Reiter RJ, Mayo JC, Tan DX, Sainz RM, Alatorre-Jimenez M, Qin L. Melatonin as an antioxidant: under promises but over delivers. J Pineal Res. 2016;61(3):253–78.

58. Manchester LC, Coto-Montes A, Boga JA, Andersen LP, Zhou Z, Galano A, et al. Melatonin: an ancient molecule that makes oxygen metabolically tolerable. J Pineal Res. 2015;59(4):403–19.

59. Volt H, Garcia JA, Doerrier C, Diaz-Casado ME, Guerra-Librero A, Lopez LC, et al. Same molecule but different expression: aging and sepsis trigger NLRP3 inflammasome activation, a target of melatonin. J Pineal Res. 2016;60(2): 193–205.

60. Gitto E, Karbownik M, Reiter RJ, Tan DX, Cuzzocrea S, Chiurazzi P, et al. Effects of melatonin treatment in septic newborns. Pediatr Res. 2001; 50(6):756–60.

61. El-Gendy FM, El-Hawy MA, Hassan MG. Beneficial effect of melatonin in the treatment of neonatal sepsis. J Matern Fetal Neonatal Med. 2018;31(17): 2299–303.

62. Effenberger-Neidnicht K, Brencher L, Broecker-Preuss M, Hamburger T, Petrat F, de Groot H. Immune stimulation by exogenous melatonin during experimental endotoxemia. Inflammation. 2014;37(3):738–44.

3

Lipopolysaccharide mediates immuno-pathological alterations in young chicken liver through TLR4 signaling

Xi-Yao Huang[1†], Abdur Rahman Ansari[1,2†], Hai-Bo Huang[1], Xing Zhao[1], Ning-Ya Li[1], Zhi-Jian Sun[1], Ke-Mei Peng[1], Juming Zhong[1,3] and Hua-Zhen Liu[1*]

Abstract

Background: Lipopolysaccharide (LPS) induces acute liver injury and the complex mechanisms include the activation of toll like receptor 4 (TLR4) signaling pathway in many species. However, immuno-pathological changes during TLR4 signaling under LPS stress in acute liver injury is poorly understood in avian species. The present investigation was therefore carried out to evaluate these alterations in TLR4 signaling pathway during acute liver injury in young chickens.

Results: After intraperitoneal injection of LPS or saline, liver samples were harvested at 0, 2, 6, 12, 24, 36, 72 and 120 h ($n = 6$ at each time point) and the microstructures were analyzed by hematoxylin and eosin (H&E) staining. Alanine aminotransferase (ALT) and caspase-3 enzyme activity was assessed by enzyme-linked immunosorbent assay (ELISA). Proliferative cell nuclear antigen (PCNA), single stranded DNA (ssDNA) and TLR4 protein expressions were determined by immunohistochemistry. Gene expressions of PCNA, caspase-3, caspase-8, TLR4 and its downstream molecules were analyzed by quantitative polymerase chain reaction (qPCR). LPS injection induced significantly higher ALT activity, severe fatty degeneration, necrotic symptoms, ballooning degeneration, congestion, enhanced inflammatory cell infiltration in liver sinusoids, decreased proliferation, increased apoptosis and significant up-regulation in TLR4 and its downstream molecules (MyD88, NF-κB, TNF-α, IL-1β and TGF-β) expression at different time points.

Conclusions: This study indicated that TLR4 signaling and its downstream molecules along with certain cytokines play a key role in acute liver injury in young chickens. Hence, our findings provided novel information about the histopathological, proliferative and apoptotic alterations along with changes in ALT and caspase-3 activities associated with acute liver injury induced by *Salmonella* LPS in avian species.

Keywords: Lipopolysaccharide, Chicken, Liver, Acute injury, Toll-like receptor 4

Background

The liver is regarded as both metabolic as well as immunological lymphoid organ [1, 2]. It harbors many kinds of resident immune cells and has capability for the production of immune related defense mediators as well as regulatory molecules [3]. It is responsible for the synthesis of cytokines, chemokines, complement components and acute phase proteins that play essential role in innate immunity [3]. It is located at hemodynamic converging place in the body and conjoins the arterial system with portal venous system causing mixing of oxygenated blood with portal venous blood. The liver sinusoids have several components of nutrients, lymphocytes and myeloid cells together with many kinds of antigens and other microbial products as derived from intestinal bacteria [4, 5]. The liver is also under constant exposure of environmental toxins, food antigens and bacterial components [6]. Lipopolysaccharide (LPS) or endotoxin is a major component of cell wall in Gram negative bacteria. Under normal physiological conditions, LPS is not detectable in systemic blood circulation. However its detectable amount (about 1.0 ng/ml) is usually present in portal venous circulation [5]. LPS stimulation has been

* Correspondence: lhz219@mail.hzau.edu.cn
†Equal contributors
[1]Department of Basic Veterinary Medicine, College of Animal Science and Veterinary Medicine, Huazhong Agricultural University, Wuhan, Hubei 430070, China
Full list of author information is available at the end of the article

widely used in several experimental models [7–9] for the understanding of mechanisms involved in endotoxin-mediated acute liver tissue damage [7]. However, LPS-induced immuno-pathological and micro-morphological alterations in chicken liver are poorly understood yet.

Toll like receptors (TLRs) are considered as evolutionary conserved pattern recognition receptors (PPRs) that act as critical mediators of host response to many pathogenic organisms [10, 11]. PPRs identify the pathogen associated molecular patterns (PAMPs) and the appropriate localization of TLRs in cells is considered to be important for the accessibility of ligand and the understanding of downstream signal transduction molecules [12]. Until now 13 functional TLRs have been reported in mouse [13] and as many as 10 in both human [12] and chicken [14]. Out of these, TLR4 plays an important role after LPS stimulation and induces host defense mechanism that leads to the activation of intracellular signaling pathways and production of co-stimulatory molecules and cytokines [9, 15]. TLR4 expression has been reported in both parenchymal and non-parenchymal liver cells in response to injury [16]. Parenchymal cells of liver undergo apoptotic changes during liver injury [17]. Deregulation of transforming growth factor β (TGF-β) is also associated with liver cancer and fibrotic liver disease. Activation of TGF-β signaling pathway leads to immune suppression, arrest of cell cycle at G1/S phase and induction of apoptosis in mouse model [18]. But the information about the changed expression of these cytokines in chicken liver under endotoxin stress is still scarce. Moreover, proliferative and apoptotic changes during TLR4 signaling need further characterization at tissue level in LPS-induced chicken liver. Therefore, the current study was designed for the better understanding of micro-morphological changes and molecular events involved in TLR4 mediated hepatic injury following intrapertoneal LPS stimulation in time series manner in young chickens.

Methods

Healthy one-day-old commercial Cobb strain (genetically Cobb 500) broiler chicks were purchased from Zhengda chicken breeding company (Wuhan, China) and chicks with uniform body weight were selected and provided with commercial chick-starter feed and water *ad libitum* along with supplementary heating without any vaccinations [19]. All the birds were intraperitoneally (i.p.) injected at the same peritoneal location by lifting the skin over mid-abdominal line, immediately anterior to the pubic bones with LPS derived from *Salmonella* enterica serovar Typhimurium (STm) (L7261; Sigma-Aldrich, St. Louis, MO, USA) at 50 mg/kg of body weight in 0.5 mL avian saline solution (0.75% NaCl) [19]. Birds in the control group were exposed to mock infection with 0.5 mL avian saline solution only.

The chickens ($n = 6$ at each time point) were euthanized by CO_2 inhalation and sacrificed by dissecting the abdominal cavity at 0, 2, 6, 12, 24, 36, 72 and 120 h. After dissection, liver samples were immediately harvested from the birds for morphological and molecular studies. A portion of liver samples were fixed in 4% paraformaldehyde solution in PBS, dehydrated and then embedded in paraffin wax for morphological analysis. After that, 4-μm tissue sections were cut using a Leica microtome (Nussloch Gmbh, Germany) and mounted on polylysine-coated slides (Boster Corporation, China). The rest of fresh liver samples were also frozen quickly in liquid nitrogen and then stored at –70 °C for qPCR and ELISA analysis.

H&E staining was performed by routinely used protocol. Stained tissue sections were examined by light microscopy (Olympus BX51, Tokyo, Japan) with a digital camera (DP72; Olympus).

The tissue sections were immunostained by following the same steps as described previously [19, 20]. In brief, serial liver tissue sections were deparaffinized twice in xylene and rehydrated in a graded series of ethanol. Heat antigen retrieval was accomplished using a microwave oven (MYA-2270 M, Haier, Qindao, China) and tissue sections were microwaved in citrate acid buffer solution (pH 6.0) for 20 min (5 min at high level i.e., 700 W and 15 min at low level i.e., 116 W). Following heat-induced antigen retrieval, tissue section were allowed to cool down at room temperature for 2–3 h. Endogenous peroxidase activity was quenched by treating tissue sections with 3% H_2O_2 for 10 min at room temperature. To block non-specific antibody binding, the tissue sections were then incubated with 5% bovine serum albumin (BSA) at 37 °C for half an hour. Liver tissue sections were then incubated with primary antibodies using rabbit anti-TLR4 antibody (1:100) and PCNA (1:200) (Santa Cruz Biotechnology, Inc., Santa Cruz, CA, USA). Subsequently, tissue sections were incubated at 37 °C with suitable horseradish peroxidase (HRP)-conjugated secondary antibodies (Boster, Wuhan, China) for 30 min. In situ detection of cell apoptosis was accomplished by using a mouse IgM anti-ssDNA monoclonal antibody (1:30; EMD Millipore, Billerica, USA), following same steps as described above with the exception of treatment of tissue sections with 0.1 mg/ml saponin and 20 μg/ml proteinase K in PBS for 20 min at 37 °C, incubation in 50% (v/v) formamide in distilled water for 20 min at 56 °C. These sections were then cooled in cold PBS for 5 min, instead of heat induced antigen retrieve in a micro oven, and employed anti-mouse IgM SABC kit (Boster, Wuhan, China) instead of other secondary antibodies kit. Immunostaining for all the tissue sections was accomplished using chromogenic marker, diaminobenzidine (DAB) (Boster, Wuhan, China) and counterstaining was performed using hematoxylin. Finally, sections were washed, dried, dehydrated, cleared, and mounted with a coverslip. In the current study, isotype serum of primary antibodies was used for both LPS stimulated and saline treated (negative control) groups.

Serial sections were examined under a light microscope (BH-2; Olympus, Japan) with a digital camera (DP72; Olympus), and the fields of vision were chosen according to different regions of the liver tissue in each section. The distribution and expression level of different proteins were measured in high-power fields selected at random. All of the images were taken using the same microscope and camera set. Image-Pro Plus (IPP) 6.0 software (Media Cybernetics, USA) was used to calculate the integral optical density (IOD) for positive staining (Additional file 1) and the graphs were prepared by Prism software version 5.0 (GraphPad Software, Inc., San Diego, USA).

The expression level of alanine aminotransferase (ALT) and caspase-3 activity of liver tissues were determined by following previously described modified ELISA method [21].

The tissue homogenate for ALT activity assay was prepared according to the manufacturer's instructions. Briefly, the samples of liver from the ultra-low temperature freezer were weighed and homogenized (0.1 g of tissue in 0.90 ml of 4 °C pre-cooled physiological saline). The homogenate was centrifuged at $1000 \times g$ for 10 min and then aliquots supernatants were stored at −70 °C. The expression level of alanine aminotransferase (ALT) of liver tissues was assessed using ALT assay kit (C009-2, Nanjing Institute of Jiancheng, China). Briefly, standards and supernatants obtained from the processed liver tissues were pipetted into the wells. The absorbencies were read at 492 nm wave length. For each set of reference standards, samples and control, the average absorbance values (A_{492}) were calculated with the help of standard curve.

The cell lysate for casepase-3 activity assay was prepared according to the manufacturer's instructions. Briefly, the 100 mg solid liver tissues were cut into small pieces and then 100 μl lysate pre-cooled working fluid was added in an ice bath and homogenized with a glass homogenizer. Centrifugation was performed at $12,000 \times g$ for 10 min at 4 °C and then the supernatant (lysate containing protein) was transferred to a new tube and placed on ice until needed. The expression level of caspase-3 activity in liver tissues was determined using caspase-3 activity assay kit (G007, Nanjing Institute of Jiancheng, China). Briefly, cell lysate obtained from the processed liver tissues and standard solutions from the kit were pipetted into the wells according to the recommended experimental setting. After 4 h incubation at 37 °C, the color changes were obvious. The absorbencies were measured at 405 nm on microplate reader. The final caspase-3 activity levels were

determined by comparing optical density (OD) values from apoptosis inducer and negative control wells.

Total RNA was extracted from liver tissues according to the manufacturer's instructions. Then total RNA were treated with RNase-free DNase I (Fermentas, Opelstrasse, Germany) to remove contaminating genomic DNA. The first strand cDNA was synthesized using the RevertAid First Strand cDNA Synthesis Kit (Fermentas, Opelstrasse, Germany). The reaction mixture (10 μl) for qPCR contained of 5 μL SYBR Select Master Mix for CFX (Applied Biosystems), 0.2 μL of each forward and reverse primer and 1 μL of template cDNA. The qPCR reactions were performed on a Bio-Rad CFX Connect real-time PCR detection system (Bio-Rad, Hercules, CA, USA). The qPCR conditions were as follows: pre-denaturation at 95 °C for 5 min, followed by 40 cycles of denaturation at 95 °C for 30 s, annealing at 60 °C for 30 s, and elongation at 72 °C for 20 s. The primer sequences used in this experiments are listed in Table 1. All samples were run in triplicate and gene expression levels were quantified (Additional file 2) using the ΔΔCt method [22].

Data were expressed as the mean ± standard deviation (SD) and the statistical analyses were performed using the GraphPad Prism version 5.0. The arithmetic mean was calculated and any significant differences between groups in the same tissue regions were analyzed using the independent-samples t test for group means (Fig. 2b, Fig. 3b and Fig. 4b). The statistical significance in the comparison of multiple sample sets versus control was performed with Bonferroni's multiple comparisons test after one-way ANO VA test (Fig. 1b, Fig. 2c, Fig. 3c,

Table 1 Primers used for Real-time PCR

Gene	Primer sequences (5'to3')	Accession no.
actin beta	f-TTGTTGACAATGGCTCCGGT r-TCTGGGCTTCATCACCAACG	NM_205518.1
TLR4	f-TGAAAGAGCTGGTGGAACCC r-CCAGGACCGAGCAATGTCAA	NM_001030693.1
MyD88	f-AGGATGGTGGTCGTCATTTC r-TTGGTGCAAGGATTGGTGTA	NM_001030962.2
NF-κB	f-CTACTGATTGCTGCTGGAGTTG r-CTGCTATGTGAAGAGGCGTTGT	M86930.1
TNF-α	f-CAGATGGGAAGGGAATGAAC r-CACACGACAGCCAAGTCAAC	AY765397.1
IL-1β	f-ACCTACAAGCTAAGTGGGCG r-ATACCTCCACCCCGACAAGG	NM_204524.1
TGF-β	f-ATGTGTTCCGCTTTAACGTGTC r-GCTGCTTTGCTATATGCTCATC	NM_205454.1
caspase-3	f- TCCACCGAGATACCGGACTG r- ACAAAACTGCTTCGCTTGCT	NM_204725.1
caspase-8	f- CGGATCAATCGAATAGACCTTC r- CGGCATTGTAGTTTCAGGACTT	NM_204592.2
PCNA	f- TCTGAGGGCTTCGACACCTA r- AACCTTTTCCTGATTTGGTGCTT	NM_204170.2

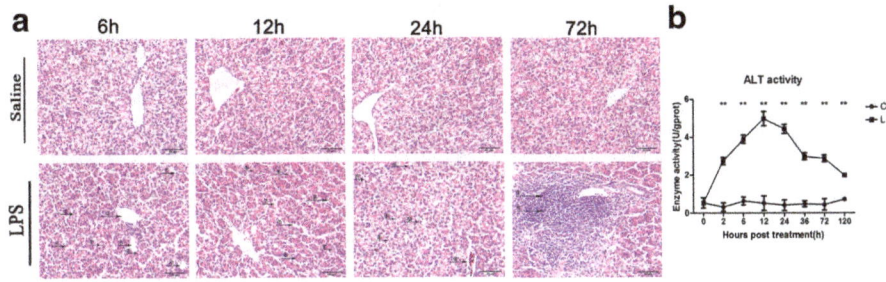

Fig. 1 Effect of lipopolysaccharide on histomorphology and ALT activity and in chicken liver. Following intraperitoneal LPS treatment in chickens at different time points, H&E staining was performed on liver serial tissue sections. Stellate macrophages (Kupffer cells) in perisinusoidal areas ①, diffuse infiltration of fat vacuoles indicating fatty infiltration ②, dilated central vein ③ and sinusoidal capillaries ④, reduction in size of a few hepatocytes ⑤, dissociated liver cells from each other in hepatic cords ⑥, dilated hepatic sinusoids along with fibrocytes proliferation in perisinusoidal areas ⑦, intracytoplasmic infiltration of variable size and shape fat vacuoles ⑧, dilated hepatic sinusoids ⑨, infiltration of oval shaped nucleated RBCs ⑩, cytoplasmic fat vacuoles have pushed hepatocyte nuclei at periphery ⑪, reduction in size of a few hepatocytes ⑫ and intense inflammatory cells infiltration around the portal area ⑬ (**a**). After LPS stimulation, alanine aminotransferase (ALT) activity was measured from liver tissues at 0 h, 2 h, 6 h, 12 h, 24 h, 36 h, 72 h and 120 h by ELISA technique (**b**). The letter C represents saline (control) group and L represents LPS group. The numbers represent the hours after stimulation. $**P < 0.01$

Fig. 4c and Fig. 5). Differences were considered significant if $P < 0.05$. $*P < 0.05$, $**P < 0.01$ and $***P < 0.001$.

Results
Acute liver injury after Salmonella lipopolysaccharide stimulation

In comparison to saline group, histopathology of liver showed prominent stellate macrophages (Kupffer cells) in peri-sinusoidal areas, diffuse infiltration of fat vacuoles indicating fatty infiltration, dilation of both central veins and sinusoidal capillaries and reduction in size of a few hepatocytes at 6 h post LPS stimulation. Liver cells were seen dissociated from each other in hepatic cords, hepatic sinusoids were dilated at many places along with fibrocyte proliferation in peri-sinusoidal areas and intra-cytoplasmic infiltration of variable size and shape fat vacuoles was seen at 12 h post LPS stimulation. Hepatic sinusoids were dilated in many areas with severe vascular congestion, cytoplasmic fat vacuoles have pushed hepatocyte nuclei at periphery at some places and reduction in size of a few hepatocytes was also seen at 24 h post LPS stimulation. Obvious pathological changes

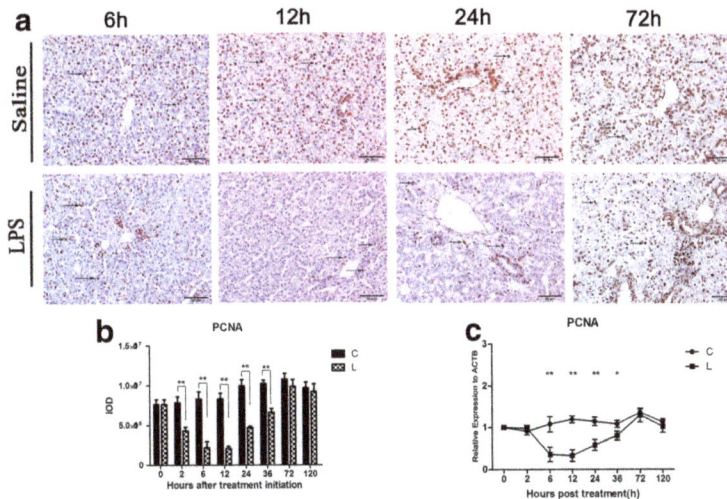

Fig. 2 Effect of LPS stimulation on hepatic cell proliferation in chicken liver. After intraperitoneal LPS injection in chicks at different time points, PCNA protein expression was assessed in liver tissue by immunohistochemistry using anti-PCNA antibody, PCNA positive product was mainly distributed around the portal and biliary epithelial cells and more concentrated expression was present on epithelial cell near portal area in saline group at 6 h, 12 h, 24 h, and 72 h as compared to LPS group (**a**). Quantification of PCNA expression from liver tissue images was accomplished by image-pro plus (IPP) computer software where IOD represents integrated optical density (**b**). The analysis of PCNA gene expression was performed by real-time quantitative RT-PCR and normalized by the expression of actin beta (ACTB) (**c**). The letter C represents saline (control) group and L represents LPS group. The numbers represent the hours after stimulation. $*P < 0.05$, $**P < 0.01$

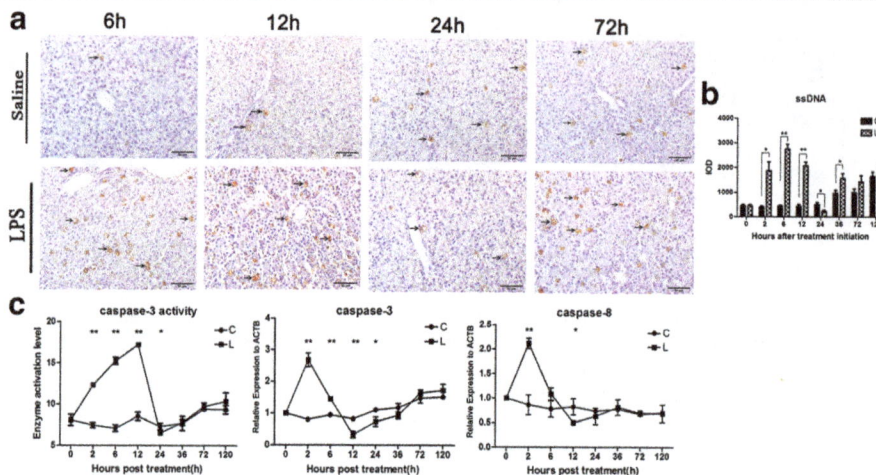

Fig. 3 Effect of LPS stimulation on hepatocyte apoptosis in chicken liver. Following intraperitoneal LPS injection in chicks at different time points, single stranded DNA (ssDNA) protein expression was assessed in liver tissues by immunohistochemistry using anti-ssDNA antibody, ssDNA positive product was extensively distributed in biliary epithelial cells and hepatic sinosoidal endothelial cells in LPS group at 6 h, 12 h, 24 h, and 72 h as compared to PBS (saline) group (**a**). Quantification of ssDNA expression from liver tissue images was accomplished by image-pro plus (IPP) computer software where IOD represents integrated optical density (**b**). The activity of caspase-3 enzyme was measured by ELIZA technique and the expressions of caspase-3 and caspase-8 genes were also determined by quantitative RT-PCR and normalized by the expression of actin beta (ACTB) (**c**). The letter C represents saline (control) group and L represents LPS group. The numbers represent the hours after stimulation. *$P < 0.05$, **$P < 0.01$

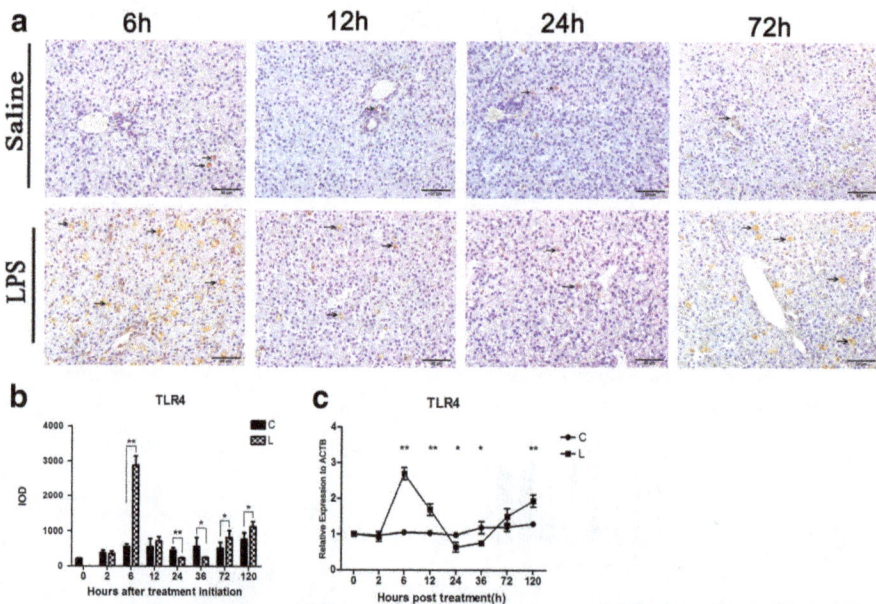

Fig. 4 Effect of LPS stimulation on TLR4 expression in chicken liver. After intraperitoneal LPS injection in chicks at different time points, TLR4 protein expression was assessed in liver tissue by immunohistochemistry using anti-TLR4 antibody, TLR4 positive product was mainly distributed on hepatocytes. In LPS group, strong TLR4 expression was present at 6 h, 12 h, 24 h, and 72 h as compared to saline group (**a**). Quantification of TLR4 expression from liver tissue images was accomplished by image-pro plus (IPP) computer software where IOD represents integrated optical density (**b**). The analysis of TLR4 gene expression was performed by quantitative RT-PCR and normalized by the expression of actin beta (ACTB) (**c**). The letter C represents saline (control) group and L represents LPS group. The numbers represent the hours after stimulation. *$P < 0.05$, **$P < 0.01$

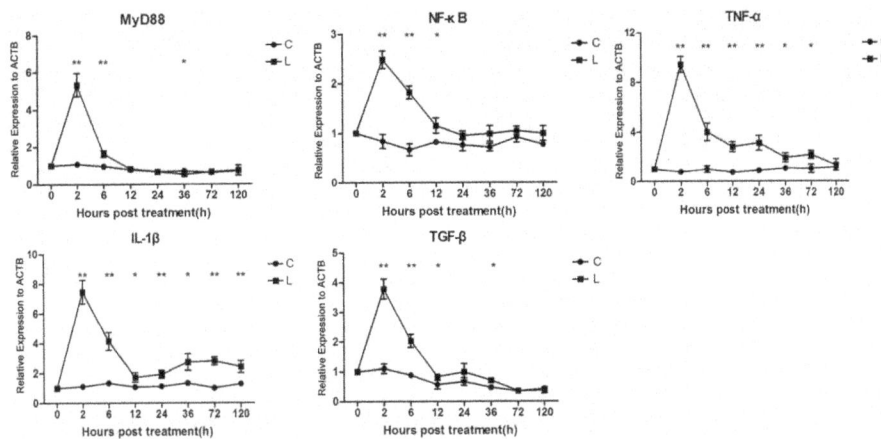

Fig. 5 Effect of LPS stimulation on downstream molecules of TLR4 signaling and cytokines in chicken liver. Following intraperitoneal LPS stimulation in chicks at 0 h, 2 h, 6 h, 12 h, 24 h, 36 h, 72 h and 120 h, the expressions of MyD88, NF-κB, TNF-α, TGF-β and IL-1β genes were determined by real-time quantitative PCR (qRT-PCR) and normalized by the expression of actin beta (ACTB). The letter C represents saline (control) group and L represents LPS group. The numbers represent the hours after stimulation. *$P < 0.05$, **$P < 0.01$

(inflammatory cell infiltration around the portal area) were present at 72 h post LPS stimulation (Fig. 1a; Additional file 3). Following LPS treatment, ALT activity was significantly higher than that of control group. It reached the peak at 12 h after LPS stimulation, and then gradually returned to normal level (Fig. 1b).

PCNA expression was remarkably decreased after LPS stimulation in chicken liver

In the control (saline) group, the PCNA positive products showed brownish shades under microscope and mainly distributed around the portal and biliary epithelial cells and more concentrated expression was present on epithelial cell near portal area (Fig. 2a). PCNA expression was remarkably decreased after LPS stimulation ($P < 0.01$) at 6 h, 12 h, 24 h, and 36 h as compared to saline group (Fig. 2b). Consistent with the results of PCNA by immunohistochemistry, mRNA expression of PCNA following LPS stimulation exhibited first decrease and then slightly returned towards the normal level and showed significant difference at 6 h, 12 h, 24 h ($P < 0.05$) and 36 h ($P < 0.01$) as compared to control group (Fig. 2c).

Effect of LPS stimulation on hepatocyte apoptosis

The single stranded DNA (ssDNA) positive products showed brownish shades under microscope and mainly distributed in the hepatocytes, biliary epithelial cells and hepatic sinosoidal endothelial cells (Fig. 3a). IPP analysis indicated that ssDNA expression changed after LPS stimulation and showed significant up-regulation ($P < 0.05$ or $P < 0.01$) at 2 h, 6 h, 12 h and 36 h, while significant down regulation ($P < 0.05$) at 24 h as compared to control group (Fig. 3b). The activity of caspase-3 as measured by ELISA, was considerably enhanced at 2 h, 6 h

and 12 h ($P < 0.01$) in LPS stimulated group as compared to control group. The levels of mRNA expression of caspase-3 following LPS stimulation exhibited first increased, then decreased and again a little increased trends and showed significant increase at 2 h, 6 h ($P < 0.01$) and significant decrease at 12 h and 24 h ($P < 0.05$ or $P < 0.01$) as compared to control group. The statistical analysis of mRNA expression of caspase-8 following LPS stimulation exhibited similar events as of caspase-3 i.e., first increased, then slightly decreased and again a little increased trends and showed significant increase at 2 h ($P < 0.01$) and significant decrease at 12 h ($P < 0.05$) as compared to control group (Fig. 3c).

Effect of LPS stimulation on TLR4 expression in chicken liver

TLR4 protein expression in chicken liver tissue sections was determined by immunoperoxidase–hematoxylin staining. In TLR4-positive hepatocytes, the cytoplasm and plasma membrane were stained light brown by DAB and nucleus was stained blue with hematoxylin. In control group, the weak TLR4 expression was only present in portal bile duct epithelial cells. After LPS stimulation TLR4 expression was more concentrated and presented in hepatocytes in the liver (Fig. 4a). IPP analysis showed that TLR4 expression was remarkably increased after LPS stimulation at 6 h, 72 h and 120 h ($P < 0.05$ or $P < 0.01$)) while significantly decreased at 24 h and 36 h ($P < 0.05$) as compared to control group (Fig. 4b). The statistics of mRNA expression of TLR4 following LPS stimulation exhibited first increase, then decrease and again increase trends and showed significant increase at 6 h, 12 h and 120 h ($P < 0.01$) and significant decrease at 24 h and 36 h ($P < 0.05$) as compared to control group (Fig. 4c).

Effect of LPS stimulation on downstream molecules of TLR4 signaling pathway and cytokines in chicken liver

Following LPS stimulation in chickens, the statistics of mRNA expression of MyD88 exhibited first drastic increase, then considerable decrease and again slight increase trends and showed very significant increase at 2 h and 6 h ($P < 0.01$) and significant decrease at 36 h ($P < 0.05$) while NF-κB demonstrated increasing trends at all the time points and showed significant difference at 2 h, 6 h and 12 h ($P < 0.05$ or $P < 0.01$) as compared to control group. The gene expressions of cytokines (TNF-α, TGF-β and IL-1β) exhibited increasing trends at all the time points after LPS stimulation illustrating significant difference ($P < 0.05$ or $P < 0.01$) at several time points as compared to saline group (Fig. 5).

Discussion

Alanine aminotransferase (ALT) is an important liver enzyme and exists in cytosol of hepatocytes. ALT activity has been reported about 3000 times in liver tissues than that in serum. Increased level of ALT is present during acute hepatocellular injury, therefore the direct measurement of ALT activity is more efficient and accurate for the damaged liver tissue [23]. Bacterial LPS is well known and critical cofactor that is usually implicated in liver injury [24]. In previous studies, LPS stimulation was found to be linked with considerable increase in serum ALT release in both mice [25] and chicken [26]. In the current investigation, we found significantly higher ALT release in liver tissue after intraperitoneal LPS stimulation that attained its peak at 12 h of treatment in young chicken as compared to control group. All these facts indicated that LPS could disrupt liver function particularly at early stages of pathological stimulation.

LPS administration has been found to disrupt liver architecture and leads to significant alteration in histological organization along with fatty degenerations and irregular and loose arrangement of hepatic cells in mice [25]. In the present study, liver showed fatty degeneration, necrotic symptoms, ballooning degeneration, congestion and enhanced inflammatory cell infiltration at different time points of LPS treatment as compared to saline injected control group in young chickens. In a previous study, LPS treatment exhibited considerable morphological changes such as necrosis, lymphocytic infiltration, Kupffer cell hyperplasia and portal triaditis in murine experimental models [27]. Hence, it seems that LPS stimulation may cause similar histo-pathological alteration in both murine and chicken liver. However underlying molecular mechanism needs further investigation.

In this study, both mRNA levels and cellular expression of proliferative cell nuclear antigen (PCNA) by immunohistochemistry were remarkably decreased at certain time points after LPS stimulation. In a prior report, LPS stimulation also showed decreased expression of PCNA in murine model with acute liver damage [28]. It is also reported that LPS treatment can trigger the activation of apoptosis related genes and the activated caspase-3 ultimately causes the cell apoptosis [29, 30]. Herein, we found significant up regulation in the expression of apoptosis related genes, caspase-3 and caspase-8 at different time points after LPS stimulation. Moreover, single stranded DNA (ss-DNA) protein expressions by immunohistochemistry were also decreased significantly after LPS treatment in the current investigation. Previously hepatocyte apoptosis has been observed after intravenous treatment of LPS in experimental shock models and the activated caspase-3 in liver tissue corresponds to apoptotic index in hepatocytes [31, 32]. Hence, it is concluded that decreased proliferation and increased apoptosis are associated with LPS induced acute liver injury in young chickens.

Complex mechanisms are involved in LPS induced acute liver damage [33]. High expression of TLR4 and down streaming molecules such as MyD88 play an essential role in progression of LPS induced acute liver injury and act as powerful mediator of inflammatory process and innate immune activation [34–36]. Herein, strong TLR4 expression was present on hepatocytes in liver and both protein and mRNA expressions levels of TLR4 were remarkably increased at certain time points after LPS stimulation. Previously, liver mRNA of chicken was sequenced for the determination of the entire chTLRs (chicken TLRs) sequences [8]. The expression of TLR4 has been reported in activated hepatic stellate cells (HSCs) as well as on parenchymal and non-parenchymal hepatic cells during acute liver damage [16]. In the current study, mRNA expressions of MyD88 and NF-κB are significantly increased at certain time points following LPS stimulation in chicken liver. During TLR4 signaling, both myeloid differentiation primary response gene 88 (MyD88)-dependent and MyD88-independent pathways are activated upon LPS stimulation in mammals and MyD88-dependent pathway leads to production of transcription factors such as nuclear factor kappaB (NF-kB) along with expressions of tumor necrosis factor (TNF) and interleukin (IL) while MyD88-independent pathway arbitrates the induction of type-I interferones and interferon-inducible genes [37–39]. In contrast, only MyD88-dependent signaling is involved in response to TLR4-MD2 complex activation under LPS stress in chicken [9]. Therefore, it is concluded that LPS/TLR4-MyD88-dependent signaling along with its downstream molecules is involved in acute liver injury in young chickens.

Determination of cytokine expressions during bacterial infection not only helps in the understanding of appropriate induction of immune response but also assists in the devising innovative therapeutic strategies [40]. In the present investigation, the statistical analysis of mRNA expression of different inflammatory cytokines such as TNF-α, IL-1β and TGF-β showed significant increase at different time points after LPS treatment in young chicken liver. In a previous study, several inflammatory cytokines such as interleukin-1 (IL-1), tumor necrosis factor-α (TNF-α) along with reactive oxygen intermediates are produced by liver in response to LPS exposure and play critical roles in its injury [24]. Hepatic injury in response to LPS exposure is also caused by TNF-α that is secreted from Kupffer cells [31]. Taken together, it is concluded that LPS/TLR4 signaling along with its downstream molecules and cytokines may play key role in acute liver injury in avian species.

Conclusions

This study demonstrated that LPS is involved in acute liver injury and significantly altered the liver's structure and function in young chickens. It was found that TLR4 signaling and its downstream molecules along with certain cytokines play a key role in hepatocyte apoptosis during acute liver injury in young chickens. Hence, our findings provided novel information about the histopathological, proliferative and apoptotic alterations along with changes in ALT and caspase-3 activities associated with acute liver injury induced by Salmonella LPS in avian species.

Abbreviations
ALT: Alanine aminotransferase; BSA: Bovine serum albumin; CFU: Colony forming unit; DAB: 3,3'-diaminobenzidine; ELIZA: Enzyme-linked immunosorbent assay; G1: Growth 1 phase; H&E: Hematoxylin and Eosin; h: Hour/hours; HRH: Horseradish peroxidase; IHC: Immunohistochemistry; IL: Interleukin; IOD: Integrated optical density; IPP: Image-Pro-plus; LPS: Lipopolysaccharide; MyD88: Myeloid differentiation primary response gene 88; NF-kB: Nuclear factor-kB; PAMPs: Pathogen associated molecular patterns; PBS: Phosphate buffered saline; PCNA: Proliferating cell nuclear antigen; PRRs: Pattern recognition receptors; qRT-PCR: Quantitative real time polymerase chain reaction; S phase: DNA synthesis phase; SABC: StreptAvidin-Biotin Complex; SD: Standard deviation; ssDNA: Single stranded DNA; STm: Salmonella enterica serovar Typhimurium; TLRs: Toll like receptors; TNF-α: Tumour necrosis factor-alpha

Acknowledgements
None.

Funding
This work was supported by the Fundamental Research Funds for the Central Universities (2662016PY011, 2014PY046), grants from the National Natural Science Foundation of China (30800808).

Authors' contributions
HZL and KMP and JMZ planned and conceived the experiments. XYH, ARA, HBH, NYL and ZJS performed the experiments and carried out other laboratory works. HZL, XYH and ARA analyzed data, designed the figures and wrote the manuscript. HZL, JMZ and KMP performed the proof reading. XYH and ARA have contributed equally as first-coauthors. All the authors read and approved the final manuscript.

Competing interests
The authors declare that they have no competing interests.

Author details
[1]Department of Basic Veterinary Medicine, College of Animal Science and Veterinary Medicine, Huazhong Agricultural University, Wuhan, Hubei 430070, China. [2]Section of Anatomy and Histology, Department of Basic Sciences, College of Veterinary and Animal Sciences (CVAS) Jhang, University of Veterinary and Animal Sciences (UVAS), Lahore, Pakistan. [3]Department of Anatomy, Physiology and Pharmacology, College of Veterinary Medicine, Auburn University, Auburn, USA.

References
1. Nemeth E, Baird AW, O'Farrelly C. Microanatomy of the liver immune system. Semin Immunopathol. 2009;31(3):333–43.
2. Knolle PA, Wohlleber D. Immunological functions of liver sinusoidal endothelial cells. Cell Mol Immunol. 2016;13(3):347–53.
3. Robinson MW, Harmon C, O'Farrelly C. Liver immunology and its role in inflammation and homeostasis. Cell Mol Immunol. 2016;13(3):267–76.
4. Racanelli V, Rehermann B. The liver as an immunological organ. Hepatology. 2006;43 Suppl 1:S54–62.
5. Crispe IN. The liver as a lymphoid organ. Annu Rev Immunol. 2009;27:147–63.
6. Gao B. Basic liver immunology. Cell Mol Immunol. 2016;13(3):265–6.
7. Masaki T, Chiba S, Tatsukawa H, Yasuda T, Noguchi H, Seike M, Yoshimatsu H. Adiponectin protects LPS-induced liver injury through modulation of TNF-α in KK-Ay obese mice. Hepatology. 2004;40(1):177–84.
8. Fukui A, Inoue N, Matsumoto M, Nomura M, Yamada K, Matsuda Y, Toyoshima K, Seya T. Molecular cloning and functional characterization of chicken toll-like receptors: a single chicken toll covers multiple molecular patterns. J Biol Chem. 2001;276(50):47143–9.
9. Keestra AM, van Putten JPM. Unique properties of the chicken TLR4/MD-2 complex: selective lipopolysaccharide activation of the MyD88-dependent pathway. J Immunol. 2008;181(6):4354–62.
10. Akira S, Takeda K, Kaisho T. Toll-like receptors: critical proteins linking innate and acquired immunity. Nat Immunol. 2001;2(8):675–80.
11. Medzhitov R. Toll-like receptors and innate immunity. Nat Rev Immunol. 2001;1(2):135–45.
12. Kawai T, Akira S. The role of pattern-recognition receptors in innate immunity: update on Toll-like receptors. Nat Immunol. 2010;11(5):373–84.
13. Reuven EM, Fink A, Shai Y. Regulation of innate immune responses by transmembrane interactions: lessons from the TLR family. Biochim Biophys Acta. 2014;1838(6):1586–93.
14. Kannaki T, Reddy M, Verma P, Shanmugam M. Differential Toll-Like receptor (TLR) mRNA expression patterns during chicken embryological development. Anim Biotechnol. 2015;26(2):130–5.
15. Karnati HK, Pasupuleti SR, Kandi R, Undi RB, Sahu I, Kannaki T, Subbiah M, Gutti RK. TLR-4 signalling pathway. MyD88 independent pathway up-regulation in chicken breeds upon LPS treatment. Vet Res Commun. 2010;39(1):73–8.
16. Guo J, Friedman SL. Toll-like receptor 4 signaling in liver injury and hepatic fibrogenesis. Fibrogenesis Tissue Repair. 2010;3:21.
17. Schuppan D, Kim YO. Evolving therapies for liver fibrosis. J Clin Invest. 2013;123(5):1887–901.
18. Muñoz NM, Katz LH, Shina J-H, Gi YJ, Menon VK, Gagea M, Rashid A, Chen J, Mishra L. Generation of a mouse model of T-cell lymphoma based on

chronic LPS challenge and TGF-β signaling disruption. Genes Cancer. 2014; 5(9–10):348–52.

19. Ansari AR, Ge X-H, Huang H-B, Huang X-Y, Zhao X, Peng K-M, Zhong J-M, Liu H-Z. Effects of lipopolysacharide on the histomorphology and expression of toll like receptor 4 in the chicken trachea and lung. Avian Pathol. 2016;45(5): 530–7.

20. Ansari AR, Ge X-H, Huang H-B, Wang J-X, Peng K-M, Yu M, Liu H-Z. Expression patterns of Toll-Like receptor 4 in pig uterus during pregnancy. Pak Vet J. 2015; 35(4):466–9.

21. Ehrnhoefer DE, Skotte NH, Savill J, Nguyen YTN, Ladha S, Cao L-P, Dullaghan E, Hayden MR. A quantitative method for the specific assessment of caspase-6 activity in cell culture. PLoS One. 2011;6:e27680.

22. Livak KJ, Schmittgen TD. Analysis of relative gene expression data using real-time quantitative PCR and the 2-ΔΔCT method. Methods. 2001;25(4): 402–8.

23. Kim W, Flamm SL, Di Bisceglie AM, Bodenheimer HC. Serum activity of alanine aminotransferase (ALT) as an indicator of health and disease. Hepatology. 2008; 47(4):1363–70.

24. Su GL. Lipopolysaccharides in liver injury: molecular mechanisms of Kupffer cell activation. Am J Physiol Gastrointest Liver Physiol. 2002;283(2):G256–65.

25. Gao L-N, Yan K, Cui Y-L, Fan G-W, Wang Y-F. Protective effect of Salvia miltiorrhiza and Carthamus tinctorius extract against lipopolysaccharide-induced liver injury. World J Gastroenterol. 2015;21(30):9079–92.

26. GUO F-x, LIU T-f, GENG Z-x, JIANG F, YU Z-g. Immunoregulatory effects of compound ammonium glycyrrhizin soluble powder on liver injury induced by enrofloxacin and LPS in chickens. Sci Agric Sin. 2013. http://en.cnki.com. cn/Article_en/CJFDTOTAL-ZNYK201312020.htm. Accessed 15 May 2016.

27. Bharrhan S, Chopra K, Rishi P. Vitamin E supplementation modulates endotoxin-induced liver damage in a rat model. Am J Biomed Sci. 2010;2(1):51–62.

28. Cai Y, Zou Z, Liu L, Chen S, Chen Y, Lin Z, Shi K, Xu L, Chen Y. Bone marrow-derived mesenchymal stem cells inhibits hepatocyte apoptosis after acute liver injury. Int J Clin Exp Pathol. 2015;8(1):107–16.

29. Xiao K, Zou W-H, Yang Z, ur Rehman Z, Ansari AR, Yuan H-R, Zhou Y, Cui L, Peng K-M, Song H. The role of visfatin on the regulation of inflammation and apoptosis in the spleen of LPS-treated rats. Cell Tissue Res. 2015;359(2): 605–18.

30. Hongmei Z. Extrinsic and intrinsic apoptosis signal pathway review. Apoptosis and Medicine, InTech. 2012. http://www.intechopen.com/books/ apoptosis-and-medicine/extrinsic-and-intrinsic-apoptosis-signal-pathway-review. Accessed 09 Sept 2016.

31. Hamada E, Nishida T, Uchiyama Y, Nakamura J-i, Isahara K, Kazuo H, Huang T-P, Momoi T, Ito T, Matsuda H. Activation of Kupffer cells and caspase-3 involved in rat hepatocyte apoptosis induced by endotoxin. J Hepatol. 1999;30:807–18.

32. Wang JH, Redmond HP, Watson R, Bouchier-Hayes D. Role of lipopolysaccharide and tumor necrosis factor-alpha in induction of hepatocyte necrosis. Am J Physiol. 1995;269(2):G297–304.

33. Yao H, Hu C, Yin L, Tao X, Xu L, Qi Y, Han X, Xu Y, Zhao Y, Wang C. Dioscin reduces lipopolysaccharide-induced inflammatory liver injury via regulating TLR4/MyD88 signal pathway. Int Immunopharmacol. 2016;36:132–41.

34. Zhao Y, Liu Q, Yang L, He D, Wang L, Tian J, Li Y, Zi F, Bao H, Yang Y. TLR4 inactivation protects from graft-versus-host disease after allogeneic hematopoietic stem cell transplantation. Cell Mol Immunol. 2013;10(2):165–75.

35. Wang Y, Tu Q, Yan W, Xiao D, Zeng Z, Ouyang Y, Huang L, Cai J, Zeng X, Chen Y-J. CXC195 suppresses proliferation and inflammatory response in LPS-induced human hepatocellular carcinoma cells via regulating TLR4-MyD88-TAK1-mediated NF-κB and MAPK pathway. Biochem Biophys Res Commun. 2015;456(1):373–9.

36. Imamura M, Tsutsui H, Yasuda K, Uchiyama R, Yumikura-Futatsugi S, Mitani K, Hayashi S, Akira S, Taniguchi S-i, Van Rooijen N. Contribution of TIR domain-containing adapter inducing IFN-β-mediated IL-18 release to LPS-induced liver injury in mice. J Hepatol. 2009;51(2):333–41.

37. Lu Y-C, Yeh W-C, Ohashi PS. LPS/TLR4 signal transduction pathway. Cytokine. 2008;42(2):145–51.

38. Janeway Jr CA, Medzhitov R. Innate immune recognition. Annu Rev Immunol. 2002;20:197–216.

39. Kawai T, Kawasaki T. Toll-like receptor signaling pathways. Front Immunol. 2014;5:461.

40. Im YB, Jung M, Shin M-K, Kim S, Yoo HS. Expression of cytokine and apoptosis-related genes in bovine peripheral blood mononuclear cells stimulated with Brucella abortus recombinant proteins. Vet Res. 2016;47:30.

4

Rapid loss of early antigen-presenting activity of lymph node dendritic cells against Ag85A protein following *Mycobacterium bovis* BCG infection

Zhengzhong Xu[1], Aihong Xia[1], Xin Li[1], Zhaocheng Zhu[1], Yechi Shen[2], Shanshan Jin[2], Tian Lan[2], Yuqing Xie[2], Han Wu[2], Chuang Meng[1], Lin Sun[1], Yuelan Yin[2], Xiang Chen[1,3]* and Xinan Jiao[2,3]*

Abstract

Background: Control of *Mycobacterium tuberculosis* (*Mtb*) infection requires CD4$^+$ T-cell responses and major histocompatibility complex class II (MHC II) presentation of *Mtb* antigens (Ags). Dendritic cells (DCs) are the most potent of the Ag-presenting cells and are central to the initiation of T-cell immune responses. Much research has indicated that DCs play an important role in anti-mycobacterial immune responses at early infection time points, but the kinetics of Ag presentation by these cells during these events are incompletely understood.

Results: In the present study, we evaluated in vivo dynamics of early Ag presentation by murine lymph-node (LN) DCs in response to *Mycobacterium bovis* bacillus Calmette–Guérin (BCG) Ag85A protein. Results showed that the early Ag-presenting activity of murine DCs induced by *M. bovis* BCG Ag85A protein in vivo was transient, appearing at 4 h and being barely detectable at 72 h. The transcription levels of CIITA, MHC II and the expression of MHC II molecule on the cell surface increased following BCG infection. Moreover, BCG was found to survive within the inguinal LN DC pool, representing a continuing source of mycobacterial Ag85A protein, with which LN DCs formed Ag85A peptide-MHCII complexes in vivo.

Conclusions: Our results demonstrate that a decrease in Ag85A peptide production as a result of the inhibition of Ag processing to is largely responsible for the short duration of Ag presentation by LN DCs during BCG infection in vivo.

Keywords: Ag-presenting activity, Dendritic cell, *M. bovis* BCG, Major histocompatibility complex class II, In vivo

Background

Tuberculosis (TB), caused by infection with *Mycobacterium tuberculosis* (*Mtb*), remains a major disease worldwide and is the leading infectious disease in terms of mortality, being responsible for an estimated 1.3 million deaths globally in 2016. Moreover, in the same year, there were an estimated 10.4 million new cases of active TB worldwide. *Mycobacterium bovis* bacillus Calmette–Guérin (BCG) is the only TB vaccine for humans in current use, but its efficacy is insufficient to prevent pulmonary TB in adults and reactivation of latent *Mtb* infection [1]. BCG vaccination mainly induces effector, rather than central, memory T cells, which are maintained for a shorter period, explaining the limited duration of protection afforded [2, 3].

CD4$^+$ T-cell responses and the production of interferon gamma (IFN-γ) are particularly important to the containment of *Mtb* infection [4, 5]. Dendritic cells (DCs) represent the bridge between the innate and adaptive immune responses and specifically strengthen the cellular immune response against mycobacterial infections [6, 7]. Thus, the mechanisms involved in major

* Correspondence: chenxiang@yzu.edu.cn; jiao@yzu.edu.cn
[1]Jiangsu Key Laboratory of Zoonosis, Yangzhou University, No. 48 Wenhui East Road, Yangzhou 225009, Jiangsu, China
[2]Key Laboratory of Prevention and Control of Biological Hazard Factors (Animal Origin) for Agrifood Safety and Quality, MOA of China, Yangzhou University, Yangzhou, China
Full list of author information is available at the end of the article

histocompatibility complex class II (MHC II) antigen (Ag) processing and presentation, which are required for CD4[+] T-cell activation, are crucial for controlling *Mtb* infection [8]. Much research has indicated that DCs play an important role in anti-mycobacterial immune responses in the early stages of infection, but little is known of the kinetics of Ag presentation by these cells soon after *M. bovis* BCG exposure. Indeed, efforts to understand the basis of protective immunity against *Mtb* have led us the examinntion of even earlier infection time points. We previously investigated the Ag-presenting cell (APC) functions of murine DCs during the first 2 weeks following intravenous administration of recombinant BCG (rBCG) expressing the *Escherichia coli* MalE protein as a reporter Ag [9]. However, this process has not yet been directly examined in lymph node (LN) DCs using an endogenous *M. bovis* BCG Ag.

In the present study, we evaluated the in vivo dynamics of early Ag presentation by murine inguinal LN DCs in response to *M. bovis* BCG. The results showed that the early Ag-presenting activity of murine DCs induced by *M. bovis* BCG Ag85A protein in vivo was transient and that the inhibition of Ag processing due to the decreased production of Ag85A peptide is the primary reason for the rapid loss of Ag85A peptide-MHC II complexes.

Results

Stimulation of Ag85A-specific IFN-γ production in BCG-infected mice

In order to evaluate the kinetics of the Ag85A-specific T-cell immune response to BCG infection, mononuclear cells isolated from BCG-immunized mice were stimulated in vitro with Ag85A peptide, Ag85A protein, or bovine purified protein (PPD), and concentrations of IFN-γ in culture supernatants were measured. The result showed a significant increase in Ag85A-specific IFN-γ production by inguinal LN mononuclear cells 3 days after BCG injection, with an even greater increase after

6 days (Fig. 1). Ag85A-specific T lymphocytes in both the spleen (Fig. 1a) and inguinal LN (Fig. 1b) produced high levels of IFN-γ when stimulated with Ag85A, although IFN-γ production was 10-fold higher in the LN group. This suggests that the Ag85A-specific T-cell immune response was initiated in the inguinal LN 6 days following BCG infection. Differences in IFN-γ production in the murine spleen and LN may be a consequence of differences in the frequency of T cells among mononuclear cells.

Dynamics of DC ag-presenting activity in vivo

To investigate the dynamics of inguinal LN DC Ag presentation, we tested their capacity to stimulate DE10 T-cell hybridomas at several time points after subcutaneous injection of mice with BCG. The inguinal LN DCs (CD11c[high]) were sorted by auto-MACS with a purity of 94.7% (Fig. 2a). When mice were infected with BCG, LN DCs collected at early time points invoked a response from DE10 hybridomas, with IL-2 being detected following stimulation with those harvested 4 h post-injection, and the highest IL-2 production being observed in response to DCs from mice infected for 12 h. However, IL-2 was only minimally produced in response to DCs from mice infected for 72 h (Fig. 2b). Interestingly, when mice were s.c. injected with heat-killed BCG, Ag-presenting activity markedly decreased from 12 h to 96 h post-injection, suggesting that live BCG is necessary for efficient Ag presentation by DCs in vivo (Fig. 2c). Together, these results indicate that the MHC II presentation of mycobacteria-derived peptides by inguinal LN DCs is only transient, with Ag85A peptide-MHC II complexes on the surfaces of inguinal LN DCs disappearing rapidly.

Analysis of MHC II, CIITA and T-cell costimulatory molecules on DCs following BCG infection

We measured the expression of cell surface markers involved in Ag presentation and T-cell interaction. Sorted

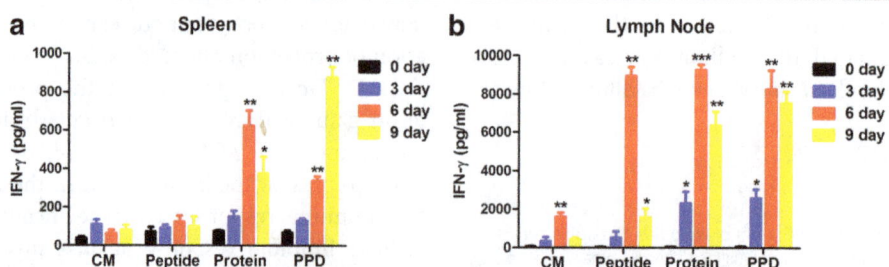

Fig. 1 Detection of IFN-γ production following BCG infection. Four groups of C57BL/6 mice ($n = 6$) s.c. vaccinated with 1×10^8 CFU BCG were sacrificed at different time points, and their spleens and inguinal LNs were removed. Increased IFN-γ levels were detected in the culture supernatants of splenocytes (**a**) and inguinal LN cells (**b**). Results are representative of three independent experiments and presented as means ± SEM. Statistical significance was determined using Student's *t*-test (*$P < 0.05$, **$P < 0.01$, ***$P < 0.001$). CM, culture medium

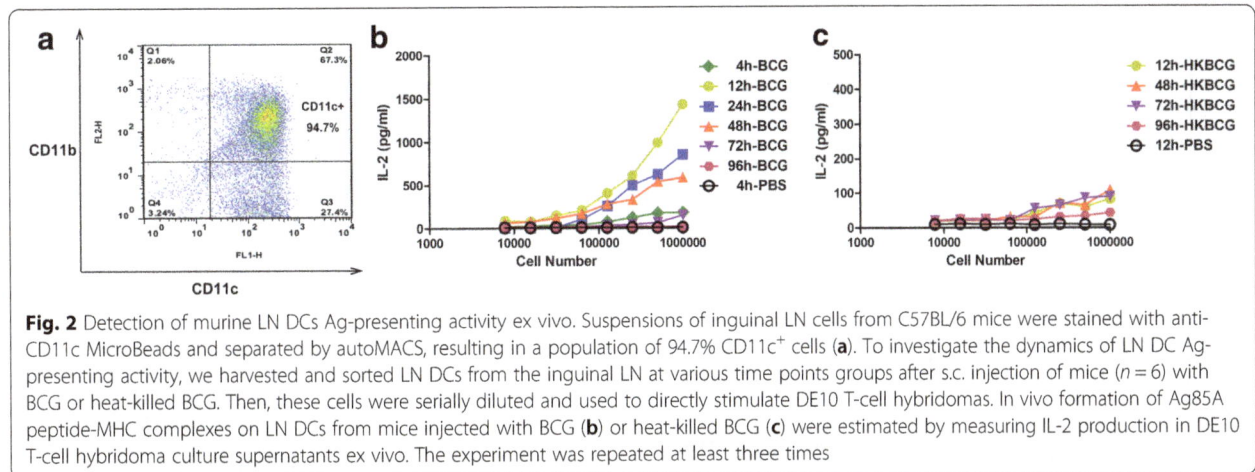

Fig. 2 Detection of murine LN DCs Ag-presenting activity ex vivo. Suspensions of inguinal LN cells from C57BL/6 mice were stained with anti-CD11c MicroBeads and separated by autoMACS, resulting in a population of 94.7% CD11c⁺ cells (**a**). To investigate the dynamics of LN DC Ag-presenting activity, we harvested and sorted LN DCs from the inguinal LN at various time points groups after s.c. injection of mice (*n* = 6) with BCG or heat-killed BCG. Then, these cells were serially diluted and used to directly stimulate DE10 T-cell hybridomas. In vivo formation of Ag85A peptide-MHC complexes on LN DCs from mice injected with BCG (**b**) or heat-killed BCG (**c**) were estimated by measuring IL-2 production in DE10 T-cell hybridoma culture supernatants ex vivo. The experiment was repeated at least three times

inguinal LN DCs were stained with a panel of monoclonal antibodies (mAbs) to detect CD40, CD54, CD80, and CD86 by Flow Cytometry (FACS). No obvious regulation of CD40 or CD54 on DCs was observed during infection (Fig. 3a, b). High levels of CD80 and CD86 were noted at 12 h, but the presence of these markers had decreased by 72 h and 96 h (Fig. 3c, d). These results indicate that inguinal LN DCs undergo functional activation in the early stages of BCG infection.

We next investigated transcription levels of MHC II and CIITA transcription in inguinal LN DCs during BCG infection using real-time PCR. MHC II expression was found to be increased by BCG infection at a relatively slow rate, while total CIITA transcription was rapidly induced, and expression of CIITA type I declined between 48 and 96 h (Fig. 3e). In addition, to evaluate the expression of MHC II molecules involved in Ag presentation, sorted inguinal LN DCs were stained with mAbs for FACS analysis. All sorted DCs demonstrated up-regulation of MHC II molecules following the initiation of infection (Fig. 3f). The fact that the transcription and expression of MHC II proteins on the cell surface did not decline following BCG infection suggests that the expression and trafficking of MHC class II molecules may be not associated with the rapid loss of Ag85A peptide-MHC II complexes. As a result, it can be deduced that LN DCs do not provide a continuous source of mycobacterial Ag85A peptides for the formation of peptideMHC II complexes.

BCG infection kinetics of murine LN DCs

In order to monitor the presence of BCG bacilli in inguinal LN DCs following s.c. infection of mice and thus evaluate the infection rate of these immune cells, rBCG-GFP cells were used in combination with FACS. As might be expected, 0.4% of LN DCs exhibited green fluorescence after 12 h of infection, and this figure had increased to 2% by 96 h post-injection (Fig. 4a). We next

determined whether BCG survives and multiplies within DCs over the course of infection. CFUs appeared at 4 h and had increased significantly by 12 h after s.c. administration of BCG to mice, and numbers remained elevated until the end of the experiment (Fig. 4b). These results suggest that BCG infected the inguinal LN DC 12 h post-infection and that it survives within the inguinal LN DC pool, representing a continuing source of mycobacterial Ag85A protein, with which LN DCs can form Ag85A peptide-MHCII complexes in vivo.

Discussion

CD4⁺ T-cell responses and the production of IFN-γ are particularly important to the containment of *Mtb* infection. In mice, between 1 and 3 weeks after initial infection, *Mtb*-specific T cells appear in the lungs, IFN-γ is expressed, and the bacterial burden is controlled [10]. Production of IFN-γ by splenocytes in response to Ag restimulation is observed within 6 days after i.v. *Mtb* infection [11]. To determine when the T-cell response is initiated, we obtained splenocytes and inguinal LN cells from mice 3, 6, and 9 days after s.c. BCG injection. Inguinal LN cells collected 6 days after infection produced IFN-γ in response to Ag85A restimulation. Thus, the T-cell immune response appears to have been initiated in the inguinal LN day 6 following BCG infection.

The mechanisms involved in MHC class II Ag processing and presentation, which are required for CD4⁺ T-cell activation, are crucial for controlling *Mtb* infection. Previous research investigated the kinetics of Ag-presenting activity by harvesting spleens following i.v. administration of rBCG expressing the *E. coli* MalE protein as a reporter Ag. The formation of MalE peptide-MHC complexes in splenic DCs was detected at 2, 4, and 12 h after rBCG infection, while MalE was barely detectable at 48 h [9]. However, this process has not yet been directly examined in LN DCs and by using an endogenous *M. bovis* BCG Ag. To investigate the

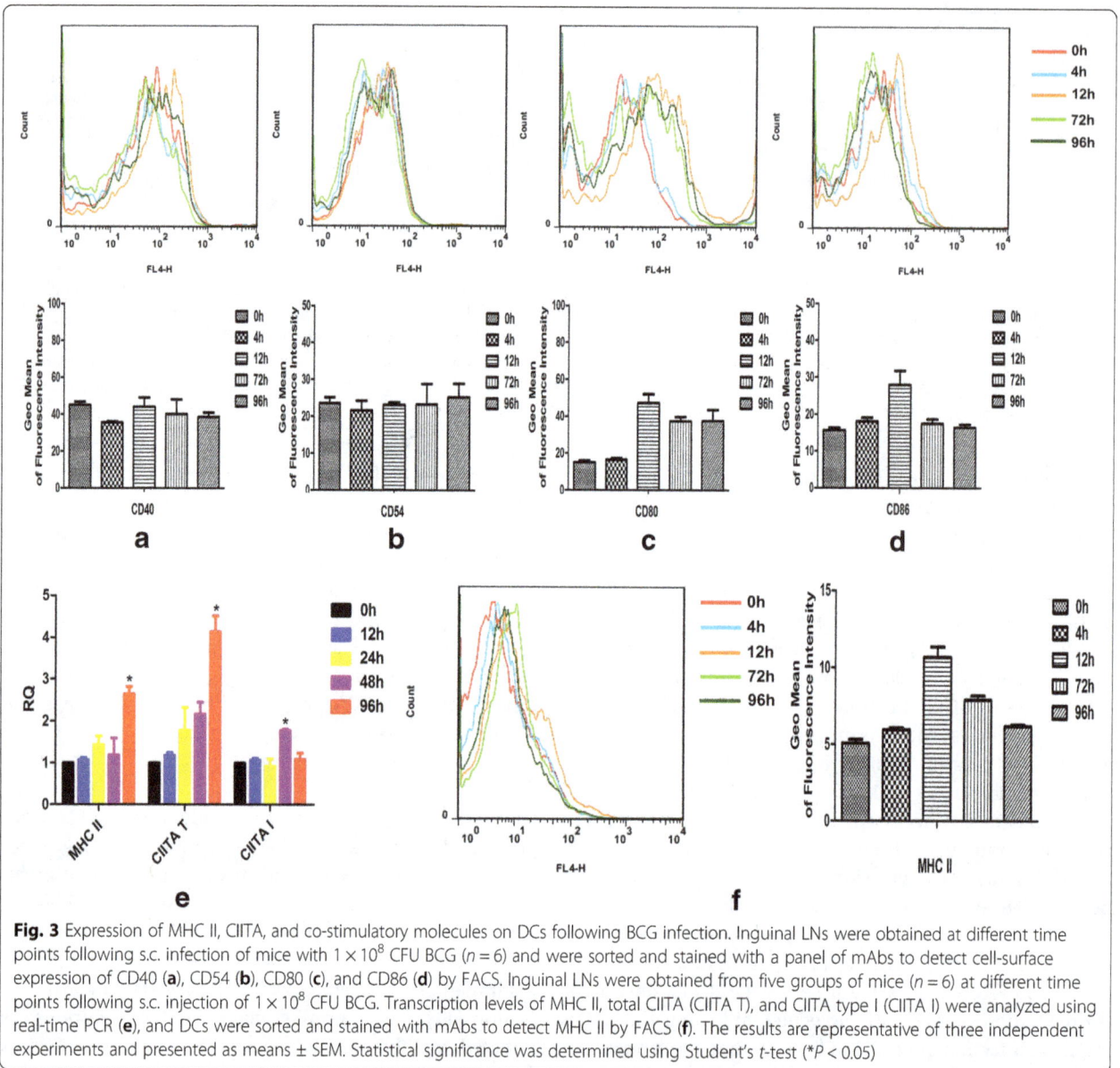

Fig. 3 Expression of MHC II, CIITA, and co-stimulatory molecules on DCs following BCG infection. Inguinal LNs were obtained at different time points following s.c. infection of mice with 1×10^8 CFU BCG ($n = 6$) and were sorted and stained with a panel of mAbs to detect cell-surface expression of CD40 (**a**), CD54 (**b**), CD80 (**c**), and CD86 (**d**) by FACS. Inguinal LNs were obtained from five groups of mice ($n = 6$) at different time points following s.c. injection of 1×10^8 CFU BCG. Transcription levels of MHC II, total CIITA (CIITA T), and CIITA type I (CIITA I) were analyzed using real-time PCR (**e**), and DCs were sorted and stained with mAbs to detect MHC II by FACS (**f**). The results are representative of three independent experiments and presented as means ± SEM. Statistical significance was determined using Student's t-test ($*P < 0.05$)

dynamics of LN DCs Ag presentation, we harvested and sorted these cells from inguinal LNs at several time points after s.c. injection of mice with Ag85A protein or BCG and tested their capacity to stimulate DE10 T-cell hybridomas, which are specific for an immunodominant Ag85A peptide. In this manner, in vivo formation of Ag85A peptide-MHC complexes on DCs from BCG-injected mice was detected by measuring IL-2 production in DE10 T-cell hybridoma culture supernatants ex vivo. Ag85A peptide-MHC complexes on LN DCs appeared rapidly after inoculation, with IL-2 production being detected in response to DCs collected 4 h after BCG infection and the highest production in response to those harvested at 12 h. By contrast, IL-2 levels following exposure to

DCs harvested 72 h after infection were barely detectable. Together, these results indicate that the MHC II presentation of mycobacteria-derived peptides by inguinal LN DCs is only transient, with Ag85A peptide-MHC II complexes on the surfaces of inguinal LN DCs disappearing rapidly. Some reports have shown that peptide-MHC complexes have a half-life of 25 h [12]. Thus, it can be concluded that the synthesis of Ag85A peptide-MHC II complexes on inguinal LN DCs was interfered.

Several reports have shown that *Mtb* and *M. bovis* inhibit intracellular processes associated with Ag presentation, including Ag processing, MHC class II expression, the trafficking of MHC class II molecules, and peptide-MHC class II binding [13, 14]. CIITA is the

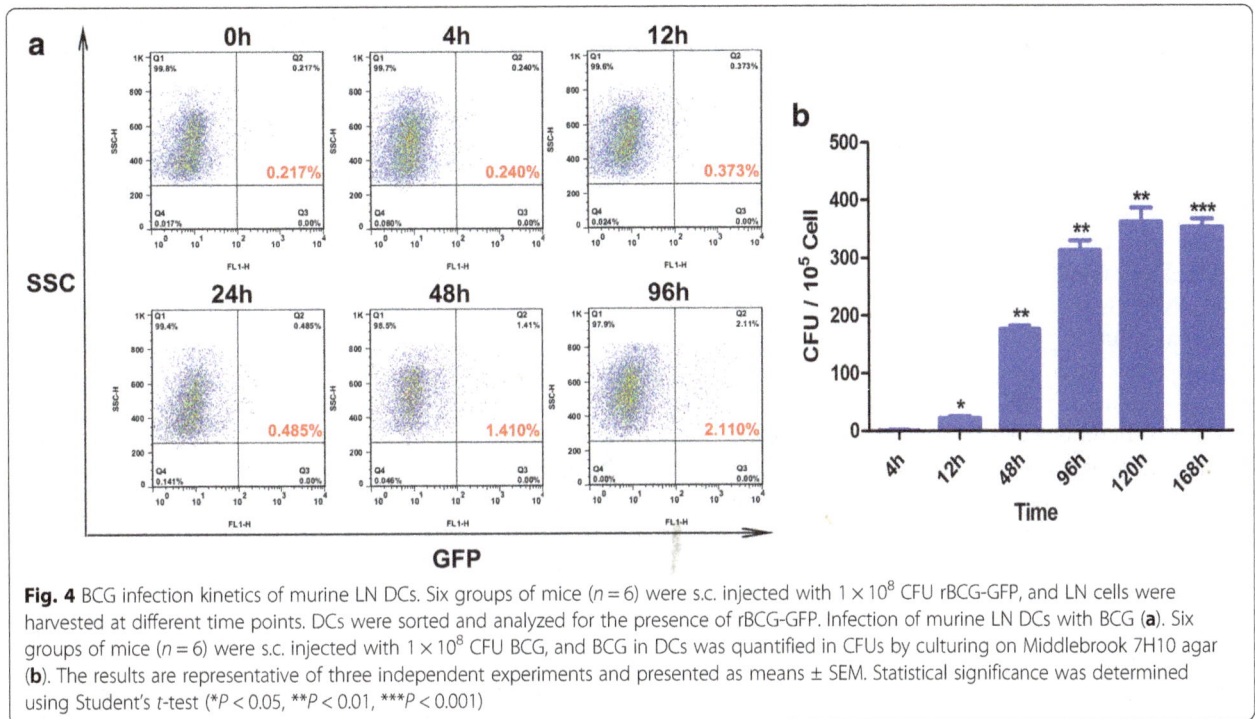

Fig. 4 BCG infection kinetics of murine LN DCs. Six groups of mice (*n* = 6) were s.c. injected with 1 × 10^8 CFU rBCG-GFP, and LN cells were harvested at different time points. DCs were sorted and analyzed for the presence of rBCG-GFP. Infection of murine LN DCs with BCG (**a**). Six groups of mice (*n* = 6) were s.c. injected with 1 × 10^8 CFU BCG, and BCG in DCs was quantified in CFUs by culturing on Middlebrook 7H10 agar (**b**). The results are representative of three independent experiments and presented as means ± SEM. Statistical significance was determined using Student's *t*-test (*P < 0.05, **P < 0.01, ***P < 0.001)

master transcriptional regulator of MHC class II molecules [15]. The transcription of CIITA itself is regulated by the three unique promoters pI, pIII, and pIV, which drive the expression of CIITA types I, III, and IV, respectively. pI is constitutively active in DCs [14]. In the current investigation, LN DCs exhibited the up-regulation of cell-surface MHC II molecules from 4 to 96 h following infection. Using real-time PCR, we analyzed the transcription levels of MHC II, total CIITA, and CIITA type I in DCs in response to BCG. Expression of MHC II was found to be induced by BCG infection relatively slowly, while total CIITA transcription was rapidly induced. This indicates that the transcription and expression of MHC II proteins on the cell surface did not declined following BCG infection, suggesting that the expression and trafficking of MHC class II molecules may be not associated with the rapid loss of Ag85A peptide-MHC II complexes. As a result, it can be deduced that LN DCs do not provide a continuing source of mycobacterial Ag85A peptides for the formation of peptide-MHC II complexes.

Considerable evidence shows that DCs can phagocytose mycobacteria and may be the first cells to encounter such pathogens, therefore, DCs are likely to be responsible for initiating the subsequent immune response. The survival of mycobacteria within DCs has been assessed previously in vitro using the BCG vaccine strain and virulent *M. bovis*, both of which were shown to be phagocytosed by DCs after 24 h of infection [16]. *Mtb* cells disseminate to draining LNs within 8 days following respiratory infection [17]. Approximately 2% of the splenic DC population (CD11c$^+$ cells) was found to contain BCG at 4 h following i.v. infection [9]. In the present study, the presence of rBCG-GFP bacilli in inguinal LN DCs following s.c. inoculation of mice was monitored by FACS. As expected, the percentage of infected DCs increased to 2% after 96 h of infection. We then examined whether mycobacteria survive and multiply within DCs during infection. Following s.c. administration of BCG to mice, CFUs appeared at 4 h, increased significantly by 12 h, remaining elevated until the last time point. These results suggest that BCG survives within the inguinal LN DC pool, representing a continuing source of mycobacterial Ag85A protein with which LN DCs can form Ag85A peptide-MHCII complexes in vivo. Some reports have shown that live *Mtb* can alter phagosome maturation and decrease Ag processing, providing a mechanism for *Mtb* to evade immune surveillance and enhance its survival within the host [18–20]. Based on our findings, we conclude that the inhibition of Ag processing due to the reduced production of Ag85A peptide is the primary reason for the rapid loss of Ag85A peptide-MHC II complexes.

Conclusions

In the present study, we evaluated the in vivo dynamics of early Ag presentation by murine LN DCs in response to *M. bovis* BCG Ag85A protein. Our results showed that the early Ag-presenting activity of murine DCs induced by *M. bovis* BCG Ag85A protein in vivo was transient and that the inhibition of Ag processing induced by a decrease in the production of Ag85A peptide is the primary reason for the rapid loss of Ag85A peptide-MHC II complexes and the short duration of Ag presentation by LN DCs during BCG infection in vivo.

Methods

Experimental animals

Six-week-old female C57BL/6 mice were purchased from Vital River (Beijing, China). The mice were housed, handled, and immunized at our animal biosafety facilities, and all procedures were approved by the Institutional Animal Experimental Committee of Yangzhou University. All experiments were performed according to the national guidelines for animal welfare. The mice were euthanized by cervical dislocation under isoflurane, and spleens and inguinal LNs were collected for analysis.

Bacterial strains and culture conditions

M. bovis BCG Pasteur 1173P2 and rBCG expressing GFP (rBCG-GFP) were kindly provided by Dr. Xiaoming Zhang (Institut Pasteur of Shanghai, Chinese Academy of Sciences, Shanghai, China). Both strains were grown with gentle agitation (80 rpm) in Middlebrook 7H9 medium (Difco, Detroit, MI, USA) supplemented with 0.05% Tween 80 and 10% albumin-dextrose-catalase (ADC) enrichment or on solid Middlebrook 7H10 medium (Difco) supplemented with 0.05% Tween 80 and 10% oleic-ADC enrichment.

T-cell hybridoma and Ags

MHC II-restricted DE10 T-cell hybridomas specific for the Mtb Ag85A peptide comprising amino acids 241 to 260 [21] were kindly provided by Dr. Claude Leclerc (Institut Pasteur, Paris, France). The Ag85A protein was constructed and expressed in our laboratory, and the Ag85A peptide (amino acids 241–260) was synthesized by SciLight Biotechnology (Beijing, China).

Detection of IFN-γ production following BCG infection

C57BL/6 mice were s.c. vaccinated with 1×10^8 CFU BCG and sacrificed 3, 6, and 9 days later, at which point, spleens and inguinal LNs were removed aseptically and transferred to complete RPMI-1640 medium for preparation of single-cell suspensions. The mononuclear cells, isolated using Histopaque 1083 (Sigma, St. Louis, MO, USA), were seeded at 1×10^6 cells/well in 96-well plates containing complete RPMI-1640 medium. They were subsequently stimulated with 10 μg/ml Ag85A peptide, 10 μg/ml Ag85A protein, or 5 μg/ml bovine PPD (Prionics, Schlieren, Switzerland) and incubated at 37 °C in an atmosphere of 5% CO_2 in air. Supernatants were then harvested at 48 h post-stimulation, frozen, and later tested for IFN-γ concentration by sandwich enzyme-linked immunosorbent assay (ELISA, BD Biosciences, Franklin Lakes, NJ, USA).

Ag presentation assay

C57BL/6 mice were s.c. injected with 1×10^8 CFU BCG or heat-killed BCG in 200 μl PBS or with PBS alone. Mice were sacrificed at various time points, and their inguinal LNs removed and perfused with 400 U/ml collagenase type IV (Invitrogen, Carlsbad, CA, USA) containing 50 μg/ml DNase I (Invitrogen). Single LN-cell suspensions were prepared, and DCs were sorted with an autoMACS separator (Miltenyi Biotec, Bergisch Gladbach, Germany) using CD11c as a cell marker. Specifically, LN cells were first incubated with anti-CD11c MicroBeads (Miltenyi Biotec) before autoMACS separation, resulting in a population of CD11c^high cells (DCs). The purity of these murine LN DCs was then analyzed using a FACSCalibur instrument (BD Biosciences). For the ex vivo Ag presentation assay itself, the purified LN DCs were transferred to 96-well microplates and serially diluted in complete RPMI-1640 medium. DE10 T-cell hybridomas at a density of 1×10^5/well were then added, and after incubation for 24 h, supernatants were collected, frozen, and later tested for IL-2 content by sandwich ELISA (BD Biosciences).

Cell phenotype analysis

C57BL/6 mice were s.c. injected with 1×10^8 CFU BCG in 200 μl PBS or with PBS alone. The mice were sacrificed after various periods for the preparation of single inguinal LN-cell suspensions and sorting of DCs by autoMACS. FITC-conjugated anti-CD11c, and biotinylated anti-I-Ad, anti-CD40, anti-CD54, anti-CD80, and anti-CD86 antibodies were used to label cells. Allophycocyanin-conjugated streptavidin was employed to visualize biotin conjugates. A FACSCalibur and FlowJo software (FlowJo LLC, Ashland, OR, USA) were then used for multicolor staining analysis of the labeled cells. DCs were sorted using the autoMACS system before being pelleted and resuspended in lysis buffer. Cellular RNA was purified with an RNeasy kit (Qiagen, Valencia, CA, USA) according to the manufacturer's instructions, and total RNA was reverse-transcribed into cDNA using SuperScript reverse transcriptase (Thermo Fisher Scientific, Waltham, MA, USA).

In vivo infection assay

C57BL/6 mice were s.c. injected with 1×10^8 CFU BCG or rBCG-GFP in 200 μl PBS or with PBS alone. Mice were sacrificed at various time points, and single inguinal LNs were removed aseptically and transferred to complete RPMI-1640 medium. Single-cell suspensions were prepared, and DCs were sorted with an autoMACS

Rapid loss of early antigen-presenting activity of lymph node dendritic cells against Ag85A protein...

39

separator as above. The percentage of DCs infected with rBCG-GFP was analyzed using a FACSCalibur instrument and FlowJo software. BCG-infected DCs were pelleted and resuspended in lysis buffer. Ten-fold serial dilutions of these suspensions were then plated on solid Middlebrook 7H10 medium, and colonies were counted after incubation at 37 °C for 2–3 weeks.

Statistical analysis

All data are expressed as means ± SE. Statistical analysis was performed by Student's *t*-test using GraphPad Prism software. *P* values < 0.05 were considered statistically significant.

Abbreviations

ADC: Albumin-dextrose-catalase; APC: Antigen-presenting cell; BCG: Bacillus Calmette–Guérin; CIITA: MHC class II transactivator; DC: Dendritic cell; LN: Lymph node; MHC II: Major histocompatibility complex class II; *Mtb*: *Mycobacterium tuberculosis*; PPD: Purified protein derivative; rBCG: Recombinant BCG; TB: Tuberculosis

Acknowledgements

The authors are grateful to Dr. Claude Leclerc (Institut Pasteur, Paris, France) and Dr. Xiaoming Zhang (Institut Pasteur of Shanghai, Chinese Academy of Sciences, Shanghai, China).

Funding

This work was supported in part by the National Key Research and Development Program of China (2017YFD0500300), the National Natural Science Foundation of China (31602031), the Science and Technology Program of Jiangsu (BK20160466, 16KJB230003, BK20171285 and BK20170493), and the Qinglan Project, Six Talent Peaks Project and Priority Academic Development Program of Jiangsu Higher Education Institutions (PADP).

Authors' contributions

ZZ X, XC and XA J designed the experiments. ZZ X, AH X, XL, ZC Z, YC S, SS J, TL, YQ X, HW, and CM performed the experiments and analyzed the data. LS, YL Y, XC, and XA J contributed reagents/materials/analysis tools. ZZ X, XC, and XA J wrote and revised the paper. All authors read and approved the final manuscript.

Competing interests

The authors declare that they have no competing interests.

Author details

[1]Jiangsu Key Laboratory of Zoonosis, Yangzhou University, No. 48 Wenhui East Road, Yangzhou 225009, Jiangsu, China. [2]Key Laboratory of Prevention and Control of Biological Hazard Factors (Animal Origin) for Agrifood Safety and Quality, MOA of China, Yangzhou University, Yangzhou, China. [3]Jiangsu Co-Innovation Center for Prevention and Control of Important Animal Infectious Diseases and Zoonoses, Yangzhou University, Yangzhou, China.

References

1. Aguilo N, Gonzalo-Asensio J, Alvarez-Arguedas S, Marinova D, AB Gomez S, Uranga R, Spallek M, Singh M, Audran R, Spertini F, et al. Reactogenicity to major tuberculosis antigens absent in BCG is linked to improved protection against Mycobacterium tuberculosis. Nat Commun. 2017;8:16085.
2. Kaveh DA, Bachy VS, Hewinson RG, Hogarth PJ. Systemic BCG immunization induces persistent lung mucosal multifunctional CD4 T(EM) cells which expand following virulent mycobacterial challenge. PLoS One. 2011;6: e21566.
3. Vogelzang A, Perdomo C, Zedler U, Kuhlmann S, Hurwitz R, Gengenbacher M, Kaufmann SH. Central memory CD4+ T cells are responsible for the recombinant Bacillus Calmette-Guerin DeltaureC::hly vaccine's superior protection against tuberculosis. J Infect Dis. 2014;210: 1928–37.
4. Kaufmann E, Spohr C, Battenfeld S, De Paepe D, Holzhauser T, Balks E, Homolka S, Reiling N, Gilleron M, Bastian M. BCG vaccination induces robust CD4+ T cell responses to Mycobacterium tuberculosis complex-specific Lipopeptides in Guinea pigs. J Immunol. 2016;196:2723–32.
5. Lindestam Arlehamn CS, McKinney DM, Carpenter C, Paul S, Rozot V, Makgotlho E, Gregg Y, van Rooyen M, Ernst JD, Hatherill M, et al. A quantitative analysis of complexity of human pathogen-specific CD4 T cell responses in healthy M. Tuberculosis infected south Africans. PLoS Pathog. 2016;12:e1005760.
6. Griffiths KL, Ahmed M, Das S, Gopal R, Horne W, Connell TD, Moynihan KD, Kolls JK, Irvine DJ, Artyomov MN, et al. Targeting dendritic cells to accelerate T-cell activation overcomes a bottleneck in tuberculosis vaccine efficacy. Nat Commun. 2016;7:13894.
7. Lozza L, Farinacci M, Bechtle M, Staber M, Zedler U, Baiocchini A, Del Nonno F, Kaufmann SH. Communication between human dendritic cell subsets in tuberculosis: requirements for naive CD4(+) T cell stimulation. Front Immunol. 2014;5:324.
8. Torres M, Ramachandra L, Rojas RE, Bobadilla K, Thomas J, Canaday DH, Harding CV, Boom WH. Role of phagosomes and major histocompatibility complex class II (MHC-II) compartment in MHC-II antigen processing of Mycobacterium tuberculosis in human macrophages. Infect Immun. 2006; 74:1621–30.
9. Jiao X, Lo-Man R, Guermonprez P, Fiette L, Deriaud E, Burgaud S, Gicquel B, Winter N, Leclerc C. Dendritic cells are host cells for mycobacteria in vivo that trigger innate and acquired immunity. J Immunol. 2002;168:1294–301.
10. Harding CV, Boom WH. Regulation of antigen presentation by Mycobacterium tuberculosis: a role for toll-like receptors. Nat Rev Microbiol. 2010;8:296–307.
11. Tian T, Woodworth J, Skold M, Behar SM. In vivo depletion of CD11c+ cells delays the CD4+ T cell response to Mycobacterium tuberculosis and exacerbates the outcome of infection. J Immunol. 2005;175:3268–72.
12. Lanzavecchia A, Reid PA, Watts C. Irreversible association of peptides with class II MHC molecules in living cells. Nature. 1992;357:249–52.
13. Chang ST, Linderman JJ, Kirschner DE. Multiple mechanisms allow Mycobacterium tuberculosis to continuously inhibit MHC class II-mediated antigen presentation by macrophages. Proc Natl Acad Sci U S A. 2005;102:4530–5.
14. Srivastava S, Grace PS, Ernst JD. Antigen export reduces antigen presentation and limits T cell control of M. Tuberculosis. Cell Host Microbe. 2016;19:44–54.
15. Ghorpade DS, Holla S, Sinha AY, Alagesan SK, Balaji KN. Nitric oxide and KLF4 protein epigenetically modify class II transactivator to repress major histocompatibility complex II expression during Mycobacterium bovis bacillus Calmette-Guerin infection. J Biol Chem. 2013;288:20592–606.
16. Hope JC, Thom ML, McCormick PA, Howard CJ. Interaction of antigen presenting cells with mycobacteria. Vet Immunol Immunopathol. 2004; 100:187–95.
17. Chackerian AA, Alt JM, Perera TV, Dascher CC, Behar SM. Dissemination of Mycobacterium tuberculosis is influenced by host factors and precedes the initiation of T-cell immunity. Infect Immun. 2002;70:4501–9.

18. Ramachandra L, Noss E, Boom WH, Harding CV. Processing of
     Mycobacterium tuberculosis antigen 85B involves intraphagosomal
     formation of peptide-major histocompatibility complex II complexes and is
     inhibited by live bacilli that decrease phagosome maturation. J Exp Med.
     2001;194:1421–32.
19. Sendide K, Deghmane AE, Pechkovsky D, Av-Gay Y, Talal A, Hmama Z.
     Mycobacterium bovis BCG attenuates surface expression of mature class II
     molecules through IL-10-dependent inhibition of cathepsin S. J Immunol.
     2005;175:5324–32.
20. Singh CR, Moulton RA, Armitige LY, Bidani A, Snuggs M, Dhandayuthapani
     S, Hunter RL, Jagannath C. Processing and presentation of a mycobacterial
     antigen 85B epitope by murine macrophages is dependent on the
     phagosomal acquisition of vacuolar proton ATPase and in situ activation of
     cathepsin D. J Immunol. 2006;177:3250–9.
21. Johansen P, Fettelschoss A, Amstutz B, Selchow P, Waeckerle-Men Y, Keller
     P, Deretic V, Held L, Kundig TM, Bottger EC, et al. Relief from Zmp1-
     mediated arrest of phagosome maturation is associated with facilitated
     presentation and enhanced immunogenicity of mycobacterial antigens. Clin
     Vaccine Immunol. 2011;18:907–13.

5

MiR-18a and miR-17 are positively correlated with circulating PD-1$^+$ICOS$^+$ follicular helper T cells after hepatitis B vaccination in a chinese population

Xiaojia Xu[1†], Yulian Li[2†], Yaping Liang[1], Mingjuan Yin[1], Zuwei Yu[2], Yan Zhang[1], Lingfeng Huang[1] and Jindong Ni[1*]

Abstract

Background: While vaccination remains the most effective method to control hepatitis B virus (HBV) infection, 5–10% of recipients exhibit non-responsiveness to the HB vaccine. Immunological analysis of strong, weak or absent protective antibody responses to the HB vaccine should provide insights into the mechanisms that contribute to non-responsiveness.

Results: We investigated the potential involvement of follicular helper T (Tfh) cells in the immune response to HB vaccine, and associations between the miR-17–92 cluster and Tfh cells. We recruited 12 adults who had completed the HB vaccination course during childhood. Following a booster dose of HB vaccine, hepatitis B surface antibody (HBsAb) titers, percentage of PD-1+ICOS+ circulating Tfh (cTfh) and plasma cells, and expression of miR-17–92 were assessed at baseline (before immunization) and after vaccination on days 7 and 14. Notably, the HBsAb level gradually increased after HB vaccination while the proportion of PD-1+ICOS+ cTfh cells was significantly increased on day 7 relative to baseline, so as plasma cells. Expression of miR-18a and miR-17 within the miR-17–92 cluster and HBsAb titers in CD4+ T cells were positively correlated with the PD-1+ICOS+ cTfh cells proportions after HB vaccination.

Conclusions: The increase in HBsAb titers was positively associated with expression of all the components of the miR-17–92 cluster except miR-19a. Our findings indicate that the miR-17–92 cluster contributes to antibody production, and miR-18a and miR-17 are involved in Tfh cells differentiation after HB vaccination.

Keywords: Follicular helper T cells, MiR-17–92, Hepatitis B vaccine

Background

Hepatitis B is a major public health priority worldwide with more than 350 million chronic hepatitis B virus (HBV) carriers, accounting for approximately 686,000 deaths per year [1]. The hepatitis B (HB) vaccination is currently the most effective and economical measure to prevent HBV infection. However, 5–10% patients exhibit non-responsiveness to the vaccine and remain susceptible to infection. Immunological assessment of strong, weak or absent protective antibody responses to the HB vaccine should provide further insights into the precise mechanisms underlying non-responsiveness to hepatitis B vaccine.

CD4$^+$ T cells play a crucial role in assisting B cells with antibody production. T helper (Th) cells, mainly Th1 and Th2, are widely recognized as key cells that regulate the immune response to HB vaccine whereas Th cells play a regulatory role only in B cell activation [2, 3]. Recent studies have demonstrated that the follicular helper T (Tfh) subset of CD4$^+$ T cells plays a major role in B cell-mediated production of high-affinity, class-switched antibodies, and generation of high-affinity memory B cells through germinal center (GC) reaction during

* Correspondence: nijd-gw@gdmu.edu.cn

†Xiaojia Xu and Yulian Li contributed equally to this work.

[1]Department of Environmental and Occupational Health, Dongguan Key Laboratory of Environmental Medicine, School of Public Health, Guangdong Medical University, Dongguan 523808, China

Full list of author information is available at the end of the article

infection and vaccination [4, 5]. The transcriptional repressor, Bcl-6, is essential for Tfh cell differentiation and IL-21 induces B cell proliferation and differentiation [6]. Tfh cells are characterized by expression of chemokine (C-X-C) receptor 5 (CXCR5), co-stimulatory molecules (ICOS) and programmed death 1 (PD-1), which are critical for their function [7]. CXCR5+CD4+ T cells in peripheral blood are known as circulating Tfh (cTfh) cells. In healthy adults subjects cTfh cells resemble Tfh cells in their capacity to produce IL-21 and induce B cell differentiation [8–10]. Researchers generally utilize cTfh for study instead of Tfh due to the difficulty in obtaining lymphoid T cells in humans. Accumulating studies suggest that the antibody response to vaccination in humans is correlated with cTfh cells [11, 12]. However, the issue of whether Tfh cells are involved in immune response to the HB vaccine is unknown at present.

MiRNA-mediated post-transcriptional regulation plays a key role in the differentiation and function of Tfh cells [13]. Tfh cells display a characteristic miRNA expression profile, compared to other effector Th cells [6, 14] and differentiation fails in the absence of miRNA [15]. Several miRNAs and miRNA clusters reported to be involved in the regulation of Tfh cells [16]. Recent progress in clarifying the mechanisms by which Tfh cells are affected has revealed important roles of posttranscriptional control of gene expression mediated by miRNAs, including miR-17-92, miR-155 and miR-146a [17, 18]. The miRNA cluster, miR-17–92, is encoded by a polycistronic miRNA that generates a single precursor transcript for six distinct mature miRNAs: miR-17, miR-18a, miR-19a, miR-19b-1, miR-20a and miR-92a-1 [19]. Expression of miR-17–92 is induced early during T cell activation and suppressed after completion of Tfh cell differentiation [20], suggesting a role in the immune response to HB vaccine.

To explore the pathways underlying the immune response to HB vaccine, we investigated the involvement of cTfh cells. Furthermore, we identified the relationship between miR-17–92 and Tfh cells after HB vaccination. Data from our study provide novel insights into the roles of miR-17–92 and cTfh cells in the immune response to the HB vaccine.

Results

Dynamic changes in HBsAb titers, PD-1+ICOS+ cTfh cells, plasma cells and miR-17–92 after HB vaccination

Serum samples were obtained from 12 adult subjects at baseline, 7 and 14 days after HB vaccination. The gating

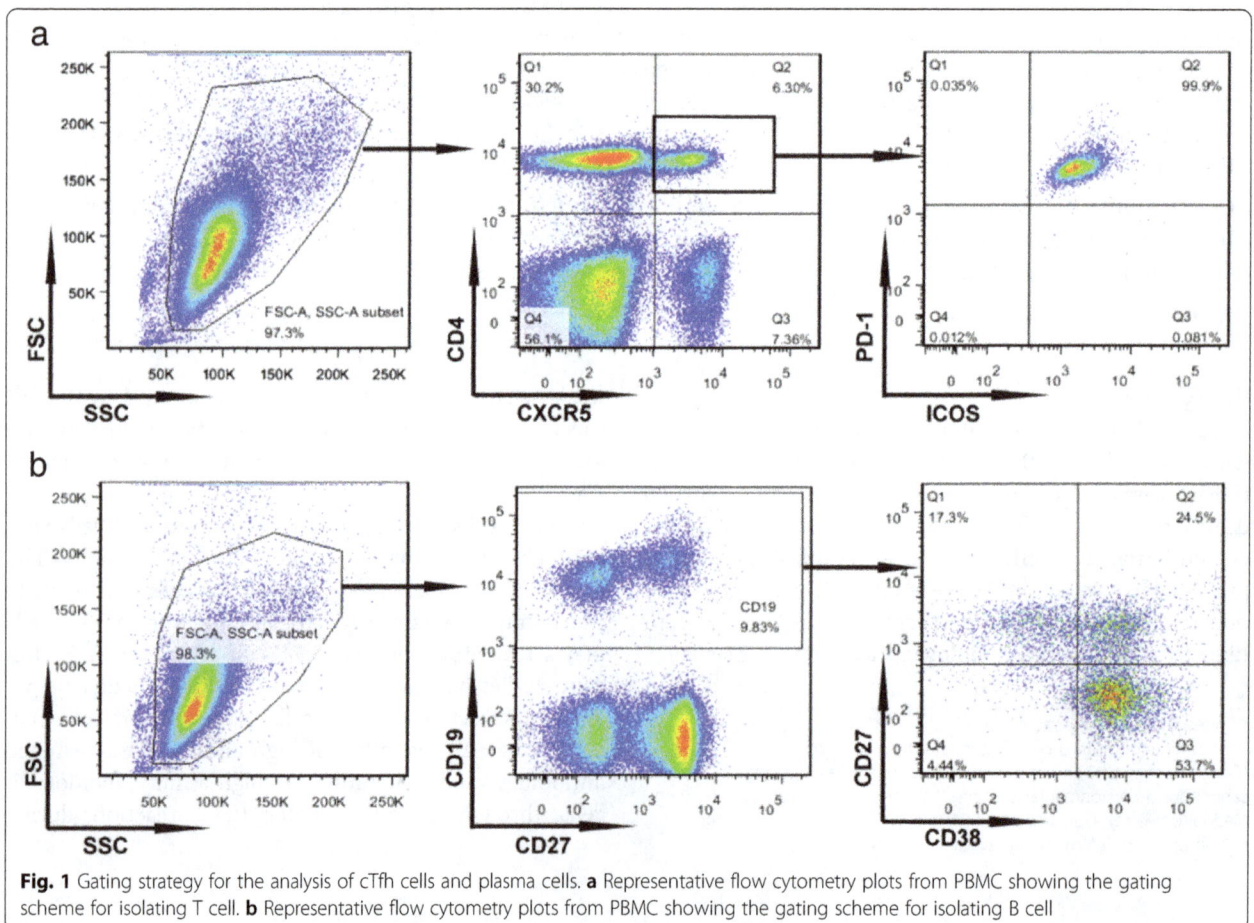

Fig. 1 Gating strategy for the analysis of cTfh cells and plasma cells. **a** Representative flow cytometry plots from PBMC showing the gating scheme for isolating T cell. **b** Representative flow cytometry plots from PBMC showing the gating scheme for isolating B cell

strategy for analysis of cTfh and plasma cells is shown in Fig. 1. We observed alterations in the level of HBsAb titers levels at three time-points after vaccination (days 0, 7 and 14) (Table 1), which was higher on day 14, compared to day 7 (Fig. 2a). The percentage of PD-1$^+$ICOS$^+$ cTfh cells was significantly increased on day 7, compared to that at baseline ($P < 0.01$) (Fig. 2b), and higher than that day on 14. Furthermore, the percentage of CD38$^+$CD27$^+$CD19$^+$ B (plasma) cells was markedly increased on day 7, compared to that at baseline ($P < 0.05$) (Fig. 2c). Expression of miR-92a-1, miR-20a, miR-19a and miR-19b-1 in CD4$^+$ T cells was significantly upregulated on day 14, compared to day 7 ($P < 0.05$) (Fig. 2d-g). In addition, both miR-18a and miR-17 levels in CD4$^+$ T cells were markedly increased on day 14, compared to day 7 and baseline ($P < 0.05$) (Fig. 2f-h).

MiR-18 and miR-17 in CD4$^+$ T cells are positively correlated with the PD-1$^+$ICOS$^+$ cTfh cell population after HB vaccination

Analysis of combined data for all three time-points, revealed that the miR-17 level is correlated with percentage of PD-1$^+$ICOS$^+$ cTfh cells ($r = 0.372$, $P = 0.047$) (Fig. 3a). Moreover, the miR-18a level in CD4$^+$ T cells showed a strong positive correlation with the percentage of PD-1$^+$ICOS$^+$ cTfh cells ($r = 0.452$, $P = 0.014$) (Fig. 3b). Unexpectedly, the other miRNAs within the cluster failed to show a similar association ($P > 0.05$) (Table 2).

HBsAb titers are correlated with the PD-1$^+$ICOS$^+$ cTfh cells population and the miR-17-92 cluster except miR-19a

Data from the correlation analysis revealed that the HBsAb titer is positively correlated with percentage of PD-1$^+$ICOS$^+$ cTfh cells (Fig. 4a). Furthermore, increased HBsAb titers are positively correlated with expression of all miRNAs from the miR-17-92 cohort, expect miR-19a (Fig. 4b–f) (Table 3).

Discussion

Recent studies have reported that blood memory Tfh cells contain three subsets, among which PD-1$^+$ICOS$^+$ Tfh cells are an activated subset [21, 22]. To our knowledge, this is the first report to explore the potential relationship between the miR-17–92 cohort and PD-1$^+$ICOS$^+$ cTfh cells after HB vaccination in a Chinese population.

In our experiment, the percentage of PD-1$^+$ICOS$^+$ cTfh cells was significantly increased on day 7 relative to baseline after HB vaccination ($P < 0.01$). These observations suggest that PD-1$^+$ICOS$^+$ cTfh cells are involved in the immune response to HB vaccine. Intriguingly, however, emergence of PD-1$^+$ICOS$^+$ cTfh and plasma cells in blood peaked on day 7 after HB vaccination, suggesting similar kinetics of development for both cell types. Similarly, a recent study showed that emergence of plasmablasts and ICOS$^+$CXCR3$^+$CXCR5$^+$CD4$^+$ T cells in blood peaked on day 7 after influenza vaccination [23]. Therefore, induction of these T cells may be an effecting factor for generation of plasma cells and plasmablasts and identification of the pathways or adjuvants that promote their generation is critical.

Another important finding is that the expression of miR-18a and miR-17 in CD4$^+$ T cells are positively correlated with the percentage of PD-1$^+$ICOS$^+$ cTfh cells after HBV vaccination. In combination with previous results, our data suggest that miR-17–92 promotes the differentiation of Tfh cells and maintains the fidelity of cell identity by suppressing non-Tfh cell-related genes both directly and indirectly [15]. The miR-17–92 cluster is reported to positively regulate differentiation of Tfh cells by driving the migration of CD4$^+$ T into B cell follicles through modulation of ICOS signaling [24]. MiR-17, as the member of the cluster, it can protected CD4$^+$T cells from excessive activation-induced cell death to targeted transforming growth factor-β receptor II(TgfbrII) and cAMP-responsive element-binding protein 1 (Creb1) [25]. Also, the cluster member of miR-18a, it was the

Table 1 The result of one way repeated measures analysis

	Day 0	Day 7	Day 14	F	P
HBsAb titers (IU/ml)	57.87 ± 37.93	249.16 ± 125.95	667.39 ± 312.78	48.60	< 0.001
The percentage of PD-1$^+$ICOS$^+$ cTfh cells	6.17 ± 1.17	7.68 ± 1.62	7.46 ± 2.20	5.62	0.014
The percentage of Plasma cells	20.82 ± 5.03	22.31 ± 6.07	21.66 ± 6.04	2.54	0.114
The expression of miR-92a-1	18.63 ± 0.91	18.35 ± 0.96	19.55 ± 0.76	3.36	0.076
The expression of miR-20a	12.32 ± 0.90	12.01 ± 1.02	13.11 ± 0.68	3.42	0.067
The expression of miR-19a	13.19 ± 1.83	11.11 ± 1.05	12.50 ± 0.75	3.94	0.048
The expression of miR-19b-1	19.18 ± 1.25	18.52 ± 1.06	19.91 ± 0.92	3.37	0.069
The expression of miR-18a	17.84 ± 0.63	17.86 ± 0.96	19.38 ± 0.93	10.37	0.002
The expression of miR-17	10.55 ± 0.70	10.37 ± 0.72	11.44 ± 0.77	5.25	0.023

F: The statistics of one way repeated measures analysis

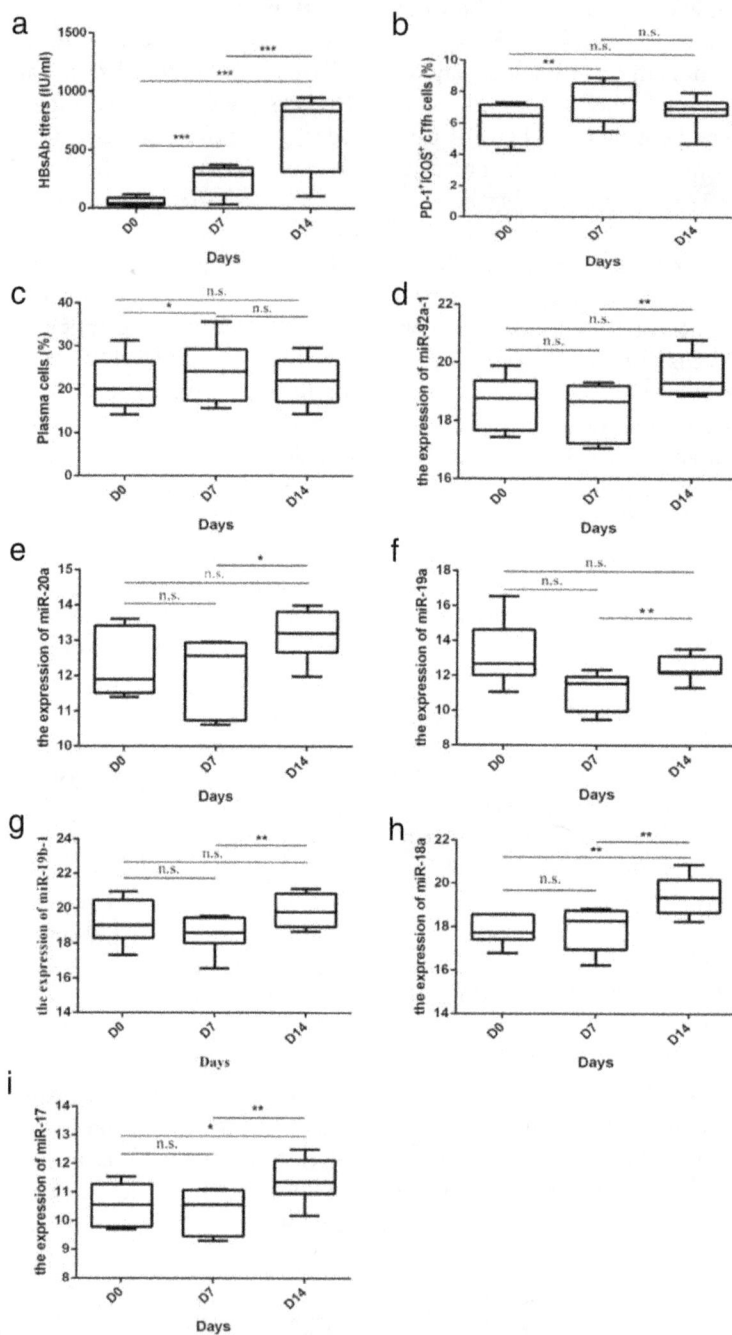

Fig. 2 Dynamic changes of HBsAb titers, PD-1+ICOS+ cTfh cells, plasma cells and miR-17~ 92 after HBV vaccination. **a** The level of HBsAb titers in different points (day 0, 7, 14). **b** The percentage of PD-1+ICOS+ cTfh cells. **c** The percentage of plasma cells. **d** The level of miR-92a-1 in CD4+ T cells. **e** The level of miR-20a in CD4+ T cells. **f** The level of miR-19a in CD4+ T cells. **g** The level of miR-19b-1 in CD4+ T cells. **h** The level of miR-18 in CD4+ T cells. **i** The level of miR-17 in CD4+ T cells.*, $P < 0.05$; **, $P < 0.01$; ***, $P < 0.001$; n.s., no significant differences

most dynamically upregulated microRNA of the miR-17–92 cluster in activated T cells [26]. According, miR-18a and miR-17 may regulate PD-1+ICOS+ cTfh cell differentiation after HB vaccination.

In addition, we observed a positive correlation between the percentage increase in PD-1+ICOS+ cTfh cells and HBsAb titers. This finding is consistent with recent data showing that increased generation of ICOS+PD-1+CXCR3+ Tfh cells are positively correlated with induction of protective antibody responses in response to influenza vaccination [11]. Similarly, in a study on seasonal influenza vaccines, the increase in the ICOS +PD-1 + CCR7lo subpopulation of Tfh1 cells were positively correlated with generation of the protective

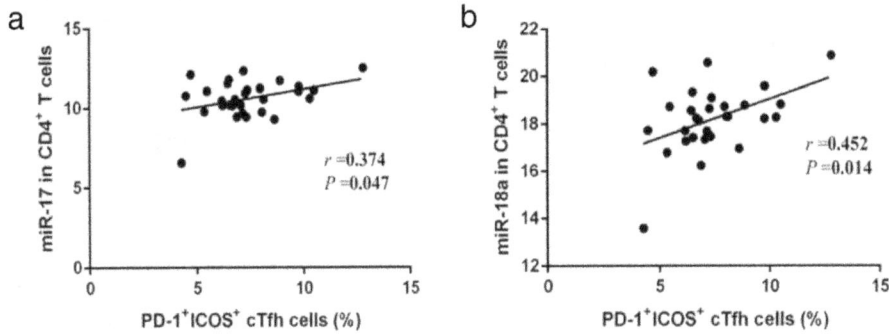

Fig. 3 The correlation between PD-1$^+$ICOS$^+$ cTfh cells and miRNA in CD4$^+$ T cells. **a** The correlation of PD-1$^+$ICOS$^+$ cTfh cells with the level of miR-17 was analyzed. **b** The correlation of PD-1$^+$ICOS$^+$ cTfh cells with the level of miR-18a was analyzed

antibody response [27]. These findings clearly suggest that cTfh cells contribute to the generation of antibody responses to HB vaccination.

HBsAb titers were significantly correlated with miR-18a and miR-17 expression in CD4$^+$ T cells inour study. Based on the collective results, we propose that miR-18a and miR-17 induce production of HBsAb by regulating cTfh cell differentiation. Furthermore, miR-92a-1, miR-20a and miR-19b-1 were positively correlated with HBsAb titers. In contrast, miR-19a was not associated with the HBsAb titer. Clayton A White et al. have also been shown that miR-19a irrelevant to plasma cell differentiation in vitro [28]. So we suggesting that individual miRNAs interact with each other and exert their functions through regulation of different signaling networks. This finding is consistent with the recent report that overexpression of the miR-17–92 cluster in T cells leads to production of autoantibodies in mice [29]. The combined data support the possibility that miR-17–92 regulates differentiation of cTfh cells and induces the antibody production after HB vaccination.

Conclusions

Our results provide preliminary evidence that the percentage of PD-1$^+$ICOS$^+$ cTfh cells are positively correlated with expression of miR-18a and miR-17 in CD4$^+$ T cells after HB vaccination, which may aid in the

Table 2 miR-17~ 92 correlated with the percentage of PD-1$^+$ICOS$^+$ cTfh cells

	r	P
PD-1$^+$ICOS$^+$ cTfh cells and miR-92a-1	0.228	0.254
PD-1$^+$ICOS$^+$ cTfh cells and miR-20a	0.197	0.306
PD-1$^+$ICOS$^+$ cTfh cells and miR-19a	−0.022	0.910
PD-1$^+$ICOS$^+$ cTfh cells and miR-19b-1	0.160	0.408
PD-1$^+$ICOS$^+$ cTfh cells and miR-18a	0.452	0.014
PD-1$^+$ICOS$^+$ cTfh cells and miR-17	0.372	0.047

strengthening the rationale for design of improved vaccines. Future studies should focus on establishing the mechanisms by which miR-18a and miR-17 regulate cTfh cell differentiation.

Methods
Subjects and samples
The present study was conducted in a Chinese Han population. A cohort of 12 healthy adults was voluntarily recruited from the community health service center of Dalang, Dongguan (Table 4).The HB vaccine (20 μg) was administered via intramuscular injection of the deltoid according to a 0-, 1-, and 6-month standard schedule (recombinant hepatitis B vaccine, Engerix-B, GlaxoSmithKline, Brentford, UK) [30].None of the subjects had a history of infection with HBV, hepatitis C virus or human immunodeficiency virus, and none were immunodeficient. There were no smokers among the study subjects. We administered a booster HB vaccine via intramuscular injection in the upper arm deltoid and collected 25 mL peripheral venous blood at baseline before and after vaccination on days 7 and 14.

Cell isolation and purification
Peripheral blood mononuclear cells (PBMCs) were isolated by whole blood. Whole blood was diluted with equal volume PRMI Medium 1640 (Life, USA) and then added to a SEPMATE-50 tube containing density gradient (Lymphoprep)medium (StemCell Technologies, Vancouver, BC) and centrifuged at 1200×g for10 min. The top-layer or supernatant is enriched for PBMCs which were collected, washed 2 × with PRMI Medium 1640 [31]. CD4$^+$ T cells were isolated from PBMCs using EasySep™ human CD4$^+$ T-cell enrichment kit (StemCell Technologies, Vancouver, BC).

Flow cytometry analysis
All antibodies were purchased from eBioscience (Thermo Fisher Scientific, Massachusetts, USA) and BD

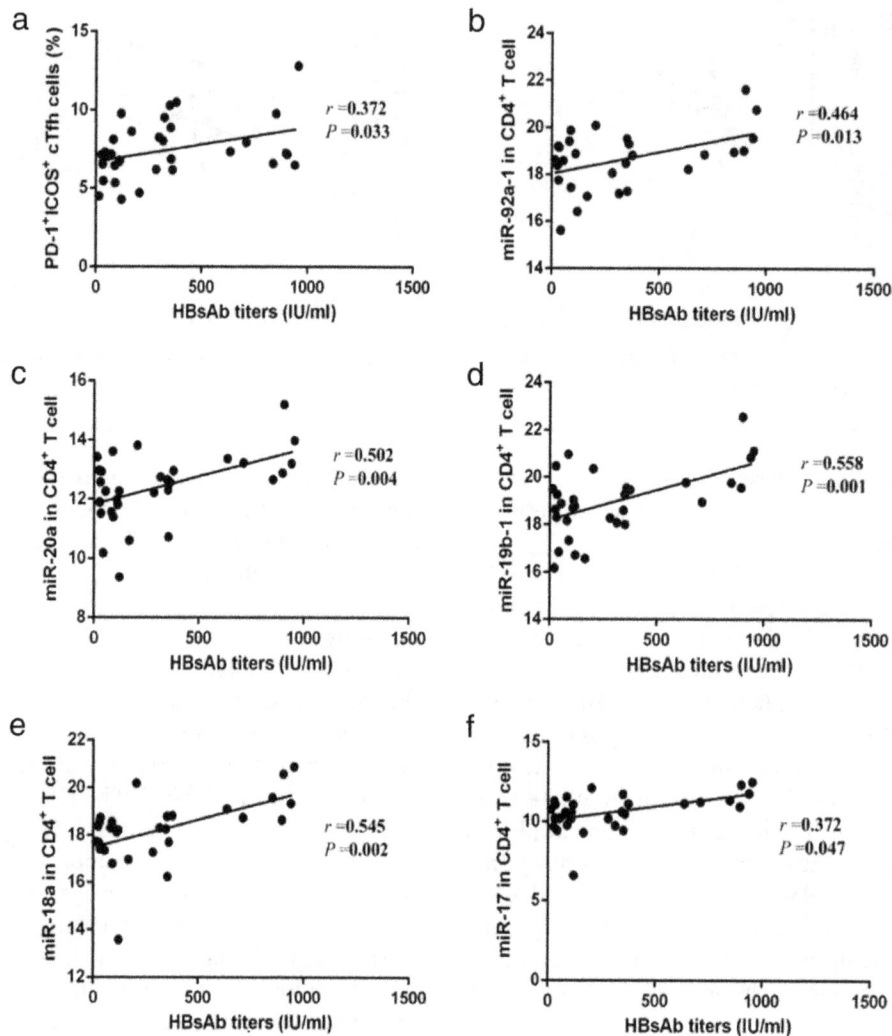

Fig. 4 The correlation between the HBsAb titers and PD-1+ICOS+ cTfh cells, miR17~ 92 in CD4+ T cells. **a** The correlation of HBsAb titers with PD-1+ICOS+ cTfh cells was analyzed. **b** The correlation of HBsAb titers with miR-92a-1was analyzed. **c** The correlation of HBsAb titers with miR-20a was analyzed. **d** The correlation of HBsAb titers with miR-19b-1 was analyzed. **e** The correlation of HBsAb titers with miR-18a was analyzed. **f** The correlation of HBsAb titers with miR-17 was analyzed

Table 3 HBsAb titers correlated with cTfh cells and miR-17~ 92

	r	P
HBsAbtiters and PD-1+ICOS+cTfh cells	0.372	0.033
HBsAb titers and miR-92a-1	0.464	0.013
HBsAb titers and miR-20a	0.502	0.004
HBsAb titers and miR-19a	0.156	0.401
HBsAb titers and miR-19b-1	0.558	0.001
HBsAb titers and miR-18a	0.545	0.002
HBsAb titers and miR-17	0.492	0.006

Biosciences (New York, USA). PBMCs were incubated with the relevant mouse anti-human antibodies for 30 min, followed by surface staining for the indicated markers. The antibodies used to analyze B cells were PE-labeled mouse anti-human CD19, FITC-labeled mouse anti-human CD27, BV421-labeled mouse anti-human CD38 (BD Biosciences) and those for T cells were PerCP-Cyanine 5.5-labeled anti-human CD4, PE-labeled anti-human CXCR5, eVolve 655-labeled anti-human PD-1

Table 4 Demographic characteristics of study cohort

N	12
Gender (M/F)	6/6
Age (years)	28.83 ± 3.95
BMI	21.81 ± 3.54

and APC-eFluor 780-labeled anti-human ICOS (eBioscience).

Antibody assays

Serum was separated for immediate testing of the anti-HBV antibody level using a commercial enzyme-linked immunosorbent assay kit (Da An Gene Co. Ltd., Guangzhou, China).

RNA isolation and real-time PCR

Total RNA was extracted with TRIzol reagent (Invitrogen, Carlsbad, CA) from CD4$^+$ T cells according to the manufacturer's instructions. Quantitative real-time PCR (qRT-PCR) was applied used to detect expression of mature miR-17–92, and first-strand cDNA generated with the transcriptor first strand cDNA synthesis kit (Roche, Mannheim, Germany) using 2 μg total RNA and miRNA-specific stem-loop reverse transcription primers. The reverse transcription primers for miR-17–92 and U6 small nuclear RNA (snRNAs) are shown in Table 5. QRT-PCR reactions were performed in triplicate in a 96-well plate containing 1 μl of synthesized cDNA,

FastStart Universal SYBR Green Master (Roche, Mannheim, Germany) on PikoReal (Thermo Scientific, USA) in a total volume of 10 μL. The reaction procedures were as follows: 95 °C for 10 min, 40 cycles at 95 °C for 15 s and 60 °C for 30 s. The expression levels of miR-NAs were normalized to U6 and calculated using the $2^{-\Delta Ct}$ method. All of primers were designed and synthesized by Generay Biotechnology (Generay Biotechnology, Shanghai).

Statistical analysis

Data are presented as means ± SD. One-Way Repeated Measures Analysis of Variance (ANOVA) was applied for comparison of the three groups. For comparison between two populations, paired two-tailed student's t test was performed. Correlations between variables were determined with Pearson's correlation coefficient. Data were analyzed with SPSS 15.0 (SPSS Inc., Chicago, IL, USA) and GraphPad Prism 5 software (GraphPad Software Inc., La Jolla, CA). The significance level was set at $P < 0.05$ for all statistical analyses. (*, $P < 0.05$; **, $P < 0.01$; ***, $P < 0.001$).

Table 5 Primers

Gene	Primer sequence (5' - 3')
U6 RT	AACGCTTCACGAATTTGCGT
U6 Forward	CTCGCTTCGGCAGCACA
U6 Reverse	AACGCTTCACGAATTTGCGT
miR-17-5p RT	CCTGTTGTCTCCAGCCACAAAAGAGCACAATATTTCAGGAGACAACAGGCTACCTG
miR-17-5p Forward	GCGGCCAAAGTGCTTACAGTG
miR-17-5p Reverse	CAGCCACAAAAGAGCACAAT
miR-18a-5p RT	CCTGTTGTCTCCAGCCACAAAAGAGCACAATATTTCAGGAGACAACAGGCTATCTG
miR-18a-5p Forward	CGGGCTAAGGTGCATCTAGTG
miR-18a-5p Reverse	CAGCCACAAAAGAGCACAAT
miR-19a-3p RT	CCTGTTGTCTCCAGCCACAAAAGAGCACAATATTTCAGGAGACAACAGGTCTAGTG
miR-19a-3p Forward	CGCCGAGTTTTGCATAGTTG
miR-19a-3p Reverse	CAGCCACAAAAGAGCACAAT
miR-19b-1-5p RT	CCTGTTGTCTCCAGCCACAAAAGAGCACAATATTTCAGGAGACAACAGGGCTGGAT
miR-19b-1-5p Forward	GCGGCAGTTTTGCAGGTTTGC
miR-19b-1-5p Reverse	CAGCCACAAAAGAGCACAAT
miR-20a-5p RT	CCTGTTGTCTCCAGCCACAAAAGAGCACAATATTTCAGGAGACAACAGGCTACCTG
miR-20a-5p Forward	CGGGCTAAAGTGCTTATAGTG
miR-20a-5p Reverse	CAGCCACAAAAGAGCACAAT
miR-92a-1-5p RT	CCTGTTGTCTCCAGCCACAAAAGAGCACAATATTTCAGGAGACAACAGGAGCATTG
miR-92a-1-5p Forward	CGCCGAGGTTGGGATCGGTTG
miR-92a-1-5p Reverse	CAGCCACAAAAGAGCACAAT

Abbreviations

(ANOVA): One-way repeated measures analysis of variance; cTfh cell: Circulating Tfh cell; CXCR5: Chemokine receptor 5; GC: Germinal center; HB: Hepatitis B; HBsAb: Hepatitis B surface antibody; HBV: Hepatitis B virus; ICOS: Co-stimulatory molecules; PBMCs: Peripheral blood mononuclear cells; PD-1: Programmed death 1; qRT-PCR: Quantitative real-time PCR; Tfh cell: Follicular helper T cell; Th cell: T helper cell

Acknowledgements

We would like to express special gratitude to all the personnel who supported or helped with this study.

Funding

This work was supported by grants from Natural Science Foundation of Guangdong Province, China, grant number 2015A030313516, and fund for social science and technology development project of Dongguan, grant number 2014108101040.

Authors' contributions

JDN designed the study. XJX, YLL, YPL, MJY, ZWY, YZ, LFH performed the experiments. XJX, YLL analyzed the data and wrote the manuscript. YPL, MJY provided the required equipments and materials. ZWY, YZ, LFH helped perform the analysis with constructive discussions. JDN revised the manuscript and edited the English language. All authors read and approved the final manuscript.

Competing interest

The authors declare that they have no competing interest.

Author details

[1]Department of Environmental and Occupational Health, Dongguan Key Laboratory of Environmental Medicine, School of Public Health, Guangdong Medical University, Dongguan 523808, China. [2]Dalang Community Health Service Centers, Dongguan 523770, China.

References

1. Zhang Q, Liao Y, Chen J, et al. Epidemiology study of HBV genotypes and antiviral drug resistance in multi-ethnic regions from western China[J]. Sci Rep. 2015;5:17413.
2. Sage PT, Sharpe AH. T follicular regulatory cells in the regulation of B cell responses[J]. Trends Immunol. 2015;36(7):410–8.
3. Crotty S. T follicular helper cell differentiation, function, and roles in disease[J]. Immunity. 2014;41(4):529–42.
4. Crotty S. Follicular helper CD4 T cells (TFH)[J]. Annu Rev Immunol. 2011;29: 621–63.
5. Victora GD, Nussenzweig MC. Germinal centers[J]. Annu Rev Immunol. 2012; 30:429–57.
6. Yu D, Rao S, Tsai LM, et al. The transcriptional repressor Bcl-6 directs T follicular helper cell lineage commitment[J]. Immunity. 2009;31(3):457–68.
7. Jogdand GM, Mohanty S, Devadas S. Regulators of Tfh cell differentiation[J]. Front Immunol. 2016;7:520.
8. Chevalier N, Jarrossay D, Ho E, et al. CXCR5 expressing human central memory CD4 T cells and their relevance for humoral immune responses[J]. J Immunol. 2011;186(10):5556–68.
9. Ma CS, Deenick EK. Human T follicular helper (Tfh) cells and disease[J]. Immunol Cell Biol. 2014;92(1):64–71.
10. Morita R, Schmitt N, Bentebibel SE, et al. Human blood CXCR5(+)CD4(+) T cells are counterparts of T follicular cells and contain specific subsets that differentially support antibody secretion[J]. Immunity. 2011;34(1):108–21.
11. Bentebibel SE, Lopez S, Obermoser G, et al. Induction of ICOS+CXCR3 +CXCR5+ TH cells correlates with antibody responses to influenza vaccination[J]. Sci Transl Med. 2013;5(176):132r–76r.
12. Bentebibel SE, Khurana S, Schmitt N, et al. ICOS(+)PD-1(+)CXCR3(+) T follicular helper cells contribute to the generation of high-avidity antibodies following influenza vaccination[J]. Sci Rep. 2016;6:26494.
13. Krol J, Loedige I, Filipowicz W. The widespread regulation of microRNA biogenesis, function and decay[J]. Nat Rev Genet. 2010;11(9):597–610.
14. Kuchen S, Resch W, Yamane A, et al. Regulation of microRNA expression and abundance during lymphopoiesis[J]. Immunity. 2010;32(6):828–39.
15. Baumjohann D, Kageyama R, Clingan JM, et al. The microRNA cluster miR-17 approximately 92 promotes TFH cell differentiation and represses subset-inappropriate gene expression[J]. Nat Immunol. 2013;14(8):840–8.
16. Baumjohann D, Ansel KM. MicroRNA regulation of the germinal center response[J]. Curr Opin Immunol. 2014;28:6–11.
17. Jiang SH, Shen N, Vinuesa CG. Posttranscriptional T cell gene regulation to limit Tfh cells and autoimmunity[J]. Curr Opin Immunol. 2015;37:21–7.
18. Maul J, Baumjohann D. Emerging roles for MicroRNAs in T follicular helper cell differentiation[J]. Trends Immunol. 2016;37(5):297–309.
19. Olive V, Jiang I, He L. Mir-17-92, a cluster of miRNAs in the midst of the cancer network[J]. Int J Biochem Cell Biol. 2010;42(8):1348–54.
20. Kang SG, Liu WH, Lu P, et al. MicroRNAs of the miR-17 approximately 92 family are critical regulators of T(FH) differentiation[J]. Nat Immunol. 2013; 14(8):849–57.
21. Locci M, Havenar-Daughton C, Landais E, et al. Human circulating PD-1 +CXCR3-CXCR5+ memory Tfh cells are highly functional and correlate with broadly neutralizing HIV antibody responses[J]. Immunity. 2013;39(4):758–69.
22. He J, Tsai LM, Leong YA, et al. Circulating precursor CCR7(lo)PD-1(hi) CXCR5(+) CD4(+) T cells indicate Tfh cell activity and promote antibody responses upon antigen reexposure[J]. Immunity. 2013;39(4):770–81.
23. Wrammert J, Smith K, Miller J, et al. Rapid cloning of high-affinity human monoclonal antibodies against influenza virus[J]. Nature. 2008;453(7195): 667–71.
24. de Kouchkovsky D, Esensten JH, Rosenthal WL, et al. microRNA-17-92 regulates IL-10 production by regulatory T cells and control of experimental autoimmune encephalomyelitis[J]. J Immunol. 2013;191(4):1594–605.
25. Jiang S, Li C, Olive V, et al. Molecular dissection of the miR-17-92 cluster's critical dual roles in promoting Th1 responses and preventing inducible Treg differentiation[J]. Blood. 2011;118(20):5487–97.
26. Montoya MM, Maul J, Singh PB, et al. A distinct inhibitory function for miR-18a in Th17 cell differentiation[J]. J Immunol. 2017;199(2):559–69.
27. Schmitt N, Bentebibel SE, Ueno H. Phenotype and functions of memory Tfh cells in human blood[J]. Trends Immunol. 2014;35(9):436–42.
28. White CA, Pone EJ, Lam T, et al. Histone deacetylase inhibitors upregulate B cell microRNAs that silence AID and Blimp-1 expression for epigenetic modulation of antibody and autoantibody responses[J]. J Immunol. 2014; 193(12):5933–50.
29. Xiao C, Srinivasan L, Calado DP, et al. Lymphoproliferative disease and autoimmunity in mice with increased miR-17-92 expression in lymphocytes[J]. Nat Immunol. 2008;9(4):405–14.
30. Yang L, Yao J, Li J, et al. Suitable hepatitis B vaccine for adult immunization in China[J]. Immunol Res. 2016;64(1):242–50.
31. Belle K, Shabazz FS, Nuytemans K, et al. Generation of disease-specific autopsy-confirmed iPSCs lines from postmortem isolated peripheral blood mononuclear cells[J]. Neurosci Lett. 2017;637:201–6.

In vitro evidence of efficacy and safety of a polymerized cat dander extract for allergen immunotherapy

María Morales[1], Mayte Gallego[1], Victor Iraola[1], Marta Taulés[2], Eliandre de Oliveira[3], Raquel Moya[1] and Jerónimo Carnés[1*]

Abstract

Background: Allergy to cat epithelia is highly prevalent, being the major recommendation for allergy sufferers its avoidance. However, this is not always feasible. Allergen specific immunotherapy is therefore recommended for these patients. The use of polymerized allergen extracts, allergoids, would allow to achieve the high allergen doses suggested to be effective while maintaining safety.

Results: Cat native extract and its depigmented allergoid were manufactured and biochemically and immunochemically characterized. Protein and chromatographic profiles showed significant modification of the depigmented allergoid with respect to its corresponding native extract. However, the presence of different allergens (Fel d 1, Fel d 2, Fel d 3, Fel d 4 and Fel d 7) was confirmed in the allergoid. Differences in IgE-binding capacity were observed as loss of biological potency and lower stability of the IgE-allergen complex on surface plasmon resonance. The allergoid induced production of IgG antibodies able to block IgE-binding to native extract. Finally, studies carried out with peripheral-blood mononuclear cells from cat allergic patients showed that the allergoid induced IFN-γ and IL-10 production similar to that induced by native extract.

Conclusions: Cat depigmented allergoid induced production of cytokines involved in a Th1 and Treg response, was able to induce production of IgG-antibodies that blocks IgE-binding to cat native extract, and showed reduced interaction with IgE, suggesting greater safety than native extract while maintaining in vitro efficacy.

Keywords: Cat, Immunotherapy, Surface plasmon resonance, Cell studies, Dander

Background

Sensitization to cat dander presents a high prevalence, affecting more than 25% of the population in Western countries [1] and more than 15% in the US [2]. Around half of sensitized patients may present symptoms [3], being rhinoconjunctivitis the most frequent symptom.

Apart from avoidance strategies or symptomatic treatment, cat allergy is currently treated with immunotherapy consisting of the administration of native extracts (NE) either via subcutaneous or sublingual routes of administration. The use of cat native extracts has demonstrated clinical efficacy and safety profile in several clinical trials [4, 5], being the efficacy related to Fel d 1 content [6], and the amount of extract used is in turn related to adverse reactions [7]. The development of chemically modified allergen extracts by polymerization with glutaraldehyde has been postulated as an alternative in immunotherapy, maintaining/increasing the efficacy while reducing the risk of adverse reactions [8]. The resulting products are high molecular weight allergen chains which contain all the allergens present in NE in a polymerized form. An intermediate patented process known as "depigmentation" [9] consist on the purification of the NE for the removal of irrelevant allergenic substances with the objective to increase the concentration of the individual allergens. To date, this method has yielded good results in other aeroallergens, including mites and pollens [10, 11]. Other alternatives based on immunologically active peptides are

* Correspondence: jcarnes@leti.com
[1]Research & Development, Laboratorios LETI, S.L., Calle del Sol n° 5, 28760 Madrid, Tres Cantos, Spain
Full list of author information is available at the end of the article

currently under investigation [12, 13]. In addition, monomeric carbamylated allergoid sublingual immunotherapy also present good results [14].

In recent years, different techniques have been implemented in characterization of active substances used in immunotherapy, providing a clear advantage not only in the quality of immunotherapy treatments already in the market but also supporting and providing useful information for immunotherapeutic design and for the early stages of the development process. Measurement of IgE interaction with allergens by surface plasmon resonance (SPR) analysis has been postulated as an indicator of safety [15], while cellular assays based on cytokine release or quantification of IgE-blocking IgG-antibodies indicate immunological response suggesting efficacy. The design of immunotherapy based on immunological principles seems logical to guarantee the success of new products.

Based on these concepts, the objective of this study was to design and produce a depigmented allergoid of cat epithelium to be used in immunotherapy based on safety and efficacy data.

Methods
Allergen extract preparation
Two hundred grams of cat dander (Allergon, Sweden) were extracted in Phosphate Buffered Saline 0.01 M under continuous magnetic stirring, for 4 h at 4 °C. The resulting product was called native extract (NE). The NE was depigmented after a mild acid treatment (pH 2) followed by dialysis against bi-distilled water with a cut-off membrane of 3.5 kDa (Cellu Sep Membrane, Seguin, TX, USA) with the objective to remove the low molecular weight components. Finally the pH was adjusted to seven. The resulting depigmented extract was polymerized with glutaraldehyde at a concentration of 5 mg/ml and extensively dialyzed against bi-distilled water in 100 kDa dialysis membranes (Millipore, Bedford, USA) to remove non-polymerized compounds. Finally, the polymerized product was freeze-dried, obtaining the cat depigmented-polymerized extract (CDA). All extracts were manufactured in strict compliance with GMP principles, following internal procedures (Laboratorios LETI, Spain, [9]).

Serum samples and PBMC
A pool of four sera was used to evaluate IgE-binding to allergen extracts. In that sense, sera from cat-sensitized individuals were purchased from Plasmalab International (WA, USA), which operates in full compliance with U.S. Food and Drug Administration regulations. Specific IgE titer to cat dander in the pool of sera were 66.4 KU/l, to Fel d 1 55.3 KU/l, to Fel d 2 6.43KU/l, and to Fel d 4 9.60 KU/l, performed in ImmunoCAP system (Thermo

Fisher Scientific, MA USA). The pool of sera was negative for bromelain (0.05 KU/l).

Polyclonal antibodies were used for IgG-binding assays to allergen extracts. Specific antibodies were induced in two New Zealand white rabbits after three immunizations with 200 µg of CDA adsorbed onto 3% aluminium hydroxide. All procedures were approved by the Biolab Institutional Review Board (Biolab, S.L., Colmenar Viejo, Spain), and followed local ethics rules for animal experimentation.

Peripheral-blood mononuclear cell (PBMC) culture supernatants (Sanguine BioSciences, CA, USA, compliant with FDA regulations) from three asthmatic cat-atopic donors not previously treated with immunotherapy were used to evaluate the capacity to stimulate cytokine production.

Allergen extract characterization
Protein content
The protein content of NE and CDA extracts was measured using the Lowry–Biuret method (Sigma Diagnostics, St. Louis, USA) following the manufacturer's instructions.

Protein profile
One hundred micrograms of NE and CDA extracts were loaded in SDS–PAGE gels with 2.67% C, 15% T acrylamide under reducing conditions and stained with Biosafe Coomassie (Bio-Rad Laboratories, Hercules, CA, USA).

Allergenic profile
Proteins from previously prepared SDS–PAGE gels (see above) were transferred to an Immobilon®-P membrane (Millipore, Bedford, Mass., USA). Thereafter, the membrane was incubated overnight with a pool of sera from cat-sensitized individuals. Afterwards, the membrane was washed and finally incubated with monoclonal α-human-IgE-PO (Ingenasa, Madrid, Spain). Finally the reaction was developed with Immun-Star™ Western Kit (BioRad).

Fel d 1, the major allergen from cat, was identified using a similar methodology but using as a primary antibody α-Fel d 1 monoclonal antibody-biotin (Indoor Biotech, VA, USA). After washing, the membrane was incubated with streptavidin-peroxidase and finally developed with Immun-Star™ Western Kit.

Major allergen quantification
Major allergen, Fel d 1, was quantified in NE extract using a specific commercial kit (EL-FD1) following manufacturer's instructions (Indoor Biotech, VA, USA). Data were adjusted to a four-parameter logistic curve by the least-squares method. Determination of Fel d 1 in CDA was estimated based on NE determination and yield.

Polymerization profile

CDA molecular weight distribution was determined by SDS-PAGE (AnyKD TGX Precast Gels, BioRad Laboratories, CA, USA) using a high-molecular weight standard (Thermo Fisher Scientific Inc, MA USA), and by high-performance size exclusion chromatography (SEC) using a Bio SEC-3 Column (Agilent Technologies, CA, USA) in a 1200 series HPLC system (Agilent), at 1 ml/min 150 mM phosphate buffer, pH 7. Detection was performed at UV-280 nm.

Allergen identification

The presence of relevant allergens in NE and CDA was determined by mass spectrometry. Briefly, extracts were digested with trypsin and the peptide mixture was analyzed in a nanoAcquity liquid chromatography system (Waters Corporation, MA, USA) coupled to a LTQ-Orbitrap Velos (Thermo) mass spectrometer. Raw data were collected with ThermoXcalibur software (Thermo). A database search was performed through the Mascot search engine using Thermo Proteome Discover against the Uniprot database.

In vitro safety

IgE affinity by Surface Plasmon Resonance SPR measurements were performed on a Biacore T100 system (Biacore, Uppsala, Sweden). Briefly, α-human-IgE was immobilized through amine coupling onto a C1 chip (GE Healthcare, NJ, USA) and the reference flow cell was treated using the same chemicals but in the absence of antibodies. The pool of sera from cat-sensitized individuals was diluted 1:2 and injected to capture IgE. Finally, NE and CDA (0.4 mg/ml) were injected to determine the stability of the IgE-NE or IgE-CDA complexes by measuring the dissociation rate (k_d) and half-life ($t\frac{1}{2} = \ln2/k_d$) of the complex.

IgE binding capacity by determination of biological potency Biological potency of the extracts was calculated by ELISA competition assays, as previously described [16]. Briefly, each extract is compared with the In House Reference Preparation (IHRP), previously in vivo standardized. Nunc microplates (Thermo Scientific) were coated with anti-IgE (Ingenasa, Madrid, Spain). A pool of sera from cat sensitized patients was incubated in the plate. Dilutions of the sample and IHRP were incubated with the allergen labelled with peroxidase. The mixture was added to the coated plate and incubated. Afterwards, development solution (chromogen) was added, stopped with sulfuric acid and measured at OD 450 nm. Percentage of loss of potency was calculated as difference of biological potency between NE and CDA divided by NE potency.

In vitro efficacy

IgE Blocking antibodies The capacity of CDA to induce allergen-specific polyclonal IgG antibodies able to block IgE binding sites to the allergen was evaluated by ELISA inhibition, as previously described [17]. Briefly, microplates were coated with NE (2 µg/well). After incubation with the generated polyclonal antibodies against CDA, plates were incubated with the pool of sera from cat-sensitized individuals. A secondary antibody anti-human-IgE-PO (Ingenasa, Madrid, Spain) was used for detection at 405 nm. Percent of inhibition was calculated by comparing IgE binding after incubation with preimmune or final bleeding polyclonal antibodies. Briefly, CDA capacity to induce sIgG with capacity to inhibit IgE binding of patients serum to a cat epithelia NE was evaluated. Percentage of inhibition was calculated as follows: percentage of IgE binding $= 100 - (ODf/OD\,P) \times 100$. ODf and OD$P$ correspond to the optical densities after the preincubation of serum with the rabbit's final sera and the corresponding preimmune sera, respectively.

Cytokine production The capacity to stimulate cytokine production in PBMCs was evaluated using a quantitative ELISA-based Q-Plex™ test (Quansys Biosciences, UT, USA), performed in accordance with the manufacturer's instructions. PBMCs (2×10^5 cells per well) from cat sensitized patients were stimulated in triplicate with NE or CDA extract (100 µg/ml), and the production of IL-4, IFN-γ, IL-10 and IL-17 cytokines was measured in culture supernatants at 24 and 72 h. Phosphate buffered saline (PBS, 50 ng/ml) and concanavalin A (Con A, 5 µg/ml) were used as negative and positive controls, respectively.

Results
Protein and major allergen content
Protein content estimated by the Lowry-Biuret method was 216 µg prot/mg in NE and 254 µg prot/mg in CDA. NE contained approximately 25 µg of Fel d 1/mg. The estimated Fel d 1 content in CDA was 48 µg/mg.

Protein and allergen profile
The protein profile of NE (Fig. 1a) showed different bands of a wide range of molecular weight. The most prominent bands showed a low molecular weight (mainly 8 and 6 kDa). On the contrary, CDA showed higher molecular weight bands.

Allergenic profile was significantly different between NE and CDA (Fig. 1b), showing the most intense IgE-recognized band at 18 kDa in NE, coincident with Fel d 1 heterodimer (constituted by two subunits, of 4 and 14 kDa). Fel d 1 can also be found in a 36 kDa tetramer form. Fel d 1 band identity was confirmed by immunoblot using α-Fel d 1 monoclonal antibody (Fig. 1c). IgE binding to Fel d 1 was not observed in CDA (Fig. 1b),

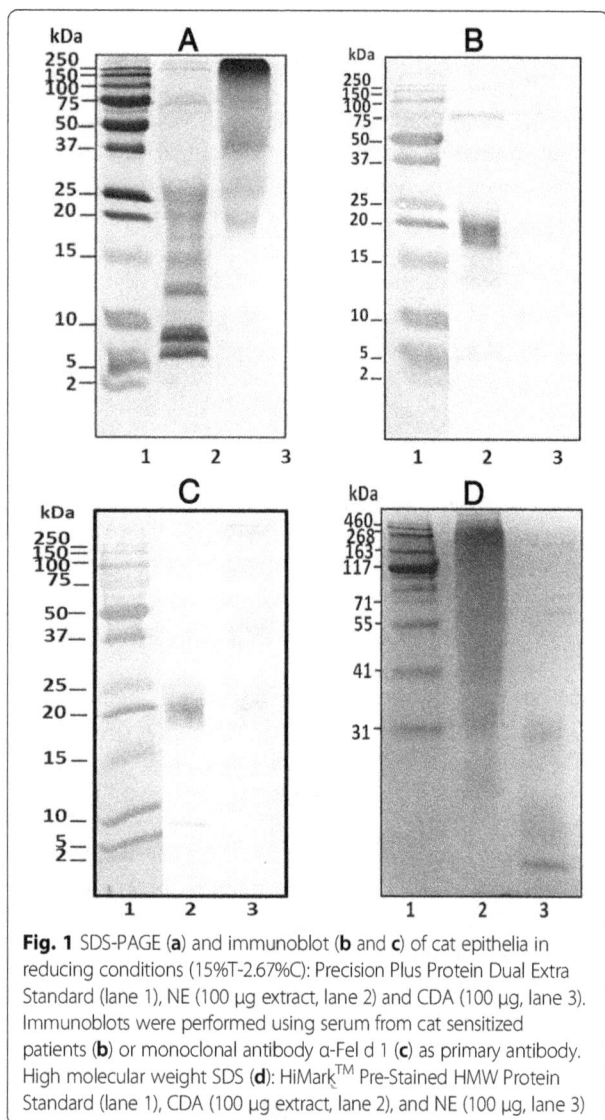

Fig. 1 SDS-PAGE (**a**) and immunoblot (**b** and **c**) of cat epithelia in reducing conditions (15%T-2.67%C): Precision Plus Protein Dual Extra Standard (lane 1), NE (100 µg extract, lane 2) and CDA (100 µg, lane 3). Immunoblots were performed using serum from cat sensitized patients (**b**) or monoclonal antibody α-Fel d 1 (**c**) as primary antibody. High molecular weight SDS (**d**): HiMark™ Pre-Stained HMW Protein Standard (lane 1), CDA (100 µg extract, lane 2), and NE (100 µg, lane 3)

and Fel d 7. The sequence coverage was 59% for chain 1 Fel d 1 (compared to Uniprot sequence code P30438), 40% for chain 2 Fel d 1 (Uniprot P30440), 51% for Fel d 2 (Uniprot M3WFW6), 69% for Fel d 3 (Uniprot Q8WNR9), for 37% Fel d 4 (Uniprot Q5VFH6) and 48% for Fel d 7 (Uniprot E5D2Z5). CDA sequencing showed the same allergens identified in NE.

CDA sequencing showed the same allergens identified in NE. Sequences coverage were 59% for chain 1 Fel d 1 (compared to Uniprot sequence code P30438), 26% for chain 2 Fel d 1 (Uniprot P30440), 45% for Fel d 2 (Uniprot P49064), 47% for Fel d 3 (Uniprot Q8WNR9), 29% for Fel d 4 (Uniprot Q5VFH6) and 52% for Fel d 7 (Uniprot E5D2Z5).

In vitro safety

In vitro safety was evaluated as the reduced IgE binding capacity of CDA compared to NE. Two assays were planned. The first one was IgE binding to evaluate dissociation constant and half-life of the complex IgE-extract by Surface Plasmon Resonance. The second one was the loss of biological potency after polymerization. This was performed by ELISA competition assays comparing IgE binding capacity of NE and CDA to a IHRP.

The stability of the complex Antigen-IgE, measured by SPR, showed that the k_d of IgE-CDA was $8.0*10^{-3} s^{-1}$ and the $t_{1/2}$ was 87.22 s. In contrast, the k_d of IgE-NE was $1.9*10^{-3} s^{-1}$, and the $t_{1/2}$ was 360.2 s. The IgE-CDA complex was 4.1 times less stable than IgE-NE regarding half life of the complex. In line with these results, polymerization induced a loss of biological potency higher than 95%. CDA presented a biological potency of 15 HEPL/mg, that represented a 99% of loss of biological potency compared to the NE (1035 HEPL/mg).

In vitro efficacy

CDA extract induced the production of IgG antibodies able to block up to IgE-binding sites. Specific IgE titers serums showed a low titer of sIgG titer (consequence of natural exposure to this allergen) lower than final bleeding samples. There was a 90% increase of induced inhibition comparing final and preimmune bleeding polyclonal samples (Fig. 3).

Cellular studies showed a similar production of IFN-γ and IL-10 (Fig. 4) by NE and CDA extracts. After 72 h, NE induced levels of 258.1 pg IFN-γ/ml and 648.7 pg IL-10/ml, while CDA induced 394.7 pg IFN-γ/ml and 520.7 pg IL-10/ml. IL-17 and IL-4 were not detected in any case (values below the limit of quantification).

Discussion

Cat allergy is one of the most prevalent allergic diseases in Western countries [1, 2]. Although limited clinical studies and numerous clinical observations have

and α-Fel d 1 monoclonal antibody recognition was less intense (Fig. 1c).

Polymerization profile

Specific methods (SDS-PAGE and SEC-HPLC) for detection of high molecular weight proteins were used to evaluate CDA polymerization profile (Figs. 1d and 2). Both methods showed a significant modification of CDA protein profile with respect to its corresponding NE. Low molecular weight proteins (at 4 and 14 kDa) were observed in NE but not in CDA (Fig. 1d. Proteins of approximately 31 and 107 kDa were observed in CDA chromatogram, although a high percentage of molecules exhibited a molecular weight higher than 1500 kDa (Fig. 2).

Allergen identification

NE was sequenced by mass spectrometry, which confirmed the presence of Fel d 1, Fel d 2, Fel d 3, Fel d 4

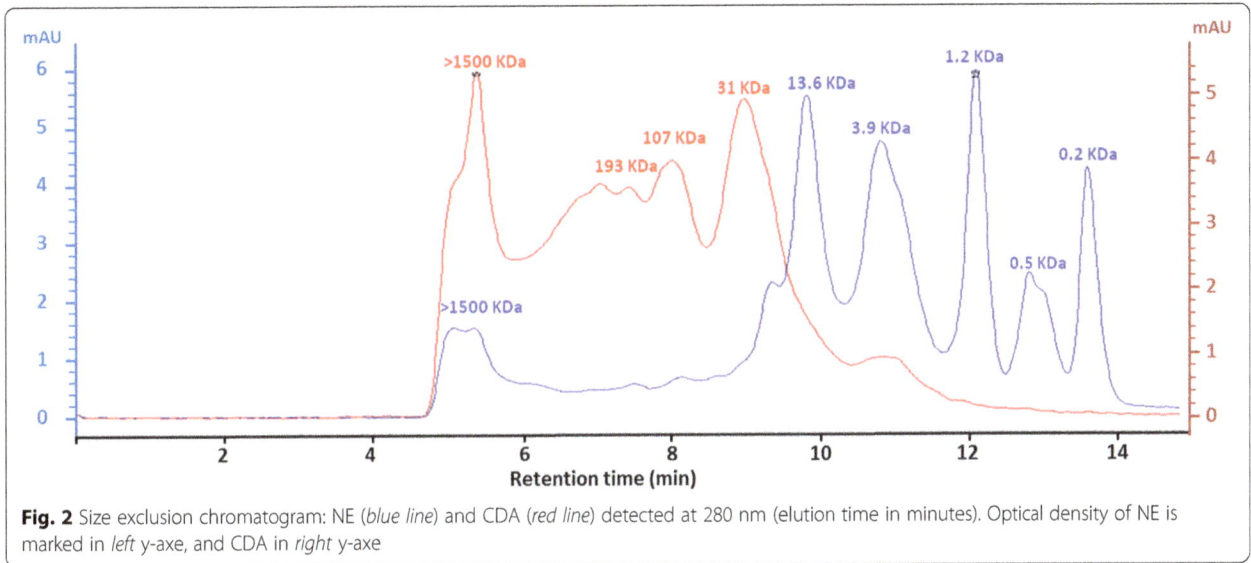

Fig. 2 Size exclusion chromatogram: NE (*blue line*) and CDA (*red line*) detected at 280 nm (elution time in minutes). Optical density of NE is marked in *left* y-axe, and CDA in *right* y-axe

demonstrated the efficacy of cat immunotherapy with native extracts [4–6, 18], the adverse reactions associated to these allergenic extracts remains being an issue to be solved. To our knowledge, this is the first time that a polymerized allergenic extract is manufactured and its safety and efficacy deeply evaluated by in vitro techniques. The manufacturing process was designed based of the reduction of the IgE binding capacity, but also to increase the immunological and clinical efficacy of the product by confirming the presence of the relevant allergens and the stimulation of the appropriate immunological pathways. The present study confirmed that CDA was immunologically active and able to induce a Th1/Treg response. Moreover, it also induced the production of IgG blocking antibodies, inhibiting the IgE binding capacity of serum obtained from allergic patients. In addition, CDA was also less allergenic, as its binding capacity to IgE was lower than that of NE.

In recent years, many studies have tried to elucidate the mechanism of action of immunotherapy. It has been suggested that successful allergen immunotherapy should be accompanied by induction of regulatory T cells (Treg) and shift from a Th2 response toward a Th1 response [19]. Additionally, recent studies have suggested that specific biomarkers for measurement of the success of immunotherapy should be related to the capacity of allergen vaccines to specifically stimulate production of IL-10 and IFN-γ, which are involved in the Th1 and Treg responses, respectively, and a reduction of IL-4 [20]. In our case, CDA stimulated the release of IL-10 and IFN-γ, suggesting a beneficial immune response that could lead to tolerance. On the contrary, IL-4 was not detected after either treatment, nor with positive control.

The clinical efficacy of immunotherapy has been also associated with the ability of the immunotherapeutic agent

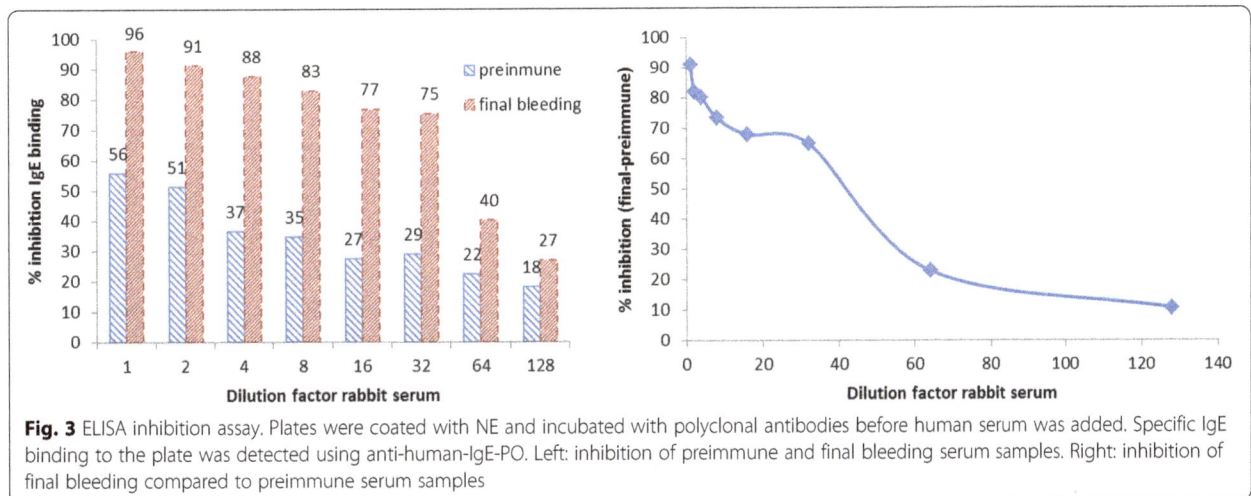

Fig. 3 ELISA inhibition assay. Plates were coated with NE and incubated with polyclonal antibodies before human serum was added. Specific IgE binding to the plate was detected using anti-human-IgE-PO. Left: inhibition of preimmune and final bleeding serum samples. Right: inhibition of final bleeding compared to preimmune serum samples

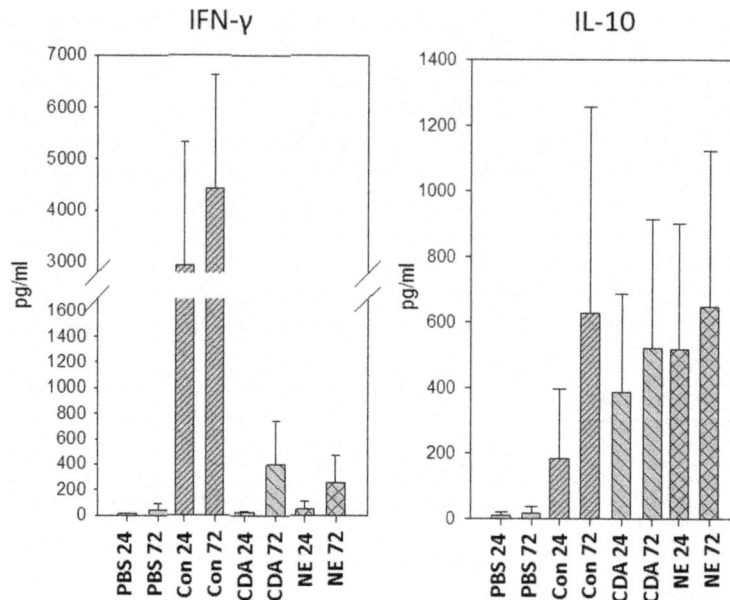

Fig. 4 Mean value of the IFN-γ (left) and IL-10 (right) induction (in pg/ml) by PBMCs from cat-allergic donors (N = 3) after 24 or 72 h of treatment with PBS (negative control), concanavalin A (positive control), cat depigmented allergoid (CDA) or native cat extracts (NE). Error bars refer to standard deviation

to induce IgG antibodies that block IgE-binding sites to the allergens (humoral response) [21]. The results obtained with CDA were positive. CDA extract administered in rabbits produced specific antibodies with capacity to block the IgE binding sites of NE epitopes. This is consistent with the detection of relevant allergens in CDA by mass spectrometry [22]. This means that CDA is captured and processed by the cells of the immune system, producing a specific response (specific IgG) against the allergens combined in the polymerized chains. These specific IgG antibodies generated after the administration of CDA are recognizing and block the natural allergens to which patients are exposed when they are in contact with the allergenic source, in this case, cats. In consequence, the treatment with CDA induces sIgG that blocks IgE binding to the allergen in patients serum [14].

On the other hand, adverse reactions and anaphylaxis as a consequence of IgE reactions remain as the major threat of immunotherapy. Several approaches have been used to reduce immunotherapy-induced side effects. These include immunotherapy with hypoallergens, T-cell epitope-containing peptides, and formulations consisting of Fel d 1 coupled to an immunomodulatory protein or carrier [23]. The polymerization process is the most common method for the reduction of allergenicity because it reduces IgE reactivity, thus improving treatment safety [11]. In our case, the CDA showed a different chromatographic profile compared to NE, characterized by proteins with higher molecular weight. Polymerization also induced a loss of IgE binding, as observed on immunoblot assays,

and loss of potency of the CDA extract compared to its corresponding NE, used as a marker of safety. In recent years, new methods based on measurement of the kinetic reaction between antigen and antibody have been postulated as a reliable alternative for the determination of the safety prior to in vivo assays [15]. CDA extract showed more than 4 times less affinity to IgE than NE confirming that the polymerized extract is safer for immunotherapy than native extracts using the same amount of material.

Conclusions

In summary, we have produced a depigmented and polymerized allergen extract of cat dander to be used as an alternative for cat allergy treatment. The new extract has been designed based on immunological efficacy and safety parameters. The results obtained demonstrate that CDA induces the production of cytokines involved in a Th1 and Treg response (induction of tolerance), is able to induce the production of IgG-blocking antibodies (humoral response), and exhibits reduced interaction with IgE, confirming in vitro efficacy and higher safety than NE. Further in vivo studies should be performed on allergic patients to prove the safety and efficacy of this extract, but the present results suggest that it is a good candidate for the treatment of allergy to cats. New in vitro methods and biomarkers should be optimized in order to design better products for treatments. This work shows the steps followed to evaluate efficacy and safety in vitro during the development of a cat allergoid, which would decrease risks in future clinical trials.

Abbreviations
CDA: Cat depigmented-polymerized extract; NE: Native Extract;
PBMC: Peripheral-blood mononuclear cell; SPR: Surface plasmon resonance

Acknowledgements
We thank Tamara Aranda, Beatriz Rojas and Beatriz Martínez for their
technical support in in vitro analysis.

Funding
This study was funded by Laboratorios Leti, Spain.

Authors' contributions
MM, MG and RM made biochemical and immunological characterizations,
VI coordinated cellular assays. MT made Biacore assays. EO made protein
sequencing. JC supervised all experiments and designed the study. MM,
VI and JC wrote the manuscript. All authors read and approved the final
manuscript.

Authors' Information
MM, MG, VI, RM and JC are employees of Laboratorios Leti, Tres Cantos,
Spain. MT is employee of the Universitat de Barcelona, Barcelons, Spain. EO is
employeed of Plataforma de Proteòmica, Parc Científic de Barcelona,
Barcelona, Spain.

Competing interests
Authors declare no competing financial interests. MM, MG, VI, RM and JC are
employees of Laboratorios Leti, Spain. MT and EO are supported by the
Universidad de Barcelona, Spain.

Author details
[1]Research & Development, Laboratorios LETI, S.L., Calle del Sol n° 5, 28760
Madrid, Tres Cantos, Spain. [2]Centres Científics i Tecnològics, Universitat de
Barcelona, Barcelona, Spain. [3]Plataforma de Proteòmica, Parc Científic de
Barcelona, Barcelona, Spain.

References
1. Heinzerling LM, Burbach GJ, Edenharter G, Bachert C, Bindslev-Jensen C, Bonini S, Bousquet J, Bousquet-Rouanet L, Bousquet PJ, Bresciani M, Bruno A, Burney P, Canonica GW, Darsow U, Demoly P, Durham S, Fokkens WJ, Giavi S, Gjomarkaj M, Gramiccioni C, Haahtela T, Kowalski ML, Magyar P, Murakozi G, Orosz M, Papadopoulos NG, Rohnelt C, Stingl G, Todo-Bom A, von Mutius E, Wiesner A, Wohrl S, Zuberbier T. Ga (2) len skin test study i: Ga (2) len harmonization of skin prick testing: Novel sensitization patterns for inhalant allergens in europe. Allergy. 2009;64:1498–506.
2. Arbes Jr SJ, Gergen PJ, Elliott L, Zeldin DC. Prevalences of positive skin test responses to 10 common allergens in the us population: Results from the third national health and nutrition examination survey. J Allergy Clin Immunol. 2005;116:377–83.
3. Stemeseder T, Klinglmayr E, Moser S, Lueftenegger L, Lang R, Himly M, Oostingh GJ, Zumbach J, Bathke AC, Hawranek T, Gadermaier G: Cross-sectional study on allergic sensitization of austrian adolescents using molecule-based ige profiling. Allergy. 2016. doi: 10.1111/all.13071. [Epub ahead of print]
4. Alvarez-Cuesta E, Berges-Gimeno P, Gonzalez-Mancebo E, Fernandez-Caldas E, Cuesta-Herranz J, Casanovas M. Sublingual immunotherapy with a standardized cat dander extract: Evaluation of efficacy in a double blind placebo controlled study. Allergy. 2007;62:810–7.
5. Varney VA, Edwards J, Tabbah K, Brewster H, Mavroleon G, Frew AJ. Clinical efficacy of specific immunotherapy to cat dander: A double-blind placebo-controlled trial. Clin Exp Allergy. 1997;27:860–7.
6. Ewbank PA, Murray J, Sanders K, Curran-Everett D, Dreskin S, Nelson HS. A double-blind, placebo-controlled immunotherapy dose–response study with standardized cat extract. J Allergy Clin Immunol. 2003;111:155–61.
7. Demoly P, Calderon MA. Dosing and efficacy in specific immunotherapy. Allergy. 2011;66 Suppl 95:38–40.
8. Ibarrola I, Sanz ML, Gamboa PM, Mir A, Benahmed D, Ferrer A, Arilla MC, Martinez A, Asturias JA. Biological characterization of glutaraldehyde-modified *Parietaria judaica* pollen extracts. Clin Exp Allergy. 2004;34:303–9.
9. 9 Carnés Sánchez J: Process for producing an allergen extract. WO 2011/098569; PCT/EP2011/052049
10. Gallego MT, Iraola V, Himly M, Robinson DS, Badiola C, Garcia-Robaina JC, Briza P, Carnes J. Depigmented and polymerised house dust mite allergoid: Allergen content, induction of IgG4 and clinical response. Int Arch Allergy Immunol. 2010;153:61–9.
11. Pfaar O, Sager A, Robinson DS. Safety and effect on reported symptoms of depigmented polymerized allergen immunotherapy: A retrospective study of 2927 paediatric patients. Pediatr Allergy Immunol. 2015;26:280–6.
12. Gronlund H, Saarne T, Gafvelin G, van Hage M. The major cat allergen, Fel d 1, in diagnosis and therapy. Int Arch Allergy Immunol. 2010;151:265–74.
13. Couroux P, Patel D, Armstrong K, Larche M, Hafner RP. Fel d 1-derived synthetic peptide immuno-regulatory epitopes show a long-term treatment effect in cat allergic subjects. Clin Exp Allergy. 2015;45:974–81.
14. Siman IL, de Aquino LM, Ynoue LH, Miranda JS, Pajuaba AC, Cunha-Junior JP, Silva DA, Taketomi EA. Allergen-specific IgG antibodies purified from mite-allergic patients sera block the IgE recognition of *Dermatophagoides pteronyssinus* antigens: An in vitro study. Clin Dev Immunol. 2013;2013: 657424.
15. Iraola V, Gallego MT, Taules M, Carnes J. Measurement of immunoglobulin e interaction with allergen extracts by surface plasmon resonance biosensor analysis. Ann Allergy Asthma Immunol. 2013;111:228–9.
16. Casanovas M, Maranon F, Bel I. Comparison of skin-prick test assay and reverse enzyme immunoassay competition (REINA-C) for biological activity of allergens. Clin Exp Allergy. 1994;24:134–9.
17. Lopez-Matas MA, Gallego M, Iraola V, Robinson D, Carnes J. Depigmented allergoids reveal new epitopes with capacity to induce IgG blocking antibodies. Biomed Res Int. 2013;2013:284615.
18. Van Metre Jr TE, Marsh DG, Adkinson Jr NF, Kagey-Sobotka A, Khattignavong A, Norman Jr PS, Rosenberg GL. Immunotherapy for cat asthma. J Allergy Clin Immunol. 1988;82:1055–68.
19. Jutel M, Akdis CA. Immunological mechanisms of allergen-specific immunotherapy. Allergy. 2011;66:725–32.
20. Matsuoka T, Shamji MH, Durham SR. Allergen immunotherapy and tolerance. Allergol Int. 2013;62:403–13.
21. James LK, Shamji MH, Walker SM, Wilson DR, Wachholz PA, Francis JN, Jacobson MR, Kimber I, Till SJ, Durham SR. Long-term tolerance after allergen immunotherapy is accompanied by selective persistence of blocking antibodies. J Allergy Clin Immunol. 2011;127:509–16. e501-505.
22. Carnes J, Himly M, Gallego M, Iraola V, Robinson DS, Fernandez-Caldas E, Briza P. Detection of allergen composition and in vivo immunogenicity of depigmented allergoids of *Betula alba*. Clin Exp Allergy. 2009;39:426–34.
23. Andersson TN, Ekman GJ, Gronlund H, Buentke E, Eriksson TL, Scheynius A, Van Hage-Hamsten M, Gafvelin G. A novel adjuvant-allergen complex, CBP-rFel d 1, induces up-regulation of CD86 expression and enhances cytokine release by human dendritic cells in vitro. Immunology. 2004;113:253–9.

7

Characterization of anti-EBA175RIII-V in asymptomatic adults and children living in communities in the Greater Accra Region of Ghana with varying malaria transmission intensities

L. E. Amoah[1*], H. B. Abagna[1], K. Akyea-Mensah[1], A. C. Lo[1,2], K. A. Kusi[1] and B. A. Gyan[1]

Abstract

Background: Antibodies against Region III-V of the erythrocyte binding antigen (EBA) 175 (EBA175RIII-V) have been suggested to provide protection from malaria in a natural infection. However, the quality and quantity of naturally induced antibodies to EBA175RIII-V has not been fully characterized in different cohorts of Ghanaians. This study sought to determine the characteristics of antibodies against EBA175RIII-V in asymptomatic adults and children living in two communities of varying *P. falciparum* parasite prevalence in southern Ghana.

Methods: Microscopic evaluation of thick and thin blood smears was used to identify asymptomatic *Plasmodium falciparum* carriage and indirect enzyme linked immunosorbent (ELISA) used to assess antibody concentrations and avidity.

Results: Parasite carriage estimated by microscopy in Obom was 35.6% as opposed to 3.5% in Asutsuare. Levels of IgG, IgG1, IgG2, IgG3 and IgG4 against EBA175RIII-V in the participants from Obom were significantly higher ($P < 0.05$, Dunn's Multiple Comparison test) than those in Asutsuare. However the relative avidity of IgG antibodies against EBA175RIII-V was significantly higher ($P < 0.0001$, Mann Whitney test) in Asutsuare than in Obom.

Conclusions: People living in communities with limited exposure to *P. falciparum* parasites have low quantities of high avidity antibodies against EBA175RIII-V whilst people living in communities with high exposure to the parasites have high quantities of age-dependent but low avidity antibodies against EBA175RIII-V.

Introduction

The asexual stages of *Plasmodium falciparum* (*P. falciparum*) are partly responsible for the pathology associated with malaria and subsequently are the focus of malaria treatment regimens as well as the focus of malaria vaccine research. The merozoite is the only extracellular stage of the parasites erythrocytic life-cycle, making merozoite surface antigens promising malaria vaccine candidates. One such candidate is the erythrocyte binding antigen (EBA) 175 (EBA 175, Pf3D7_0731500), PfEBA-175 has been shown to play a

key role during the fast cascade of interactions between the parasite and host molecules before the merozoite completely invades the erythrocyte by binding to sialic acid residues on glycophorin A on the red blood cell during merozoite invasion [1]. Of the 6 extracellular domains of EBA175, region 2 (RII), which comprises of two cysteine rich domains F1 and F2 [2] as well as RIII-V, which comprises of the dimorphic region 3 (RIII) as well as the highly conserved regions 4 (RIV) and 5 (RV) [2] have been implicated as vaccine candidate antigens.

Antibodies induced against diverse antigenic components of the erythrocytic parasite are important mediators of anti-disease immunity [3]. Some known functions of antibodies induced against the asexual parasite

* Correspondence: lamoah@noguchi.ug.edu.gh
[1]Noguchi Memorial Institute for Medical Research, University of Ghana, Accra, Ghana
Full list of author information is available at the end of the article

include preventing merozoites from invading new erythrocytes (inhibition of invasion), preventing cytoadherence of infected erythrocytes to endothelial cells as well as interfering with the normal function of monocytes and macrophages [4, 5]. Targeting the merozoite before they invade erythrocytes can serve as a means to truncate the infection. The ability of antibodies against the merozoite to prevent erythrocyte invasion has been demonstrated through in vivo human passive transfer assays [6, 7] and in vitro erythrocyte invasion inhibition assays [8] several years ago. Antibodies specific for EBA175 RIII-V have been shown to be associated with protection from malaria in symptomatic cases [9]. Also, Healer et al., [10] in immunization studies have shown that antibodies induced by a recombinant RIII-V inhibit merozoites invasion.

Repeated exposure to malaria parasites has been suggested as a necessary requirement for the maintenance of anti-parasite immunity as it has been demonstrated in a number of studies that antibodies against merozoite antigens are relatively short-lived in the absence of a new infections [11–14]. This has been confirmed in some community studies where people with current infections had higher merozoite antibody levels than those without [15–17]. However, a few studies including one by Wipasa et al., noticed that both antibody and memory B cell responses to malaria antigens remained steady over long periods in the absence of an infection [18]. Some studies have suggested that merozoite antibody levels show a direct correlation with malaria transmission intensity in malaria endemic settings and are higher in high transmission settings [19, 20].

The cytophilic immunoglobulins, IgG1 and IgG3 have been associated with parasite repression directly, or opsonization indirectly [21]. IgG1 and IgG3 antibodies to merozoite antigens generally have short half-lives [12]. The half-lives of IgG subclass responses against EBA175 are generally short lived, however, the half-lives of IgG1 and IgG3 have been noted to be longer lived and more prevalent than those of IgG2 and IgG4 [21, 22]. IgG1 and IgG3 responses against EBA175 have also been associated with lower parasitaemia in a high transmission setting [21] as well as a seasonal transmission setting of Papua New Guinea [23].

The process of antibody selection that occurs during humoral immune response maturation, results in the production of antibodies with increased avidity [24, 25]. Antibody properties, including high avidity, have been suggested to key determinants of protective immunity against malaria [26–28]. High Avidity to whole schizont extract as well as to a number of specific *P. falciparum* antigens, have been shown to correlate with protection from malaria [29–31]. The avidity of antibodies against MSP1 has been observed to increase after a recent *P.*

falciparum infection [29], however some reports have implicated reduced antibody affinity maturation and antibody avidity to a recent malaria infection [32] and excessive stimulation of B cells in high parasite prevalence settings [33]. The avidity of antibodies to *P. falciparum* antigens has been found to be lower in areas of high malaria transmission intensity than in areas with lower transmission [34].

This study sought to determine differences in the characteristics of antibody responses to EBA175RIII-V in adults and children living in high and low malaria parasite prevalence settings.

Methods

Ethical consideration
Ethical approval for the study (#089/14–15) was obtained from the Institutional Review Board of the Noguchi Memorial Institute for Medical Research. Written informed consent, assent and parental consent were obtained for all participants recruited into the study.

Study site and population
The cross-sectional study conducted in June 2016, recruited adults and children aged between 2 and 75 years from two semi-rural communities, Obom and Asutsuare, both within the Greater Accra Region of Ghana as part of a large study which aims to identify a number of factors that influence asymptomatic *P. falciparum* carriage in high and low malaria transmission settings in Ghana. This study only recruited people in the two communities who did not exhibit any sign or symptom of clinical malaria and provided written informed consent for either themself or a dependent. Obom is a high *P. falciparum* prevalence community in the Ga South Municipality and Asutsuare is a low *P. falciparum* prevalence community, with noted low malaria transmission [35] in the Shai Osudoku District (Fig. 1). The major malaria season in the Greater Accra Region is from June to August, with a peak in July [36].

Sample collection and processing
After obtaining written informed consent, 5 ml of venous blood was collected from each participant into acid citrate dextrose (ACD) vacutainer tubes. A drop of the whole blood was used to prepare thick and thin blood smears and the rest was separated into plasma and packed cells after centrifugation. The plasma was immediately stored at -20 °C. Demographic data from the participants including ownership of insecticide treated bed nets (ITN) was also captured.

Microscopic identification of *P. falciparum* parasites
Thin and thick blood smears were processed using a method described by the WHO [37]. Briefly thin blood

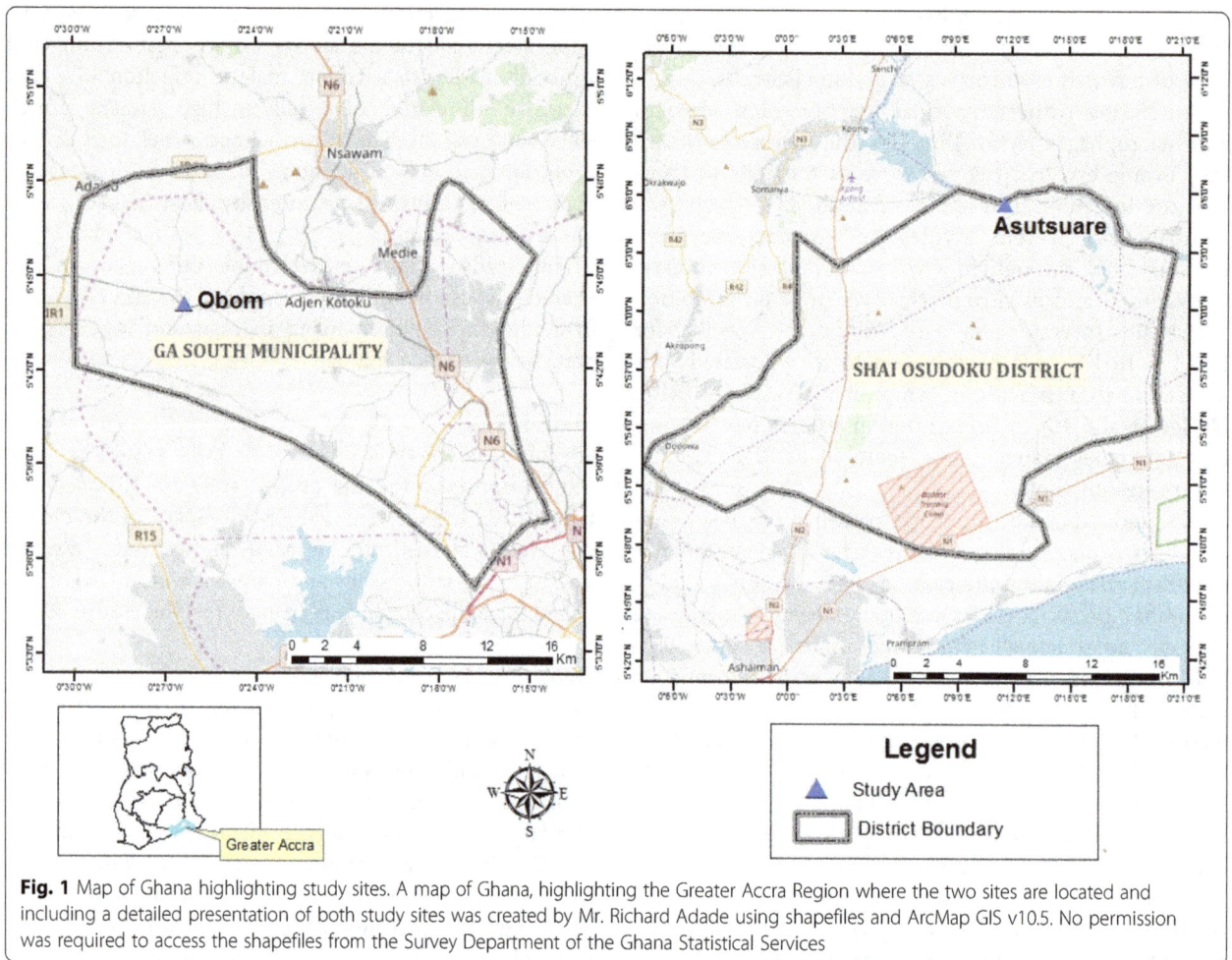

Fig. 1 Map of Ghana highlighting study sites. A map of Ghana, highlighting the Greater Accra Region where the two sites are located and including a detailed presentation of both study sites was created by Mr. Richard Adade using shapefiles and ArcMap GIS v10.5. No permission was required to access the shapefiles from the Survey Department of the Ghana Statistical Services

smears were dried, fixed in 100% methanol and then stained with 10% Giemsa after the methanol had evaporated. Thick blood smears were air-dried and stained with 10% Giemsa. The thick and thin smears were observed under an × 100 oil immersion objective by two independent microscopists. The thin smears were used to identify the infecting *Plasmodium* species [38].

Enzyme linked immunosorbent assay (ELISA)

Lactococcus lactis produced EBA175-RIII-V [39] was used in an indirect ELISA to measure total IgG and IgG subclass (IgG1, IgG2, IgG3 and IgG4) antibody responses in plasma from the study participants using a protocol similar to that previously reported by Acquah, F et al [39] for IgG and a modification of Ismail, HA et al [21] for the IgG subclasses. Briefly, 1 ng of purified antigen, EBA175-RIII-V in phosphate buffered saline (PBS, pH 7.4) was coated 100 µl /well onto NUNC Maxi-Sorp™ ELISA plates (Thermo Scientific, UK) overnight at 4 °C. Plates were blocked with 150 µl/well of 3% (*w/v*) skimmed milk powder (Marvel, UK) in PBS/T after four washes using PBS supplemented with 0.05% Tween 20

(PBS/T). Duplicate wells of the plates were then incubated with 100 µl of plasma diluted 200-fold and a reference standard, purified human polyclonal IgG [40, 41] (BP055, The Binding Site, UK) at a starting concentration of 1000 ng/µl and serially diluted 3-fold in duplicate wells was used as a standard calibrator.

Plates were incubated for an hour at room temperature and then washed four times with PBS/T. The plates were subsequently incubated with 50 µl of goat anti-human IgG-HRP (Invitrogen, USA) secondary antibodies for IgG.

For the IgG subclass ELISA, the plates were processed as for the IgG above, however the plates were incubated with 100 µl of plasma diluted 1:50 at 37 °C for 1 h and after washing, incubated with 50 µl of goat anti-human IgG1-HRP (The Binding Site, UK) and goat anti-human IgG3-HRP (The Binding Site, UK) secondary antibodies. A positive control sample was obtained by pooling a number of samples that had previously identified as containing high concentrations of EBA175-RIII-V [42]. This positive control sample was serially diluted to prepare the standard curve) at a starting concentration of 1:10 and serially diluted 2 fold. Sera from adults living in the

USA who have never been exposed to malaria (malaria naïve sera) and confirmed as having extremely low concentrations of EBA175RIII-V antibody levels were used as negative control samples. A positive and some negative control samples were used on each ELISA plate.

All plates were developed by adding 50 µl/well of 3,3′,5,5′-tetramethylbenzidine (TMB) solution for 15 min for total IgG or 20 min for the IgG subclasses and then stopped with 2 M H_2SO_4. Fluorescence was measured immediately after stopping the reactions using excitation wavelength of 450 nm.

IgG avidity ELISA

A procedure similar to the total IgG ELISA described above was used, however four replica wells were incubated with each appropriately diluted plasma sample for an hour, after which 100 µl/well of 2.4 M sodium thiocyanate (NaSCN; Sigma-Aldrich, UK) was added for an extra 10 min incubation [42–44] prior to the wash and subsequent addition of 50 µl/well of goat anti-human IgG-HRP (Invitrogen, USA).

Data analysis

A thick blood smear was classified as negative for *Plasmodium* parasites if no infected erythrocytes were observed after counting 200 WBCs by both microscopists. In instances where disparities were observed in identifying the presence of *Plasmodium* infected erythrocytes, the smear was given to a third microscopist to confirm the presence or absence of *Plasmodium* infected erythrocytes. Once a thick smear was identified as containing *Plasmodium* infected erythrocytes, the corresponding thin smear was inspected to determine the *Plasmodium* species present in the sample.

Demographic data was entered into excel and column statistics determined using GraphPad Prism v5 (GraphPad software, USA).

Optical density (OD) results from the ELISA plate reader were converted into concentrations using the four-parameter curve-fitting program known as ADAMSEL (Ed Remarque, BPRC) and the data analyzed using GraphPad Prism v5 (GraphPad software, USA). The correlation between age and EBA175RIII-V antibody (IgG, IgM, IgG1 and IgG3) concentrations were performed using Spearman non-parametric correlation matrix and Mann Whitney U tests used to determine the differences in similar antibody responses between the two sites.

Seropositivity was defined as antibody concentration higher than the average antibody concentration of the negative control samples (naïve serum) plus two standard deviations.

Relative antibody avidity was determined as the ratio of the mean IgG concentration of the SCN⁻-treated sample to the mean IgG concentration of the untreated sample multiplied by 100. (Avidity index = [antibodies following NaSCN treatment/ antibodies without NaSCN treatment] × 100).

Participants were stratified into three age groups, ≤10 (ten and below 10), 11–14 and ≥ 15 (fifteen and above) for some of the analysis. Data from seven participants from Asutsuare were excluded in age stratified analysis because their ages were not recorded. Statistical significance was defined as P value ≤0.05 unless otherwise stated.

Results

The age range for the 161 study participants from Obom was 6 to 70 years, while that of the 169 participants from Asutsuare was 2 and 75 years (Table 1). Asymptomatic *P. falciparum* parasite carriage, as determined by light microscopy, was higher in Obom (57 of the 160 participants or 35.6%) compared to Asutsuare (6 of the 169 participants, representing or 3.5%). There was thus a 10-fold difference in parasite carriage between the two study communities (Table 1). Bed net ownership was low in both communities, only 11 and 2 participants in Obom and Asutsuare respectively claimed to own bed nets.

Seroprevalence of antibodies against recombinant EBA175RIII-V$_{LI}$ antigen

The cutoff values used to calculate seroprevalence was 2581, 1773, 580 and 1198 AU for IgG1, IgG2, IgG3 and IgG4 respectively and 2137 ng/ml for IgG. The seroprevalence of IgG and IgG subclasses to EBA175RIII-V$_{LI}$ of participants from Obom (IgG, 85.6%; IgG1, 90.6%; IgG2, 51.3%; IgG3, 91.3% and IgG4, 25.0%) was significantly higher ($P < 0.05$, Mann Whitney test) than participants from Asutsuare (IgG, 58.0%; IgG1, 34.9%; IgG2, 5.9%; IgG3, 31.4% and IgG4, 16.0%). Seropositivity to the cytophilic IgG subclasses, IgG1 and IgG3 against EBA175 RIII-V$_{LI}$ in both Obom and Asutsuare was higher than seropositivity to IgG2 and IgG4.

Concentration of antibodies against recombinant EBA175RIII-V$_{LI}$ antigen

Although 161 and 169 participant samples were used for all the different ELISAs, some samples had values, which

Table 1 Characteristics of study participants

	N	% Asymptomatic infections	Median age (years)
Obom	161	35.6	15 (6–70)
Asutsuare	168	3.5	16 (2–75)

N total number of volunteers enrolled, % Asymptomatic is the % of people that tested positive for *P. falciparum* by microscopy. Median values reported with minimum and maximum age values were classified as 'Low' by the plate reader, meaning their value was similar to the blank sample and were not assigned a value. Those samples were not included in the analysis and subsequently resulted in variations in the final total number of samples, N used in the analysis.

The median antibody concentrations for both IgG and all the four IgG subclasses (IgG1, IgG2, IgG3 and IgG4) measured in participants from Obom were significantly higher than those recorded for from participants from Asutsuare ($p < 0.0001$, Mann Whitney test for each) (Figs. 2a and 3a-d). The cytophilic IgG1 and IgG3 antibody responses measured in both sites were higher than the antibody concentrations of IgG2 and IgG4 (Table 2).

Levels of IgG, IgG1, IgG2 and IgG3 antibody responses significantly correlated with age in Obom (Spearman rho: 0.2244, 0.2677, 0.2210 and 0.1724 respectively; $P < 0.05$ in

all cases). However, there was no correlation between the levels of IgG4 antibody responses in Obom or any of the antibody responses measured in samples from Asutsuare with age (Fig. 3).

Antibody avidity

The relative avidity index of IgG responses measured in participants from Obom and Asutuare both significantly correlated negatively with age, (Spearman $r = -0.2338$, $p < 0.0072$ in Obom; Spearman $r = -0.1824$, $p = 0.0394$ in Asutsuare). Although the antibody concentrations measured in volunteers from Asutsuare were significantly lower than those measured in volunteers from Obom (Fig. 2a), the relative avidities of IgG antibodies against EBA175RIII-V were higher in the volunteers from Asutsuare than from Obom (Fig. 2b). Antibody avidity index (RAI) of IgG for participants from Obom who were 10 years old and below were significantly

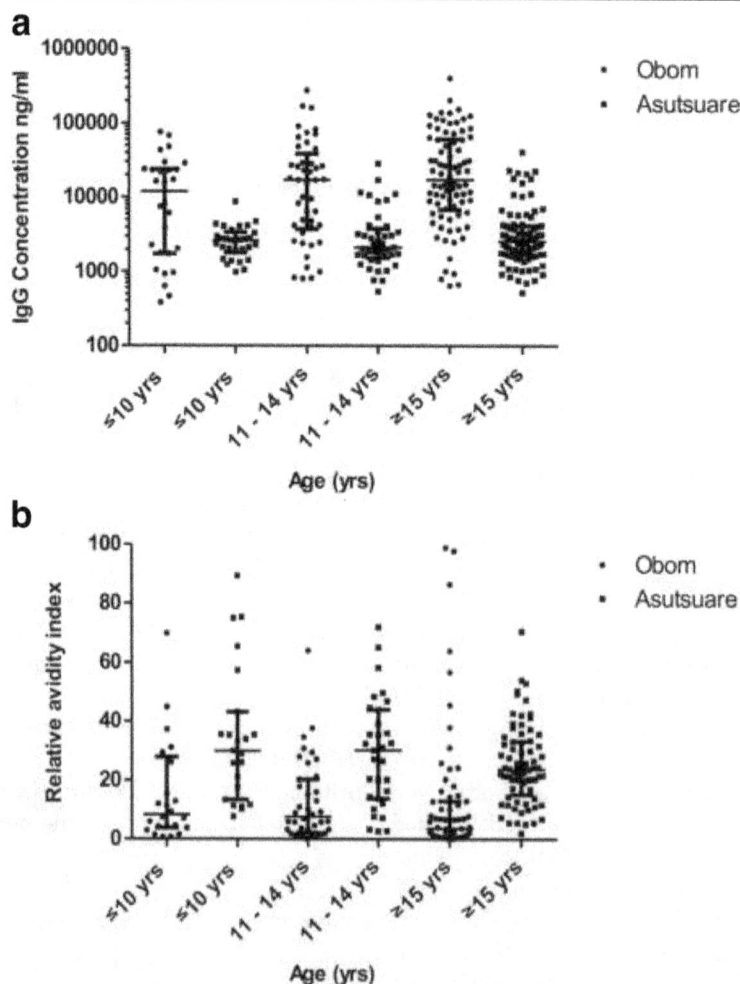

Fig. 2 Age stratified IgG concentrations and avidity. Participants in Obom (black circles) and Asutsuare (black squares) were stratified into three age groups, ≤10, 11–14 and ≤ 15 years. The concentrations (**a**) and relative avidities (**b**) of naturally induced IgG antibodies against EBA175RIII-V antigen in plasma samples obtained from whole blood collected in June 2016 was measured using ELISA as described in the methods section. The graphs represent the median concentrations with the interquartile range as the error bars

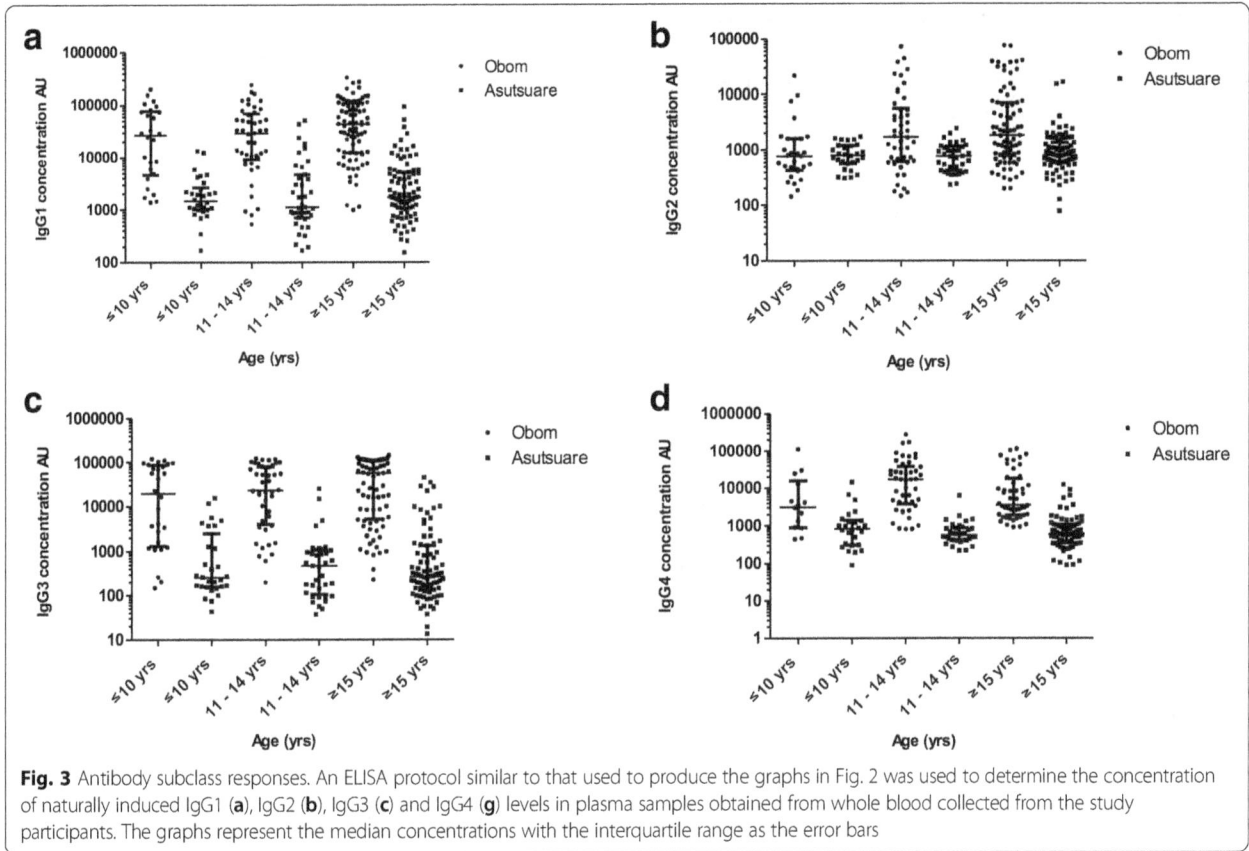

Fig. 3 Antibody subclass responses. An ELISA protocol similar to that used to produce the graphs in Fig. 2 was used to determine the concentration of naturally induced IgG1 (**a**), IgG2 (**b**), IgG3 (**c**) and IgG4 (**g**) levels in plasma samples obtained from whole blood collected from the study participants. The graphs represent the median concentrations with the interquartile range as the error bars

lower ($p < 0.05$, Dunn's multiple comparison test) than the RAI for all three categories (10 years and below, between 11 and 14 years and those 15 years and above) of participants in Asutsuare (Additional file 1). The RAI of IgG for participants from Obomaged 10 years and below was significantly higher ($p < 0.001$, Dunn's multiple comparison

test) than participants aged between 11 and 14 years as well as those 15 years and above (Additional file 1).

Discussion

Rabbit serum containing polyclonal antibodies against Region III-V of EBA175 have been found to directly inhibit *P. falciparum* merozoite invasion [10]. Naturally induced antibodies against Region III-V of EBA175 have also been suggested to be indicative of strong protection from symptomatic malaria [45], however the role antibodies against EBA175RIII-V play in asymptomatic malaria has not been fully evaluated. Data from the assessment of the magnitude and avidity of antibody responses to this antigen across different age groups will potentially be relevant for the interpretation of natural and vaccine induced immune responses to this antigen.

In order to determine possible differences in natural antibody responses to Region III-V of EBA175, a cross sectional survey was carried out in Obom, which has been reported to be a high parasite prevalence community [46] and in Asutsuare, where parasite prevalence and malaria transmission intensity is known to be very low [35]. The study enrolled a range of children and adults to determine possible differences in age related

Table 2 IgG and IgG subclass antibody concentrations

		N	Min	Median	Max
IgG	Obom	156	380.5	16,006	403,567
(ng/ml)	Asutsuare	168	518.8	2411	40,686
IgG1	Obom	153	526.8	33,041	331,686
(AU)	Asutsuare	165	154.2	1660	93,998
IgG2	Obom	158	142.2	1409	75,188
(AU)	Asutsuare	162	76.67	770	16,397
IgG3	Obom	156	146.8	40,009	141,652
(AU)	Asutsuare	156	13.4	270.7	45,058
IgG4	Obom	88	76.98	3152	113,147
(AU)	Asutsuare	143	89.89	605.8	14,617

N total number of samples used in the analysis, *Min* minimum concentration, *Max* maximum concentration. Total IgG was measured in ng/ml, whilst the IgG subclasses were measured in arbitrary units (AU)

antibody responses. This study confirmed the existence of very low *P. falciparum* parasite prevalence in Asutsuare (Table 1) as has previously been reported [35]. The number of asymptomatic individuals in Asutsuare however may be higher than the 3.5% if *Plasmodium* parasites were detected by molecular methods. Especially as a higher number of submicroscopic parasite infections are detected in asymptomatic individuals due to the increased sensitivity of the detection technique [47]. Bed net ownership was generally low in both communities. Ownership in Obom was higher than in Asutsuare, most likely because residents of Asutsuare encounter very low frequencies of malaria that they no longer think it is important to implement personal malaria control interventions relative to inhabitants of Obom, where malaria transmission is high.

Although only 3.5% of the participants from Asutsuare had microscopic densities of parasites, almost 60% of them were seropositive for anti-EBA175RIII-V antibodies. Similarly, although only about 35% of the participants from Obom were identified by microscopy as harboring *P. falciparum* parasites, over 80% had IgG antibodies against EBA175RIII-V. These collectively suggest the possible presence of parasites at densities below the detection limit of microscopy in some of the participants or that some of the participants had just recently cleared a *P. falciparum* infection, as antibodies against EBA175 have been suggested to be relatively short-lived [21].

The significantly higher IgG responses recorded in Obom than in Asutsuare (Fig. 2a) is indicative of the possible requirement of an active infection to induce antibodies against EBA175RIII-V as has been previously suggested, especially as these antibodies are relatively short-lived [21]. IgG subclass responses in both sites were predominantly cytophilic (IgG1 and IgG3) (Fig. 3), which supports a number of previous reports [9, 21, 48, 49]. However responses to IgG2 and IgG4 existed, although at much lower quantities and has been suggested to be due to the much shorter half-lives of IgG2 and IgG4 compared to IgG1 and IgG3 [21]. IgG subclass antibody levels were significantly higher in Obom than in Asutsuare, which was not surprising as total IgG levels were also significantly higher in Obom than in Asutsuare.

In Obom, the high transmission setting, IgG, IgG1 and IgG3 responses to EBA175RIII-V positively correlated with age (Figs. 2a, 3a&c). This supports data from a previous study conducted in a high transmission setting in Nigeria [21] and that of another study in highly asymptomatic children from a moderately seasonal setting Papua New Guinea [9]. High IgG1 and IgG3 responses for other merozoite antigens such as MSP1 [50] and MSP2 [51] have also been documented. A previous study did not find any correlation between IgG2 and IgG4 responses against EBA175 and age [21], however in this study, IgG2 responses correlated positively (Fig. 3b) with age in responses measured in the high transmission setting, Obom. The lack of age associated antibody responses in Asutsuare (Figs. 2a & 3) may be due to the very low prevalence of parasites observed in the community (Table 1) as parasite exposure has been found to be necessary for mounting immune responses against malaria antigens.

The relative antibody avidities measured in the participants from Asutsuare, the low transmission setting were significantly higher than those measured in Obom (Fig. 2b). A similar observation has been reported for antibody responses to this same antigen conducted in children living in the same high transmission setting and a different low transmission setting in Ghana [42] as well as for antibody responses to a different merozoite antigen, MSP1$_{19}$ [34] and could be due to the presence of fewer and less diverse parasite clones circulating in low transmission zones [52]. Although high parasite diversity and frequency of infection is anticipated in high transmission settings, the diversity of RIII-V of EBA175 was recently suggested to be relatively similar in parasites circulating in Obom (the high transmission setting) and Abura [42], a community with low parasite transmission intensity, similar to Asutsuare. Generally, an increase in exposure to diverse parasites strains/isolates will result in heterologous exposure, which could lead to reduced affinity maturation and the production of antibodies with lower avidities as measured in antibody responses in Obom. A recent report on the avidity of naturally induced antibodies against EBA175RIII-V in children living in southern Ghana similarly reported reduced avidity of antibodies from children living in the high transmission setting compared to the low transmission setting [42].

The likely short longevity of naturally induced antibodies against EBA175RIII-V is contrary to the dynamics of antibodies against MSP1−$_{19}$, which have been found to persist for several years after the clearance of *P. falciparum* parasites [53, 54] and thus may be a suitable candidate to use as a serological marker to monitor changes in malaria transmission intensity.

Conclusion

People living in communities with limited exposure to *P. falciparum* parasites have low quantities of high avidity antibodies against EBA175RIII-V whilst people living in communities with high exposure to the parasites have high quantities of age dependent but low avidity antibodies against EBA175RIII-V.

Abbreviations
ACD: Acid citrate dextrose; AU: Antibody unit; DBS: Dried blood spot; EBA 175: Erythrocyte binding antigen 175; ELISA: Enzyme linked immunosorbent assay; IgG: Immunoglobulin; OD: Optical density

Acknowledgements
The authors are grateful to all the study participants and to Mr. Abdul Haruna and Mr. Eric Kyei-Baffour both of the University of Ghana for help with reading the thick and thin blood smears. We also thank Mr. Richard Adade, GIS & Remote Sensing Unit, Department of Fisheries and Aquatic Science, Center for Coastal Management, University of Cape Coast, Cape Coast, Ghana for creating the map of the study sites.

Funding
This project was supported in part by the Ghana government Book and Research allowance to LEA and the Bill and Melinda Gates foundation through the NMIMR Postdoctoral Fellowship awarded to AL. *"The funders had no role in study design, data collection and analysis, decision to publish, or preparation of the manuscript"*.

Authors' contributions
'LEA, BG and AL designed the study; LEA, HBA, BG and KAK wrote the manuscript and performed the statistical analysis; LEA and AL provided reagents, AL and KA-M collected the samples; HA performed the experiments. All authors read and approved the final manuscript.'

Competing interests
The authors declare that they have no competing interests.

Author details
[1]Noguchi Memorial Institute for Medical Research, University of Ghana, Accra, Ghana. [2]Present address: University Cheikh Anta DIOP, Dakar, Senegal.

References
1. Okenu DM, Riley EM, Bickle QD, Agomo PU, Barbosa A, Daugherty JR, Lanar DE, Conway DJ. Analysis of human antibodies to erythrocyte binding antigen 175 of Plasmodium falciparum. Infect Immun. 2000;68(10):5559–66.
2. Sim B. EBA-175: an erythrocyte-binding ligand of Plasmodium falciparum. Parasitol Today. 1995;11(6):213–7.
3. Turner L, Wang CW, Lavstsen T, Mwakalinga SB, Sauerwein RW, Hermsen CC, Theander TG. Antibodies against PfEMP1, RIFIN, MSP3 and GLURP are acquired during controlled Plasmodium falciparum malaria infections in naive volunteers. PLoS One. 2011;6(12):e29025.
4. Wipasa J, Elliott S, Xu H, Good MF. Immunity to asexual blood stage malaria and vaccine approaches. Immunol Cell Biol. 2002;80(5):401–14.
5. Beeson JG, Osier FH, Engwerda CR. Recent insights into humoral and cellular immune responses against malaria. Trends Parasitol. 2008;24(12): 578–84.
6. Cohen S, Mc GI, Carrington S. Gamma-globulin and acquired immunity to human malaria. Nature. 1961;192:733–7.
7. Sabchareon A, Burnouf T, Ouattara D, Attanath P, Bouharoun-Tayoun H, Chantavanich P, Foucault C, Chongsuphajaisiddhi T, Druilhe P. Parasitologic and clinical human response to immunoglobulin administration in falciparum malaria. Am J Trop Med Hyg. 1991;45(3):297–308.
8. Brown GV, Anders RF, Mitchell GF, Heywood PF. Target antigens of purified human immunoglobulins which inhibit growth of Plasmodium falciparum in vitro. Nature. 1982;297(5867):591–3.
9. Richards JS, Stanisic DI, Fowkes FJ, Tavul L, Dabod E, Thompson JK, Kumar S, Chitnis CE, Narum DL, Michon P, et al. Association between naturally acquired antibodies to erythrocyte-binding antigens of Plasmodium falciparum and protection from malaria and high-density parasitemia. Clin Infect Dis. 2010;51(8):e50–60.
10. Healer J, Thompson JK, Riglar DT, Wilson DW, Chiu YH, Miura K, Chen L, Hodder AN, Long CA, Hansen DS, et al. Vaccination with conserved regions of erythrocyte-binding antigens induces neutralizing antibodies against multiple strains of Plasmodium falciparum. PLoS One. 2013;8(9):e72504.
11. Langhorne J, Ndungu FM, Sponaas AM, Marsh K. Immunity to malaria: more questions than answers. Nat Immunol. 2008;9(7):725–32.
12. Kinyanjui SM, Conway DJ, Lanar DE, Marsh K. IgG antibody responses to Plasmodium falciparum merozoite antigens in Kenyan children have a short half-life. Malar J. 2007;6:82.
13. Kusi KA, Bosomprah S, Kyei-Baafour E, Dickson EK, Tornyigah B, Angov E, Dutta S, Dodoo D, Sedegah M, Koram KA. Seroprevalence of antibodies against Plasmodium falciparum Sporozoite antigens as predictive disease transmission markers in an area of Ghana with seasonal malaria transmission. PLoS One. 2016;11(11):e0167175.
14. Kusi KA, Bosomprah S, Dodoo D, Kyei-Baafour E, Dickson EK, Mensah D, Angov E, Dutta S, Sedegah M, Koram KA. Anti-sporozoite antibodies as alternative markers for malaria transmission intensity estimation. Malar J. 2014;13:103.
15. Jakobsen PH, Kurtzhals JA, Riley EM, Hviid L, Theander TG, Morris-Jones S, Jensen JB, Bayoumi RA, Ridley RG, Greenwood BM. Antibody responses to Rhoptry-associated Protein-1 (RAP-1) of Plasmodium falciparum parasites in humans from areas of different malaria endemicity. Parasite Immunol. 1997; 19(9):387–93.
16. Al-Yaman F, Genton B, Anders RF, Falk M, Triglia T, Lewis D, Hii J, Beck HP, Alpers MP. Relationship between humoral response to Plasmodium falciparum merozoite surface antigen-2 and malaria morbidity in a highly endemic area of Papua New Guinea. Am J Trop Med Hyg. 1994;51(5):593–602.
17. Soares IS, da Cunha MG, Silva MN, Souza JM, Del Portillo HA, Rodrigues MM. Longevity of naturally acquired antibody responses to the N- and C-terminal regions of Plasmodium vivax merozoite surface protein 1. Am J Trop Med Hyg. 1999;60(3):357–63.
18. Wipasa J, Suphavilai C, Okell LC, Cook J, Corran PH, Thaikla K, Liewsaree W, Riley EM, Hafalla JC. Long-lived antibody and B cell memory responses to the human malaria parasites, Plasmodium falciparum and Plasmodium vivax. PLoS Pathog. 2010;6(2):e1000770.
19. Fruh K, Doumbo O, Muller HM, Koita O, McBride J, Crisanti A, Toure Y, Bujard H. Human antibody response to the major merozoite surface antigen of Plasmodium falciparum is strain specific and short-lived. Infect Immun. 1991;59(4):1319–24.
20. Cavanagh DR, Elhassan IM, Roper C, Robinson VJ, Giha H, Holder AA, Hviid L, Theander TG, Arnot DE, McBride JS. A longitudinal study of type-specific antibody responses to Plasmodium falciparum merozoite surface protein-1 in an area of unstable malaria in Sudan. J Immunol. 1998;161(1):347–59.
21. Ahmed Ismail H, Tijani MK, Langer C, Reiling L, White MT, Beeson JG, Wahlgren M, Nwuba R, Persson KE. Subclass responses and their half-lives for antibodies against EBA175 and PfRh2 in naturally acquired immunity against Plasmodium falciparum malaria. Malar J. 2014;13:425.
22. Weaver R, Reiling L, Feng G, Drew DR, Mueller I, Siba PM, Tsuboi T, Richards JS, Fowkes FJ, Beeson JG. The association between naturally acquired IgG subclass specific antibodies to the PfRH5 invasion complex and protection from Plasmodium falciparum malaria. Sci Rep. 2016;6:33094.
23. Richards JS, Arumugam TU, Reiling L, Healer J, Hodder AN, Fowkes FJ, Cross N, Langer C, Takeo S, Uboldi AD, et al. Identification and prioritization of merozoite antigens as targets of protective human immunity to Plasmodium falciparum malaria for vaccine and biomarker development. J Immunol. 2013;191(2):795–809.
24. Perciani CT, Peixoto PS, Dias WO, Kubrusly FS, Tanizaki MM. Improved method to calculate the antibody avidity index. J Clin Lab Anal. 2007; 21(3):201–6.

25. Tutterrow YL, Salanti A, Avril M, Smith JD, Pagano IS, Ako S, Fogako J, Leke RG, Taylor DW. High avidity antibodies to full-length VAR2CSA correlate with absence of placental malaria. PLoS One. 2012;7(6):e40049.

26. Nogaro SI, Hafalla JC, Walther B, Remarque EJ, Tetteh KK, Conway DJ, Riley EM, Walther M. The breadth, but not the magnitude, of circulating memory B cell responses to *P. falciparum* increases with age/exposure in an area of low transmission. PLoS One. 2011;6(10):e25582.

27. Groux H, Gysin J. Opsonization as an effector mechanism in human protection against asexual blood stages of Plasmodium falciparum: functional role of IgG subclasses. Res Immunol. 1990;141(6):529–42.

28. Hill DL, Eriksson EM, Li Wai Suen CS, Chiu CY, Ryg-Cornejo V, Robinson LJ, Siba PM, Mueller I, Hansen DS, Schofield L. Opsonising antibodies to *P. falciparum* merozoites associated with immunity to clinical malaria. PLoS One. 2013;8(9):e74627.

29. Ferreira MU, Kimura EA, De Souza JM, Katzin AM. The isotype composition and avidity of naturally acquired anti-Plasmodium falciparum antibodies: differential patterns in clinically immune Africans and Amazonian patients. Am J Trop Med Hyg. 1996;55(3):315–23.

30. Leoratti FM, Durlacher RR, Lacerda MV, Alecrim MG, Ferreira AW, Sanchez MC, Moraes SL. Pattern of humoral immune response to Plasmodium falciparum blood stages in individuals presenting different clinical expressions of malaria. Malar J. 2008;7:186.

31. Reddy SB, Anders RF, Beeson JG, Farnert A, Kironde F, Berenzon SK, Wahlgren M, Linse S, Persson KE. High affinity antibodies to Plasmodium falciparum merozoite antigens are associated with protection from malaria. PLoS One. 2012;7(2):e32242.

32. Cadman ET, Abdallah AY, Voisine C, Sponaas AM, Corran P, Lamb T, Brown D, Ndungu F, Langhorne J. Alterations of splenic architecture in malaria are induced independently of toll-like receptors 2, 4, and 9 or MyD88 and may affect antibody affinity. Infect Immun. 2008;76(9):3924–31.

33. Anders RF. Multiple cross-reactivities amongst antigens of Plasmodium falciparum impair the development of protective immunity against malaria. Parasite Immunol. 1986;8(6):529–39.

34. Ssewanyana I, Arinaitwe E, Nankabirwa JI, Yeka A, Sullivan R, Kamya MR, Rosenthal PJ, Dorsey G, Mayanja-Kizza H, Drakeley C, et al. Avidity of anti-malarial antibodies inversely related to transmission intensity at three sites in Uganda. Malar J. 2017;16(1):67.

35. Dadzie SK, Aboagye-Antwi F, Kyerematen R, Ononye NC. Characterization of malaria transmission and insecticide susceptibility status of *Anopheles gambiae* Sensu Lato Gilles (Diptera: Culicidae) in Shai-Osudoku District of southern Ghana. Ghana: University of Ghana; 2015.

36. Donovan C, Siadat B, Frimpong J. Seasonal and socio-economic variations in clinical and self-reported malaria in Accra, Ghana: evidence from facility data and a community survey. Ghana Med J. 2012;46(2):85–94.

37. WHO. Giemsa Staining of Malaria Blood Films. In: malaria microscopy standard operating procedure - MM-SOP-07A; 2016.

38. W.H.O. Malaria parasite counting. In: Malaria Microscopy Standard Operating Procedure - MM-SOP-09; 2016.

39. Acquah FK, Obboh EK, Asare K, Boampong JN, Nuvor SV, Singh SK, Theisen M, Williamson KC, Amoah LE. Antibody responses to two new Lactococcus lactis-produced recombinant Pfs48/45 and Pfs230 proteins increase with age in malaria patients living in the central region of Ghana. Malar J. 2017; 16(1):306.

40. Dodoo D, Aikins A, Kusi KA, Lamptey H, Remarque E, Milligan P, Bosomprah S, Chilengi R, Osei YD, Akanmori BD, et al. Cohort study of the association of antibody levels to AMA1, MSP119, MSP3 and GLURP with protection from clinical malaria in Ghanaian children. Malar J. 2008;7:142.

41. Jepsen MP, Roser D, Christiansen M, Olesen Larsen S, Cavanagh DR, Dhanasarnsombut K, Bygbjerg I, Dodoo D, Remarque EJ, Dziegiel M, et al. Development and evaluation of a multiplex screening assay for Plasmodium falciparum exposure. J Immunol Methods. 2012;384(1–2):62–70.

42. Abagna HB, Acquah FK, Okonu R, Aryee NA, Theisen M, Amoah LE. Assessment of the quality and quantity of naturally induced antibody responses to EBA175RIII-V in Ghanaian children living in two communities with varying malaria transmission patterns. Malar J. 2018;17(1):14.

43. Wilson KM, Di Camillo C, Doughty L, Dax EM. Humoral immune response to primary rubella virus infection. Clin Vaccine Immunol. 2006;13(3):380–6.

44. Ibison F, Olotu A, Muema DM, Mwacharo J, Ohuma E, Kimani D, Marsh K, Bejon P, Ndungu FM. Lack of avidity maturation of merozoite antigen-specific antibodies with increasing exposure to Plasmodium falciparum amongst children and adults exposed to endemic malaria in Kenya. PLoS One. 2012;7(12):e52939.

45. Chiu CY, White MT, Healer J, Thompson JK, Siba PM, Mueller I, Cowman AF, Hansen DS. Different regions of Plasmodium falciparum erythrocyte-binding antigen 175 induce antibody responses to infection of varied efficacy. J Infect Dis. 2016;214(1):96–104.

46. Amoah LE, Opong A, Ayanful-Torgby R, Abankwa J, Acquah FK. Prevalence of G6PD deficiency and Plasmodium falciparum parasites in asymptomatic school children living in southern Ghana. Malar J. 2016;15(1):388.

47. Lo E, Zhou G, Oo W, Afrane Y, Githeko A, Yan G. Low parasitemia in submicroscopic infections significantly impacts malaria diagnostic sensitivity in the highlands of Western Kenya. PLoS One. 2015;10(3):e0121763.

48. Stanisic DI, Fowkes FJ, Koinari M, Javati S, Lin E, Kiniboro B, Richards JS, Robinson LJ, Schofield L, Kazura JW, et al. Acquisition of antibodies against Plasmodium falciparum merozoites and malaria immunity in young children and the influence of age, force of infection, and magnitude of response. Infect Immun. 2015;83(2):646–60.

49. Toure FS, Deloron P, Migot-Nabias F. Analysis of human antibodies to erythrocyte binding antigen 175 peptide 4 of Plasmodium falciparum. Clin Med Res. 2006;4(1):1–6.

50. Da Silveira LA, Dorta ML, Kimura EA, Katzin AM, Kawamoto F, Tanabe K, Ferreira MU. Allelic diversity and antibody recognition of Plasmodium falciparum merozoite surface protein 1 during hypoendemic malaria transmission in the Brazilian amazon region. Infect Immun. 1999;67(11): 5906–16.

51. Taylor RR, Smith DB, Robinson VJ, McBride JS, Riley EM. Human antibody response to Plasmodium falciparum merozoite surface protein 2 is serogroup specific and predominantly of the immunoglobulin G3 subclass. Infect Immun. 1995;63(11):4382–8.

52. Adjah J, Fiadzoe B, Ayanful-Torgby R, Amoah LE. Seasonal variations in Plasmodium falciparum genetic diversity and multiplicity of infection in asymptomatic children living in southern Ghana. BMC Infect Dis. 2018; 18(1):432.

53. Drakeley CJ, Corran PH, Coleman PG, Tongren JE, McDonald SL, Carneiro I, Malima R, Lusingu J, Manjurano A, Nkya WM, et al. Estimating medium- and long-term trends in malaria transmission by using serological markers of malaria exposure. Proc Natl Acad Sci U S A. 2005;102(14):5108–13.

54. Zoghi S, Mehrizi AA, Raeisi A, Haghdoost AA, Turki H, Safari R, Kahanali AA, Zakeri S. Survey for asymptomatic malaria cases in low transmission settings of Iran under elimination programme. Malar J. 2012;11:126.

8

Pharmacologically upregulated carcinoembryonic antigen-expression enhances the cytolytic activity of genetically-modified chimeric antigen receptor NK-92MI against colorectal cancer cells

Masayuki Shiozawa[1], Chuan-Hsin Chang[2,3], Yi-Chun Huang[3], Yi-Ching Chen[2,3], Mau-Shin Chi[2,4], Hsu-Chao Hao[5], Yue-Cune Chang[6], Satoru Takeda[1], Kwan-Hwa Chi[2,7,8*†] and Yu-Shan Wang[2,3,4*†]

Abstract

Background: The natural killer cell line, NK-92MI, is cytotoxic against various types of cancer. The aim of this study was to develop chimeric antigen receptor-modified (CAR) NK-92MI cells targeting carcinoembryonic antigen-expressing (CEA) tumours and increase killing efficacy by pharmacologically modifying CEA-expression.

Result: We generated anti-CEA-CAR NK-92MI cells by retroviral vector transduction. This genetically-modified cell line recognised and lysed high CEA-expressing tumour cell lines (LS174T) at $47.54 \pm 12.60\%$ and moderate CEA-expressing tumour cell lines (WiDr) at $31.14 \pm 16.92\%$ at a 5:1 effector: target (E/T) ratio. The cell line did not lyse low CEA-expressing tumour cells (HCT116) as they did their parental cells (NK-92MI cells). The histone deacetylase-inhibitor (HDAC) sodium butyrate (NaB) and the methylation-inhibitor 5-azacytidine (5-AZA), as epigenetic modifiers, induced CEA-expression in HCT116 and WiDr cells. Although the IC_{50} of 5 fluorouracil (5-FU) increased, both cell lines showed collateral sensitivity to anti-CEA-CAR NK-92MI cells. The cytolytic function of anti-CEA-CAR NK-92MI cells was increased from $22.99 \pm 2.04\%$ of lysis background to $69.20 \pm 11.92\%$ after NaB treatment, and $69.70 \pm 9.93\%$ after 5-AZA treatment, at a 10:1 E/T ratio in HCT116 cells. The WiDr cells showed similar trend, from $22.99 \pm 4.01\%$ of lysis background to $70.69 \pm 10.19\%$ after NaB treatment, and $59.44 \pm 10.92\%$ after 5-AZA treatment, at a 10:1 E/T ratio.

Conclusions: This data indicates that the effector-ability of anti-CEA-CAR NK-92MI increased in a CEA-dependent manner. The combination of epigenetic-modifiers like HDAC-inhibitors, methylation-inhibitors, and adoptive-transfer of ex vivo-expanded allogeneic-NK cells may be clinically applicable to patients with in 5-FU resistant condition.

Keywords: Natural killer cell, NK-92MI, Chimeric antigen receptor (CAR), Carcinoembryonic antigen (CEA), Cellular immunotherapy

* Correspondence: m006565@ms.skh.org.tw; yusam.wang@gmail.com
†Kwan-Hwa Chi and Yu-Shan Wang contributed equally to this work.
[2]Department of Radiation Therapy and Oncology, Shin Kong Wu Ho-Su Memorial Hospital, No.95, Wenchang Road, Shilin District, Taipei, Taiwan
Full list of author information is available at the end of the article

Background

Human natural killer cells (NK) play an important role in innate immune defence against viral infections and malignant cells [1, 2]. NK cells do not require antigen representation for target recognition. They show tumour cytotoxicity in a major histocompatibility complex-unrestricted (MHC-unrestricted) manner [1, 2]. Cancers induce NK cell dysfunction, resulting in reduced proliferation of NK cells, decreased infiltration of tumours, and/or defective cytokine production. Cancer cells also evade NK cell attack via lowering expressions of activating receptors and intracellular signalling molecules, and/or overexpression of inhibitory receptors [3].

The adoptive transfer of NK cells has been used widely in clinical trials [4]. Sources of NK cells used in adoptive transfer include primary autologous (patients) [5], allogeneic (healthy donor) [6], umbilical cord blood [7], induced pluripotent stem cells (iPSC) [8], and NK cell lines [9]. NK-92 cells have undergone extensive preclinical development [10] and have completed phase I trials in cancer patients [9]. Unlike primary NK cells, NK-92 cells express almost no inhibitory killer cell immunoglobulin-like receptors (KIRs) [11]. NK-92MI is an interleukin-2-independent (IL-2-independent) cell line derived from NK-92 by transfection of human IL-2 cDNA. It has the same characteristics as activated-NK cells and its parental NK-92 cells [12]. It has been shown that both NK-92 and NK-92MI cells are highly cytotoxic to human melanoma cells both in vitro and in vivo [13, 14]. Genetically-modified effector cells with a chimeric antigen receptor (CAR) were chosen with the intention of enhancing their reactivity against antigen-expressing tumour cells [15–17]. However, chimeric antigen receptor T-cell (CAR-T) treatments are associated with adverse events, mostly commonly eliciting Cytokine Release Syndrome (CRS), a systemic inflammatory response that can lead to widespread organ dysfunction and death [18, 19]. NK cell lines may be alternative cytotoxic effectors for CAR-driven tumour cell-specific cytolysis [20, 21]. The limited life span of NK cells may make them safer than T cells [15]. In recent years several CAR-modified NK-92 and NK-92MI cells have been developed. They were highly cytotoxic both in vitro and in vivo [22–27]. However, developments in anti-CEA-CAR-modified NK-92 and NK-92MI cells have not been well-characterized. CEA is expressed in various cancers and has been used in CEA-CAR-T therapy [28]. CEA-overexpression may contribute to human cancer progression by inhibiting cell-differentiation, apoptosis, and anoikis [29, 30]. CEA-expression level per cell may be a suitable biomarker for predicting tumour response to chemotherapy in colorectal cancer [32]. We proposed that CEA-targeted adoptive immunotherapy is a good example of collateral sensitivity to 5-FU-resistant CEA-expression in tumours.

In this study, we successfully transduced NK-92MI cells with an anti-CEA-specific single-chain variable antibody fragment (scFv). The anti-CEA-CAR-modified NK-92MI specifically recognized and efficiently eradicated CEA-expressing tumour cells. Furthermore, by pharmacologically-inducing CEA-upregulation, the cytotoxicity of these modified-NK cells was enhanced. These observations show the promise for anti-CEA-CAR-modified NK-92MI cells in clinical therapy for terminal-stage colorectal cancer treatment.

Methods
Cell and culture media

NK-92MI cells were incubated in an alpha modification of Eagle's Minimum Essential Medium (α-MEM) from Gibco Laboratories (Gaithersburg, MD, USA) supplemented with 1.5 g L^{-1} sodium bicarbonate, 0.2 mM inositol, 0.02 mM folic acid, 0.01 mM 2-mercaptoethanol, 12.5% foetal bovine serum (FBS) (Invitrogen, Grand Island, NY, USA), and 12.5% horse serum (Sigma-Aldrich Corp., St. Louis, MO, USA). The human colorectal carcinoma cell lines used in this study were HCT116 (ATCC CCL-247), WiDr (ATCC CCL-218), and LS174T (ATCC CL-188). They were obtained from the Bioresource Collection and Research Center, Taiwan (BCRC). The HCT116 cells were cultured in McCoy's 5A medium (Gibco Laboratories) containing 1.5 g L^{-1} sodium bicarbonate, 4.5 g L^{-1} glucose, 10 mM HEPES, 1.0 mM sodium pyruvate (90%), and 10% FBS (Invitrogen, Grand Island, NY). The WiDr- and LS174T cells were maintained in α-MEM (Gibco Laboratories) supplemented with 1.5 g L^{-1} sodium bicarbonate and 10% FBS. K562 cells were grown in Iscove's Modified Dulbecco's Medium (Invitrogen, Grand Island, NY) containing 1.5 g L^{-1} sodium bicarbonate and 10% FBS. All cells were grown in a humidified incubator at 37 °C under a 5% CO_2 atmosphere.

Generation of anti-CEA-CAR NK-92MI cells

It has been shown that mouse monoclonal antibody (mAb) T84.66 scFv binds to CEA with high specificity and affinity [33]. The coding domain sequences for the variable regions of the mAb T84.66 heavy (V_H) and light (V_L) chains [34] were amplified separately and assembled with a linker using an overlapping polymerase chain reaction (PCR). The cDNA encoding of CEA-specific scFv of mAb T84.66 was isolated by PCR using gene-specific primers. The V_L region was amplified by PCR using the primer T84.66-V_L- (forward: 5'-GGGG CCCAGCCGGCCTCAGAGATGGAGACAGACACAC-3'; reverse: 5'-CGCCAGATCCGGGCTTGCCGGATCCAGAG GTGGAGCCTTTTATTTCCAGCTTGGTCC-3') and the V_H region was amplified by using the primer T84.66-V_H (forward: 5'-CGGCAAGCCCGGATCTGGCGAGGGATCCACC AAGGGCGAGGTTCAGCTGCAGCAGT-3'; reverse:

5'-CCGCTCGAGCGGTGAGGAGACGGTGACTGAG GTTC). The construct was generated by cloning the sequences encoding anti-CEA scFv fragment and the hinge region of CD8α (amino acids 105–165) into the plasmid pcDNA3.1/V5-HIS©TOPO®TA vector (Invitrogen, Groningen, Netherlands). The CD3ζ chain (amino acids of the transmembrane and intracellular domains) was cloned into the plasmid GEM®-T vector (Promega, Madison, WI, USA). The complete CAR sequence was derived from the resulting pcDNA3.1-scFv (anti-CEA)-CD8α-CD3ζ construct and cloned into the SfiI- and ClaI restriction sites of a modified retroviral pLNCX vector kindly provided by S. R. Roffler, Institute of Biomedical Sciences (Academia Sinica, Taipei, Taiwan). The pLNCX contained a leader sequence and an HA tag. It was sequenced for identification and yielded pLNCX-scFv (anti-CEA antibody)-CD8α-CD3ζ. Both the recombinant retroviral vector pLNCX-scFv (anti-CEA antibody)-CD8α-CD3ζ and the pVSV-G plasmid (envelope plasmid) (Clontech Laboratories, Inc., Mountain View, CA, USA) were co-transfected into packaging cell line 293 (Clontech Laboratories) with lipofectamine 2000 (Invitrogen, Carlsbad, CA, USA). Retroviral supernatants were generated from the GP2–293 cell line in DMEM supplemented with 10% FBS. After a 48 h incubation at 37 °C, the supernatants were harvested and then filtered through a 0.45-μm low-protein-binding filter (Minisart NML; Sartorius Lab Instruments GmbH, Göttingen, Germany). They were then used to transduce NK-92MI cells for 24 h. The transduced NK-92MI cells were further screened by neomycin sulphate-G418 (500 μg mL^{-1}).

Cell treatments

HCT116 and WiDr human colorectal cancer cells were seeded in 6-cm tissue culture dishes at a density of 2.5×10^5 cells/ml under normal culture condition for 24 h. The cells were subjected to increasing concentrations of either the HDAC-inhibitor, sodium butyrate (NaB) (0.1-1 mM) or the DNA methylation inhibitor 5-azacytidine (5-AZA) (1 μM) for 10 h and 72 h, respectively. A 1 μM 5-FU treatment for 24 h was established as positive control. Total CEA protein was detected by western blot and surface CEA-expression was detected by flow cytometry. Non-cytotoxic concentration-levels which induced higher CEA-expression levels were selected for NaB and 5-AZA, at 0.1 mM and 1 μM, respectively. These induced cultures were then used to determine the cytotoxicity of anti-CEA-CAR NK-92MI cells.

Western blot

HCT116 and WiDr cells were treated with NaB (0.1 mM) for 10 h or 5-AZA (1 μM) for 72 h. These groups, along with an untreated control group, were lysed in a radioimmunoprecipitation assay (RIPA) buffer

(Sigma-Aldrich Corp., St. Louis, MO, USA) containing EDTA-free Protease-Inhibitor Cocktail Tablets and Phosphatase-Inhibitor Cocktail Tablets (Roche Diagnostics, Monza, Italy). Total protein concentrations in the lysates was measured using a bicinchoninic acid protein concentration assay (Pierce Biotechnology, Rockford, IL, USA). Total protein (20 μg) was electrophoresed on 10% polyacrylamide gels, transferred onto Immobilon-P polyvinylidene fluoride membranes (EMD Millipore, Bedford, MA, USA), and blocked with Tris-buffered saline (TBS)-0.05% Tween 20 containing 5% non-fat milk at room temperature (25 °C) for 1 h. Filters were probed with anti-human CEA (Santa Cruz Biotechnology, Dallas, TX, USA) or anti-β-actin antibodies (Sigma-Aldrich Corp., St. Louis, MO, USA) at 4 °C in the same buffer overnight. After wash, the filter was probed with horseradish peroxidase-conjugated secondary antibodies (Jackson ImmunoResearch Laboratories, West Grove, PA, USA) at room temperature (25 °C) in the same buffer for 1 h. Blots were developed using a chemiluminescent detection system (ECL; GE Life Science, Buckinghamshire, UK). Proteins were visualised using enhanced chemiluminescence detection. This process was performed in triplicate, and quantitation of immunoblots was performed using Adobe Photoshop 7.0.

Binding assay

CEA-binding activity was examined by western blotting. In brief, either anti-CEA-CAR NK-92MI or NK-92MI cells were incubated with recombinant human CEA protein (rCEA) (0.8 μg) for 4 h. The cells were washed in PBS then lysed with 1 mL ice-cold RIPA (Boston Bioproducts, Worcester, MA, USA) containing protease inhibitors (Roche Applied Science, Vilvoorde, Belgium). The ability of the chimeric anti-CEA receptors on the NK cells to bind with human rCEA was determined by immunoblotting. The membrane was hybridised with mouse anti-human CEA antibody supernatant (Santa Cruz Biotechnology) and horseradish peroxidase-conjugated secondary antibodies (Jackson ImmunoResearch Laboratories). Proteins were visualised using enhanced chemiluminescence detection. This process was performed in triplicate, and quantitation of immunoblots was performed using Adobe Photoshop 7.0.

Phenotype analysis of cell surface CEA-CAR expression of NK-92MI cells

Flow cytometer was used to analyse the cell surface expression of human influenza hemagglutinin (HA)-tagged CEA-CAR in transduced anti-CEA-CAR NK-92MI cells. To evaluate the cell surface expression of HA-tagged CEA-CAR, transduced anti-CEA-CAR NK-92MI cells were labelled with anti-HA antibody (Abcam, Cambridge, UK) or IgG isotype antibody as control. For surface CEA staining, cancer cells were harvested and stained with mouse anti-human CEA-FITC (BD Biosciences, San Jose, CA, USA). Cells were analysed with a FACSCalibur flow cytometer (Becton Dickinson, Franklin Lakes, NJ, USA). The fluorescence intensities of at least 10^5 cells were recorded and analysed using CellQuest Pro software (Becton Dickinson). Geometric mean was established as the mean fluorescence intensity (MFI).

Phenotype analysis of NK cell surface marker expression of NK-92MI cells

The phenotypes of NK cell surface marker expression on transduced anti-CEA-CAR NK-92MI and parental NK-92MI cells were determined using a FACSCalibur flow cytometer (Becton Dickinson). The cells were stained with FITC-labelled NKG2D, CD45, and CD56 antibodies (BioLegend, San Diego, CA, USA). The fluorescence intensities of $\geq 10^5$ cells were recorded and analysed with CellQuest Pro software (Becton Dickinson). Geometric mean was established as the MFI.

Cytotoxicity assay

The cytotoxic effects of anti-CEA-CAR NK-92MI cells were investigated with a CytoTox96® Non-Radioactive Cytotoxicity Assay (Promega, Madison, WI, USA) according to the manufacturer's protocols. This technique is the colorimetric alternative to the standard 4-h ^{51}Cr release assay. Briefly, target cells were co-cultured with anti-CEA-CAR NK-92MI cells at various effector/target ratios (E/T) including 10:1, 5:1, 1:1, or 0.5:1. They were planted into a round-bottom 96-well culture plate. Each well contained a final volume of 100 μL. The contents were mixed gently and centrifuged at 250×g for 5 min and then incubated at 37 °C under a 5% CO_2 atmosphere for 24 h. Fifty microlitres of the supernatant in each well was then transferred to the corresponding well of a flat-bottom 96-well enzymatic assay plate. Fifty microlitres of CytoTox96® Reagent was added to each well and the plate was incubated at room temperature (25 °C) and protected from light for 30 min. Fifty microlitres of Stop Solution was then added to each well and the absorbances were measured at $\lambda = 490$ nm. The percentage of cytotoxicity for each E/T was calculated as (experimental culture medium background) - (effector cell spontaneous release - culture medium background) - (target spontaneous release - culture medium background) / (target maximum release - volume correction control - target spontaneous release - culture medium background) × 100.

Cell proliferation assay

Cell viability was determined by a CellTiter96 aqueous one-solution cell proliferation assay according to the manufacturer's instructions (Promega, Madison, WI, USA).

In brief, 5×10^3 cells were seeded into a flat-bottom 96-well enzymatic assay plate for 1 day before exposure to the various compounds. HCT116 and WiDr cells were treated with NaB (0.1 mM) for 10 h or 5-AZA (1 μM) for 72 h. The treated groups were used to determine the effect of CEA-overexpression in correlation with 5-FU resistance. Cells were simultaneously co-treated with either NaB (0.1 mM) or 5-AZA (1 μM) at various 5-FU concentrations (0 μM, 2.4 μM, 4.8 μM, 9.6 μM, 19.2 μM, and 38.4 μM) for 72 h. The IC_{50} values were defined as 50% cell growth inhibitory concentrations of the 5-FU treatment groups and MTS assay was performed to determine IC_{50}. After 72 h, 20 μL CellTiter96 aqueous one-solution was added to each well. After 4 h, the UV-absorbance of each solution was measured at $\lambda = 492$ nm. This process was performed in triplicate.

Animal study

Nine-week-old female SCID mice were subcutaneously injected with 2×10^6 WiDr cells in their right-side dorsa. When the tumours reached a volume range of 100-200 mm^3, the mice were segregated into five groups (control, NaB, NK-92MI, anti-CEA-CAR NK-92MI, and anti-CEA-CAR NK-92MI + NaB). NaB 200 mg/kg was injected intraperitoneally 5 days per week and 10^7 anti-CEA-CAR NK-92MI cells were injected intraperitoneally twice per week for 2 cycles. Tumour sizes were measured weekly. Mice were sacrificed either after 15 days of treatment or when the tumour reached the maximum allowed volume of 1,000mm^3. Tumours were stored at – 80 °C for western blot analysis.

Statistical analysis

All experiments were performed at a minimum of 3 times and the data were expressed as means ± standard error of the mean (SEM). Statistical significance was determined using Student's t test. All data was processed with Prism v. 5.0 (GraphPad Software, San Diego, CA, USA). A multiple linear regression analysis was used to compare the differences among the three groups after adjusting for the effects of cell generation, a potential confounding variable. To take into the repeated measurements' dependence, multiple linear regression by GEE method was used to further compare the difference of tumour volumes between the various control groups (control, NaB, and NK-92MI) and the CAR-NK cell therapies group (anti-CEA-CAR NK-92MI and anti-CEA-CAR NK-92MI + NaB). Statistical significance was defined as $P < 0.05$.

Results

Expression of anti-CEA-CAR in NK-92MI cells

To construct the anti-CEA specific CAR, the cDNAs of variable heavy-chain (V_H) and light-chain (V_L) domains of the humanised-monoclonal-anti-CEA antibody, the human influenza hemagglutinin (HA)-tag sequence, the CD8α hinge region, and the transmembrane and intracellular domains of CD3ζ were assembled stepwise into a pGEM-1 plasmid (Promega, Madison, WI, USA). The cDNAs were used to produce a scFv of the anti-CEA antibody. The complete CAR sequence was derived from the pcDNA3.1–1-anti-CEA scFv-CD8α-CD3ζ construct and cloned into pLNCX, a modified retroviral expression vector, to yield the pLNCX-based pL-anti-CEA scFv-CD8α-CD3ζ construct (Fig. 1a). NK-92MI cells were transduced with the anti-CEA scFv-CD8α-CD3ζ specific construct to generate anti-CEA-CAR NK-92MI cells and were repeatedly selected with G418 (500 μg mL^{-1}). The cell surface expression of the anti-CEA-CAR in the transduced NK-92MI cells was investigated by staining with human influenza hemagglutinin (HA) tag-specific antibody recognising the HA-tag epitope incorporated into

the extracellular domain of the chimeric receptor (Fig. 1b). The binding ability of the anti-CEA chimeric antigen receptor to recombinant human CEA protein was verified by western blotting. Transduced anti-CEA-CAR NK-92MI cells were cultured with 0.8 μg recombinant human CEA (rCEA) for 4 h. Lysate of the transduced NK-92MI cells cultured with rCEA was collected and analysed by immunoblotting (Fig. 1c, lane 3). Specificity was verified in parallel using a commercially available rCEA (Fig. 1c, lane 1).

Phenotype of the anti-CEA-CAR NK-92MI cells

We investigated whether expression of the chimeric scFv receptor affected the NK-92MI phenotype. Flow cytometry was used to compare adhesion molecules (CD45 and CD56) and activation receptors (NKG2D) expressed by the anti-CEA-CAR NK-92MI cells with those of the parental NK-92MI. Separate experiments revealed no

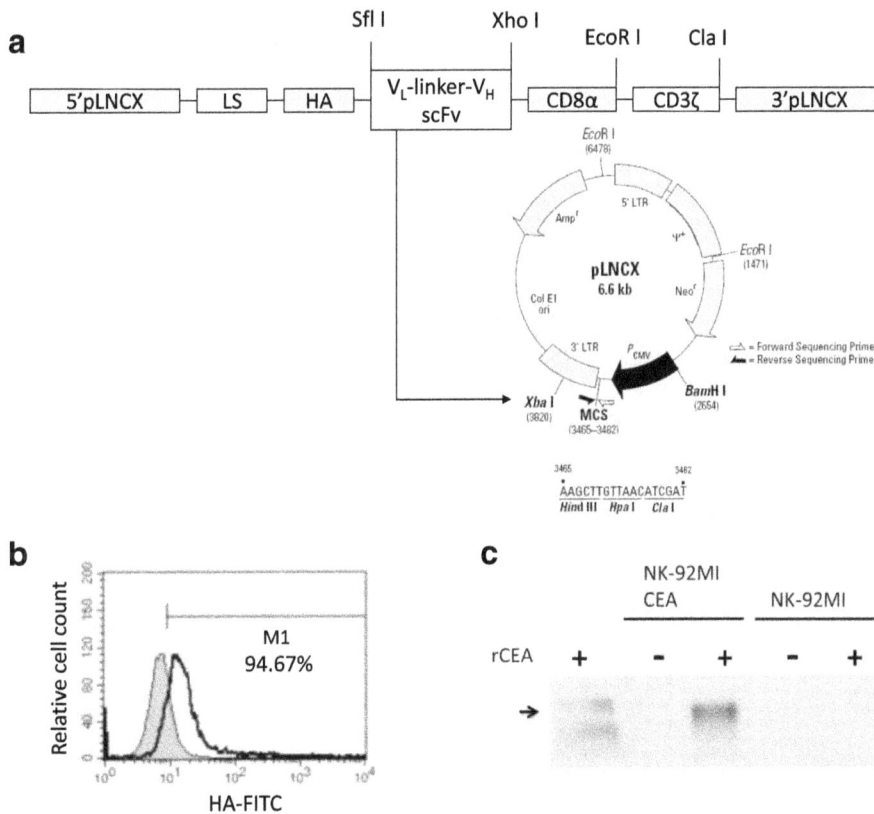

Fig. 1 Genetic modification of NK-92MI cells with anti-CEA-CD8α-CD3ζ chimeric receptor. **a** Schematic image of the chimeric receptor anti-CEA-CD8α-CD3ζ. The chimeric receptor consisted of the V$_L$ and V$_H$ regions of the anti-CEA mAb joined to a CD8α and fused to the transmembrane and intracellular regions of human TCR-CD3ζ. Map of destination vector pLNCX wherein the cDNA for the fusion protein anti-CEA-CD8α-CD3ζ was cloned into SfiI and ClaI restriction enzyme sites of modified retroviral pLNCX vector containing leader sequence and HA tag and sequenced for identification. The product was pLNCX- anti-CEA scFv-CD8α-CD3ζ. Transfected cells expressing the transgene of interest were selected on cytocidal concentrations of neomycin sulphate (G418). **b** Surface expression of chimeric anti-CEA scFv-CD8α-CD3ζ. NK-92MI cells were analysed following staining with FITC-labelled HA tag Ab. Briefly, CAR expression was determined by flow cytometry with HA-tagged- and recognised anti-CEA chimeric receptor (green open area). Parental NK-92MI cells served as control (blue filled area). **c** Ability of anti-CEA chimeric receptor to recognise recombinant human CEA was determined by immunoblotting. Lysates of NK-92MI (lane 4) and transduced anti-CEA NK-92MI cells (lane 2) were separated by SDS-PAGE. Transduced anti-CEA NK-92MI or parental NK-92MI co-cultured with rCEA (lanes 3 and 5) were analysed by immunoblot analysis

differences between the NK-92MI cells and the anti-CEA-CAR NK-92MI cells in terms of the expression levels of NK-92MI cell markers CD45, CD56, and NKG2D (Fig. 2). This data indicates that transduction of NK-92MI cells with scFv chimeric receptor did not phenotypically alter the expression levels of several important NK-92MI cell-associated markers.

Detection of CEA-expression levels in various cancer cells lines

To assess the surface CEA-expression on various human colorectal cancer cell lines (HCT116, WiDr, and LS174T), intact cells were stained with a human CEA-specific antibody followed by flow cytometry. LS174T was shown to have highest CEA-expression levels, whereas expression levels were moderate in WiDr, and low in HCT116 (Fig. 3a). Relative differences in total CEA protein levels were confirmed by immunoblotting analysis. Human CEA-expressed protein was detectable in both WiDr and LS174T cells (Fig. 3b). Surface CEA-expression and CEA-secretion levels were found to have positive correlation (Fig. 3a). In contrast, CEA protein was almost undetectable in HCT116 cancer cells.

Enhanced cytotoxicity of anti-CEA-CAR NK-92MI is correlated to surface CEA-expression on target cells

NK-92 cell lines are highly cytotoxic against various malignant cells such as those found in leukaemia, lymphoma, and myeloma [35]. To determine whether genetic manipulation altered intrinsic NK cytotoxicity, the cell-killing activities of anti-CEA scFv-CD8α-CD3ζ NK-92MI and parental NK-92MI cells against different tumour cell lines were compared. The cytotoxicity of the transduced anti-CEA-CAR NK-92MI cells against the NK cell-sensitive target cell line K562 did not significantly differ from that of parental NK-92MI (Fig. 4a).

This result shows that the process of transduction and gene modification does not diminish the native-cytotoxicity of parental NK-92MI cells. Anti-CEA-CAR NK-92MI cells failed to lyse low CEA-expressing HCT116 cells even at a high E/T ratio (specific lysis $23.71 \pm 5.23\%$ at $E/T = 10{:}1$) (Fig. 4b). Moderate CEA-expressing WiDr cells were found to sustain high cytotoxicity (specific lysis $57.51 \pm 4.95\%$ at $E/T = 10{:}1$; $31.14 \pm 16.92\%$ at $E/T = 5{:}1$). High CEA-expressing LS174T cells sustained even greater cytotoxicity (specific lysis $64.68 \pm 9.01\%$ at $E/T = 10{:}1$; $47.54 \pm 12.60\%$ at $E/T = 5{:}1$) (Fig. 4c and d). Even with E/T ratio decreased to 1:1, anti-CEA-CAR NK-92MI cells specifically and efficiently lysed LS174T cells (specific lysis $27.34 \pm 7.68\%$ at E/T 1:1), evidently due to high CEA-expression (Fig. 4d). Specific lysis at these conditions, however, was significantly reduced for moderate CEA-expressing WiDr cells (specific lysis $11.13 \pm 1.378\%$ at $E/T = 1{:}1$) (Fig. 4c). In contrast, all test groups were slightly sensitive, or insensitive altogether, to parental NK-92MI. These results suggest that after gene-modification, NK-92MI gain the capability to recognize and kill CEA-expressing cancer cells in a CEA-dependent manner.

NaB and 5-AZA induced CEA-expression in human colorectal cancer cells

To further confirm whether CEA-specific anti-CEA-CAR NK-92MI cell cytotoxicity was CEA-dependent, we pharmacologically-induced CEA-expression in either low-CEA-expressing HCT116 cells or moderate-CEA-expressing WiDr cells. HCT116 and WiDr cell lines were independently treated with NaB (0.1 mM) for 10 h or 5-AZA (1 μM) for 72 h. Both HCT116 groups treated either with NaB or separately treated with 5-AZA showed significantly increased CEA-secretion (Fig. 5b), and surface CEA-expression (Fig. 5d). Both WiDr groups treated either with NaB or separately treated with 5-AZA showed

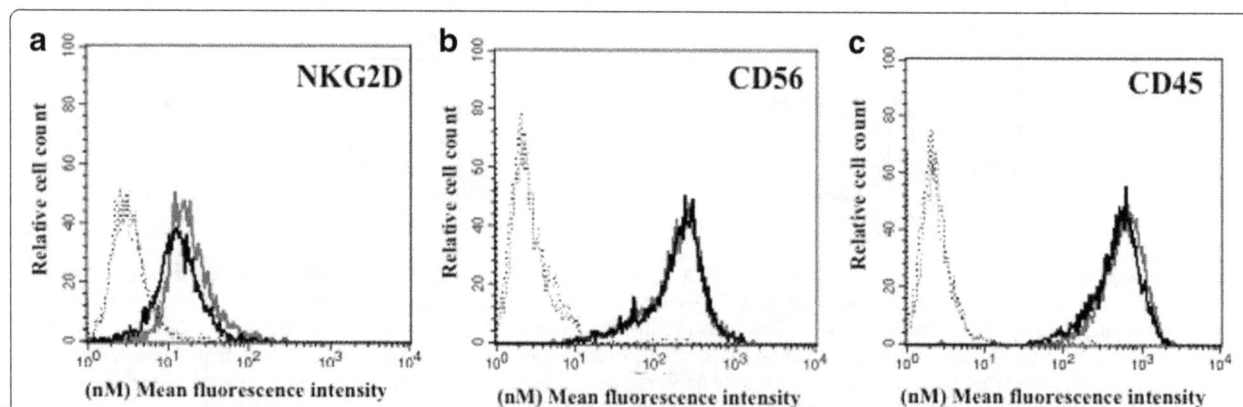

Fig. 2 Phenotypic characterization of genetically-modified NK-92MI cells. Surface expression levels of various NK-92MI activation receptors were measured by flow cytometry. There was no significant difference between anti-CEA-CAR NK-92MI and parental NK-92MI cells in terms of (**a**) NKG2D, (**b**) CD56, and (**c**) CD45. Black line represents transfected anti-CEA-CAR NK-92MI cells. Grey line represents non-transfected NK-92MI cells. Dotted lines represent cells stained with isotype control

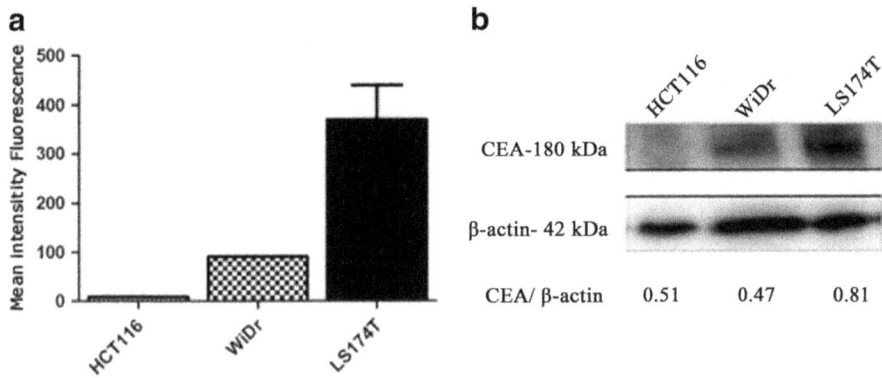

Fig. 3 CEA-expression on colorectal carcinoma cell lines HCT116, WiDr, and LS174T. **a** Surface CEA-expression levels in colorectal carcinoma cell lines HCT116, WiDr, and LS174T were monitored by flow cytometry. **b** Determination of CEA protein expression by immunoblotting analysis in colorectal carcinoma cell lines

increased CEA-secretion (Fig. 5a), and surface CEA-expression (Fig. 5c).

CEA-expression induced by NaB and 5-AZA enhanced cytotoxicity mediated by anti-CEA-CAR NK-92MI cells

Previously, experiments had shown that anti-CEA-CAR NK-92MI cytotoxicity was CEA-dependent. Follow-up experiments then showed that nontoxic doses of NaB and 5-AZA induced total CEA-expression in both HCT116 and WiDr colorectal cancer cells (Fig. 5). We hoped to further investigate the effects of anti-CEA-CAR NK-92MI cytotoxicity on pharmacologically-induced CEA-expression colorectal cancer cells. HCT116 cell line, with its inherent low CEA-expression, was found that have significantly increased CEA-expression after treatment with NaB (0.1 mM) for 10 h or 5-AZA (1μM) for 72 h. These groups were then co-cultured with anti-CEA-CAR NK-92MI cells. Relative to the parental HCT116 treated by anti-CEA-CAR NK-92MI (specific lysis $22.99 \pm 2.04\%$ at $E/T = 10:1$; $10.71 \pm 1.75\%$ at $E/T = 5:1$) as control, we found pharmacologically-induced groups to have significantly-increased cell death levels.

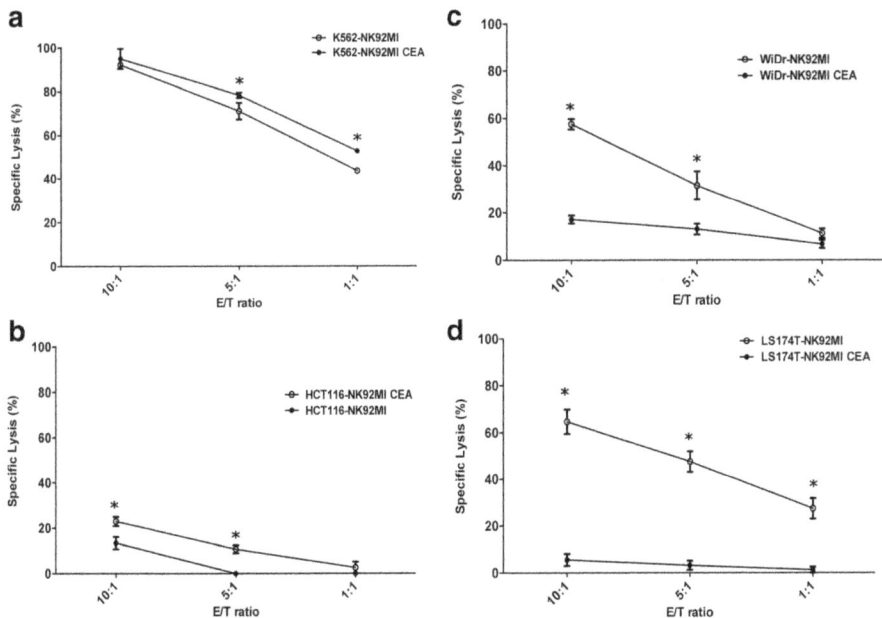

Fig. 4 Anti-CEA-CAR NK-92MI recognise and kill CEA-expressing cells. Cytotoxicity of parental NK-92MI (●) or anti-CEA-CAR NK-92MI (○) against (**a**) human K562 erythroleukemia cells, (**b**) low-CEA-expressing HCT116 cells, (**c**) mildly CEA-expressing WiDr cells, and (**d**) highly CEA-expressing LS174T cells. Cells were incubated either with parental or anti-CEA-CAR NK-92MI at various effector/target (E/T) ratios for 4 h. Tumour lysis was determined from the release of LDH and measured by CytoTox96® non-radioactive cytotoxicity assay. Representative data from experiments conducted independently in triplicate are shown. *$P < 0.05$

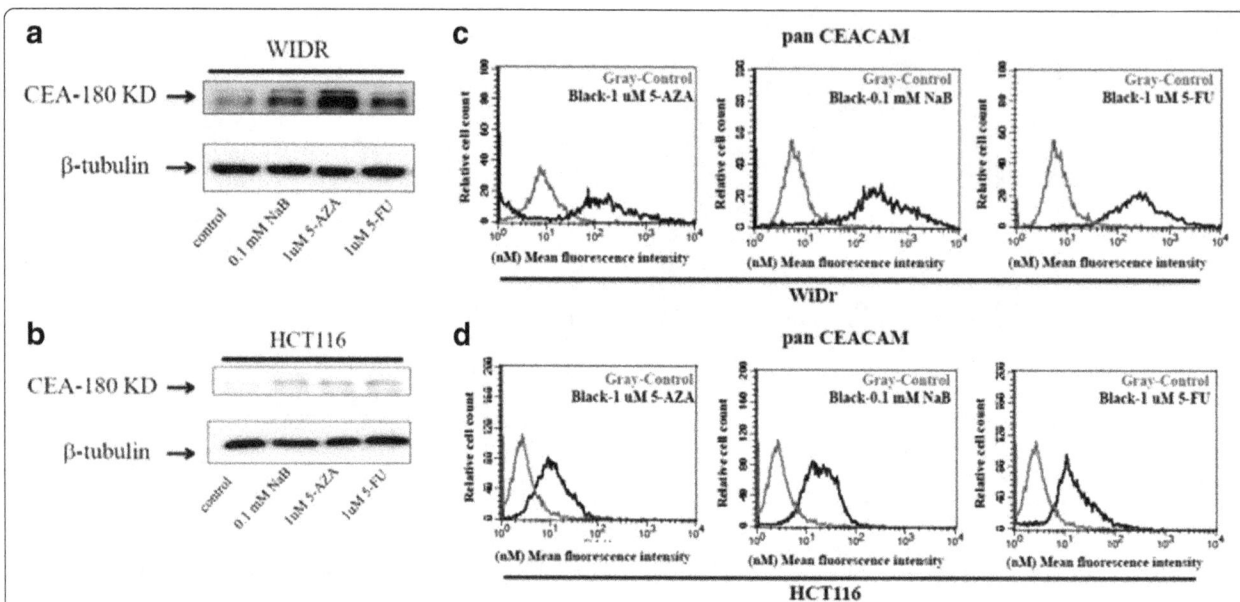

Fig. 5 Quantification of surface and total CEA-expression in HCT116 and WiDr colorectal cancer cells after NaB and 5-AZA treatments. Low-CEA-expressing HCT116 cells and moderate-CEA-expressing colorectal cancer cells were treated with NaB (0.1 mM) for 10 h and 5-AZA (1 µM) for 72 h. Treatment with 5-FU (1 µM) for 24 h was used as positive control. Treatments with either NaB or 5-AZA induced the expressions of total CEA protein (**a** and **b**) and surface CEA (**c** and **d**) in both HCT116 and WiDr cells

NaB-induced HCT116 groups had specific lysis of 69.20 ± 11.92% at E/T = 10:1 and 29.08 ± 6.81% at E/T = 5:1. The 5-AZA-induced groups had specific lysis of 69.70 ± 9.93% at E/T = 10:1 and 43.52 ± 2.67% at E/T = 5:1 (Fig. 6a and b). The WiDr cell line showed similar effects. NaB-induced

WiDr group had specific lysis of 70.69 ± 10.19% at E/T = 10:1 and 39.56 ± 8.54% at E/T = 5:1. The 5-AZA-induced groups had specific lysis of 59.44 ± 10.92% at E/T = 10:1 and 42.37 ± 8.73% at E/T = 5:1 (Fig. 7a and b). On the other hand, there were no significant differences between the

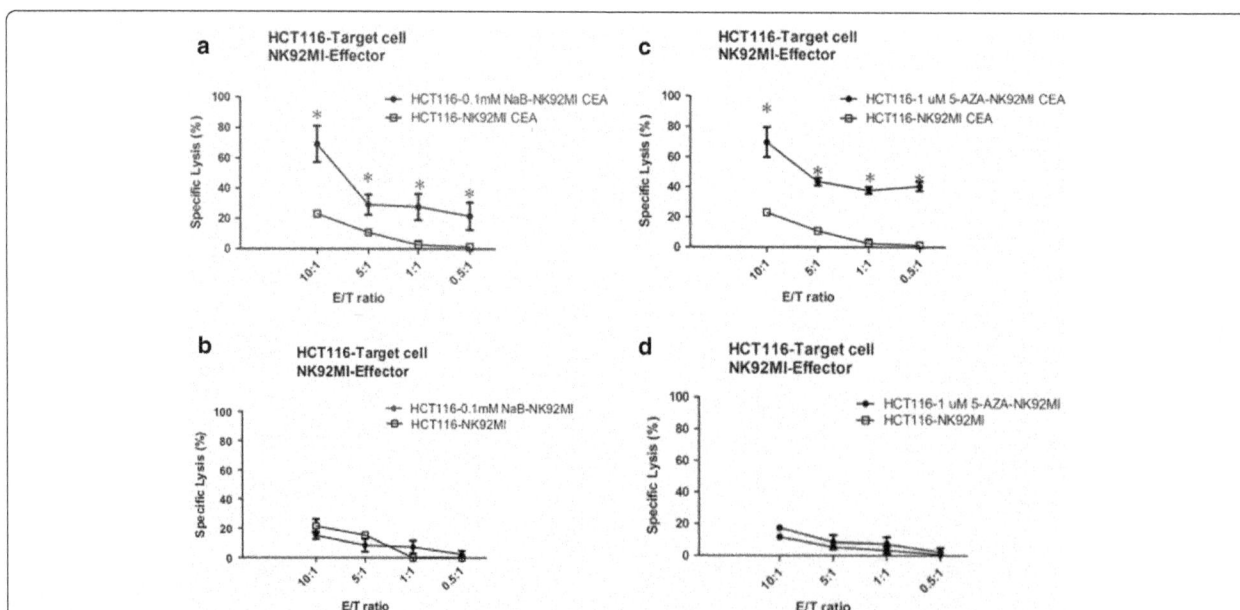

Fig. 6 Increased specific lysis of HCT116 colorectal cancer cells by anti-CEA-CAR NK-92MI after treatments with NaB and 5-AZA. Retrovirally transduced anti-CEA-CAR NK-92MI were co-cultivated with HCT116 cells. Either NaB (0.1 mM) (**a**) or 5-AZA (1 µM) (**c**) treatment significantly enhanced the antigen-specific killing power of anti-CEA-CAR NK-92MI in HCT116 cells. HCT116 cells were also co-cultured with parental NK-92MI cells after treatment with either NaB (0.1 mM) for 10 h (**b**) or (1 µM) for 72 h (**d**). Representative data from experiments conducted independently in triplicate are shown. *$P < 0.05$

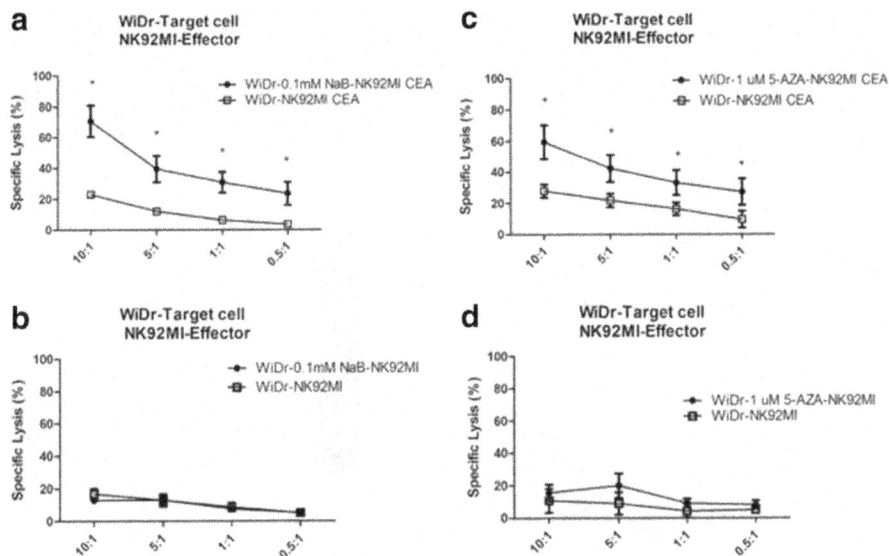

Fig. 7 Increased specific lysis of WiDr colorectal cancer cells by anti-CEA CAR NK-92MI after NaB and 5-AZA treatments. Retrovirally transduced anti-CEA CAR NK-92MI cells were co-cultivated with WiDr cells. Either NaB (0.1 mM) (**a**) or 5-AZA (1 μM) (**c**) treatment significantly enhanced the antigen-specific killing power of anti-CEA CAR NK-92MI in WiDr cells. WiDr cells were also co-cultured with parental NK-92MI cells after treatment with either NaB (0.1 mM) for 10 h (**b**) or 5-AZA (1 μM) for 72 h (**d**). Representative data from experiments conducted independently in triplicate are shown. *$P < 0.05$

drug-treated groups (NaB 0.1 mM and 5-AZA 1μM) and the non-pharmacologically-treated control groups in terms of the cytotoxicity of parental NK-92MI cells against colorectal cancer cells (Figs. 6b, d, 7b, d). Whereas pharmacologically-enhanced CEA-expression had limited effect on parental NK-92MI cytotoxicity, NaB and 5-AZA sensitized and/or enhanced cytotoxicity of anti-CEA-CAR NK-92MI. This further confirms our previous findings that cancer cell killing effect of anti-CEA-CAR NK-92MI is positively-correlated to CEA-expression.

Increased CEA-expression induced by NaB and 5-AZA correlated with 5-FU resistance

It has been reported CEA-expression levels are positively correlated to colorectal cancer cell resistance to 5-FU chemotherapy [31]. The effect of pharmacologically-enhanced CEA overexpression on 5-FU resistance was investigated.

HCT116 and WiDr cells were treated with NaB (0.1 mM) or 5-AZA (1μM) plus various 5-FU concentrations (1.2 μM, 2.4 μM, 4.8 μM, 9.6 μM, and 19.2 μM) for 72 h. We treated HCT116 cells independently with 5-FU, and found IC$_{50}$ 4.39 ± 3.10 μM. We then applied 5-FU with NaB or 5-FU with 5-AZA, and found increased IC$_{50}$, to 9.40 ± 6.03 μM and 11.76 ± 9.05 μM, respectively (Table 1). Levels measured by MTS Assay.

WiDr cells showed similar pattern, IC$_{50}$ 4.67 ± 0.55 μM when treated with 5-FU. The groups treated with 5-FU and NaB or 5-FU and 5-AZA, IC$_{50}$ was 9.20

± 2.74 μM and 10.81 ± 3.34 μM, respectively (Table 1). Levels measured by MTS Assay.

In vivo evaluation of the therapeutic efficacy of combination of anti-CEA-CAR NK-92MI cells and NaB

The therapeutic effect of anti-CEA-CAR NK-92MI cells was further confirmed by in vivo xenogeneic mice model. Tumour growth curves and sizes by Day 15 are shown (Fig. 8). There was no therapeutic effect in groups treated with NK-92MI or with NaB alone. However, anti-CEA-CAR NK-92MI cell therapy, with or without NaB, showed significant tumour growth-inhibition ($P < 0.05$) (Fig. 8a). The Day 15 tumours treated with anti-CEA-CAR NK-92MI cells were significantly smaller (508.19 ± 58.64 mm^3) than the control groups

Table 1 NaB and 5-AZA-induced resistance to anti-cancer drug-5-FU in HCT116 and WiDr cells

Cell line	Treatment	IC50 of 5-FU (uM) Mean ± SD*	P-value**
HCT116	5-FU	4.39 ± 3.10	
	0.1 mM NaB+5-FU	9.40 ± 6.03	<0.05(0.036)
	1 μM 5-AZA+5-FU	11.76 ± 9.05	<0.05(0.020)
WiDr	5-FU	4.67 ± 0.55	
	0.1 mM NaB+5-FU	9.20 ± 2.74	<0.001
	1 μM 5-AZA+5-FU	10.81 ± 3.34	<0.001

*Results are presented as mean± SD of three independent experiments, each done in triplicate.

**The groups treated with 5-FU and NaB or 5-FU and 5-AZA were significantly increase IC50 comparing to 5-FU alone treatment group in HCT116 and WiDr cells

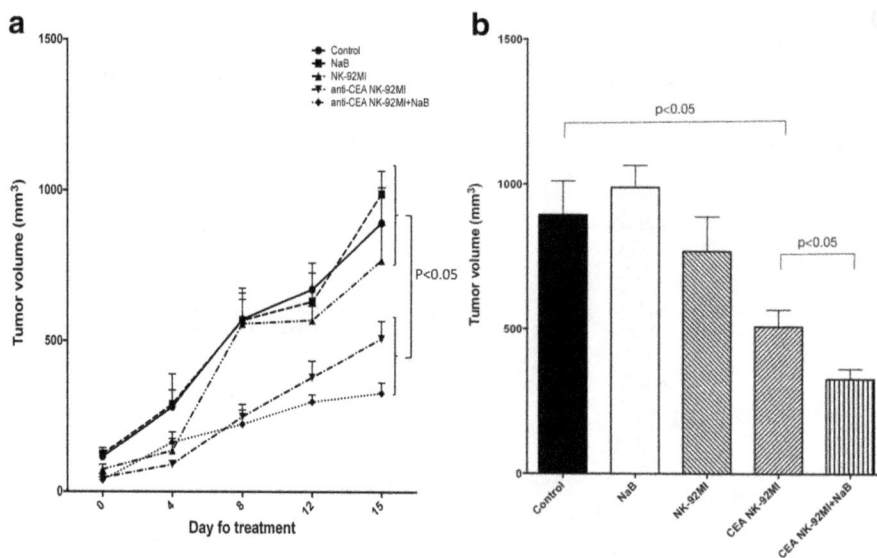

Fig. 8 WiDr-injected SCID mice were treated with NaB, NK-92MI, anti-CEA CAR NK-92MI, and anti-CEA CAR NK-92MI + NaB for 15 days. Tumours were measured at Days 0, 4, 9, 12 and 15 after treatment. **a** Tumour growth curves show that the anti-CEA CAR NK-92MI and anti-CEA CAR NK-92MI + NaB treatments inhibit tumour growth significantly better than the control, NaB alone, or NK-92MI alone. **b** Treatment with NaB or NK-92MI did not significantly inhibit tumour growth relative to the control. Tumour size was significantly reduced by treatment with anti-CEA CAR NK-92MI and even more so in response to the combination of anti-CEA CAR NK-92MI and NaB

(untreated, with NaB-alone, or with NK-92MI-alone) $(893.7 \pm 116.7 \text{ mm}^3)$ $(P < 0.05)$. Combination treatment of anti-CEA-CAR NK-92MI cells with NaB showed even smaller tumour volumes $(328.7 \pm 34.92 \text{ mm}^3)$, with relative significance to control $(P < 0.05)$.

In Table 2, multiple linear regression by GEE method showed that tumour volume in the control groups, had significant tumour volume increases, with averages of 142.59, 457.89, 523.35, 792.51, and 1138.87(mm^3) at Days 4, 8, 12, 15, and 19, respectively. In the anti-CEA-CAR NK-92MI cell therapy groups, tumour

volume growth was significantly smaller, with average decrease to controls of 57.67, 262.75, 225.25, 415.92, and 582.99(mm^3) less than those of the various control groups at Days 4, 8, 12, 15, and 19, respectively. The differences reached significance at Day 8. All p-values< 0.001.

Discussion

In this study, we determined that anti-CEA-CAR NK-92MI cells target CEA-positive tumour cells in a CEA-expression-dependent manner. Epigenetic modifiers

Table 2 Comparing the differences of the tumor volumes between the various control groups and the CEA CAR-NK cell therapies group

Parameter	B	Std. Error	95% Wald Confidence Interval		Hypothesis Test		
			Lower	Upper	Wald Chi-Square	df	Sig.
(Intercept)	109.135	10.4772	88.600	129.670	108.502	1	< 0.001
Group 1 vs. 0	−67.294	12.6052	−91.999	−42.588	28.500	1	< 0.001
Day 19 vs. 0	1138.866	120.2273	903.225	1374.508	89.730	1	< 0.001
Day 15 vs. 0	792.512	54.7220	685.259	899.766	209.743	1	< 0.001
Day 12 vs. 0	523.350	43.5205	438.052	608.649	144.609	1	< 0.001
Day 8 vs. 0	457.892	37.7332	383.936	531.848	147.258	1	< 0.001
Day 4 vs. 0	142.592	37.5555	68.984	216.199	14.416	1	< 0.001
Group x Day 19	−582.990	147.3587	− 871.808	−294.172	15.652	1	< 0.001
Group x Day 15	−415.924	68.5264	− 550.233	−281.615	36.839	1	< 0.001
Group x Day 12	−225.254	51.5495	−326.289	−124.219	19.094	1	< 0.001
Group x Day 8	−262.753	47.9948	− 356.821	− 168.685	29.971	1	< 0.001
Group x Day 4	−57.667	44.7379	−145.352	30.017	1.662	1	0.197

Group = 0 Various Controls Group; =1 CEA CAR-NK Cell Therapies Group

which increased CEA-expression further enhanced cytotoxicity. High-expression CEA cells are generally resistant to 5-FU chemotherapy. To our knowledge, this is first demonstration of a collateral sensitivity strategy to salvage 5-FU-resistant CEA-expressing cells by utilization of CEA-targeting immunotherapy.

CAR-T-cell therapy has emerged as a potentially effective approach for the treatment of metastatic colorectal cancer [36, 37]. However, CAR-T treatments are associated with adverse events [18] and off-target effects [38], mostly commonly eliciting Cytokine Release Syndrome (CRS), a systemic inflammatory response that can lead to widespread organ dysfunction and death. The off-target effects generally associated with CAR-T were not observed in our study with NK or NK-92 cells, which lead us to believe NK and NK-92MI, specifically, to have less off-target concerns. References also show when compared to CAR-T, "CAR-NK-92 show 'on-tumour' in the absence of 'off-target' effects," and "No concern about persisting CAR associated side effects" [15, 39]. Moreover, in clinical trials, patients with metastatic colorectal cancer receiving adoptively transferred autologous CEA-specific CAR-T experienced dose-limiting toxicity and severe transient inflammatory colitis. This reaction could be attributed to the intense immune response of T-cells [37]. Therefore, NK cells may be alternative cytotoxic effectors of CAR-driven cytolysis for the following reasons [15]: (1) NK cells may be safer and more effective CAR effectors than T-cells. T-cells induce proinflammatory cytokines (including tumour necrosis factorα (TNFα), interleukin (IL)-1, IL-6, and others) which could trigger cytokine storms, (2) NK kill target cells using specific natural receptors or transduced CAR, (3) each NK cell can kill four target cells on average, and [40] (4) CAR-NK have a shorter lifespan and, therefore, possibly lower residing toxicity than CAR-T. In contrast to CAR-T, the short-lived NK lines have no need for a suicide gene system [21, 41].

There are several limitations of the adoptive transfer of primary NK cells. These include (1) autologous NK cells may be silenced when their inhibitory receptors interact with self-MHC antigens [42], and (2) NK cells constitute only 10% of all lymphocytes, so primary NK cell adoption is limited by hindrances to ex vivo expansion and variations among patients in terms of their NK cell activity [14]. To overcome these limitations, established NK cell lines are used instead of primary NK cells [14, 43]. Clonal NK cell lines may be an attractive option as effector cells for immunotherapy. It is relatively easier and more cost-effective to use them in clinical trials under GMP conditions [44]. The United States Food and Drug Administration (USFDA) has approved NK-92 for use in clinical trials. NK-92 has undergone extensive preclinical development and completed phase I trials in

cancer patients. Several CAR-modified NK-92 cells have been developed and demonstrated strong cytotoxicity in preclinical models [9, 22–24, 42, 43, 45–47]. The NK-92MI cells used in the present study are highly cytotoxic to human melanoma cells, as are their parental NK-92 cells [12, 13]. We obtained a satisfactory transfection efficiency of NK-92MI to CAR NK-92MI.

CEA is expressed in colorectal as well several other cancer types. CEA is considered a valuable target according to immunotherapy literature [48–50]. In the present study, genetically-modified NK-92MI-scFv cells harboured the scFv sequence specific for CEA mAb T84.66 on their plasma membranes and, therefore, had a high affinity and specificity for CEA [49, 51, 52]. We also showed that our stably transfected anti-CEA-CAR NK-92MI retains its intrinsic characteristics of adhesion and an activation marker of NK-92MI cells. NK-92MI cells also retain their cytolytic activity against the K562 human erythroleukemic cell line. Transduced anti-CEA-CAR NK-92MI exerted significantly elevated cytotoxicity against CEA-positive colon cancer cell lines relative to parental NK-92MI cells. Consequently, the anti-tumour activity of anti-CEA-CAR NK-92MI was also significantly increased in high CEA-expressing LS174T colon cancer cells. In contrast, HCT116 cells expressing only low CEA levels remained insensitive. There is, then, obvious target selection, and it occurs in a CEA-dependent manner.

It has been reported that membrane CEA-expression is ≥2× higher than that of the released CEA [53]. Our in vivo and in vitro data (Fig. 4) demonstrated that the cytotoxicity of transduced anti-CEA-CAR NK-92MI was higher than that of parental NK-92MI. Therefore, surface CEA-expression is highly important. CEA-secretion levels may have only a very minor effect. The level of CEA-secretion may be associated with poor tumour responses to chemoradiotherapy and increased risks of relapse [31, 54]. Drug-resistant human colorectal adenocarcinoma tumours produce abnormally high levels of CEA per cell [55]. It has been reported that several anticancer drugs (cisplatin, aspirin, and 5-FU) induced CEA-expression. Upon treatment, drug-resistant LoVo colon cancer cells produced higher CEA levels than non-resistant cells [55]. Therefore, chemotherapy-induced CEA-expression levels may indicate more chemo-resistant status. We explored whether epigenetic modifiers like DNA methyltransferase-inhibitors and HDAC-inhibitors induced higher CEA-expression levels and, therefore, increased CEA vulnerability to targeted immunotherapy. The results showed that NaB and 5-AZA induced CEA-expression in both WiDr and HCT116 colon cancer cells (Fig. 5). They also increased IC_{50} of 5-FU for both cell lines (Tables 1). Anti-CEA-CAR NK-92MI cells recognized low-CEA HCT116 colon cancer cells more efficiently after drug treatment in vitro. We also demonstrated tumour growth delay in a WiDr mouse model after treatment with anti-CEA-CAR NK-92MI plus NaB.

Conclusion

We successfully transduced NK-92MI with a retroviral vector encoding an anti-CEA-specific chimeric receptor. The chimeric receptor expression, phenotype, and anti-CEA-CAR NK-92MI cell line cytotoxicity were all defined. The cells specifically recognised and lysed CEA-expressing cancer cells. In addition, the epigenetic-modifiers which increased CEA-expression in cancer cells may have also increased the CEA-targeted cytotoxicity of anti-CEA-CAR NK-92MI cells. CEA-density per cell is frequently induced after chemotherapy, thereby, a collateral sensitivity strategy may apply to clinical bedside, in which CEA-targeting NK cells salvage post-chemotherapy relapses.

Abbreviations
5-AZA: 5-Azacytidine; 5-FU: 5-Fluorouracil; CAR: Chimeric Antigen Receptor; CEA: Carcinoembryonic Antigen; CRC: Colorectal Cancer; DNAM-1: DNAX Accessory Molecule-1; FBS: Foetal Bovine Serum; HA: Human Influenza Hemagglutinin; HDAC: Histone Deacetylase; IFN-γ: Interferon-γ; IL: Interleukin; KIRs: Killer Cell Immunoglobulin-Like Receptors; MHC: Major Histocompatibility Complex; NK: Natural Killer; NKG2D: NK Group 2 Member D; PCR: Polymerase Chain Reaction; RIPA: Radioimmunoprecipitation Assay; scFv: Single-Chain Variable Fragment; TCR: T-Cell Receptor; α-MEM: Alpha Modification of Eagle's Minimum Essential Medium

Acknowledgements
The authors would like to thank S. R. Roffler for providing retroviral pLNCX vector (Institute of Biomedical Sciences, Academia Sinica, Taipei, Taiwan) and Mr. Winston Han for his editing and proofing of this manuscript.

Funding
This research was funded in part by the Ministry of Science and Technology, R.O.C. (Grant No. MOST 106–2314-B-341-002-MY2).

Authors' contributions
MS and CHC performed the experiments, analysed the data, and wrote the paper. YCH, YCC, and MSC participated in the phenotype analysis and the cytotoxicity assay. ST participated in the discussion and provided critical manuscript revisions. HCH and YCC analysed the data and performed statistical analyses. KHC and YSW supervised the experiments and revised the paper. All authors read and approved the final manuscript.

Competing interests
The authors declare that they have no competing interests.

Author details
[1]Department of Obstetrics and Gynecology, Juntendo University Hospital, 3-1-3 Hongo, Bunkyo-ku, Tokyo, Japan. [2]Department of Radiation Therapy and Oncology, Shin Kong Wu Ho-Su Memorial Hospital, No.95, Wenchang Road, Shilin District, Taipei, Taiwan. [3]Department of Research and Development, Johnpro Biotech Inc., 2F., No.118, Hougang St., Shilin Dist., Taipei City, Taiwan. [4]Institute of Molecular Medicine and Bioengineering, National Chiao Tung University, Room 117 Lab Building 1, 75 Bo-Ai Street, Hsinchu, Taiwan. [5]Department of Biotechnology, Hungkuang University, No. 1018, Sec. 6, Taiwan Boulevard, Shalu District, Taichung City, Taiwan. [6]Department of Mathematics, Tamkang University, No.151, Yingzhuan Rd., Tamsui Dist., New Taipei City, Taiwan. [7]Institute of Veterinary Clinical Science, School of Veterinary Medicine, National Taiwan University, Taipei, Taiwan. [8]Department of Biomedical Imaging and Radiological Sciences, National Yang-Ming University, Taipei, Taiwan.

References
1. Zamora AE, Grossenbacher SK, Aguilar EG, Murphy WJ. Models to Study NK Cell Biology and Possible Clinical Application. Curr Protoc Immunol. 2015; 110(14 37):11–4.
2. Kumar S. Natural killer cell cytotoxicity and its regulation by inhibitory receptors. Immunology. 2018;154(3):383–93.
3. Sutlu T, Alici E. Natural killer cell-based immunotherapy in cancer: current insights and future prospects. J Intern Med. 2009;266(2):154–81.
4. Davis ZB, Felices M, Verneris MR, Miller JS. Natural killer cell adoptive transfer therapy: exploiting the first line of defense against Cancer. Cancer J. 2015; 21(6):486–91.
5. Burns LJ, Weisdorf DJ, DeFor TE, Vesole DH, Repka TL, Blazar BR, Burger SR, Panoskaltsis-Mortari A, Keever-Taylor CA, Zhang MJ, et al. IL-2-based immunotherapy after autologous transplantation for lymphoma and breast cancer induces immune activation and cytokine release: a phase I/II trial. Bone Marrow Transplant. 2003;32(2):177–86.
6. Grossenbacher SK, Canter RJ, Murphy WJ. Natural killer cell immunotherapy to target stem-like tumor cells. Journal for immunotherapy of cancer. 2016;4:19.
7. Spanholtz J, Preijers F, Tordoir M, Trilsbeek C, Paardekooper J, de Witte T, Schaap N, Dolstra H. Clinical-grade generation of active NK cells from cord blood hematopoietic progenitor cells for immunotherapy using a closed-system culture process. PLoS One. 2011;6(6):e20740.
8. Ni Z, Knorr DA, Bendzick L, Allred J, Kaufman DS. Expression of chimeric receptor CD4zeta by natural killer cells derived from human pluripotent stem cells improves in vitro activity but does not enhance suppression of HIV infection in vivo. Stem Cells. 2014;32(4):1021–31.
9. Arai S, Meagher R, Swearingen M, Myint H, Rich E, Martinson J, Klingemann H. Infusion of the allogeneic cell line NK-92 in patients with advanced renal cell cancer or melanoma: a phase I trial. Cytotherapy. 2008;10(6):625–32.
10. Aktas ON, Ozturk AB, Erman B, Erus S, Tanju S, Dilege S. Role of natural killer cells in lung cancer. J Cancer Res Clin Oncol. 2018;144(6):997–1003.
11. Moretta A, Bottino C, Vitale M, Pende D, Cantoni C, Mingari MC, Biassoni R, Moretta L. Activating receptors and coreceptors involved in human natural killer cell-mediated cytolysis. Annu Rev Immunol. 2001;19:197–223.
12. Gong JH, Maki G, Klingemann HG. Characterization of a human cell line (NK-92) with phenotypical and functional characteristics of activated natural killer cells. Leukemia. 1994;8(4):652–8.
13. Tam YK, Miyagawa B, Ho VC, Klingemann HG. Immunotherapy of malignant melanoma in a SCID mouse model using the highly cytotoxic natural killer cell line NK-92. J Hematother. 1999;8(3):281–90.
14. Tonn T, Becker S, Esser R, Schwabe D, Seifried E. Cellular immunotherapy of malignancies using the clonal natural killer cell line NK-92. J Hematother Stem Cell Res. 2001;10(4):535–44.
15. Klingemann H. Are natural killer cells superior CAR drivers? Oncoimmunology. 2014;3:e28147.
16. Zhao Y, Wang QJ, Yang S, Kochenderfer JN, Zheng Z, Zhong X, Sadelain M, Eshhar Z, Rosenberg SA, Morgan RA. A herceptin-based chimeric antigen receptor with modified signaling domains leads to enhanced survival of transduced T lymphocytes and antitumor activity. J Immunol. 2009;183(9): 5563–74.
17. Jindal V, Arora E, Gupta S. Challenges and prospects of chimeric antigen receptor T cell therapy in solid tumors. Med Oncol. 2018;35(6):87.

18. Bonifant CL, Jackson HJ, Brentjens RJ, Curran KJ. Toxicity and management in CAR T-cell therapy. Molecular therapy oncolytics. 2016;3:16011.

19. Siegler EL, Wang P. Preclinical models in chimeric antigen receptor-engineered T-cell therapy. Hum Gene Ther. 2018;29(5):534–46.

20. Klingemann H, Boissel L, Toneguzzo F. Natural killer cells for immunotherapy - advantages of the NK-92 cell line over blood NK cells. Front Immunol. 2016;7:91.

21. Koehl U, Kalberer C, Spanholtz J, Lee DA, Miller JS, Cooley S, Lowdell M, Uharek L, Klingemann H, Curti A, et al. Advances in clinical NK cell studies: donor selection, manufacturing and quality control. Oncoimmunology. 2016;5(4):e1115178.

22. Rafiq S, SL PT, Klingemann H, Brentjens RJ. NK-92 cells engineered with anti-CD33 chimeric antigen receptors (CAR) for the treatment of acute myeloid leukemia (AML). Cytotherapy. 2015;17(6):S23.

23. Boissel L, Betancur-Boissel M, Lu W, Krause DS, Van Etten RA, Wels WS, Klingemann H. Retargeting NK-92 cells by means of CD19- and CD20-specific chimeric antigen receptors compares favorably with antibody-dependent cellular cytotoxicity. Oncoimmunology. 2013;2(10):e26527.

24. Sahm C, Schonfeld K, Wels WS. Expression of IL-15 in NK cells results in rapid enrichment and selective cytotoxicity of gene-modified effectors that carry a tumor-specific antigen receptor. Cancer immunology, immunotherapy : CII. 2012;61(9):1451–61.

25. Schonfeld K, Sahm C, Zhang C, Naundorf S, Brendel C, Odendahl M, Nowakowska P, Bonig H, Kohl U, Kloess S, et al. Selective inhibition of tumor growth by clonal NK cells expressing an ErbB2/HER2-specific chimeric antigen receptor. Mol Ther. 2015;23(2):330–8.

26. Jiang H, Zhang W, Shang P, Zhang H, Fu W, Ye F, Zeng T, Huang H, Zhang X, Sun W, et al. Transfection of chimeric anti-CD138 gene enhances natural killer cell activation and killing of multiple myeloma cells. Mol Oncol. 2014; 8(2):297–310.

27. Chen Y, You F, Jiang L, Li J, Zhu X, Bao Y, Sun X, Tang X, Meng H, An G, et al. Gene-modified NK-92MI cells expressing a chimeric CD16-BB-zeta or CD64-BB-zeta receptor exhibit enhanced cancer-killing ability in combination with therapeutic antibody. Oncotarget. 2017;8(23):37128–39.

28. Zhang C, Wang Z, Yang Z, Wang M, Li S, Li Y, Zhang R, Xiong Z, Wei Z, Shen J, et al. Phase I escalating-dose trial of CAR-T therapy targeting CEA(+) metastatic colorectal cancers. Mol Ther. 2017;25(5):1248–58.

29. Camacho-Leal P, Stanners CP. The human carcinoembryonic antigen (CEA) GPI anchor mediates anoikis inhibition by inactivation of the intrinsic death pathway. Oncogene. 2008;27(11):1545–53.

30. Chan CH, Stanners CP. Recent advances in the tumour biology of the GPI-anchored carcinoembryonic antigen family members CEACAM5 and CEACAM6. Curr Oncol. 2007;14(2):70–3.

31. Eftekhar E, Jaberie H, Naghibalhossaini F. Carcinoembryonic antigen expression and resistance to radiation and 5-fluorouracil-induced apoptosis and autophagy. Int J Mol Cell Med. 2016;5(2):80–9.

32. Eftekhar E, Naghibalhossaini F. Carcinoembryonic antigen expression level as a predictive factor for response to 5-fluorouracil in colorectal cancer. Mol Biol Rep. 2014;41(1):459–66.

33. Vaquero C, Sack M, Chandler J, Drossard J, Schuster F, Monecke M, Schillberg S, Fischer R. Transient expression of a tumor-specific single-chain fragment and a chimeric antibody in tobacco leaves. Proc Natl Acad Sci U S A. 1999;96(20):11128–33.

34. Xu X, Clarke P, Szalai G, Shively JE, Williams LE, Shyr Y, Shi E, Primus FJ. Targeting and therapy of carcinoembryonic antigen-expressing tumors in transgenic mice with an antibody-interleukin 2 fusion protein. Cancer Res. 2000;60(16):4475–84.

35. Klingemann HG, Wong E, Maki G. A cytotoxic NK-cell line (NK-92) for ex vivo purging of leukemia from blood. Biol Blood Marrow Transplant. 1996;2(2): 68–75.

36. Burga RA, Thorn M, Point GR, Guha P, Nguyen CT, Licata LA, DeMatteo RP, Ayala A, Joseph Espat N, Junghans RP, et al. Liver myeloid-derived suppressor cells expand in response to liver metastases in mice and inhibit the anti-tumor efficacy of anti-CEA CAR-T. Cancer immunology, immunotherapy : CII. 2015; 64(7):817–29.

37. Zhang Q, Zhang Z, Peng M, Fu S, Xue Z, Zhang R. CAR-T cell therapy in gastrointestinal tumors and hepatic carcinoma: from bench to bedside. Oncoimmunology. 2016;5(12):e1251539.

38. Frey NV, BD AR, Chew A, Kalos M, Levine BL, Litchman M, Maude SL, Rheingold SR, Shen A, et al. T cells engineered with a chimeric antigen receptor (CAR) targeting CD19 (CTL019) produce significant in vivo proliferation, complete responses and long-term persistence without

39. GVHD in children and adults with relapsed, refractory ALL. Blood. 2013;122(21):67. http://www.bloodjournal.org/content/122/21/67?sso-checked=true.

39. Suck G, Odendahl M, Nowakowska P, Seidl C, Wels WS, Klingemann HG, Tonn T. NK-92: an 'off-the-shelf therapeutic' for adoptive natural killer cell-based cancer immunotherapy. Cancer immunology, immunotherapy : CII. 2016;65(4):485–92.

40. Bhat R, Watzl C. Serial killing of tumor cells by human natural killer cells--enhancement by therapeutic antibodies. PLoS One. 2007;2(3):e326.

41. Glienke W, Esser R, Priesner C, Suerth JD, Schambach A, Wels WS, Grez M, Kloess S, Arseniev L, Koehl U. Advantages and applications of CAR-expressing natural killer cells. Front Pharmacol. 2015;6:21.

42. Shah NN, Baird K, Delbrook CP, Fleisher TA, Kohler ME, Rampertaap S, Lemberg K, Hurley CK, Kleiner DE, Merchant MS, et al. Acute GVHD in patients receiving IL-15/4-1BBL activated NK cells following T-cell-depleted stem cell transplantation. Blood. 2015;125(5):784–92.

43. Swift BE, Williams BA, Kosaka Y, Wang XH, Medin JA, Viswanathan S, Martinez-Lopez J, Keating A. Natural killer cell lines preferentially kill clonogenic multiple myeloma cells and decrease myeloma engraftment in a bioluminescent xenograft mouse model. Haematologica. 2012;97(7): 1020–8.

44. Cheng M, Chen Y, Xiao W, Sun R, Tian Z. NK cell-based immunotherapy for malignant diseases. Cellular & molecular immunology. 2013;10(3):230–52.

45. Yan Y, Steinherz P, Klingemann HG, Dennig D, Childs BH, McGuirk J, O'Reilly RJ. Antileukemia activity of a natural killer cell line against human leukemias. Clin Cancer Res. 1998;4(11):2859–68.

46. Han J, Chu J, Keung Chan W, Zhang J, Wang Y, Cohen JB, Victor A, Meisen WH, Kim SH, Grandi P, et al. CAR-engineered NK cells targeting wild-type EGFR and EGFRvIII enhance killing of Glioblastoma and patient-derived Glioblastoma stem cells. Sci Rep. 2015;5:11483.

47. Cho FN, Chang TH, Shu CW, Ko MC, Liao SK, Wu KH, Yu MS, Lin SJ, Hong YC, Chen CH, et al. Enhanced cytotoxicity of natural killer cells following the acquisition of chimeric antigen receptors through trogocytosis. PLoS One. 2014;9(10):e109352.

48. Abdel-Nabi HH, Schwartz AN, Higano CS, Wechter DG, Unger MW. Colorectal carcinoma: detection with indium-111 anticarcinoembryonic-antigen monoclonal antibody ZCE-025. Radiology. 1987;164(3):617–21.

49. Lind P. Application of radioimmunodetection with a radiolabeled monoclonal antibody to CEA (BW 431/26) in colorectal and breast cancer. Pathologie-biologie. 1993;41(1):39.

50. Stillwagon GB, Order SE, Haulk T, Herpst J, Ettinger DS, Fishman EK, Klein JL, Leichner PK. Variable low dose rate irradiation (131I-anti-CEA) and integrated low dose chemotherapy in the treatment of nonresectable primary intrahepatic cholangiocarcinoma. Int J Radiat Oncol Biol Phys. 1991;21(6):1601–5.

51. Beatty JD, Duda RB, Williams LE, Sheibani K, Paxton RJ, Beatty BG, Philben VJ, Werner JL, Shively JE, Vlahos WG, et al. Preoperative imaging of colorectal carcinoma with 111In-labeled anticarcinoembryonic antigen monoclonal antibody. Cancer Res. 1986;46(12 Pt 1):6494–502.

52. Wong JY, Williams LE, Yamauchi DM, Odom-Maryon T, Esteban JM, Neumaier M, Wu AM, Johnson DK, Primus FJ, Shively JE, et al. Initial experience evaluating 90yttrium-radiolabeled anti-carcinoembryonic antigen chimeric T84.66 in a phase I radioimmunotherapy trial. Cancer research. 1995;55(23 Suppl):5929s–34s.

53. Shi ZR, Tsao D, Kim YS. Subcellular distribution, synthesis, and release of carcinoembryonic antigen in cultured human colon adenocarcinoma cell lines. Cancer Res. 1983;43(9):4045–9.

54. Park YA, Sohn SK, Seong J, Baik SH, Lee KY, Kim NK, Cho CW. Serum CEA as a predictor for the response to preoperative chemoradiation in rectal cancer. J Surg Oncol. 2006;93(2):145–50.

55. Lee HC, Ling QD, Yu WC, Hung CM, Kao TC, Huang YW, Higuchi A. Drug-resistant colon cancer cells produce high carcinoembryonic antigen and might not be cancer-initiating cells. Drug design, development and therapy. 2013;7:491–502.

9

Small-intestinal TG2-specific plasma cells at different stages of coeliac disease

Minna Hietikko[1], Outi Koskinen[1], Kalle Kurppa[2,3], Kaija Laurila[1], Päivi Saavalainen[4], Teea Salmi[1,5], Tuire Ilus[1,6], Heini Huhtala[7], Katri Kaukinen[1,8] and Katri Lindfors[1*] (ID)

Abstract

Background: In coeliac disease, ingestion of gluten induces the production of transglutaminase 2 (TG2)-targeted autoantibodies by TG2-specific plasma cells present at high frequency in the small intestinal mucosa in untreated disease. During treatment with a gluten-free diet (GFD), the number of these cells decreases considerably. It has not been previously investigated whether the cells are also present prior to development of villous atrophy, or in non-responsive patients and those with dietary lapses. We aimed to define the frequency of small bowel mucosal TG2-specific plasma cells in coeliac disease patients with varying disease activity, and to investigate whether the frequency correlates with serum and small intestinal TG2-targeting antibodies as well as mucosal morphology and the number of intraepithelial lymphocytes.

Results: Mucosal TG2-specific plasma cells were found in 79% of patients prior to development of mucosal damage, in all patients with villous atrophy, and in 63% of the patients after 1 year on GFD. In these disease stages, TG2-specific plasma cells accounted for median of 2.3, 4.3, and 0.7% of all mucosal plasma cells, respectively. After long-term treatment, the cells were present in 20% of the patients in clinical remission (median 0%) and in 60% of the patients with poor dietary adherence (median 5.8%). In patients with non-responsive coeliac disease despite strict GFD, the cells were found in only one (9%) subject; the cells accounted for 2.4% of all plasma cells. A positive correlation between the percentage of TG2-specific plasma cells and serum TG2 antibody levels ($r_S = 0.69$, $P < 0.001$) and the intensity of mucosal TG2-targeting IgA deposits ($r_S = 0.43$, $P < 0.001$) was observed.

Conclusions: Our results show that TG2-specific plasma cells are already detectable prior to villous atrophy, and that generally their frequency increases during overt disease. By contrast, on GFD, the percentage of these cells decreases. Overall, the presence of TG2-specific plasma cells in the small bowel mucosa mirrors the presence of gluten in the diet, but the frequency is not always parallel to the level of serum or intestinal TG2 antibodies. These findings increase the knowledge about the development of the TG2 plasma cell responses especially in the early phases of coeliac disease.

Keywords: Coeliac disease, Gluten, Transglutaminase 2, Autoantibody, Small intestine

Background

In coeliac disease, dietary gluten in wheat, rye, and barley functions as a driving antigen for an abnormal immune response that develops in genetically susceptible individuals carrying the human leukocyte antigen (HLA)-DQ2 or -DQ8 haplotypes. The disease is characterised by small-bowel mucosal damage which develops gradually from normal villous morphology to inflammation and finally to villous atrophy with crypt hyperplasia diagnostic of coeliac disease. The intestinal damage is often coupled with numerous gastrointestinal symptoms, although various extraintestinal manifestations are also prevalent. A specific characteristic of coeliac disease is the generation of immunoglobulin class A (IgA) antibodies towards the main autoantigen, transglutaminase 2 (TG2) [1]. These autoantibodies are generally found in the circulation of coeliac disease patients [2] and as deposits in the small intestinal mucosa below the subepithelial basement membrane and around blood vessels [3]. Interestingly, intestinal TG2-targeted deposits can be detected even prior to manifest mucosal damage and in the absence of serum antibodies [4–6].

* Correspondence: katri.lindfors@uta.fi
[1]Celiac Disease Research Center, Faculty of Medicine and Life Sciences, University of Tampere, P.O. Box 100, 33014 Tampere, Finland
Full list of author information is available at the end of the article

Upon removal of gluten from the diet, the only currently available treatment, the clinical symptoms and histo-pathological changes in the small intestine resolve, and both the circulating and intestinal antibodies disappear within 1 year in most patients [7]. However, a subset of patients fails to respond to the dietary treatment and the villous atrophy persists despite a strict gluten-free diet (GFD). The most common reason for persistent villous atrophy is either advertent or inadvertent gluten intake or, in rare cases, refractory coeliac disease [8].

TG2-targeting antibodies were long thought to be generated by intestinal plasma cells [9–11], but recent data suggests that they might also be produced in lymphoid tissues outside the gut [12]. In the small intestine, the TG2-specific plasma cells are present at high frequency during the active disease [10, 11], and they decrease considerably within 6–12 months after commencement of a strict GFD [11]. However, no data exist regarding the presence of these cells in the early phases of coeliac disease when the mucosal morphology is still normal. In addition, their existence in non-responding coeliac disease patients or those with dietary lapses has not been previously investigated. With this in mind, we enumerated the TG2-specific plasma cells in untreated and treated coeliac patients with varying degrees of disease activity, and investigated whether the number of these cells correlates with serum TG2 antibody levels, the intensity of mucosal TG2-targeting IgA deposits, and small intestinal mucosal morphology and inflammation.

Methods

Patients and study design

The study cohort comprised 46 coeliac disease patients who underwent upper gastrointestinal endoscopy at the Department of Gastroenterology and Alimentary Tract Surgery of Tampere University Hospital (Table 1). Fifteen of the patients were clinically suspected of having coeliac disease based on gastrointestinal symptoms and positive coeliac disease-specific autoantibodies (endomysial and/or TG2 antibodies) despite having normal small bowel mucosa (villous height crypt depth ratio (Vh/CrD) ≥ 2). These patients were prospectively followed up while they continued on a normal gluten-containing diet

Table 1 Demographic data and the small-bowel mucosal and serological findings of patients participating in the study

	Prospectively studied coeliac patients (n = 15)			Long-term treated coeliac patients (n = 31)			Disease controls (n = 25)	
	CD prior to atrophy n = 14	Overt CD n = 15	1 year GFD n = 11	Patients in remission n = 15	Non-responding CD n = 11	Patients with dietary lapses n = 5	Gluten sensitivity n = 18	Dyspepsia n = 7
Female; n (%)	10 (71)	10 (67)	7 (64)	10 (67)	7 (64)	5 (100)	16 (89)	1 (14)
Age; median (range), years	55 (16–70)	55 (17–71)	57 (28–72)	59 (24–66)	49 (40–76)	51 (31–77)	49 (24–65)	47 (24–76)
Duration of GFD; median (range), years	0	0	1 (1–1)	8 (3–34)	7 (3–24)	10 (9–17)	0	0
HLA-DQ2 or -DQ8-positive; n (%)	14 (100)	15 (100)	11 (100)	15 (100)	11 (100)	4[a] (100)	9 (50)	1 (14)
EmA; median (range), titer	1:100 (0–1:2000)	1:100 (0–1:4000)	0 (0–1:50)	0 (0)	0 (0–1:5)	1:200 (0–1:2000)	0 (0)	0 (0)
TG2 abs; median (range), U/ml	9.4 (3.3->100)	11.9 (4.2->100)	3.9 (0–8.6)	0.5 (0–2.8)	1.3 (0–9.9)	56.9 (12.9->100)	1.4 (0–4.1)	0.6 (0–2.8)
Mucosal TG2-IgA deposits present; n (%)	14 (100)	14[a] (100)	7[b] (88)	5 (33)	10[a] (100)	3[c] (100)	4 (22)	0 (100)
Vh/CrD; mean (95% CI), ratio	2.9 (2.6–3.1)	1.4 (1.1–1.7)	3.4 (2.4–4.5)	3.4 (3.2–3.6)	0.2 (0.0–0.4)	0.5 (−0.3–1.3)	3.5 (3.0–4.1)	3.5 (3.0–4.1)
CD3[+] IELs; median (range), cells/mm	54 (12–79)	67 (38–116)	39 (23–80)	42 (25–77)	60 (30–109)	50 (38–69)	21 (7–59)	26 (16–40)
αβ[+] IELs; median (range), cells/mm	30 (12–50)	43 (21–75)	22 (14–43)	31 (20–46)	44 (26–105)	38 (35–56)	16 (5–26)	22 (17–31)
γδ[+] IELs; median (range), cells/mm	18.8 (0–38.5)	23.7 (14–58.7)	v13.6 (1.4–56.3)	14.0 (7.3–27.8)	12.1 (0–37.8)	13.0 (4.4–20.5)	2.7 (0–10.2)	1.6 (0.7–16.1)

abs antibodies, *CD* coeliac disease, *CI* confidence interval, *EmA* endomysial antibodies, *GFD* gluten-free diet, *GS* gluten sensitive; *IgA* immunoglobulin A; *IELs* intraepithelial lymphocytes; TG2-abs, transglutaminase 2 antibodies; *Vh/CrD* villous height crypt depth ratio
Reference values set at 2.0 for Vh/CrD, 37 cells/mm for CD3[+] IELs, 25 cells/mm for αβ[+] IELs, and 4.3 cell/mm for γδ+ IELs (Järvinen et al., [15])
Cut-off value for TG2 antibodies ≥ 5 AU/ml
[a]Data missing from one patient
[b]Data missing from three patients
[c]Data missing from two patients

for 1 year, during which villous atrophy developed (Vh/CrD < 2) in all patients. Thereafter, the patients started a GFD, and after 1 year on the diet, their mucosal morphology had recovered. Small bowel samples from 14 of the patients at the time of the normal mucosal morphology, all 15 patients at the time of the villous atrophy, and 11 of the patients after 1 year on a GFD were available for the current study (Table 1).

Furthermore, 15 coeliac disease patients on a long-term GFD without symptoms and evincing full histological recovery, 11 non-responsive coeliac disease patients with persistent villous atrophy despite a strict GFD, and five patients with poor dietary adherence were investigated. Twenty patients with self-reported gluten sensitivity experiencing abdominal symptoms after consumption of gluten-containing products [13] and seven patients with dyspepsia served as the non-coeliac controls in the study. All controls had been excluded for coeliac disease, as demonstrated by negative serology and normal small bowel mucosal morphology. The demographic data and small-bowel mucosal and serological findings of all subjects are reported in Table 1.

The study protocol was approved by the Ethics Committee of the Pirkanmaa Hospital District, Tampere, Finland, and written informed consent was obtained from all participating subjects.

Small-intestinal mucosal morphology and inflammation

Small-intestinal mucosal biopsies were obtained upon upper gastrointestinal endoscopy. For morphological studies, one formalin-fixed biopsy sample was stained with haematoxylin and eosin to determine the villous height-crypt depth ratios (Vh/CrD) according to a previously published procedure [14]. A ratio of ≥ 2 was considered normal. One of the biopsies was submerged in optimal cutting temperature compound (OCT; Tissue-Tek, Sakura Finetek Europe, Holland), followed by snap-freezing in liquid nitrogen. Thereafter, 5-μm-thick sections were cut. According to an established protocol [15], the sections were stained for CD3$^+$, $\alpha\beta^+$, and $\gamma\delta^+$ intraepithelial lymphocyte (IEL) subsets. The reference values were 37 cells/mm, 25 cells/mm, and 4.3 cells/mm for CD3$^+$ IELs, $\gamma\delta^+$ IELs and $\alpha\beta^+$ IELs, respectively [15].

Serological measurements and HLA genotyping

Serum endomysial antibodies (EmA) in IgA class were determined by an indirect immunofluorescence method exploiting human umbilical cord as substrate. A dilution of 1:$\geq$5 was considered positive [16]. Serum IgA-class TG2 antibodies were measured by a commercially available enzyme-linked immunosorbent assay (Celikey®, Phadia, Freiburg, Germany) in samples diluted 1:100. A titre of ≥ 5 AU/ml was set as the cut-off for positivity.

SSP DQB1 low-resolution kit (Olerup SSP AB, Saltsjöbaden, Sweden), DELFIA Celiac Disease Hybridization Assay (PerkinElmer Life and Analytical Sciences, Wallac Oy, Turku, Finland) or HLA-tagging single-nucleotide peptides [17] were used for HLA genotyping.

Small-intestinal TG2-specific IgA deposits

For the determination of mucosal TG2-targeting IgA deposits, frozen sections were stained with mouse monoclonal anti-TG2 antibody (CUB7402; NeoMarkers, Fremont, California, USA), followed by detection with fluorescein isothiocyanate (FITC) -labelled rabbit anti-human IgA antibody (Dako A/S, Glostrup, Denmark) [3]. Based on their intensity along the basement membrane in the villous-crypt area, the deposits were graded blinded as a negative, or a weak, moderate, or strong positive, as described previously [6].

Small-intestinal TG2-specific plasma cells

An earlier described technique was used to detect mucosal TG2-specific plasma cells [10]. Initially, 5-μm-thick frozen sections were air-dried for 20 min at room temperature (RT). After washing in PBS, the sections were incubated with biotinylated human recombinant TG2 (2 μg/ml; T002, Zedira) for 45 min at RT. Biotinylation was performed using EZ-Link® Sulfo-NHS-LC-Biotin (Thermo Scientific, Waltham, MA, USA) according to the instructions provided by the manufacturer. Thereafter, the sections were incubated with rhodamine-labelled streptavidin (1:1000; KPL, Gaithersburg, MD, USA) for 30 min at RT. Plasma cells were identified using a mouse monoclonal CD138 antibody (1:25; B-A38, Bio-Rad), followed by goat anti-mouse IgG Alexa Fluor 488 (1:2000; A-11001, Thermo-Fisher Scientific). Stainings were analysed at 20x and 40x magnification (Olympus BX60F5, Olympus Optical Co. LTD, Japan) on two consecutive small intestinal biopsy sections and the percentage of TG2-specific cells out of all *lamina propria* plasma cells in the entire section was determined.

Statistical analyses

Data are expressed as the number of subjects (n) and percentages, or as medians and ranges. Statistical analyses were performed using the Wilcoxon test or Mann–Whitney test as appropriate. Correlation was evaluated using Spearman's correlation. Statistical testing was performed using statistical analysis software (IBM SPSS Statistics, SPSS Inc., Chicago, IL, USA). A P-value < 0.05 was considered statistically significant.

Results

Of the 15 prospectively studied coeliac disease patients, TG2-specific plasma cells were already present in 11 out of the 14 available small bowel samples (79%) from the patients before the development of villous atrophy. The median percentage of the cells was 2.3% (range 0–12.7%) of all *lamina propria* plasma cells (Fig. 1a and b). After continuing on a gluten-containing diet for 1 year and developing overt small bowel mucosal damage, all fifteen patients had intestinal TG2-specific plasma cells, and the median percentage of the cells was 4.3% (range 1.8–8.8%) ($P = 0.055$ when compared to patients with early-stage coeliac disease). By contrast, after 1 year on a GFD, the cells were found in 7 out of 11 (64%) patients with available samples, and the median percentage of the cells significantly decreased to 0.7% (range 0–2.9%, $P = 0.003$) when compared to the overt disease.

In long-term GFD-treated patients in clinical remission responding well to dietary treatment, only a few remaining TG2-specific plasma cells (median 0.0%, range 0–1.1%) were detected in 3 out of 15 (20%) of the patients (Fig. 1a and b). In non-responding coeliac disease patients on a strict GFD, the cells were mostly absent, being present in only one patient (9%) who had 2.4% of TG2-specific cells out of all *lamina propria* plasma cells. Of the coeliac disease patients with dietary lapses, three out of five (60%) had TG2-specific plasma cells, the median being 5.8% (range 0–7.0%). No TG2-specific plasma cells were found in any of the non-coeliac control patients with either gluten sensitivity or dyspepsia.

A positive correlation between the percentage of TG2-specific plasma cells and serum TG2 antibody levels ($r_S = 0.690$, $P < 0.001$, Fig. 2a) as well as EmA ($r_S = 0.712$, $P < 0.001$) was observed when data from all coeliac disease patient groups were included in the analysis. Similarly, the percentage of the TG2-specific plasma cells correlated with the intensity of the small intestinal IgA deposits in all coeliac disease patients ($r_S = 0.430$, $P < 0.001$) (Fig. 2b). However, the percentage of TG2-specific plasma cells did not correlate with serum

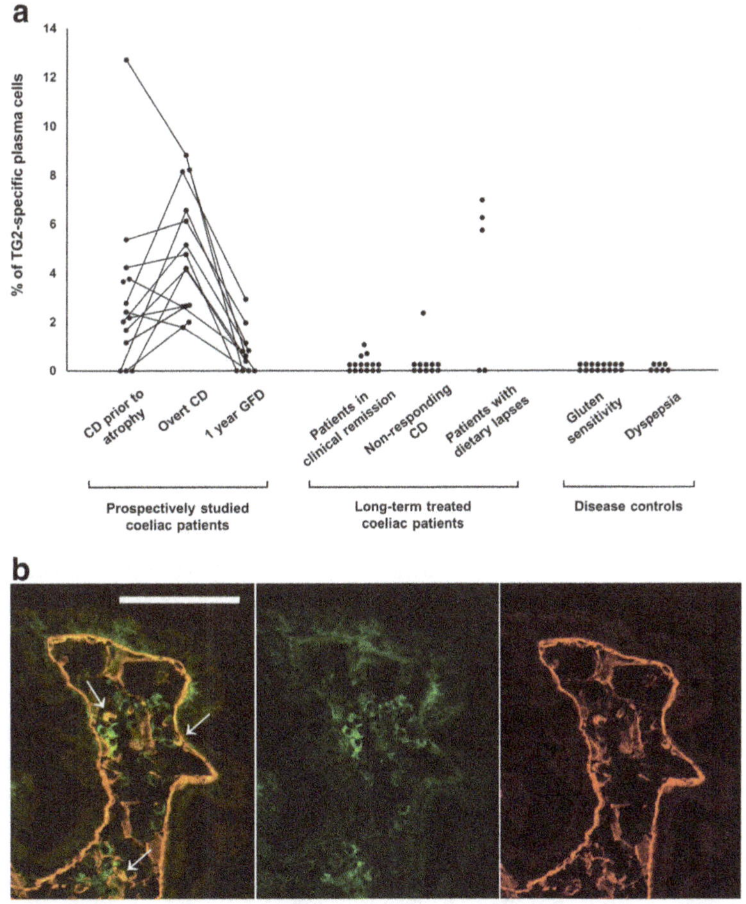

Fig. 1 a. The percentage of small-bowel mucosal transglutaminase 2 (TG2) -specific plasma cells out of all *lamina propria* plasma cells in the different patient groups. **b.** Immunofluorescence staining for transglutaminase 2 (TG2) antibodies and plasma cells in small-bowel mucosal sections. Representative picture of a coeliac disease patient prior to villous atrophy showing positive staining for TG2-specific plasma cells (arrows). Recombinant TG2 (red), plasma cell marker CD138 (green), and their colocalisation (yellow) at 20x magnification. Scale bar = 100 μm. Abbreviations: CD, coeliac disease; GFD, gluten-free diet

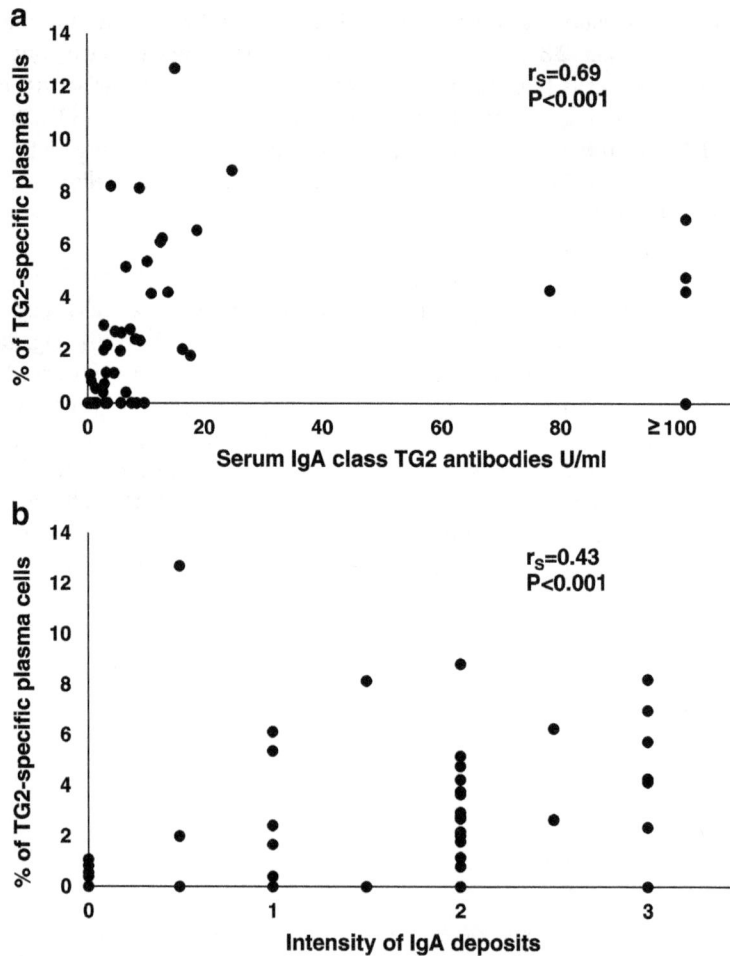

Fig. 2 Correlation between the percentage of small intestinal transglutaminase 2 (TG2) -specific plasma cells and serum IgA class TG2 antibody levels (**a**) and the intensity of small intestinal TG2-targeting immunoglobulin a (IgA) deposits (**b**) in all coeliac disease patients. Grading of IgA deposits as follows: 0 = negative, 1 = weak, 2 = moderate, 3 = strong

or mucosal TG2 antibodies in any of the individual coeliac disease patient groups (Additional file 1 Table S1). Considering all coeliac disease patients, there was no correlation between the percentage of the plasma cells and Vh/CrD. Of the IELs, there was a modest correlation between the percentage of TG2-specific plasma cells and $\gamma\delta^+$ IELs. Detailed information about the correlations is presented in Additional file 1 Table S1.

Discussion

In the current study, we have discovered that TG2-specific plasma cells are already present in most patients prior to detectable mucosal damage. Moreover, we showed that in the majority of cases the percentage of these cells increases upon continuous gluten intake and the subsequent development of villous atrophy. On a strict GFD, the percentage of these cells declines. After long-term treatment, the cells are mostly absent both in patients in clinical remission and in non-responding

patients with persistent villous atrophy. By contrast, TG2-specific plasma cells can be detected in patients with dietary lapses. In controls, even those with gluten-related symptoms, no cells were detected.

Our results from untreated and treated coeliac disease patients are in line with previous studies [10, 11], showing that the amount of TG2-specific plasma cells is elevated in the small intestinal mucosa at the time of diagnosis and this amount decreases on a GFD. It has earlier been shown that the percentage of these cells out of all *lamina propria* plasma cells accounts for up to 24% in overt disease, being on average 10% [10, 11]. However, in the current study, the corresponding percentages were lower. Our patients had been recruited to the study while still having normal mucosal morphology, and they developed overt villous atrophy within a one-year follow-up on a gluten-containing diet. Thus, it is conceivable that the patients had had flat mucosal lesion for a reasonably shorter time than in the previous studies, which might explain the lower percentages of TG2-specific plasma cells in our study.

TG2-specific plasma cells correlated positively with serum TG2 antibody levels when the data of all coeliac disease patients were analysed together. This correlation most likely mirrors the responsiveness of the plasma cells to gluten exposure which is not surprising in the light that TG2 antibodies have been suggested to arise by a hapten-carrier-like mechanism involving TG2-catalysed generation of gluten-TG2 complexes [18, 19]. On the other hand, correlations between the percentages of the plasma cells and serum antibody levels were not detected when different coeliac disease groups were analysed separately; this is in agreement with previous findings in untreated coeliac disease patients [11]. It has been proposed that the lack of correlation could be explained by the production of the antibodies also outside the gut [11]. This concept has recently been further supported by the finding that coeliac patient serum and intestinal TG2 antibodies are clonally related but have different molecular compositions, pointing to different sites of origin [12]. Such extraintestinal production of TG2 antibodies could also explain why some patients in our study had serum TG2 antibodies in the absence of intestinal TG2-specific plasma cells.

Although small intestinal TG2-specific plasma cells are not likely to be the major source of serum TG2 antibodies [12], it would be logical to assume that the TG2 antibodies bound to their antigen in the small intestinal mucosa and predicting forthcoming mucosal damage are produced locally by *lamina propria* TG2-specific plasma cells. In this study, we observed a correlation between the percentage of the plasma cells and the intensity of mucosal TG2-specific IgA deposits, which supports this hypothesis. Interestingly, however, TG2-specific plasma cells were mostly absent in non-responding coeliac patients, even though they all presented with strong TG2-targeting IgA deposits in the small intestinal mucosa despite a strict GFD. It has been proposed that the long persistence of small intestinal IgA deposits in non-responsive patients on a strict diet may be explained, for instance, by the high avidity binding of the IgA antibodies to small intestinal TG2 [6, 7]. This could explain the presence of IgA deposits in the absence of TG2 antibody-secreting plasma cells in our non-responsive patients. However, it does not provide an explanation for the presence of IgA deposits in the absence of plasma cells in the small subset of patients prior to development of villous atrophy. Similarly, it does not explain the presence of weak IgA deposits without TG2-antibody secreting plasma cells in a few gluten-sensitive control patients. Whether extraintestinal production of TG2 antibodies occurring for instance in the bone marrow, spleen and lymph nodes contributes to the appearance of mucosal IgA deposits remains to be addressed in future studies.

Conclusions

We conclude that the TG2-specific plasma cells are already present in the early phases of coeliac disease when the mucosal morphology is still normal, their percentage increases upon the development of villous atrophy and decreases on a GFD. Overall, the frequency of TG2 antibody-secreting plasma cells in the different phases of coeliac disease reflects the presence of gluten in the diet, but the frequency of these cells is not always parallel with serum TG2 antibody levels or the intensity of small intestinal TG2-targeting IgA deposits. Our findings widen the understanding of small-bowel mucosal TG2-specific plasma cells in coeliac disease and thus provide further insight into the generation of TG2 antibody responses.

Abbreviations
EmA: Endomysial antibody; GFD: Gluten-free diet; HLA: Human leukocyte antigen; IEL: Intraepithelial lymphocyte; IgA: Immunoglobulin A; RT: Room temperature; TG2: Transglutaminase 2; Vh/CrD: Villous height-crypt depth ratio

Acknowledgements
Not applicable.

Funding
This study was supported by the Academy of Finland, the Finnish Medical Foundation, the Research Fund of the Finnish Coeliac Society, the Sigrid Juselius Foundation, the Foundation for Pediatric Research, and the Competitive State Research Financing of the Expert Area of Tampere University Hospital.

Authors' contributions
Conceived and designed the study: KL, KaKa. Conceived, designed, and performed the experiments: MH, OK, KL, PS. Analysed the data: MH. Performed the statistical analysis: MH, HH. Participated in patient recruitment and material sampling: OK, KuKa, TS, TI, KaKa. All authors have read, revised, and approved the final manuscript.

Competing interests
All authors have read the journal's policy on the disclosure of potential conflicts of interest and have none to declare.

Author details

[1]Celiac Disease Research Center, Faculty of Medicine and Life Sciences, University of Tampere, P.O. Box 100, 33014 Tampere, Finland. [2]Tampere Center for Child Health Research, University of Tampere, Tampere, Finland. [3]Department of Paediatrics, Tampere University Hospital, Tampere, Finland. [4]Department of Medical and Clinical Genetics and the Research Programs Unit, Immunobiology, University of Helsinki, Helsinki, Finland. [5]Department of Dermatology, Tampere University Hospital, Tampere, Finland. [6]Department of Gastroenterology and Alimentary Tract Surgery, Tampere University Hospital, Tampere, Finland. [7]Faculty of Social Sciences, University of Tampere, Tampere, Finland. [8]Department of Internal Medicine, Tampere University Hospital, Tampere, Finland.

References

1. Dieterich W, Ehnis T, Bauer M, Donner P, Volta U, Riecken E, et al. Identification of tissue transglutaminase as the autoantigen of celiac disease. Nat Med. 1997;3:797–801.
2. Sulkanen S, Halttunen T, Laurila K, Kolho K, Korponay-Szabó IR, Sarnesto A, et al. Tissue transglutaminase autoantibody enzyme-linked immunosorbent assay in detecting celiac disease. Gastroenterology. 1998;115:1322–8.
3. Korponay-Szabo IR, Halttunen T, Szalai Z, Laurila K, Kiraly R, Kovacs JB, et al. In vivo targeting of intestinal and extraintestinal transglutaminase 2 by coeliac autoantibodies. Gut. 2004;53:641–8.
4. Kaukinen K, Peräaho M, Collin P, Partanen J, Woolley N, Kaartinen T, et al. Small-bowel mucosal transglutaminase 2-specific IgA deposits in coeliac disease without villous atrophy: a prospective and randomized clinical study. Scand J Gastroenterol. 2005;40:564–72.
5. Salmi T, Collin P, Järvinen O, Haimila K, Partanen J, Laurila K, et al. Immunoglobulin a autoantibodies against transglutaminase 2 in the small intestinal mucosa predict forthcoming coeliac disease. Aliment Pharmacol Ther. 2006;24:541–52.
6. Salmi TT, Collin P, Korponay-Szabo IR, Laurila K, Partanen J, Huhtala H, et al. Endomysial antibody-negative coeliac disease: clinical characteristics and intestinal autoantibody deposits. Gut. 2006;55:1746–53.
7. Koskinen O, Collin P, Lindfors K, Laurila K, Maki M, Kaukinen K. Usefulness of small-bowel mucosal transglutaminase-2 specific autoantibody deposits in the diagnosis and follow-up of celiac disease. J Clin Gastroenterol. 2010;44: 483–8.
8. Ilus T, Kaukinen K, Virta L, Huhtala H, Mäki M, Kurppa K, et al. Refractory coeliac disease in a country with a high prevalence of clinically-diagnosed coeliac disease. Aliment Pharmacol Ther. 2014;39:418–25.
9. Marzari R, Sblattero D, Florian F, Tongiorgi E. Not T, Tommasini a , et al. molecular dissection of the tissue transglutaminase antoantibody response in celiac disease. J Immunol. 2001;166:4170–6.
10. Di Niro R, Mesin L, Zheng N, Stamnaes J, Morrissey M, Lee J, et al. High abundance of plasma cells secreting transglutaminase 2-specific IgA autoantibodies with limited somatic hypermutation in celiac disease intestinal lesions. Nat Med. 2012;18:441–U204.
11. Di Niro R, Snir O, Kaukinen K, Yaari G, Lundin K, Gupta N, et al. Responsive population dynamics and wide seeding into the duodenal lamina propria of transglutaminase-2-specific plasma cells in celiac disease. Mucosal Immunol. 2016;9:254–64.
12. Iversen R, Snir O, Stensland M, Kroll JE, Steinsbø Ø, Korponay-Szabó IR, et al. Strong clonal relatedness between serum and gut IgA despite different plasma cell origins. Cell Rep. 2017;20:2357–67.
13. Kaukinen K, Turjanmaa K, Mäki M, Partanen J, Venäläinen R, Reunala T, et al. Intolerance to cereals is not specific for coeliac disease. Scand J Gastroenterol. 2000;35:942–6.
14. Taavela J, Koskinen O, Huhtala H, Lähdeaho M, Popp A, Laurila K, et al. Validation of morphometric analyses of small-intestinal biopsy readouts in celiac disease. PLoS One. 2013;8:e76163.
15. Järvinen TT, Kaukinen K, Laurila K, Kyrönpalo S, Rasmussen M, Mäki M, et al. Intraepithelial lymphocytes in celiac disease. Am J Gastroenterol. 2003;98: 1332–7.
16. Sulkanen S, Collin P, Laurila K, Mäki M. IgA-and IgG-class antihuman umbilical cord antibody tests in adult coeliac disease. Scand J Gastroenterol. 1998;33:251–4.
17. Koskinen L, Romanos J, Kaukinen K, Mustalahti K, Korponay-Szabo I, Barisani D, et al. Cost-effective HLA typing with tagging SNPs predicts celiac disease risk haplotypes in the Finnish, Hungarian, and Italian populations. Immunogenetics. 2009;61:247–56.
18. Sollid LM, Molberg O, McAdam S, Lundin KE. Autoantibodies in coeliac disease: tissue transglutaminase-guilt by association? Gut. 1997;41:851–2.
19. Stamnaes J, Sollid LM. Celiac disease: autoimmunity in response to food antigen. Semin Immunol. 2015;27:343–52.

10

The immunoregulatory role of alpha enolase in dendritic cell function during Chlamydia infection

Khamia Ryans[1,2], Yusuf Omosun[1]* (ID), Danielle N. McKeithen[1,2], Tankya Simoneaux[1], Camilla C. Mills[1], Nathan Bowen[2], Francis O. Eko[1], Carolyn M. Black[3], Joseph U. Igietseme[1,3] and Qing He[1]*

Abstract

Background: We have previously reported that interleukin-10 (IL-10) deficient dendritic cells (DCs) are potent antigen presenting cells that induced elevated protective immunity against *Chlamydia*. To further investigate the molecular and biochemical mechanism underlying the superior immunostimulatory property of IL-10 deficient DCs we performed proteomic analysis on protein profiles from *Chlamydia*-pulsed wild-type (WT) and IL-10$^{-/-}$ DCs to identify differentially expressed proteins with immunomodulatory properties.

Results: The results showed that alpha enolase (ENO1), a metabolic enzyme involved in the last step of glycolysis was significantly upregulated in *Chlamydia*-pulsed IL-10$^{-/-}$ DCs compared to WT DCs. We further studied the immunoregulatory role of ENO1 in DC function by generating ENO1 knockdown DCs, using lentiviral siRNA technology. We analyzed the effect of the ENO1 knockdown on DC functions after pulsing with *Chlamydia*. Pyruvate assay, transmission electron microscopy, flow cytometry, confocal microscopy, cytokine, T-cell activation and adoptive transfer assays were also used to study DC function. The results showed that ENO1 knockdown DCs had impaired maturation and activation, with significant decrease in intracellular pyruvate concentration as compared with the *Chlamydia*-pulsed WT DCs. Adoptive transfer of *Chlamydia*-pulsed ENO1 knockdown DCs were poorly immunogenic in vitro and in vivo, especially the ability to induce protective immunity against genital chlamydia infection. The marked remodeling of the mitochondrial morphology of *Chlamydia*-pulsed ENO1 knockdown DCs compared to the *Chlamydia*-pulsed WT DCs was associated with the dysregulation of translocase of the outer membrane (TOM) 20 and adenine nucleotide translocator (ANT) 1/2/3/4 that regulate mitochondrial permeability. The results suggest that an enhanced glycolysis is required for efficient antigen processing and presentation by DCs to induce a robust immune response.

Conclusions: The upregulation of ENO1 contributes to the superior immunostimulatory function of IL-10 deficient DCs. Our studies indicated that ENO1 deficiency causes the reduced production of pyruvate, which then contributes to a dysfunction in mitochondrial homeostasis that may affect DC survival, maturation and antigen presenting properties. Modulation of ENO1 thus provides a potentially effective strategy to boost DC function and promote immunity against infectious and non-infectious diseases.

Keywords: Alpha enolase, ENO1, Chlamydia, Dendritic cells, Metabolism

* Correspondence: yomosun@msm.edu; qhe@msm.edu
[1]Department of Microbiology, Biochemistry, and Immunology, Morehouse School of Medicine, 720 Westview Drive S.W., Atlanta, GA 30310, USA
Full list of author information is available at the end of the article

Background

Chlamydia trachomatis genital infection is the most frequently reported bacterial sexually transmitted infection in the United States [1]. *C. trachomatis* is an obligate intracellular pathogen that causes a broad range of female reproductive diseases including pelvic inflammatory disease (PID), ectopic pregnancy and tubal factor infertility (TFI) [2]. In a recent study about 20% of PID and 29% of TFI in women aged 16–44 years was attributed to *C. trachomatis* infections [3, 4]. Preventive strategies proposed against *C. trachomatis* include increased screening with mass treatment [5, 6]. However, recent clinical and epidemiological data suggests that the vaccine strategy would be the most reliable and cost effective preventive method with the greatest potential impact in the control of *C. trachomatis* infections and its associated complications in the human population [7, 8]. However, there is no human vaccine available for *C. trachomatis* infections; the development of an effective vaccine against *C. trachomatis* has been a challenging task due to the incomplete understanding of the complex immunological processes associated with chlamydial infection.

Studies using mouse models of genital chlamydial infection have shown that infection causes dendritic cells (DCs) to undergo maturation and strongly up-regulate major histocompatibility complex (MHC) antigens, and costimulatory molecules such as cluster of differentiation (CD) 40, CD80 and CD86, which are crucial for effective activation of the $CD4^+$ T helper cell type 1 (Th1) cell response, especially the CD4 T cells and interferon (IFN) -γ production required for host defense [9–11]. Current vaccine efforts are focusing on antigen delivery and immunomodulatory strategies to induce protective immunity and at the same time prevent detrimental immunopathologies.

DCs are potent, professional antigen-presenting cells that play very import role in primary humoral and T-cell-mediated immune responses. It is gradually becoming apparent that different stages of immune cell activation coincide with, and are underpinned by, different types of cellular metabolism that are tailored towards the bioenergetic and biosynthetic needs of these cells. Emerging data have recently demonstrated the contribution of cellular metabolic pathways to the ability of immune cells to sense their microenvironment and thereafter alter their functions [12–15]. Distinct changes in the microenvironment induce a spectrum of inducible and reversible metabolic programs that might be necessary in functional immune cell activation/polarization phenotypes. For example, after exposure to Toll-like receptor agonists, DCs undergo a metabolic transition from oxidative phosphorylation (OXPHOS) to aerobic glycolysis, which is required to meet the increased biosynthetic and bioenergetic demands of activated DCs specifically by funneling metabolites into pathways for lipid and protein synthesis [14, 16]. Cytokines such as IL-10 and IFN-γ are key regulators of immune responses whose actions are mediated via cellular process that include active metabolism. As a negative immune-modulator, IL-10 suppresses inflammatory immunostimulation by acting on both regulatory and effector immune cells but the molecular mechanisms are not completely understood. Interestingly, IL-10 deficient DCs exhibit a high efficiency in chlamydial antigen presentation and the induction of a high frequency of specific immune effectors that protect against chlamydial disease [17]. Proteomics and functional immunologic analyses revealed that the efficient APC function of IL-10 deficient DCs coincided with rapid maturation, and expression of high levels of co-stimulatory and metabolic molecules, including Leucine/glutamic acid/lysine protein 1 (LEK1), Vimentin, Arginase-1, Fatty acid binding protein and ENO1. This suggests that IL-10 deficient DCs are highly effective cellular vaccines that possess certain immunomodulatory features that provide us a suitable immunotherapeutic platform to better define the immunological and biochemical determinants and conditions for inducing adequate and long-term immunity against *Chlamydia*-induced tubal pathologies [18, 19]. Such immunostimulatory features can also be applied to improve vaccine delivery and elicitation of protective immunity against other infectious and non-infectious diseases in general [17, 20].

Proteomics data showing that ENO1 was significantly increased in IL-10$^{-/-}$ DCs suggested that it may play a role in the immunostimulatory properties of the DCs. ENO1 is a glycolytic enzyme which is expressed in cytoplasm, nucleus, and on the surface of many eukaryotic cells, such as stimulated hematopoietic (neutrophils, B & T lymphocytes and monocytes), epithelial, neuronal and endothelial cells. Its functions are related to its subcellular location, and ENO1 catalyzes the dehydration of 2-phosphoglycerate to phosphoenolpyruvate [21, 22], which is an important step in ATP generation through substrate-level phosphorylation. ENO1 has been found to play other roles in inflammation, tumor suppression, monocyte and mast cell differentiation [21, 22]. Disruption of glycolysis through the reduced expression of ENO1 has recently been linked to NLR family pyrin domain containing 3 (NLRP3) activation [23], and we have previously shown that NLRP3 inflammasome assembly was suppressed in IL-10$^{-/-}$ DCs [18]. In this study, we further analyze the molecular basis of the potent immunostimulatory action of IL-10 DC focusing on the contribution of ENO1 to immunostimulation. We used siRNA technology to knockdown ENO1 in DCs and evaluated the maturation, activation, and antigen presenting functions of DCs in vivo and in vitro. In addition, we also investigated the remodeling of DC mitochondria, which controls metabolic programs and therefore regulates DC function. We provide evidence for the role of ENO-1 in the potent immunostimulatory function of IL-10 deficient DCs, which involves the regulation of DC metabolism, DC mitochondrial modeling, DC survival and antigen presentation function.

Methods
Chlamydia stocks

Stocks of *C. muridarum*, provided by the Molecular Pathogenesis Laboratory of the Division of Scientific Resources, Centers for Disease Control and Prevention were used for stimulating DCs. They were prepared by propagating elementary bodies (EBs) in McCoy or HeLa cells. The cell lines were maintained in minimum essential medium (MEM) supplemented with 2 mM L-glutamine, 10% heat-inactivated FBS, 1 mM sodium pyruvate, 0.5% fungizone, and 1.0% penicillin/streptomycin (100U/mL; 100 µg/mL) in an incubator at 37 °C in 5% $CO2$. *Chlamydia* stock titers were expressed as inclusion forming units (IFU) per milliliter.

Animals

Six-week-old female WT mice (C57BL/6 J background) were purchased from The Jackson Laboratory (Bar Harbor, ME). The mice were fed with food and water ad libitum and maintained in laminar flow racks under pathogen-free conditions of 12 h of light and 12 h of darkness. The animal use protocols described in this proposal have been approved by the Institutional Animal Care and Use Committee of Morehouse School of Medicine (MSM-IACUC) and follow approved federal guidelines.

DC isolation and culture

Immature DCs were isolated from bone marrow collected from the femurs of WT mice and cultured by plating the cells in 100 cm^2 dishes using DC culture media containing complete RPMI 1640 medium, FBS, HEPES, glutamine, nonessential amino acids, sodium pyruvate, gentamicin, mouse recombinant interleukin-4 (IL-4) and granulocyte-macrophage colony-stimulating factor (GM-CSF) (Gemini Bioproducts, Sacramento, CA). The cells were cultured in an incubator at 37°Celsius in 5% carbon dioxide air, replacing with fresh media on day 3 and transferring cells to new dishes on day 5. After 5 days in culture, the cells were characterized as loosely adherent mononuclear cells and further purified as CD11c expressing DCs by using the Pan Dendritic Cell Isolation Kit from Miltenyi Biotec (San Diego, CA) [24]. Cells were then ready to be used in the experiments as described.

Lentiviral transfection of ENO1 small interfering RNA in dendritic cells

For ENO1 knockdown studies, a siRNA vector against mouse ENO1containing H1 promoter (piLenti-siRNA-GFP) was purchased from Applied Biological Materials (Richmond, BC, CA). The siRNA vector has an independent open reading frame of green fluorescent protein (GFP). The GFP-positive cells were monitored as a marker for transfection. The target sequences were;

5′ -ACTGTTGAGGTCGATCTGTACACCGCAAA-3′ ,
5′ -GCCCTAGAACTCCGAGACAATGATAAGAC-3′ ,
5′ -GCGCCTGCTCTGGTTAGCAAGAAAGTGAA-3′ ,
and
5′ -GCCACCAATGTGGGTGATGAGGGTGGATT-3′ .

Controls used were the scramble siRNA vector target sequence was 5′-GGGTGAACTCACGTCAGAA-3′ and WT DCs without siRNA vector. DCs were incubated overnight in 6 well plates with complete media without IL-4 and GM-CSF. Cells were transfected with 1 µg of siRNA vector and seeded at a density of 0.3×10^6 cells per well in complete media containing polybrene (8 µl/ml) and after 48 h, cell viability was checked with trypan blue. This experiment was repeated 3 times.

Proteomics assay

In the proteomic analysis of WT and IL-10$^{-/-}$ DCs, DCs were pulsed with Chlamydia for 0, 2, 4 and 8 h. Proteins were then extracted from the Chlamydia pulsed DCs using a Bio-Rad protein extraction kit (Bio-Rad, Hercules, CA) and then cleaned up with a 2-D Clean up Kit (Bio-Rad, Hercules, CA), following the manufacturer's protocol. Protein concentration was determined using 2D Quant Kit (GE Healthcare, Piscataway, NJ). Samples were labeled with Cy5 (Red-IL-10$^{-/-}$DCs) and Cy3 (Green-WT DCs) respectively, then mixed together in a rehydration buffer and subjected to two-dimensional fluorescence differential gel electrophoresis analysis (2D-DIGE). Yellow color indicated the expression of the same protein by both WT DCs and IL-10$^{-/-}$ DCs, while, green color indicated proteins expressed at a higher level in WT DCs compared to IL-10$^{-/-}$ DCs. Red color indicated proteins in IL-10$^{-/-}$ DCs that were over--expressed compared to WT DCs. The spots corresponding to differentially expressed proteins were digested and analyzed by nanocapillary LC–MS/MS (Xevo G2 Tof, 210 Waters, Milford, MA). Protein candidates were identified using automated database search against the NCBI database using MASCOT Daemon software (Matrix Science Inc., Boston, MA). This experiment was repeated 3 times.

Western blot analysis

Lysates from *Chlamydia* pulsed and nonpulsed WT, IL10$^{-/-}$ and ENO1 knockdown DCs were prepared by homogenization in lysis buffer supplemented with 1 mmol/L phenylmethylsulfonyl fluoride and protease inhibitor cocktail. 20 µg protein of *Chlamydia* pulsed and nonpulsed WT, IL10$^{-/-}$ and ENO1 knockdown DCs lysates were loaded onto 4–20% TGX gradient gel (Bio-Rad, Hercules, CA) and run for 1 h. Proteins were then transferred onto nitrocellulose paper (Bio-Rad, Hercules, CA). After 1 h, the blots were washed, blocked with 5% milk, and then incubated with desired primary monoclonal antibody against ENO1 raised in rabbit (Abcam, Cambridge, MA), overnight at 4 °C. Goat anti-rabbit Horseradish peroxidase (HRP)-conjugated secondary antibodies (Southern Biotech, Birmingham Al) were added for 1 h at room temperature, and then the blots were developed using Clarity Western enhanced chemiluminescence (ECL) substrate (Bio-Rad, Hercules, CA). Viewing and quantification was analyzed using ImageQuant LAS 4000 (GE Healthcare, Pittsburgh, PA). The experiment was repeated three times.

ENO1 has been shown to be associated with cytoskeletal proteins in cells [25], so in order to get a true and definite picture of protein expression in DCs we used the Cy5 Total Protein Normalization method [26]. In this method, chlamydia pulsed and nonpulsed WT and ENO1 knockdown DC cell lysates were stained for total protein with Amersham WB CY5 antibody (GE Healthcare, Pittsburgh, PA) for 30 min at room temperature and ran on TGX gels (Bio-Rad, Hercules, CA) for 1 h. Proteins were then transferred in seven minutes onto PVDF membrane (Bio-Rad, Hercules, CA) using the Trans-Blot Turbo Transfer System (Bio-Rad, Hercules, CA). The blots were washed, then blocked with 5% milk and incubated with primary antibody; PDH-Eα (mouse monoclonal), TOM20 (rabbit polyclonal), ANT1/2/3/4 (rabbit polyclonal) and GAPDH (rabbit polyclonal) (Santa Cruz Biotech., Dallas, TX.) overnight at 4 °C. Subsequently, blots were washed five times in TBS/Tween followed by incubation with Cy3 anti-mouse and anti-rabbit secondary antibody (GE Healthcare, Pittsburgh, PA). Blots were washed and developed using Western ECL substrate and the fluorescence was viewed using the LAS 4000 Gel Doc System (GE Healthcare, Pittsburgh, PA). Normalization was carried out with the ImageQuant TL Software 8.1 (GE Healthcare, Pittsburgh, PA). The images were saved as Tiff files. This experiment was repeated 3 times.

Confocal microscopy

WT and IL-10$^{-/-}$ DCs (1×10^6 cells/ml) were pulsed with Chlamydia (MOI of 5) for 1 and 2 h, and then fixed for 5 min at room temperature in PBS solution containing 4% formaldehyde/ 0.01% glutaraldehyde. Samples were washed twice in cold 1X PBS and the Fc receptors were blocked with Fc blocker. DCs were incubated with Anti-ENO1 (Abcam, Cambridge, MA) for 1 h at 4 °C and washed twice with 1X PBS. DRAQ5 and Alexa Fluor 488 bound secondary antibodies (Jackson ImmunoResearch Laboratories, West Grove, PA) were then added for 1 h at 4 °C. DCs were washed three times and resuspended in wash buffer overnight at 4 °C. Confocal images were obtained on the Zeiss 510 VIS 234 Confocal Microscope (Carl Zeiss Microscopy, GmbH). Images were taken from different fields on each plate. Quantitative colocalization analysis was used in analyzing the data (ImageJ Software, NIH, USA). We repeated this experiment 3 times.

Flow cytometry

WT and ENO1 knockdown DCs pulsed with *C. muriduram* at MOI of 5 were resuspended in PBS containing 2% FBS (wash buffer) and washed and incubated for 10 min at 4 °C with 5 µg/mL Fc blocker. The cells were incubated with fluorescein isothiocyanate (FITC)-, phycoerythrin (PE)-, or allophycocyanin (APC)-conjugated antibodies against surface markers CD40, CD80, CD86, MHC II, and toll like receptor 4 (TLR4) (BD Pharmingen, San Jose, CA) for 1 h at 4 °C. Thereafter, the cells were washed 3 times and resuspended in wash buffer, and then filtered into 5 ml FACS tubes, and the flow data was acquired on a BD Accuri C6 and analyzed using BD Accuri C6 software (BD, Franklin Lakes, NJ), and for each sample, at least 100,000 events were collected, and the experiment was replicated 3 times.

Apoptosis assay

The level of apoptosis in chlamydia pulsed and nonpulsed WT and ENO1 knockdown DCs was determined using Annexin V and 7-AAD flow cytometry (Biolegend, San Diego, CA). The cells were then collected at time 0 and 2 h after infection and washed with cold BioLegend Cell Staining Buffer twice and then resuspended in Annexin V binding buffer. Five microliters of fluorescein isothiocyanate (FITC)-Annexin V and 5 µl of 7-amino-actinomycin D (7-AAD), viability staining solution were added to 100 µl cell suspensions and incubated in the dark at room temperature for 15 min. 400 µl of binding buffer was added to the sample and the mixture was vortexed and then analyzed by flow cytometry using a guava easyCyte 8HT (EMD Millipore, Billerica, MA). For each sample, at least 100,000 events were collected. Data was analyzed with guavaSoft 2.7 (EMD Millipore, Billerica, MA).

Cytokine assay

WT and ENO1 knockdown DCs were plated at 1×10^6 cells/ml in culture media and then DCs pulsed with *C.*

muriduram at MOI of 5 for 1 to 2 h. Culture supernatants were collected and the amount of cytokines produced was determined using a Bio-Plex Pro Mouse Cytokine Assay kit (Bio-Rad, Hercules, CA) in accordance with the manufacturer's protocol. The mean and SD of all replicate cultures were calculated. The experiment was repeated three times.

T-cell proliferation assay

Lymphocytes were obtained from spleens of WT mice intravaginally infected *with Chlamydia* using a 40 μm filter and syringe plunger and suspended in PBS solution. The CD4$^+$ T cells were then purified using the MACS mouse Pan T Cell Isolation Kit (mouse) (Miltenyi Biotec, Inc, San Diego, CA). To assess the antigen-presenting function of WT and ENO1 knockdown DCs, 1×10^5 γ-irradiated DCs were co-cultured with 2×10^5 purified T cells in the presence or absence of UV-inactivated *C. muriduram* (MOI of 5) in 96-well tissue culture plates for 5 days. The amounts of IL-1β, IL-1α IL-5, IL-9, IL-10, IL-13, IL-17A, and RANTES in the culture supernatants were measured using the Bio-Plex Pro Mouse Cytokine 23-Plex multiplex array according to the manufacturer's guidelines (Bio-Rad) using a Luminex machine. The T cell proliferation was detected using a spectrophotometer set at 450 nm following the XTT Cell Viability Kit protocol (Cell Signaling Technology, Danvers, MA). The concentration of cytokine in each sample was obtained by extrapolation from a standard calibration curve generated simultaneously. The mean and SD of all replicate cultures were calculated. The experiment was repeated two times.

Pyruvate assay

Supernatant from DCs pulsed with *C. muriduram* at MOI of 5 (0, 0.5, 1, 2, and 4 h) were diluted with pyruvate assay buffer and the pyruvate assay was carried out following the manufacturers' protocol (Eton Bioscience, San Diego, CA). Final measurements of pyruvate concentration were done at 570 nm on a microplate reader. The mean and SD of all replicate cultures were calculated. The experiments were repeated three times.

Adoptive transfer of DCs and assessment of protective immunity in vivo

IL-10KO, WT and ENO1 knockdown DCs pulsed with *C. muriduram* at MOI of 5 were adoptively transferred through intravenous tail injection (2.5×10^7 cells/mouse) into 6–8 weeks old WT mice ($n = 4$ per group) pretreated with Depo Provera (Pfizer Inc., NY, NY), which is used to synchronize the estrous cycle. Mice were infected intravaginally 1 week later with 20 μl of 1×10^5 IFUs of *C. muriduram,* which we have shown to cause disease pathology in mice [17]. The course of the infection was determined by periodic swabbing (every three days for two weeks and later once a week for two weeks). Chlamydia culture confirmation kit (Bio-Rad, Hercules, CA) was used to determine the bacteria IFUs. The experiment was repeated three times.

Transmission electron microscopy (TEM)

WT and ENO1 knockdown DCs were pulsed with *C. muriduram* at MOI of 5 for 2 h in 24-well tissue culture plates. The cells were then washed and fixed glass slides using 2.5% (w/v) glutaraldehyde/0.1 M cacodylate buffer for 2–6 h at 25 °C. DCs were then mounted and cut into 200 mm slices with a Vibratome (EM Corp., Hatfield, PA), and post fixed in aqueous osmium tetroxide. Fixed DC slices were dehydrated using graded ethanol and propylene oxide, and embedded in Polybed 812 resin (Polysciences, Inc., Warrington, PA). Thin sections (80 nm) were then cut with a diamond knife and stained with 5% uranyl acetate and Reynold's lead citrate. A JEOL 1200EX transmission electron microscope (JEOL USA, Inc., Peabody, MA) was used to examine mitochondrial changes. The experiment was repeated three times.

Statistical analysis

The data derived from different experiments was analyzed and compared by performing a 1- or 2-tailed *t*-test. The relationship between the diverse experimental groups was evaluated by analysis of variance (ANOVA) (Microsoft Excel 2015, Redmond, WA; GraphPad Prism, La Jolla, CA). Statistical significance was determined at $P < 0.05$.

Results

Upregulation of ENO1 expression in DCs following Chlamydia pulse

Total protein extracted from *Chlamydia*-pulsed or non-pulsed WT and IL-10$^{-/-}$ DCs were labeled with Cy5 (red, IL-10$^{-/-}$ DCs) and Cy3 (green, WT DCs) and subjected to two-dimensional fluorescence differential gel electrophoresis (2D-DIGE) analysis and LC-MS/MS to identify differentially expressed molecules. Here we show a representative protein profile map revealing that some proteins were differentially expressed by IL-10$^{-/-}$ DC compared with WT DC (Fig. 1a). At least three notable categories of differentially expressed proteins were identified: 1) proteins involve in cell metabolism (i.e., ENO1, Arginase-1, Isocitrate dehydrogenase [NADP], Triosephosphate isomerase, and Fatty acid-binding protein). 2) Proteins that are members of the cell cytoskeletal network (i.e., Coactosin-like protein, Macrophage capping protein, and Vimentin). 3) Proteins involved in the process of protein folding (i.e., Peptidyl-prolyl cis-trans isomerase A and Heat shock cognate

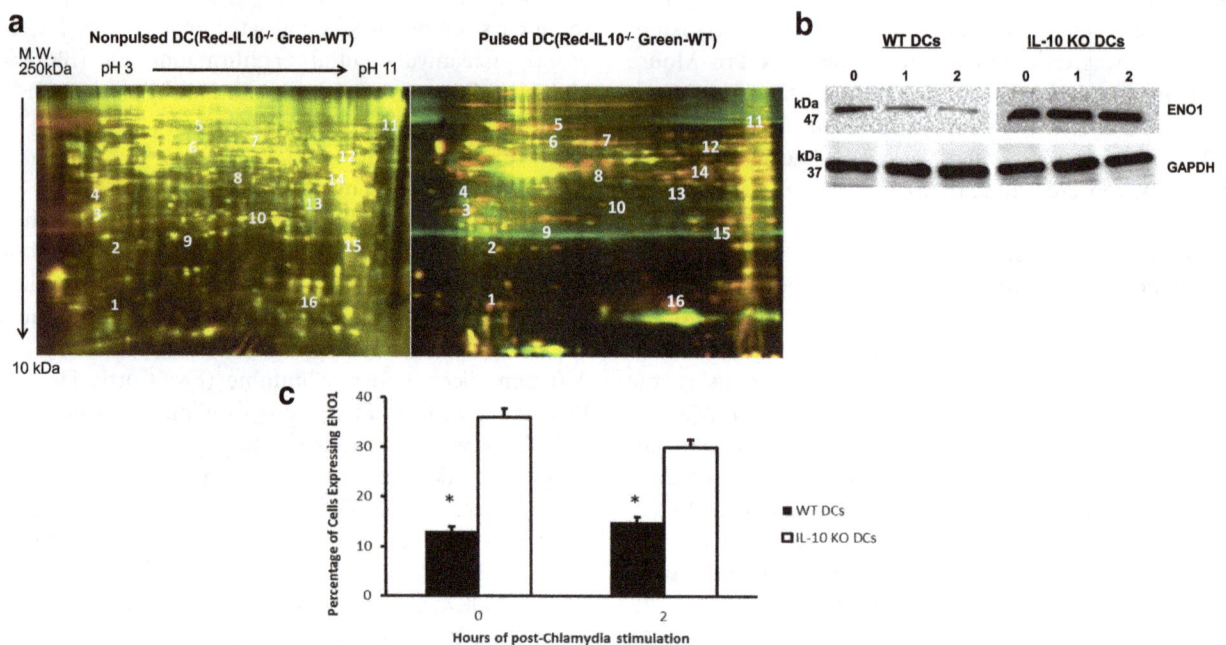

Fig. 1 Dynamic Distribution of ENO1 in DCs. **a** Dendritic Cell lysates were extracted from *Chlamydia* pulsed or nonpulsed WT DCs and IL-10$^{-/-}$ DCs. The Cy5 represents *red dye* and Cy3 represents *green dye*. The *red color* indicates high expression of protein in IL-10$^{-/-}$ DCs while the *green color* indicates high expression of protein in WT DCs. The *yellow color* indicates that the protein expression is the same for WT and IL-10 $^{-/-}$ DCs. **b** Western blot analysis of WT DCs and IL-10$^{-/-}$ DCs pulsed for 0 h, 1 h, and 2 h with *Chlamydia*. This result shows that ENO1 expression is decreased in WT DCs pulsed with *Chlamydia*. However, ENO1 expression is highly expressed in IL-10$^{-/-}$ DCs pulsed with *Chlamydia*. **c** In addition, we compared the amount of Chlamydia pulsed and nonpulsed WT and IL-10$^{-/-}$ DCs expressing ENO1 using confocal microscopic analysis. There was a significant difference in the amount of ENO1 expressing DCs in IL-10$^{-/-}$ DCs and WT DCs ($p < 0.05$). * Denotes statistical significance. We repeated this experiment 3 times

71 kDa protein). To rule out the possibility that we were working with normally overly expressed proteins, we evaluated the biological significance of the proteins, when we evaluated the metabolism related proteins by Western Blotting, ENO1 which is a key glycolytic enzyme was remarkably upregulated in IL-10$^{-/-}$ DCs compared to WT DCs (Fig. 1b). Moreover, we analyzed the percentage of IL-10$^{-/-}$ DCs expressing ENO1 using confocal microscopy (Fig. 1c). The results confirmed the upregulation of ENO1 as well as the dynamic distribution of ENO1 in IL-10$^{-/-}$ DCs after pulse with *Chlamydia*.

ENO1 Knockdown with ENO1-set siRNA Lentivector to study the role of ENO1 in DC function

Rapid and elevated T cell response is required for the clearance and establishment of long-term immunity against certain infectious and non-infectious diseases. Therefore, a better understanding of the functional aspects of the differentially expressed proteins in chlamydia-pulsed IL-10$^{-/-}$ DCs may furnish targets for modulating antigen presentation for enhanced T cell response against intracellular microbial pathogens and tumors. Using genetically engineered specific gene knockout systems and immunological and biochemical

blockers, we analyzed the effect of siRNA-mediated knockdown of ENO1 on DC functional integrity. The distribution of ENO1 in WT DCs is localized in both the nucleus and the cytoplasm, although it is more prominent in the latter, since the location of ENO1 determines its function (Fig. 2a). ENO1 expression was completely knocked down after 48 h of lentivector transfection. The control oligomer with a scrambled sequence, as described in the Methods section, did not show any reduced ENO1 expression (Fig. 2b).

ENO1 knockdown DCs have altered metabolism and mitochondrial morphology

The metabolic transition from oxidative phosphorylation (OXPHOS) to aerobic glycolysis upon exposure to microbial pathogens as the source of antigens is required for DC maturation and function. We therefore investigated the hypothesis that the suppression of ENO1 will interrupt this metabolic switch, suppress DC maturation and function upon exposure to *Chlamydia*. To confirm this hypothesis, we measured the production of pyruvate in DCs pulsed or nonpulsed with *C. muridarum*. DCs were pulsed at different time points and both the intracellular production of pyruvate and secretion of pyruvate were measured. The result showed that the secretion of

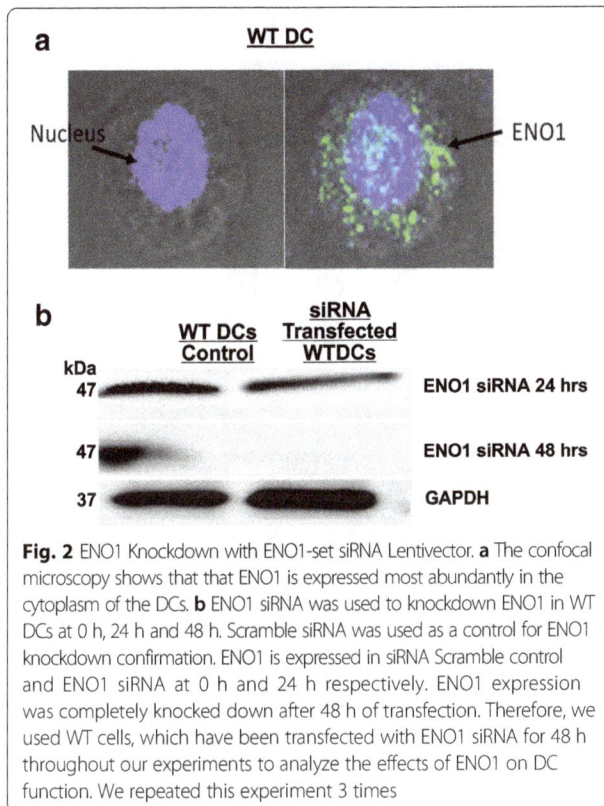

Fig. 2 ENO1 Knockdown with ENO1-set siRNA Lentivector. **a** The confocal microscopy shows that that ENO1 is expressed most abundantly in the cytoplasm of the DCs. **b** ENO1 siRNA was used to knockdown ENO1 in WT DCs at 0 h, 24 h and 48 h. Scramble siRNA was used as a control for ENO1 knockdown confirmation. ENO1 is expressed in siRNA Scramble control and ENO1 siRNA at 0 h and 24 h respectively. ENO1 expression was completely knocked down after 48 h of transfection. Therefore, we used WT cells, which have been transfected with ENO1 siRNA for 48 h throughout our experiments to analyze the effects of ENO1 on DC function. We repeated this experiment 3 times

pyruvate was significantly reduced in ENO1 knockdown DCs pulsed with *Chlamydia* at 0.5, 2, and 4 h ($P = 0.024$, 0.031, and 0.021, respectively) compared to *Chlamydia* pulsed WT DCs that had their ENO1 intact (Fig. 3a). The intracellular pyruvate production was also significantly decreased in ENO1 knockdown DCs at 0.5, 1, 2, and 4 h ($p \leq 0.05$) (Fig. 3b). We then investigated if the knockdown of ENO1 affected other enzymes involved in pyruvate metabolism further downstream. The expression of pyruvate dehydrogenase, which is involved in the conversion of pyruvate to acetyl CoA initiating the TCA (citric acid) cycle, was evaluated. Our results showed that pyruvate dehydrogenase expression was essentially indistinguishable in *Chlamydia*-pulsed and non-pulsed ENO1 knockdown DCs and WT DCs (Fig. 3c). These results suggest that the absence of ENO1 slowed the rate of production of pyruvate after pulsing the DCs with *C. muridarum* and that pyruvate dehydrogenase is not involved in this process.

Mitochondria are central to cellular energetics, metabolism, and regulation. The shape of the mitochondria and remodeling of the mitochondrial cristae instructs cell metabolic adaptation. To determine if the knockdown of ENO1 also influenced the mitochondrial phenotype we proceeded to perform transmission electron microscopy (TEM). Alteration of mitochondrial

shape as well as cristae remodeling were observed in *Chlamydia*-pulsed ENO1 knockdown DCs. There appeared to be elongated mitochondria with tubular network-like cristae in nonpulsed WT, ENO1 knockdown DCs and *Chlamydia*-pulsed WT DCs, whereas, we observed fragmented mitochondria morphology with widened intermembrane space along with short and stumpy cristae in *Chlamydia-pulsed* ENO1 knockdown DCs (Fig. 3d). This led us to investigate whether ENO1 knockdown influenced the expression of some mitochondrial-associated proteins (Tom20 and ANT1/2/3/4). Western blot analysis showed a differential expression of TOM20 and ANT 1/2/3/4 in *Chlamydia*-pulsed ENO1 knockdown DCs (Fig. 3e). These data suggest that in suppression of ENO1 expression leads to mitochondrial cristae remodeling which is coincident with metabolic reprogramming in *Chlamydia*-pulsed *D*Cs.

ENO1 affects DC apoptosis

DC survival is crucial for the APC function and we have previously reported that IL-10 deficient DCs resist apoptosis [18]. We therefore hypothesized that ENO1 upregulation may play a role in DC resistance to apoptosis and promotion of cell survival following exposure to *Chlamydia* antigen. Results from analysis of ENO1 knockdown DCs apoptosis using annexin V and 7-AAD showed that *Chlamydia*-pulsed ENO1 knockdown DCs were more apoptotic than the WT DCs ($p < 0.05$) (Fig. 4). This indicates that ENO1 is an essential anti-apoptotic molecule in DCs during chlamydia infection and that IL-10 deficiency that upregulates ENO1 in DCs decreases susceptibility to apoptosis.

ENO1 regulates DC maturation and activation

IL-10 deficient DCs exhibit rapid maturation and activation to efficiently present chlamydial antigens [17]. Therefore recent data revealing that the reprogramming of DC metabolism controls their maturation, activation and antigen presenting functions [14] would suggest that ENO1-mediated modulation of DC metabolism would affect the maturation and activation of DCs. We analyzed the effect of ENO1 knockdown on maturation and activation markers of DCs using flow cytometry. The results showed that TLR4 was significantly lower in all ENO1 knockdown DCs compared to WT DCs ($p \leq 0.05$) (Fig. 5). CD40 was upregulated in ENO1 knockdown DCs (Fig. 5). In addition, when we analyzed other maturation markers MHC II, CD80 and CD86, the results showed that all three markers had a meaningfully lower expression in *Chlamydia*-pulsed ENO1 knockdown DCs compared to *Chlamydia*-pulsed WT DCs ($p \leq 0.05$) (Figs. 5 & 6). To further determine the effect of ENO1 on the ability of DCs to activate T cells, we

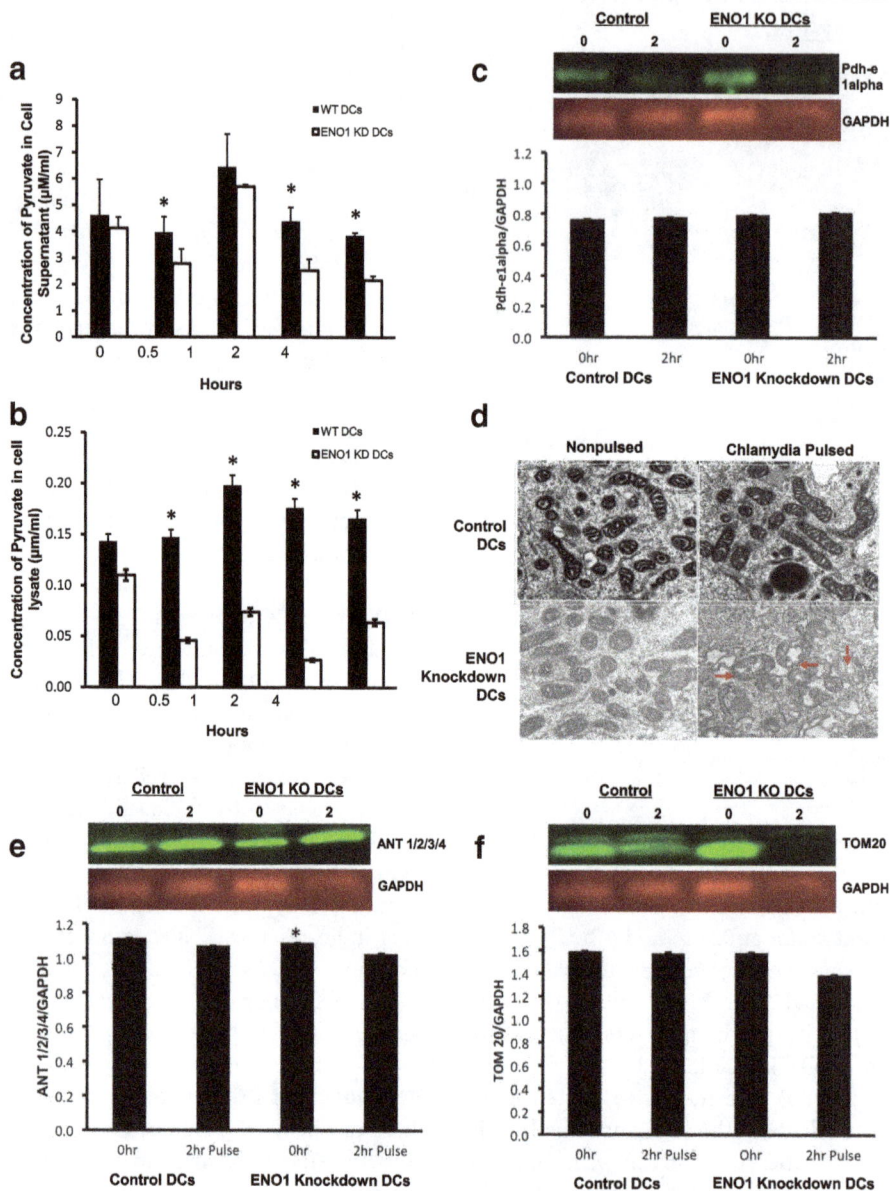

Fig. 3 ENO1 knockdown DCs have altered metabolism and mitochondrial morphology. **a & b** Pyruvate Concentration in *Chlamydia*-pulsed Dendritic Cells. Pyruvate concentration was obtained in DC lysates and supernatant. Pyruvate concentration was measured using a spectrophotometer. Pyruvate concentration was determined after pulsing with *Chlamydia* at different time points for 0, 0.5, 1, 2 and 4 h. The concentration of pyruvate was significantly higher in WT cells compared to ENO1 knockdown DCs ($p < 0.05$). * Denotes statistical significance. This experiment was repeated 3 times. **c** Pyruvate dehydrogenase expression in Chlamydia-pulsed WT and ENO1 knockdown DCs. The total protein was detected using Cy5 dye and the protein of interest, in this case pyruvate dehydrogenase, was probed using Cy3 secondary antibody from the Amersham System (GE Healthcare, Pittsburgh, PA). Proteins were normalized using ImageQuant Reader (GE Healthcare, Pittsburgh, PA). The ratio of Cy3/Cy5 indicates the differentially expressed proteins. This experiment was repeated 3 times. **d** TEM analysis of the WT and ENO1 knockdown DCs. The results indicate that there are morphological differences in the mitochondria of Chlamydia pulsed and nonpulsed WT and ENO1 knockdown DCs using TEM. This depicts the remodeling of the mitochondria to tubular and fused, with tight cristae in the WT DCs and to more circular, swollen and fissed with loose cristae in ENO1 knockdown DCs. **e & f** Expression of mitochondrial associated proteins. The blots shown are proteins associated with mitochondrial function. ANT 1/2/3/4 and TOM 20 were differentially expressed in Chlamydia pulsed ENO1 knockdown DCs. * denotes statistical significance. This experiment was repeated 3 times

evaluated the cytokine profile of DCs. Results shown that Th1 type cytokine (IL-1α, IL-1β, IL-12, and IFN-γ) production was statistically lower in *Chlamydia*-pulsed ENO1 knockdown DCs ($p \leq 0.05$), while they concomitantly expressed a higher amount of the CD4$^+$ T helper cell type 2 (Th2) cytokines IL-4, IL-10, and IL-17 compared to *Chlamydia*-pulsed WT DCs ($p \leq 0.05$) (Fig. 7a). Interestingly, tumor necrosis factor (TNF)-α, which induces apoptosis of infiltrating inflammatory cells during genital *Chlamydia* infection [27] was highly

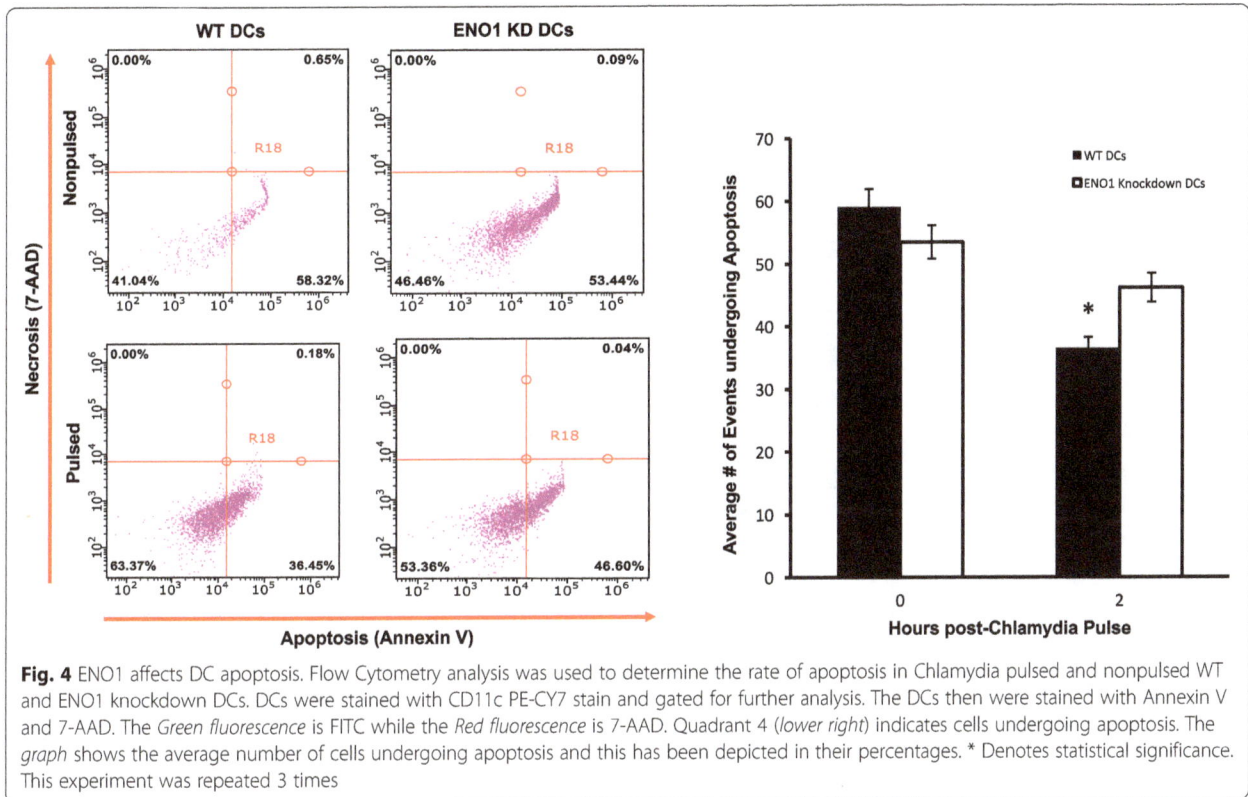

Fig. 4 ENO1 affects DC apoptosis. Flow Cytometry analysis was used to determine the rate of apoptosis in Chlamydia pulsed and nonpulsed WT and ENO1 knockdown DCs. DCs were stained with CD11c PE-CY7 stain and gated for further analysis. The DCs then were stained with Annexin V and 7-AAD. The *Green fluorescence* is FITC while the *Red fluorescence* is 7-AAD. Quadrant 4 (*lower right*) indicates cells undergoing apoptosis. The *graph* shows the average number of cells undergoing apoptosis and this has been depicted in their percentages. * Denotes statistical significance. This experiment was repeated 3 times

expressed in ENO1 knockdown DCs ($p \leq 0.05$) (Fig. 7a). We also analyzed some chemokines, and the results were mixed, with *Chlamydia*-pulsed ENO1 knockdown DCs having reduced expression of MCP-1 and Rantes and increased expression of macrophage inflammatory proteins (MIP) -1α and -1β compared to *Chlamydia*-pulsed WT DCs (Fig. 7b). Rantes and MCP-1 recruit monocytes, memory T cells, and dendritic cells to the sites of inflammation produced by infection. MIP proteins activate human granulocytes (neutrophils, eosinophils and basophils) too much of which could lead to acute neutrophilic inflammation [28, 29]. Thus overall, the suppression of ENO1 in *Chlamydia*-pulsed DCs appeared to have a deleterious effect on DCs' activating properties, by producing the inflammatory type of cytokines and chemokines, and enhancing apoptosis.

Effect of ENO1 on the antigen presenting function of DCs in vivo and in vitro

IL-10 deficient DCs exhibited efficient chlamydial antigen presentation and activated a high frequency of specific T cells and antibodies against *Chlamydia* [17, 20]. To further determine the role of ENO1 in the antigen presenting function of DCs in vivo and in vitro DCs, which were pulsed with *C. muridarum* for 2 h, were co-cultured with splenic CD4+ T cells from immune mice for 5 days. We compared the antigen presenting function of

DCs in WT and ENO1 knockdown DCs. Data showed a significant impairment in the ability of ENO1 knockdown DCs to induce antigen specific proliferation of T cells and cytokine secretion ($p \leq 0.05$) (Fig. 8a). It was not feasible to include ENO1-over-expressing WT DCs in these studies for technical reasons. Results showed a decrease in secretion of IL-1α, IL-1β, & Rantes and an increase in secretion of IL-5, IL-13, IL17A, and IL-10 in Chlamydia pulsed ENO1 knockdown DCs incubated with immune CD4+ T cells compared to the WT DCs incubated with immune T cells ($P \leq 0.01$) (Fig. 8b). This result indicates that the absence of ENO1 in DCs abrogates their capacity to present chlamydial antigen to T cells, which will lead to antigen specific Th2 immunity against *Chlamydia* infection in vivo. To further buttress our hypothesis ENO1 knockdown causes a dysregulation of DC metabolism that alters the DC function during Chlamydia infection. Chlamydia pulsed WT, IL-10$^{-/-}$ and ENO1 knockdown DCs were adoptively transferred to naive WT mice though tail vein injection. The mice were then infected intravaginally with 10^5 IFU of *C. muridarum* 1 week after adoptive transfer. The course of infection and bacterial load were monitored. WT mice that received Chlamydia pulsed ENO1 knockdown DCs experienced a longer period of bacterial shedding and higher bacterial load when compared to the Chlamydia pulsed IL-10$^{-/-}$ and WT DCs (Fig. 8c). In vivo data suggests that ENO1 knockdown DCs lose the ability

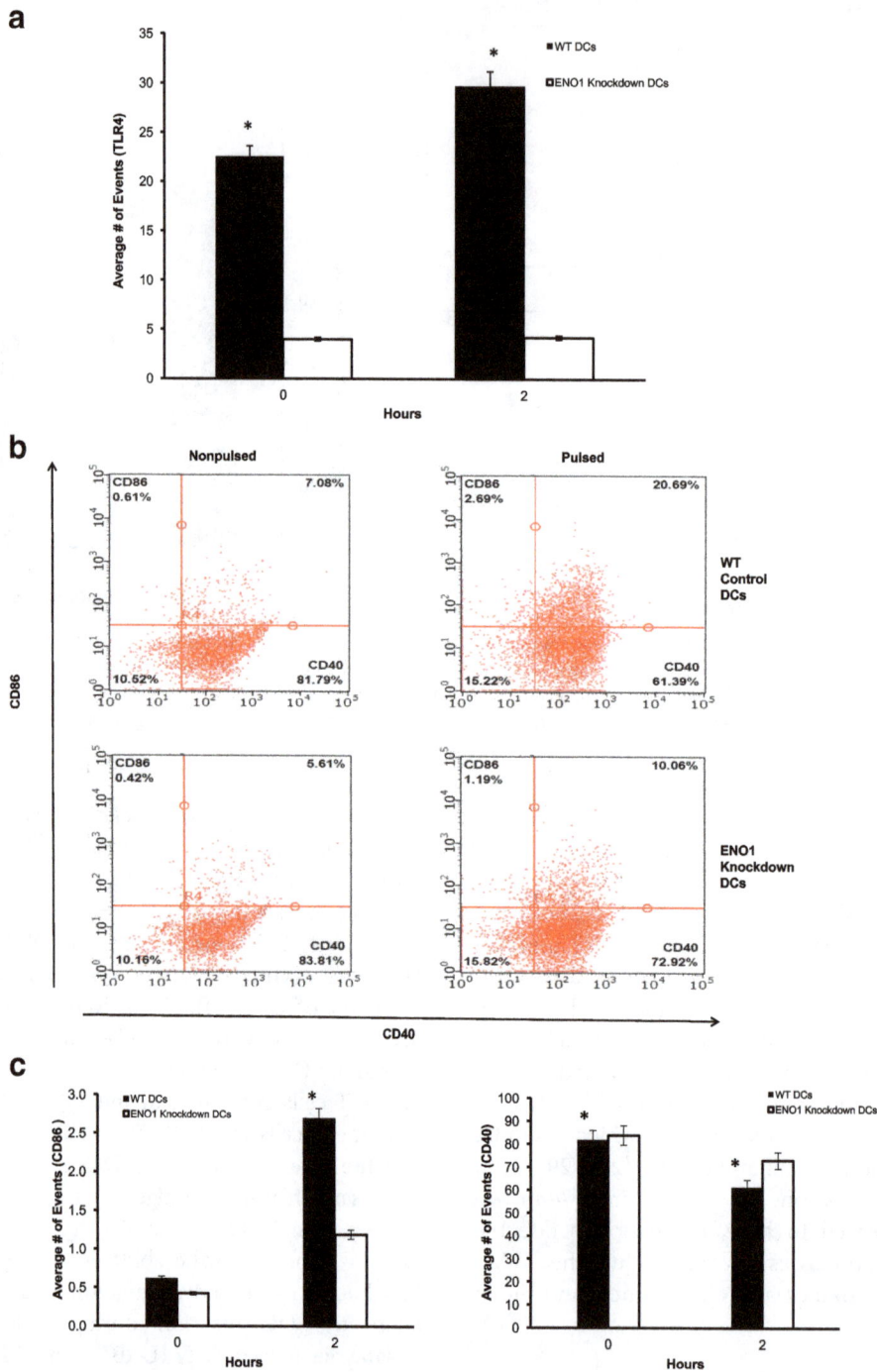

Fig. 5 ENO1 regulates DC maturation and activation (1). **a** Flow cytometry analysis using BD Accuri C6 analyzer was used to determine TLR4 expression. DCs were stained with CD11c PE-CY7 stain and gated for further analysis. Cells were then stained with FITC conjugated with TLR4. TLR4 expression was significantly lower in Chlamydia pulsed ENO1 knockdown DCs in comparison to Chlamydia pulsed WT DCs. **b** Flow Cytometry analysis was also used to determine the population of cells with the maturation and activation markers CD40 and CD86 expression in DCs. Cells were stained with FITC conjugated CD40 and PE Conjugated CD86. Samples double stained with PE and FITC were compensated. Green-B-Fluorescence indicates FITC staining and Yellow-B Fluorescence indicates PE staining. **c** The graph shows that there were significant differences between WT and ENO1 knockdown DCs ($p < 0.05$). The expression of CD86 was lower in Chlamydia pulsed ENO1 knockdown DCs compared to WT DCs. While, CD40 expression increased in Chlamydia pulsed ENO1 knockdown DCs. Experiment was repeated 3 times for each sample. * Denotes statistical significance

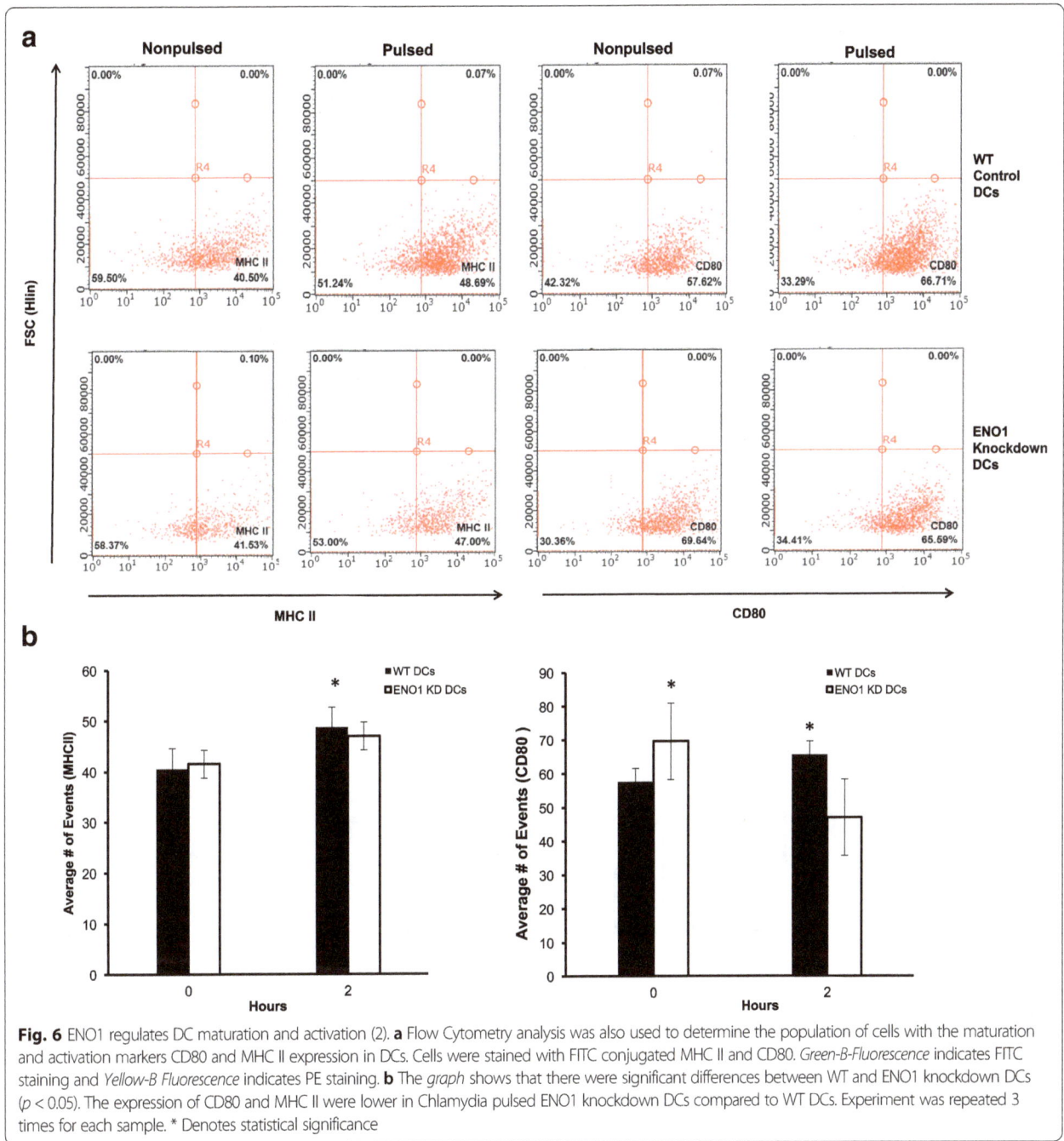

Fig. 6 ENO1 regulates DC maturation and activation (2). a Flow Cytometry analysis was also used to determine the population of cells with the maturation and activation markers CD80 and MHC II expression in DCs. Cells were stained with FITC conjugated MHC II and CD80. *Green-B-Fluorescence* indicates FITC staining and *Yellow-B Fluorescence* indicates PE staining. b The *graph* shows that there were significant differences between WT and ENO1 knockdown DCs ($p < 0.05$). The expression of CD80 and MHC II were lower in Chlamydia pulsed ENO1 knockdown DCs compared to WT DCs. Experiment was repeated 3 times for each sample. * Denotes statistical significance

to induce a robust Th1 immune response that is required for infection clearance.

Discussion

IL10$^{-/-}$ mice have been shown to clear Chlamydia infections at a faster rate than WT mice, and this protective ability of the IL-10$^{-/-}$ mice has been linked with the presence of IL-10$^{-/-}$ DCs [17, 20]. In our ongoing study of the function of IL-10$^{-/-}$ DCs during Chlamydia infection, we observed using 2-DIGE proteomics, the differential expression of the protein ENO1, which was

up regulated in IL-10$^{-/-}$ DCs compared to WT DCs. We later validated this through Western blotting and confocal microscopy analysis, where we showed that ENO1 expression decreased with time in WT DCs during Chlamydia infection, however, the levels of ENO1 in IL-10$^{-/-}$ DCs remained consistently high all through. In this study, we performed a preliminary study to elucidate a role for ENO1 in the function of DCs during Chlamydia infection. ENO1 is a glycolytic enzyme, which has been found to play other roles in inflammation, tumor suppression, monocyte and mast cell

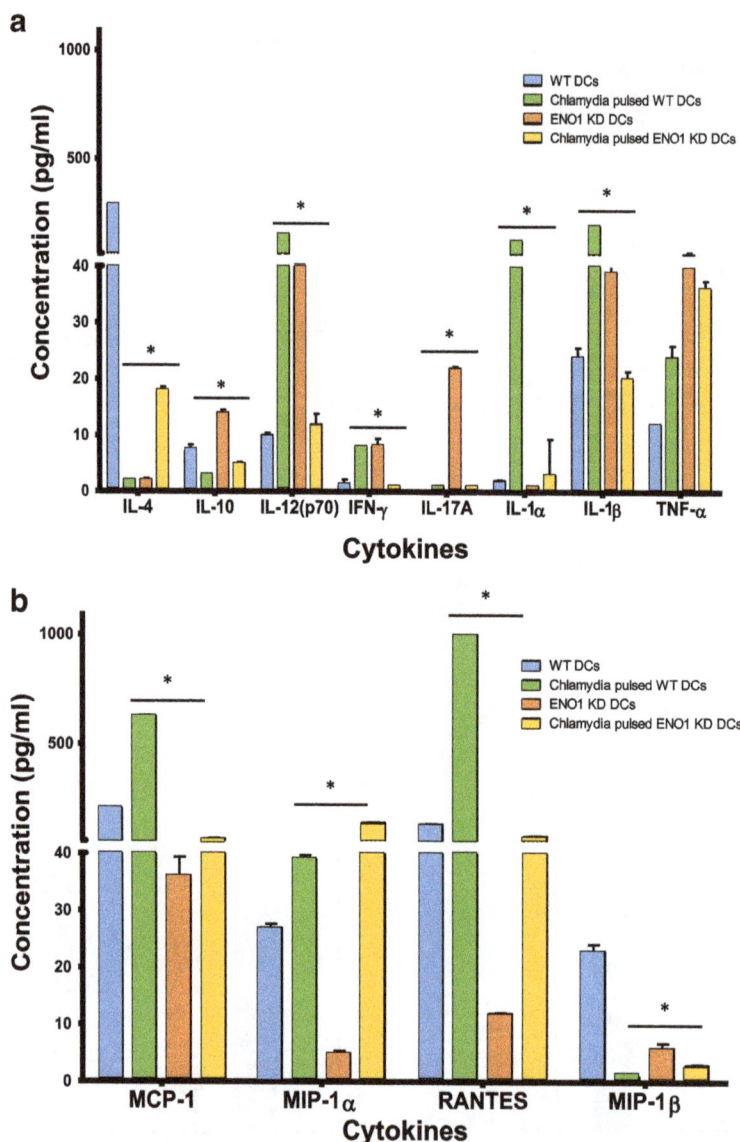

Fig. 7 ENO1 regulates DC maturation and activation (3). **a** Bio-Plex Pro Mouse Cytokine 23-Plex multiplex array (Bio-Rad, Hercules, CA) was used for cytokine analysis according to manufacturer's guidelines. The expression of Th1 type cytokines (IL-1α, IL-1β, IL-12, and IFN-γ) were low ($p \leq 0.05$), while, there was a high expression of the Th2 cytokines IL-4, IL-10, and IL-17 in Chlamydia pulsed ENO1 knockdown DCs compared to Chlamydia pulsed WT DCs ($p \leq 0.05$). TNF-α was highly expressed in ENO1 knockdown DCs ($p \leq 0.05$). Experiment was repeated 3 times. **b** Chemokine analysis showed that Chlamydia pulsed ENO1 knockdown DCs have low expression of monocyte chemoattractant protein 1 (MCP-1) and Rantes and high expression of MIP-1α and MIP-1β compared to Chlamydia pulsed WT DCs. * denotes statistical significance. Experiment was repeated 3 times

differentiation [21, 22]. To understand the role of ENO1 in DCs during chlamydia infection, we first determined its intracellular location, as this had been shown to play a role to play in its function. We determined that ENO1 was mainly located in the cytoplasm, and that this would be related to its primary role in glycolysis, the conversion of 2-phosphoglycerate to phosphoenolpyruvate [22].

To find out if ENO1 was associated with the immunoregulatory properties of DCs during chlamydia infection we first silenced ENO1 gene in DCs using siRNA lentiviral system to knockdown the gene. This knockdown

was completed at 48 h after the addition of the virus. We then determined the amount of pyruvate produced in chlamydia pulsed ENO1 knockdown and WT DCs in a time course experiment. We noticed that the amount of pyruvate produced in chlamydia pulsed ENO1 knockdown DCs was significantly lower than that produced by chlamydia pulsed WT DCs. This result was expected since ENO1 was responsible for dehydrating 2-phosphoglycerate to phosphoenolpyruvate which is then converted to pyruvate [22]. It highlighted the fact that the rate of producing pyruvate which is the final product of glycolysis was being

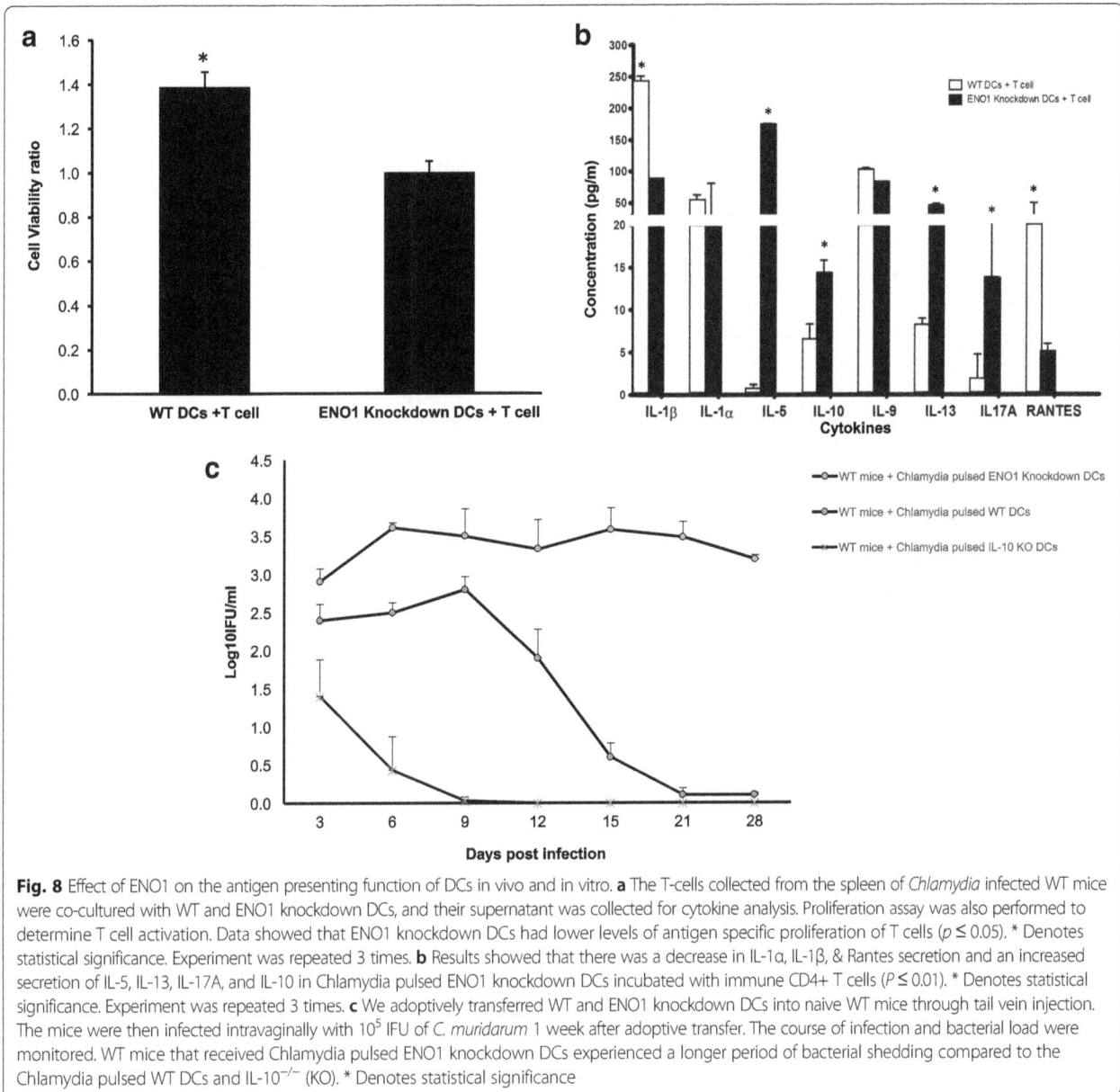

Fig. 8 Effect of ENO1 on the antigen presenting function of DCs in vivo and in vitro. **a** The T-cells collected from the spleen of *Chlamydia* infected WT mice were co-cultured with WT and ENO1 knockdown DCs, and their supernatant was collected for cytokine analysis. Proliferation assay was also performed to determine T cell activation. Data showed that ENO1 knockdown DCs had lower levels of antigen specific proliferation of T cells ($p \leq 0.05$). * Denotes statistical significance. Experiment was repeated 3 times. **b** Results showed that there was a decrease in IL-1α, IL-1β, & Rantes secretion and an increased secretion of IL-5, IL-13, IL-17A, and IL-10 in Chlamydia pulsed ENO1 knockdown DCs incubated with immune CD4+ T cells ($P \leq 0.01$). * Denotes statistical significance. Experiment was repeated 3 times. **c** We adoptively transferred WT and ENO1 knockdown DCs into naive WT mice through tail vein injection. The mice were then infected intravaginally with 10^5 IFU of *C. muridarum* 1 week after adoptive transfer. The course of infection and bacterial load were monitored. WT mice that received Chlamydia pulsed ENO1 knockdown DCs experienced a longer period of bacterial shedding compared to the Chlamydia pulsed WT DCs and IL-10$^{-/-}$ (KO). * Denotes statistical significance

hindered in the chlamydia pulsed ENO1 knockdown DCs, which might influence the function of these DCs. Checking to see if the enzyme pyruvate dehydrogenase which is responsible for converting pyruvate to acetyl CoA would be affected by the reduction in the amount of pyruvate produced, we noticed no difference in the expression of pyruvate dehydrogenase between the chlamydia pulsed or nonpulsed WT and ENO1 knockdown DCs. This meant that knockdown of ENO1 in DCs only affects pyruvate production and it does not affect the other enzymes involved in the metabolic process. It is becoming increasingly clear that DC activation and function coincide with cellular metabolism, which is tailored towards the bioenergetic and biosynthetic needs of cells [14, 15]. Notable changes during activation include enhanced glycolysis, the accumulation of

succinate and the biosynthesis of fatty acids from citrate to support lipid biosynthesis. Those alterations in metabolism are required to meet the increased biosynthetic and bioenergetic demands of activated DCs specifically by funneling metabolites into pathways for lipid and protein synthesis [14, 30–33]. Disruption of glycolysis through the reduced expression of ENO1 has recently been linked to NLRP3 activation [23], and we have previously shown that NLRP3 inflammasome assembly was suppressed in IL-10$^{-/-}$ DCs [18], which we now know to have abundantly expressed ENO1, this shows an interesting linkage of ENO1 to the inflammasome that would be explored further.

Collectively, these metabolic changes in DCs also facilitate the homeostasis of their mitochondria, which are center hubs for metabolic activity. Therefore, we evaluated the morphology of mitochondria in WT and ENO1 knockdown DCs nonpulsed or pulsed with Chlamydia. We found that the morphology of the mitochondria in the Chlamydia pulsed ENO1 knockdown DCs was markedly different from the regular mitochondrial morphology which was apparent in Chlamydia pulsed WT DCs and even to some extent in the nonpulsed ENO1 knockdown DCs. The mitochondria in Chlamydia pulsed ENO1 knockdown DCs appeared fissed, swollen and had loose cristae, which appeared, shortened, stumpy and dispersed. It seems that the reduced production of pyruvate caused by the silencing of ENO1 has led to a drastic change in mitochondrial structure causing cristae remodeling, which becomes apparent when the DC is pulsed with Chlamydia. This remodeling has been reported recently by another group specializing in effector and memory T cells; where their data indicated that mitochondria cristae remodeling and/or fission acts as a signal to drive the induction of aerobic glycolysis and subsequent cell activation [15], they also validated this in DCs and macrophages. Here we postulate that the Chlamydia pulsed WT mitochondria were still in their tubular fused form and so would function in the oxidative phosphorylation pathway, while the mitochondria in the Chlamydia pulsed ENO1 knockdown DCs were in the fissed form and so were prone to have reduced electron transport chain efficiency and promote aerobic glycolysis. To find out if underlying modifications in the expression of other mitochondrial associated proteins are associated with this change in morphology, we looked at the expression of TOM20 and ANT 1/2/3/4. There was a differential expression of TOM20 and ANT 1/2/3/4 in Chlamydia pulsed ENO1 knockdown DCs compared to Chlamydia pulsed WT DCs. Tom 20 is a central component of the translocase of the outer membrane (TOM) complex receptor, which recognizes and transports mitochondrial preproteins synthesized in the cytosol [34]. ANT is in the inner membrane of the mitochondria and is a component of the permeability transition pore complex, which has been established to play an important role in mitochondrial homeostasis [35]. Cellular models have shown that permeability transition pore complex opening dissipates the transmembrane inner potential, triggers matrix swelling, releasing cytochrome C into the cytosol, and subsequent cell apoptosis. It has been shown in ANT knockout (KO) studies that ANT not only plays an essential structural role but also has a regulatory function for permeability transition pore complex (PTPC) [36]. In this study, TOM20 and ANT1/2/3/4 expression were differentially expressed in Chlamydia pulsed ENO1 knockdown DCs with the mitochondria having progressively enlarged cristae and intermembrane spaces, suggesting that these proteins might be essential in determining the permeability of the mitochondria.

In this study, we have shown that Chlamydia pulsed ENO1 knockdown DCs have dysregulated mitochondria, which appeared swollen, fissed and have shortened/dispersed cristae. We have also shown that there are changes in proteins associated with mitochondria permeability. All these changes should inherently lead to a high level of apoptosis in these DCs. Therefore, we wanted to find out if this influenced DC survival. The results showed that there was an apparent increase in apoptosis in chlamydia pulsed ENO1 knockdown DCs compared to chlamydia pulsed WT DCs. This result implies that the alterations of DC metabolism and the mitochondria did actually have an effect on DC survival [37].

We then hypothesized that these changes in metabolism, mitochondrial structure and survival in chlamydia pulsed ENO1 knockdown DCs would have an impact on the activation and function of these DCs. We decided to look at the DCs maturation and activation markers including the cytokines produced, as well as the antigen presenting function of these DCs. Results show that Chlamydia pulsed ENO1 knockdown DCs had fewer cells expressing TLR4, CD80, CD86 and MHC II compared to Chlamydia pulsed WT DCs, thus implying that ENO1 is integral in maintaining the maturation of DCs. We further assessed the probability that this phenomenon was real, by analyzing the cytokines and chemokines produced by these DCs. There was a lower expression of the Th1 cytokine IL-12, and a higher expression of the Th2 cytokines IL-4 and IL-10 in Chlamydia pulsed ENO1 knockdown DCs compared to Chlamydia pulsed WT DCs. This result could be interpreted to mean that when ENO1 is silenced, the DCs become less inclined to fight off Chlamydia infection, since we know that the immune response against Chlamydia requires a Th1 and not Th2 response. Amongst the cytokines we evaluated, we observed that IFN-γ expression was decreased in Chlamydia pulsed ENO1 knockdown DCs compared to Chlamydia pulsed WT DCs. We know that IFN-γ is an activator of T-bet and an inhibitor of GATA-3, which are transcription factors regulating Th1 and Th2 differentiation respectively [38]. This result implies that IFN-γ would not be available to inhibit GATA-3, thus leading to a tilt towards the Th2 phenotype. The pro-inflammatory cytokines IL-1α and IL-1β were expressed at lower levels in Chlamydia pulsed ENO1 knockdown DCs compared to Chlamydia pulsed WT DCs, however TNF-α another pro-inflammatory cytokine was highly expressed in ENO1 knockdown DCs. We know that having a good boost of early IL-1 production is good for priming the innate immune system [18, 39], thus the reduced production of IL-1 in Chlamydia pulsed ENO1 knockdown DCs constitutes an immune deficiency in the clearance of Chlamydia. Increased production of TNF-α has been associated with inflammatory conditions that might lead to pathogenesis of the local area of infection [40]. In addition to the cytokine we also studied the chemokine produced by the DCs. We had mixed results with Chlamydia pulsed ENO1 knockdown DCs having reduced expression of MCP-1 and Rantes and increased expression of MIP-1α and MIP-1β compared to Chlamydia pulse WT DCs. It has been shown MCP-1 and Rantes are important in signaling cells of the innate immune and adaptive immunity to migrate towards the site of infection [28, 29]. In a bid to further determine the role of ENO1 in activation of T cells we performed T cell proliferation assays and the results showed that T cell proliferation was significantly lower in ENO1 knockdown DCs compared to WT DCs, in addition, cytokine assay results showed that Th2 enhancing cytokines IL-5, IL-10 and IL-13 expression, were increased in cultures with Chlamydia pulsed ENO1 knockdown DCs. This result further buttresses the fact that Chlamydia pulsed ENO1 knockdown DCs were more inclined to balance the immune system towards the Th2 phenotype, which would be unable to clear a Chlamydia infection. This is in addition to the fact that the expression of the chemokine Rantes was also lowered in the co-cultures with Chlamydia pulsed ENO1 knockdown DCs. This would lead to a reduction in the migration of cells to the point of infection. Our results has been corroborated by some recent studies that have established that ENO1 is able to activate CD14-dependent TLR4 pathway on monocytes, which involves a dual mechanism firstly pro-inflammatory and secondly anti-inflammatory [41]; and that ENO1 has also been linked to the regulation of differentiation of mast cells [42].

Furthermore, we wanted to show in vivo that ENO1 is important in clearing Chlamydia infection, so we carried out an adoptive transfer experiment. The results showed that WT mice that were adoptively transferred with Chlamydia pulsed IL-10$^{-/-}$ and WT DCs were better able to clear their Chlamydia infection compared to mice that were adoptively transferred with Chlamydia pulsed ENO1 knockdown DCs. This consolidated our previous results showing that the Chlamydia pulsed ENO1 knockdown DCs were not able to function optimally in clearing the Chlamydia in the mice because of the absence of ENO1, which we believe is regulated by IL-10. This result has implication in the use of ENO1 as a therapeutic treatment during Chlamydia infection; in addition, it has been shown that ENO1 deoxyribonucleic acid elicits humoral and cellular immune responses against pancreatic tumors, delays tumor progression [43].

Conclusions

In summary, we have concluded that ENO1 is important in the functioning of DCs during chlamydia infection.

We first observed this possibility by the high levels of ENO1 produced in IL-10$^{-/-}$ DCs, and we were inclined to find out if indeed this phenomenon had a real bearing in the Chlamydia clearing ability of IL-10$^{-/-}$ DCs. Results showed that the reduction in ENO1 expression in WT DCs happened after a period and that this led to a reduction in pyruvate which we believe is central to all the various factors involved in the process of metabolism and the eventual maturation and activation of the DCs. New studies show that immune cell activation coincides with cellular metabolism that is tailored towards the bioenergetic and biosynthetic needs of these cells. Studies have demonstrated the contribution of cellular metabolic pathways to the ability of immune cells to sense the microenvironment and to alter their function [12–15]. Changes in the microenvironment induce a broad spectrum of inducible and reversible metabolic programs, which in turn forms the basis of the inducible and reversible spectrum of functional immune cell activation/polarization phenotypes. This alteration in glycolytic metabolism and mitochondrial morphology, which we have observed in this study, might be required to meet the increased biosynthetic and bioenergetic demands of the Chlamydia, activated DCs [14]. The findings in this study suggest that ENO1 can be used as an immunotherapeutic strategy for inducing adequate and long-term immunity against Chlamydia-induced tubal pathologies. This because there are presently no Food and Drug Administration (FDA) approved, commercially available vaccines with built-in biologically safe immunomodulators, so if successful, our findings could have important implications for the rational design of next-generation vaccines for boosting vaccine efficacy. Modulation of alpha enolase thus provides a potentially effective strategy to boost DC function and promote immunity against intracellular microbial pathogens.

Abbreviations

2D-DIGE: Two-dimensional fluorescence differential gel electrophoresis analysis; 7-AAD: 7-amino-actinomycin D; ANT: Adenine nucleotide translocator; APC: Allophycocyanin; CD: Cluster of differentiation; DCs: Dendritic cells; EBs: Elementary bodies; ENO1: Alpha enolase; FDA: Food and Drug Administration; FITC: Fluorescein isothiocyanate; GM-CSF: Granulocyte-macrophage colony-stimulating factor; IFN-γ: Interferon gamma; IFU: Inclusion forming units; IL: Interleukin; IL-10$^{-/-}$: IL-10 knockout; LEK1: Leucine/glutamic acid/lysine protein 1; MCP-1: Monocyte chemoattractant protein 1; MEM: Minimum essential medium; MHC: Major histocompatibility complex; MIP-1α: Macrophage Inflammatory Protein -alpha; MIP-1β: Macrophage Inflammatory Protein -beta; NLRP3: NLR family pyrin domain containing 3; OXPHOS: Oxidative phosphorylation; PE: Phycoerythrin; PTPC: Permeability transition pore complex; TEM: Transmission electron microscopy; TFI: Tubal factor infertility; Th1: CD4$^+$ T helper cell type 1; Th2: CD4$^+$ T helper cell type 2; TLR4: Toll like receptor 4; TNF-α: Tumor necrosis factor- alpha; WT: Wild type

Acknowledgements
We thank Andrew Shaw of Georgia Institute of Technology Microscopy and Microanalysis Core for assistance provided with the Confocal Microscopy. We would also like to thank Mr. Brako of the Morehouse School of Medicine Core labs for assistance provided with the Transmission Electron Microscopy.

Funding
This work was supported by NIH grant 8G12MD007602 from the NIMHD, 1SC2HD086066-01A1 from NICHD to Dr. Omosun and 1SC1AII03041-01A1 from NIGMS to Dr. Qing He.

Authors' contributions
KR, YO, DM, KS, CCM and QH performed the experiments; KR, YO, DM, KS and QH performed the animal work; KR, YO and QH assisted with data analysis; KR, YO, NB, FE, CB, JUI and QH contributed to the study design and participated in the manuscript preparation. All authors read and approved this manuscript for publication.

Competing interests
The authors declare that they have no competing interests.

Author details
[1]Department of Microbiology, Biochemistry, and Immunology, Morehouse School of Medicine, 720 Westview Drive S.W., Atlanta, GA 30310, USA. [2]Department of Biology, Clark Atlanta University, Atlanta, GA 30314, USA. [3]Centers for Disease Control & Prevention (CDC), Atlanta, GA 30333, USA.

References
1. Torrone E, Papp J, Weinstock H. Prevalence of Chlamydia trachomatis genital infection among persons aged 14–39 years - United States, 2007–2012. MMWR Morb Mortal Wkly Rep. 2014;63(38):834–8.
2. Darville T, Pelvic Inflammatory Disease Workshop Proceedings C. Pelvic inflammatory disease: identifying research gaps–proceedings of a workshop sponsored by Department of Health and Human Services/National Institutes of Health/National Institute of Allergy and Infectious Diseases, November 3–4, 2011. Sex Transm Dis. 2013;40(10):761–7.
3. Price MJ, Ades AE, Welton NJ, Simms I, Macleod J, Horner PJ. Proportion of pelvic inflammatory disease cases caused by Chlamydia trachomatis: consistent picture from different methods. J Infect Dis. 2016;214(4):617–24.
4. Price MJ, Ades AE, Soldan K, Welton NJ, Macleod J, Simms I, DeAngelis D, Turner KM, Horner PJ. The natural history of Chlamydia trachomatis infection in women: a multi-parameter evidence synthesis. Health Technol Assess. 2016;20(22):1–250.
5. Turner K, Adams E, Grant A, Macleod J, Bell G, Clarke J, Horner P. Costs and cost effectiveness of different strategies for chlamydia screening and partner notification: an economic and mathematical modelling study. BMJ. 2011;342:c7250.
6. Regan DG, Wilson DP, Hocking JS. Coverage is the key for effective screening of Chlamydia trachomatis in Australia. J Infect Dis. 2008;198(3):349–58.
7. Hafner LM, Wilson DP, Timms P. Development status and future prospects for a vaccine against Chlamydia trachomatis infection. Vaccine. 2014;32(14):1563–71.
8. Poston TB, Darville T. Chlamydia trachomatis: protective adaptive responses and prospects for a vaccine. Curr Top Microbiol Immunol. 2016. [Epub ahead of print].
9. Eko FO, Mania-Pramanik J, Pais R, Pan Q, Okenu DM, Johnson A, Ibegbu C, He C, He Q, Russell R, et al. Vibrio cholerae ghosts (VCG) exert immunomodulatory effect on dendritic cells for enhanced antigen presentation and induction of protective immunity. BMC Immunol. 2014;15:584.
10. Rey-Ladino J, Koochesfahani KM, Zaharik ML, Shen C, Brunham RC. A live and inactivated Chlamydia trachomatis mouse pneumonitis strain induces the maturation of dendritic cells that are phenotypically and immunologically distinct. Infect Immun. 2005;73(3):1568–77.
11. Wang S, Fan Y, Brunham RC, Yang X. IFN-gamma knockout mice show Th2-associated delayed-type hypersensitivity and the inflammatory cells fail to localize and control chlamydial infection. Eur J Immunol. 1999;29(11):3782–92.
12. Pearce EL, Poffenberger MC, Chang CH, Jones RG. Fueling immunity: insights into metabolism and lymphocyte function. Science. 2013;342(6155):1242454.
13. Pearce EL, Pearce EJ. Metabolic pathways in immune cell activation and quiescence. Immunity. 2013;38(4):633–43.
14. Everts B, Amiel E, Huang SC, Smith AM, Chang CH, Lam WY, Redmann V, Freitas TC, Blagih J, van der Windt GJ, et al. TLR-driven early glycolytic reprogramming via the kinases TBK1-IKKvarepsilon supports the anabolic demands of dendritic cell activation. Nat Immunol. 2014;15(4):323–32.
15. Buck MD, O'Sullivan D, Klein Geltink RI, Curtis JD, Chang CH, Sanin DE, Qiu J, Kretz O, Braas D, van der Windt GJ, et al. Mitochondrial dynamics controls T cell fate through metabolic programming. Cell. 2016;166(1):63–76.
16. Krawczyk CM, Holowka T, Sun J, Blagih J, Amiel E, DeBerardinis RJ, Cross JR, Jung E, Thompson CB, Jones RG, et al. Toll-like receptor-induced changes in glycolytic metabolism regulate dendritic cell activation. Blood. 2010;115(23):4742–9.
17. He Q, Moore TT, Eko FO, Lyn D, Ananaba GA, Martin A, Singh S, James L, Stiles J, Black CM, et al. Molecular basis for the potency of IL-10-deficient dendritic cells as a highly efficient APC system for activating Th1 response. J Immunol. 2005;174(8):4860–9.
18. Omosun Y, McKeithen D, Ryans K, Kibakaya C, Blas-Machado U, Li D, Singh R, Inoue K, Xiong ZG, Eko F, et al. Interleukin-10 modulates antigen presentation by dendritic cells through regulation of NLRP3 inflammasome assembly during Chlamydia infection. Infect Immun. 2015;83(12):4662–72.
19. Yang X, Gartner J, Zhu L, Wang S, Brunham RC. IL-10 gene knockout mice show enhanced Th1-like protective immunity and absent granuloma formation following Chlamydia trachomatis lung infection. J Immunol. 1999;162(2):1010–7.
20. Igietseme JU, Ananaba GA, Bolier J, Bowers S, Moore T, Belay T, Eko FO, Lyn D, Black CM. Suppression of endogenous IL-10 gene expression in dendritic cells enhances antigen presentation for specific Th1 induction: potential for cellular vaccine development. J Immunol. 2000;164(8):4212–9.
21. Pancholi V. Multifunctional alpha-enolase: its role in diseases. Cell Mol Life Sci. 2001;58(7):902–20.
22. Diaz-Ramos A, Roig-Borrellas A, Garcia-Melero A, Lopez-Alemany R. alpha-Enolase, a multifunctional protein: its role on pathophysiological situations. J Biomed Biotechnol. 2012;2012:156795.
23. Sanman LE, Qian Y, Eisele NA, Ng TM, van der Linden WA, Monack DM, Weerapana E, Bogyo M. Disruption of glycolytic flux is a signal for inflammasome signaling and pyroptotic cell death. Elife. 2016;5:e13663.
24. Inaba K, Inaba M, Romani N, Aya H, Deguchi M, Ikehara S, Muramatsu S, Steinman RM. Generation of large numbers of dendritic cells from mouse bone marrow cultures supplemented with granulocyte/macrophage colony-stimulating factor. J Exp Med. 1992;176(6):1693–702.
25. He Q, Eko FO, Lyn D, Ananaba GA, Bandea C, Martinez J, Joseph K, Kellar K, Black CM, Igietseme JU. Involvement of LEK1 in dendritic cell regulation of T cell immunity against Chlamydia. J Immunol. 2008;181(6):4037–42.
26. Hagner-McWhirter A, Laurin Y, Larsson A, Bjerneld EJ, Ronn O. Cy5 total protein normalization in Western blot analysis. Anal Biochem. 2015;486:54–61.
27. Perfettini JL, Darville T, Gachelin G, Souque P, Huerre M, Dautry-Varsat A, Ojcius DM. Effect of Chlamydia trachomatis infection and subsequent tumor necrosis factor alpha secretion on apoptosis in the murine genital tract. Infect Immun. 2000;68(4):2237–44.
28. Belay T, Eko FO, Ananaba GA, Bowers S, Moore T, Lyn D, Igietseme JU. Chemokine and chemokine receptor dynamics during genital chlamydial infection. Infect Immun. 2002;70(2):844–50.
29. Sakthivel SK, Singh UP, Singh S, Taub DD, Igietseme JU, Lillard Jr JW. CCL5 regulation of mucosal chlamydial immunity and infection. BMC Microbiol. 2008;8:136.
30. Chang CH, Pearce EL. Emerging concepts of T cell metabolism as a target of immunotherapy. Nat Immunol. 2016;17(4):364–8.

31. Pollizzi KN, Powell JD. Integrating canonical and metabolic signalling programmes in the regulation of T cell responses. Nat Rev Immunol. 2014;14(7):435–46.

32. Tannahill GM, Curtis AM, Adamik J, Palsson-McDermott EM, McGettrick AF, Goel G, Frezza C, Bernard NJ, Kelly B, Foley NH, et al. Succinate is an inflammatory signal that induces IL-1beta through HIF-1alpha. Nature. 2013;496(7444):238–42.

33. Narayanan S, Nieh AH, Kenwood BM, Davis CA, Tosello-Trampont AC, Elich TD, Breazeale SD, Ward E, Anderson RJ, Caldwell SH, et al. Distinct roles for intracellular and extracellular lipids in hepatitis C virus infection. PLoS One. 2016;11(6):e0156996.

34. Yamamoto H, Itoh N, Kawano S, Yatsukawa Y, Momose T, Makio T, Matsunaga M, Yokota M, Esaki M, Shodai T, et al. Dual role of the receptor Tom20 in specificity and efficiency of protein import into mitochondria. Proc Natl Acad Sci U S A. 2011;108(1):91–6.

35. Vieira HL, Belzacq AS, Haouzi D, Bernassola F, Cohen I, Jacotot E, Ferri KF, El Hamel C, Bartle LM, Melino G, et al. The adenine nucleotide translocator: a target of nitric oxide, peroxynitrite, and 4-hydroxynonenal. Oncogene. 2001;20(32):4305–16.

36. Jacotot E, Ferri KF, El Hamel C, Brenner C, Druillennec S, Hoebeke J, Rustin P, Metivier D, Lenoir C, Geuskens M, et al. Control of mitochondrial membrane permeabilization by adenine nucleotide translocator interacting with HIV-1 viral protein rR and Bcl-2. J Exp Med. 2001;193(4):509–19.

37. Joffre OP, Segura E, Savina A, Amigorena S. Cross-presentation by dendritic cells. Nat Rev Immunol. 2012;12(8):557–69.

38. Heckman KL, Radhakrishnan S, Peikert T, Iijima K, McGregor HC, Bell MP, Kita H, Pease LR. T-bet expression by dendritic cells is required for the repolarization of allergic airway inflammation. Eur J Immunol. 2008;38(9):2464–74.

39. Murphy KM, Reiner SL. The lineage decisions of helper T cells. Nat Rev Immunol. 2002;2(12):933–44.

40. Murthy AK, Li W, Chaganty BK, Kamalakaran S, Guentzel MN, Seshu J, Forsthuber TG, Zhong G, Arulanandam BP. Tumor necrosis factor alpha production from CD8+ T cells mediates oviduct pathological sequelae following primary genital Chlamydia muridarum infection. Infect Immun. 2011;79(7):2928–35.

41. Guillou C, Freret M, Fondard E, Derambure C, Avenel G, Golinski ML, Verdet M, Boyer O, Caillot F, Musette P, et al. Soluble alpha-enolase activates monocytes by CD14-dependent TLR4 signalling pathway and exhibits a dual function. Sci Rep. 2016;6:23796.

42. Ryu SY, Hong GU, Kim DY, Ro JY. Enolase 1 and calreticulin regulate the differentiation and function of mouse mast cells. Cell Signal. 2012;24(1):60–70.

43. Cappello P, Rolla S, Chiarle R, Principe M, Cavallo F, Perconti G, Feo S, Giovarelli M, Novelli F. Vaccination with ENO1 DNA prolongs survival of genetically engineered mice with pancreatic cancer. Gastroenterology. 2013; 144(5):1098–106.

11

Giardia-specific cellular immune responses in post-giardiasis chronic fatigue syndrome

Kurt Hanevik[1,2]* (iD), Einar Kristoffersen[1,3], Kristine Mørch[1,2], Kristin Paulsen Rye[1], Steinar Sørnes[1], Staffan Svärd[4], Øystein Bruserud[1] and Nina Langeland[1,2]

Abstract

Background: The role of pathogen specific cellular immune responses against the eliciting pathogen in development of post-infectious chronic fatigue syndrome (PI-CFS) is not known and such studies are difficult to perform. The aim of this study was to evaluate specific anti-*Giardia* cellular immunity in cases that developed CFS after *Giardia* infection compared to cases that recovered well. Patients reporting chronic fatigue in a questionnaire study three years after a *Giardia* outbreak were clinically evaluated five years after the outbreak and grouped according to Fukuda criteria for CFS and idiopathic chronic fatigue. *Giardia* specific immune responses were evaluated in 39 of these patients by proliferation assay, T cell activation and cytokine release analysis. 20 *Giardia* exposed non-fatigued individuals and 10 healthy unexposed individuals were recruited as controls.

Results: Patients were clinically classified into CFS ($n = 15$), idiopathic chronic fatigue ($n = 5$), fatigue from other causes ($n = 9$) and recovered from fatigue ($n = 10$). There were statistically significant antigen specific differences between these *Giardia* exposed groups and unexposed controls. However, we did not find differences between the *Giardia* exposed fatigue classification groups with regard to CD4 T cell activation, proliferation or cytokine levels in 6 days cultured PBMCs. Interestingly, sCD40L was increased in patients with PI-CFS and other persons with fatigue after *Giardia* infection compared to the non-fatigued group, and correlated well with fatigue levels at the time of sampling.

Conclusion: Our data show antigen specific cellular immune responses in the groups previously exposed to *Giardia* and increased sCD40L in fatigued patients.

Keywords: *Giardia*, T cell, Chronic fatigue syndrome, Antigen-specific, Immune response, sCD40L

Background

The causes and underlying mechanisms for development of chronic fatigue syndrome (CFS) remain unresolved. In some cases the condition is elicited by an infection, with mononucleosis due to Epstein Barr infection (EBV) being the most well-known [1]. However, it is also described to occur following a number of other infections [1]. When the onset of CFS is associated with an acute infection, it can be termed post-infectious (PI) and many researchers have focused on measures of the immune system in the quest to understand mechanisms and identify biomarkers [2–6].

It is likely that the nature of the host reaction to the specific eliciting pathogens is implicated in development of PI-CFS. This is inherently difficult to study, as patients often present at a late stage where it is difficult to ascertain the specific eliciting pathogen and it is challenging to gather enough patients of a specific etiology to perform such studies.

An opportunity to investigate potential differences in the magnitude or quality of host responses towards the eliciting pathogen arose when a fraction of *Giardia* assemblage B infected persons developed post-infectious chronic fatigue (CF) after a large waterborne outbreak in Bergen, Norway in 2004 [7]. Most of these individuals also had co-morbid functional gastrointestinal disorders (FGID) elicited by the *Giardia* infection. Post-giardiasis chronic fatigue had not previously been described in the literature. It was the clinical follow-up of referred patients with persisting symptoms after successful

---

* Correspondence: kurt.hanevik@med.uib.no
[1]Department of Clinical Science, Lab-building 8.floor, University of Bergen, N-5021 Bergen, Norway
[2]Center for Tropical Infectious Diseases, Haukeland University Hospital, Bergen, Norway
Full list of author information is available at the end of the article

Giardia treatment that informed the choice of questionnaires which were sent to all laboratory-confirmed cases two years after the outbreak [8], and at three years when we also included a control group [9]. Severity of the primary *Giardia* illness was a risk factor for developing both FGID and CF [10]. It became clear that chronic fatigue symptoms were four times more prevalent in the *Giardia* exposed group compared to controls [9]. Five years after the outbreak, PI-CFS was found in 42% (22/53) among patients who had reported chronic fatigue in the questionnaire three year after the outbreak [11].

In the present study we aimed to evaluate if *Giardia* specific immune responses such as proliferative capacity, CD4 T cell activation and cytokine profiles, were associated with development of CFS in this group of carefully clinically characterized persons. Responses were compared with a *Giardia* exposed group without fatigue, and with *Giardia*-naïve controls, in order to allow interpretation of the data with respect to *Giardia* exposure and specificity of the responses.

Methods

Study populations

Participants were recruited based on responses to a questionnaire mailed three years (in 2007) after the outbreak to all persons with laboratory confirmed giardiasis during the outbreak [9]. Patients who reported chronic fatigue in

this questionnaire were invited to participate in a thorough clinical evaluation and screening two years later (in 2009). Fifty-three individuals agreed to participate, and went through a clinical evaluation by specialists in internal medicine, psychiatry and neurology. They were evaluated for CFS or idiopathic chronic fatigue (ICF) according to the 1994 Fukuda criteria [12]. Those fulfilling the criteria, and had an onset of symptoms related to the *Giardia* infection, were categorized as PI-CSF or PI-ICF. Patients with sleep apnea syndrome, significant depression or anxiety disorders that could plausibly explain their fatigue were termed "fatigue other cause". Individuals who had recovered well from the fatigue condition they had reported in the questionnaire two years previously were termed "fatigue recovered". Five patients were excluded from this study after clinical evaluation (Fig. 1).

Two control groups were recruited; 22 individuals with normal fatigue score (=11) in the 2007 questionnaire (exposed, no-PI-fatigue group), and 10 healthy individuals not affected by the outbreak and without particular fatigue or abdominal symptoms (unexposed healthy controls) (Fig. 1). All participants were HIV negative and were not taking immunomodulatory medications or antibiotics.

Sampling and questionnaires

Participants were screened with a battery of routine blood tests and a magnetic resonance imaging (MRI)

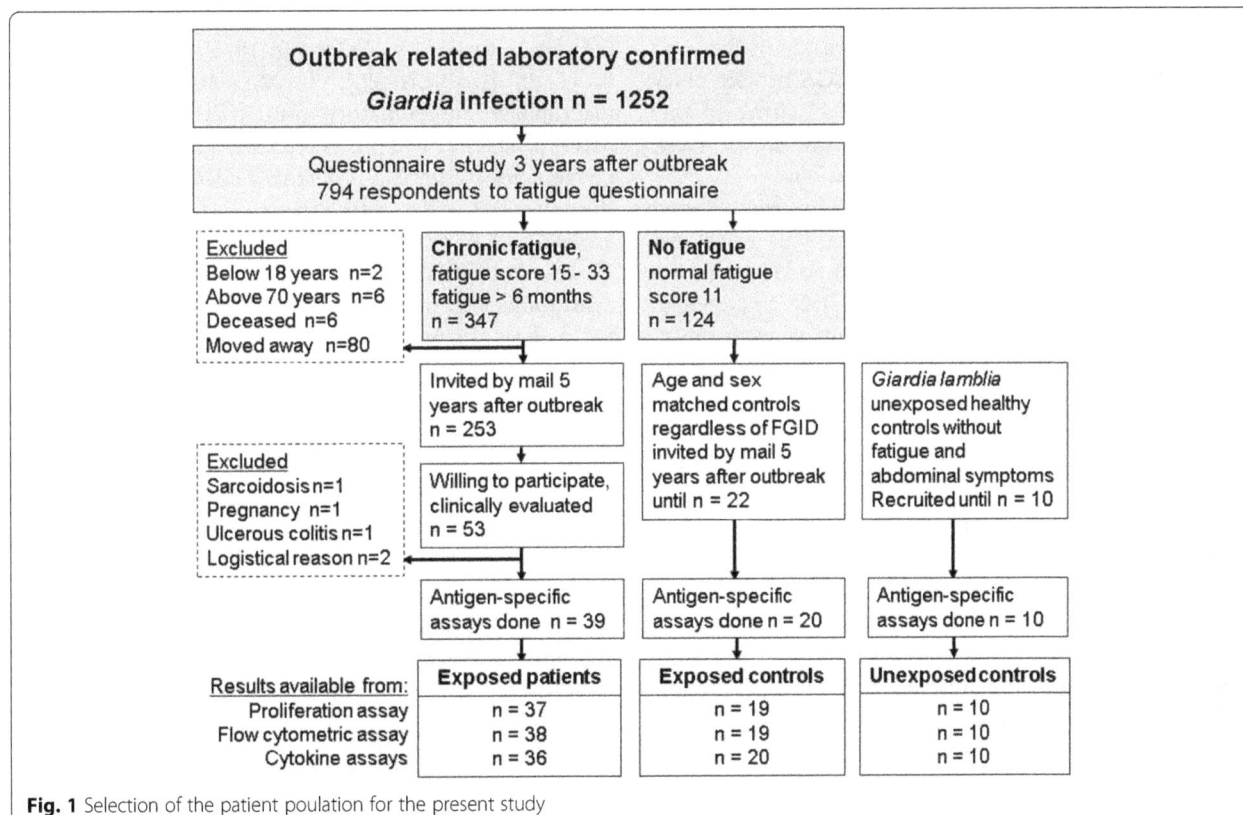

Fig. 1 Selection of the patient poulation for the present study

brain scan. Blood samples were taken between 08 am and 09 am after overnight fast and analyzed in parallel during the same period. Immunophenotyping results from these investigations have been reported previously [13]. Fecal samples were obtained and screened with microscopic examination and *Giardia* 18S PCR [14] of feces to rule out chronic giardiasis.

A total of 69 of the study participants underwent clinical characterization and were subject to one or more of the *Giardia*-specific immune response analyses presented in this paper. Some assays could not be done in all patients due to limited cell numbers (Fig. 1). Sampling and assays were stratified across groups and samples were blinded to laboratory personnel to avoid analytical bias. The severity of fatigue at the time of sampling was evaluated in all participants by the Fatigue Questionnaire [15], a validated set of 11 questions addressing different aspects of fatigue. Comorbid abdominal symptoms were recorded by the commonly used Rome II questionnaire [16].

Antigens
The Giardia antigens used in this study were made from culturing *Giardia* assemblage A strain WB-C6 (ATCC 50803) and assemblage B strain GS/M (ATCC 50581) in Diamond's TYI-S-33 medium supplemented with bile as described previously[17]. Trophozoites were washed in PBS, treeze-thawed, then sonicated for 1 min at 20 W. After sentrifugation at 13000 x g, the supernatant containing soluble *Giardia* proteins was removed, and protein content was measured by the BCA protein assay kit (Pierce). Pilot testing showed that 10ug/mL of this mixed soluble *Giardia* antigens resulted in robust T cell responses and little background stimulation.

For the proliferation assay also a sterile filtered *Candida albicans* protein extract (403 skin prick test [Allergopharma]; 10 000 BU/mL), were added as an exploratory antigen and anti-CD3 + anti-CD28 as a control of T cell activation. Positive antigen controls were tuberculin purified protein derivate (PPD) (Statens Serum Institut) and *Salmonella typhi* LPS in all assays. Several concentrations were tested in pilot studies of all stimulation antigens and positive controls to optimize the assay.

PBMC acquisition and antigen-specifc immunity assays
Peripheral blood mononuclear cells (PBMC) were isolated from BD Vacutainer Na-citrate CPT tubes (BD, Franklin Lakes, NJ, USA) by density gradient separation. After harvesting, the PBMC were washed twice in PBS and were cultured in the presence or absence of investigational or control antigens at 37 °C in a humidified atmosphere of 5% $CO_2$for six days in X-vivo 15 serum-free culture medium supplemented with L-glutamin, gentamicin, and phenol red (BioWhittaker).Proliferative

responses were measured in triplicates of stimulated cultured cells by adding ^{3}H-thymidine (Amersham International) after five days, and harvesting 18 h later. IIncorporated radioactivity was analysed by liquid scintillation counting in a β-counter. Proliferation in stimulated and unstimulated cultures was determined as median counts per minute (cpm) of each triplicate.

Activation of T cells was evaluated after six days in culture. 100 μL supernatants were carefully harvested from wells of unstimulated and stimulated PBMCs and frozen at –80 °C for later cytokine analysis. The cultured cells were then analysed by flow cytometric measurement of activated T cell subsets as published previously [17]. Briefly, after washing with PBS, the cultured cell suspensions (50 μL) were stained for 30 min in the dark with combination of 5 fluorescent dyes: CD3-ECD (Beckman Coulter), CD8a-FITC and CD4-PerCP/Cy5.5 and the activation markers CD26-PE and CD25-PE/Cy7 (BioLegend). After staining, cells were washed once, resuspended in PBS-paraformaldehyde solution (1%) and analyzed the same day using a Beckman Coulter Cytomics FC 500 MPL flow cytometer. In a typical acquisition 7×10^4 lymphocytes (min 2.3 $\times10^4$, max 1.7 $\times10^5$) were collected. The collected data were analyzed with FlowJo 7.6 software (Tree Star Inc, Ashland, OR, USA). Background responses in unstimulated cultures were adjusted for by subtracting these from responses in stimulated cultures.

Supernatants were kept frozen until analysis in three Bio-Plex assays (Bio-Rad Laboratories Inc., Hercules, CA, USA) for IFN-γ, TNF-α, IL-1β, IL-2, IL-4, IL-6, IL-9, IL-10, IL-13, IL-17A, IL-22, soluble (s) sCD40L, macrophage inflammatory protein 1 alpha (MIP-1α), MIP-1β, TGFβ1, TGFβ2, TGFβ3 and granulocyte macrophage colony-stimulation factor (GM-CSF) according to the manufacturer's instructions. The cytokines TGFβ1, TGFβ2, TGFβ3 were analyzed in unstimulated and *Giardia* antigen stimulated cultures only. Observed concentrations (pg/ml) within the standard range were used for analysis. Values above the limit of quantitation were set to the highest value in the standard range, and values below this range were set to zero. For analytes where less than 50% of values were within range, further analyses were not done.

For both flow cytometric and cytokine assays, background responses in unstimulated cultures were subtracted from those in stimulated cultures for each participant. In some cases this gave negative values in the cytokine assay which were kept in the statistical analyses and interpreted as stimulant-induced decrease in production or increase in consumption of the relevant analyte.

Statistical analysis
Unless otherwise stated the data are presented as median (standard deviation (SD)). Chi-squared tests

were used for categorical comparisons between groups. Linear regression analysis was used for correlation between response parameters as well as fatigue scores and sCD40L data. Comparison of T cell activation, proliferation and cytokine data between exposed and unexposed groups was done using the Mann Whitney U test. The significance level was set at $p <0.05$. To reduce false positive findings due to multiple comparisons within the exposed groups, we used the Kruskal-Wallis test across all exposed groups first, and further testing between the no PI-fatigue and PI-CFS/PI-ICF groups with Mann Whitney U test was only performed for variables with a p value less than 0.05. IBM SPSS Statistics version 23 (IBM Corp, Armonk, USA) was used for statistical analysis.

Results

Patient characteristics

Patients and controls were grouped according to their clinical condition at the time of sampling. Data from 39 patients (median age 40.9 years (11.2) range 19–62, females 74%), 20 exposed controls (median age 39.5 (9.3) range 27–66, females 75%) and 10 unexposed controls (median age 43.3 (14.3) range 22–63, females 70%) were analyzed in this study. There were no significant differences in age ($p = 0.06$) or sex distribution ($p = 0.61$). Fatigued patients were categorized according to their clinical categories for analyses of antigen specific immune responses (Table 1). ICF and CFS were combined in the further analyses as they were seen as a common phenotype with difference only in severity of symptoms. The fatigue scores generally reflected the categorization obtained by careful clinical evaluation with the cases of CSF scoring higher than the ICF and fatigue by other cause groups. The patients who had recovered well still

had a modestly elevated fatigue score compared to recruited exposed and unexposed controls.

Giardia-induced proliferation of immunocompetent cells

PMBC proliferated well in response to all stimuli included in this assay. A marked memory response was seen in the *Giardia* exposed groups that showed significantly stronger proliferation in response to the *Giardia* lysates compared to the unexposed group (Table 2). However, the proliferative responses to *Giardia* antigens did not differ significantly between the fatigue categories within the exposed group (Table 2). For the other specific antigen controls we found neither a difference with regard to previous exposure to *Giardia*, nor according to fatigue sequels. There was a trend towards decreased proliferation induced by the strong T cells activator anti-CD3antiCD28 among the fatigued groups compared to the no fatigued controls, but this did not attain significance (Table 2).

Giardia-induced T cell expression of activation markers

Levels of activated CD4 T cells expressing CD25 and CD26 were significantly elevated in *Giardia* exposed groups compared to unexposed patients when stimulated with both *Giardia* assemblage A and assemblage B lysates (Table 3). The PPD and LPS control antigens induced similar levels of activated CD4 T cells in both exposed and unexposed groups. None of these stimuli induced differences between the exposed participants with or without fatigue sequels. The flow cytometric responses correlated well with proliferation responses to the same antigens with $p <0.001$ for assemblage A stimulation and $p = 0.001$ for assemblage B stimulated cultures.

Giardia-induced release of soluble mediators

In Table 4 the results of cytokines and sCD40L are given for levels of an array of cytokines and sCD40L in supernatants of PBMC stimulated for six days with *Giardia* assemblage B lysate. There were significant differences for most of these, except IL-4, IL-2, TGFβ2 and TGFβ3 between the *Giardia* exposed and unexposed participants. The same pattern was seen, but with weaker differences in responses to *Giardia* assemblage A. For PPD there were smaller, but significant differences only for IFNγ and sCD40L between exposed and unexposed groups, while for LPS stimulated supernatants no difference was found (Additional file 1: Table S1).

In the analysis of *Giardia* antigen induced differences in cytokine profiles with regard to fatigue outcome we found only sCD40L to be significantly different within exposed groups (KruskalWallis $p = 0.03$) and the PI-CFS/PI-ICF groups having significantly elevated levels of sCD40L compared to the no PI-fatigue groups (Table 4). Also a significant difference was found when comparing

Table 1 Characteristics of participant groups

	Age, median (SD)	Females, n (%)	Fatigue score in 2009, median (SD)	Total participants, n
Giardia exposed				
No PI-fatigue controls	39.5 (9.3)	15 (75)	11 (1.3)	20
PI-CFS	47.0 (8.6)	11 (73)	22.0 (5.3)	15
PI-ICF	35.0 (8.9)	4 (80)	20.0 (3.1)	5
Fatigue other cause	51.0 (15.6)	9 (100)	18.0 (5.1)	9
Recovered from fatigue	31.0 (5.8)	5 (50)	17.0 (3.3)	10
Giardia unexposed				
Healthy controls	39 (11.1)	7 (70)	11 (2.1)	10

Abbreviations: *PI* post-infectious, *CFS* chronic fatigue syndrome, *ICF* idiopathic chronic fatigue

Table 2 Immune responses against *Giardia* and control antigens as measured by ^{3}H-thymidine proliferation assay

Stimulation agent	Exposed				Unexposed	p-values	
	No PI-fatigue controls (n = 19)	PI-CFS & ICF (n = 19)	Fatigue other cause (n = 9)	Recovered from fatigue (n = 9)	Healthy controls (n = 10)	Exposed n = 56)vs unexposed (n = 10)	No PI-fatigue controls (n= 19) vs PI-CFS/ICF (n = 19)
Giardia ass A 10 µg/ml	12.8 (13.0)	15.3 (19.9)	20.3 (10.9)	15.1 (65.0)	3.5 (6.2)	0.001	ns*
Giardia ass B 10 µg/ml	12.2 (13.9)	13.3 (15.3)	23.3 (13.4)	15.3 (39.0)	3.5 (4.7)	<0.001	ns*
Tuberculin (PPD)10 µg/ml	26.3 (34.1)	34.0 (47.5)	54.9 (84.5)	42.5 (23.2)	27.7 (27.0)	ns	ns*
LP S Stypi 1 µg/ml	21.5 (18.6)	14.4 (13.2)	38.2 (34.3)	21.9 (19.5)	17.7 (10.5)	ns	ns*
C albicans 10 µg/ml	7.0 (9.1)	5.8 (11.9)	10.0 (32.0)	14.6 (6.0)	11.0 (9.4)	ns	ns*
aCD3aCD28(pos ctr)	70.6 (35.4)	51.4 (33.0)	51.8 (44.1)	51.8 (63.9)	60.1 (39.8)	ns	ns*

*KruskalWallis test across all exposed groups was not significant (below $p = 0.05$). ns = not significant
Proliferation responses are expressed as median stimulation indices (counts per minute(cpm) in stimulated triplicate cultures divided by cpm in unstimulated triplicate cultures) followed by standard deviation

the no-PI-fatigue group with the PI-CFS group ($n = 14$) alone, and with the fatigue other cause group ($p = 0.038$), but not with the recovered group. Interestingly, sCD40L levels in supernatants correlated well with fatigue scores ($p = 0.001$), shown in Fig. 2.

The antigen-specific immune responses were also explored with regard to co-morbidity with functional gastrointestinal disorders, but significant correlations were not found (data not shown).

Discussion

The data presented in this study confirm previous finding of long term T cell memory responses towards *Giardia* [17], and bring new data on cytokines profiles elicited in this response. However, in the present study, performed in a well-defined group of patients with clinically observed post-infectious FGID and CFS five years after a common eliciting infection, we did not identify any differences in the antigen-specific cellular immunity against the culprit infectious agent, in this case *G. lamblia*. The higher levels of sCD40L in supernatants in *Giardia* stimulated PBMCs from persons with PI-CFS correlated well with fatigue scores, but could be unspecific for PI-CFS as it was also found in persons reporting

fatigue that could be explained by other conditions. An alternative explanation could be that also these could have a component of *Giardia* induced fatigue, but they did not fulfil the Fukuda criteria due to their other illness. As such, further investigation is warranted to evaluate whether sCD40L might be a marker of fatigue in general or a marker for PI-CFS. Alternatively, this may be an effect related to *Giardia* exposure in all the fatigued patients. Since we did not include a control group of fatigued patients without *Giardia* exposure, we cannot conclude firmly on these options.

The present study thus underlines the need to include patient control groups where fatigue is a common symptom in all studies looking for biomarkers of CFS. Our study design, which included exposed groups with fatigue, but not fulfilling the criteria for CFS/ICF allowed for a more cautious interpretation. A previous study has found that an increase in serum sCD40L eight hours after exertion correlated with increases in physical fatigue 48 h post-exertion [18]. Our data support that CD40L, a co-stimulatory molecule which is found on a variety of cells and promotes B cell maturation, could be a marker of fatigue. Another study has suggested that sCD40L can increase blood brain permeability in vivo,

Table 3 Immune responses against *Giardia* and control antigens as measured by the percentage of CD25CD26 positive CD4 T cells by flow-cytometry

Stimulation agent	Exposed				Unexposed	p-values	
	No PI-fatigue controls (n = 19)	PI-CFS & ICF (n = 18)	Fatigue other cause (n = 9)	Recovered from fatigue (n = 10)	Healthy controls (n = 10)	Exposed (n = 56) vs unexposed (n = 10)	No PI-fatigue controls (n = 19) vs PI-CFS/ICF (n = 19)
Giardia ass A 10 µg/ml	8.6 (5.8)	10.3 (7.7)	8.8 (5.0)	12.4 (8.1)	1.8 (3.9)	0.001	ns*
Giardia ass B 10 µg/ml	3.1 (2.2)	4.3 (7.3)	3.7 (3.9)	7.9 (5.7)	1.9 (1.6)	0.009	ns*
Tuberculin (PPD)10 µg/ml	6.6 (5.4)	11.3 (11.1)	9.2 (11.4)	13.6 (5.2)	10.0 (13.6)	ns	ns*
LPS S. typi 1 µg/ml	5.2 (5.5)	5.2 (9.6)	4.5 (2.5)	5.1 (2.9)	3.0 (14.6)	ns	ns*

The values are percentages of activated CD4 T cells out of all CD4 T cells in stimulated cultures subtracted by the percentage of activated CD4 T cells in unstimulated culture
*KruskalWallis test across all exposed groups was not significant (below $p = 0.05$). ns = not significant

Table 4 Analyses of cytokines and sCD40L in supernatants of PBMC cultured for six days after stimulation with *Giardia* assemblage B lysate in persons exposed to this pathogen in the Bergen 2004 outbreak with or without fatigue sequels, and in unexposed controls

| Analyte | Exposed | | | | Unexposed | p-values | |
	No PI-fatigue controls (n = 20)	PI-CFS & ICF (n = 19)	Fatigue other cause (n = 8)	Fully recovered (n = 9)	Healthy controls (n = 10)	Exposed (n = 56) vs unexposed (n = 10)	No PI-fatigue controls (n = 20) vs PI-CFS/ICF (n = 19)
IL-1b	8.4 (63.5)	23.7 (211)	10.0 (37.0)	37.3 (207)	0.8 (8.8)	<0.001	ns*
IL-4	4.1 (6.6)	4.9 (4.8)	-0.7 (7.4)	7.7 (5.6)	4.0 (29.4)	0.838	ns*
IL-6	496 (8364)	781 (18566)	957 (659)	741 (991)	85.3 (310)	<0.001	ns*
IL-10	19.7 (23.3)	25.2 (354)	22.7 (13.2)	25.1 (5.9)	7.1 (25.3)	<0.001	ns*
IFNy	1009 (3656)	1627 (4637)	775 (2569)	2577 (2322)	31.6 (956)	<0.001	ns*
sCD40L	7.5 (25.0)	35.6 (59.0)	26.6 (27.3)	19.5 (53.5)	0.0 (43.2)	0.003	0.005
TNFa	192 (407)	346 (713)	213 (990)	395 (787)	7.6 (166)	<0.001	ns*
IL-2	5.9 (9.3)	7.1 (8.1)	15.7 (15.1)	6.1 (8.9)	4.7 (4.6)	0.107	ns*
IL-9	11.7 (39.7)	23.5 (155)	20.3 (22.9)	23.6 (115)	2.8 (14.5)	0.018	ns*
IL-13	230 (203)	262 (212)	248 (371)	441 (272)	72.8 (100)	0.002	ns*
MIPa	51.1 (657)	112 (645)	252 (427)	692 (540)	15.5 (399)	0.034	ns*
MIPb	1691 (1856)	2306 (1939)	1754 (1618)	2862 (4195)	258 (1765)	0.034	ns*
TGFb1	-959 (2759)	-2083 (2243)	-1914 (1869)	-2749 (3429)	-3680 (1438)	0.033	ns*
TGFb2	-43.2 (61.7)	5.7 (46.4)	7.5 (111)	21.0 (45.0)	-34.7 (61.1)	0.132	ns*
TGFb3	4.7 (23.0)	-10.5 (19.3)	-7.2 (8.3)	-20.5 (15.3)	-10.3 (43.0)	0.869	ns*

*KruskalWallis test across all exposed groups was not significant (below $p = 0.05$)
Values are pg/mL, median (SD) in stimulated cultures after subtracting measurements in unstimulated cultures. Values are given for analyte measurements that were of sufficient quality for further analysis

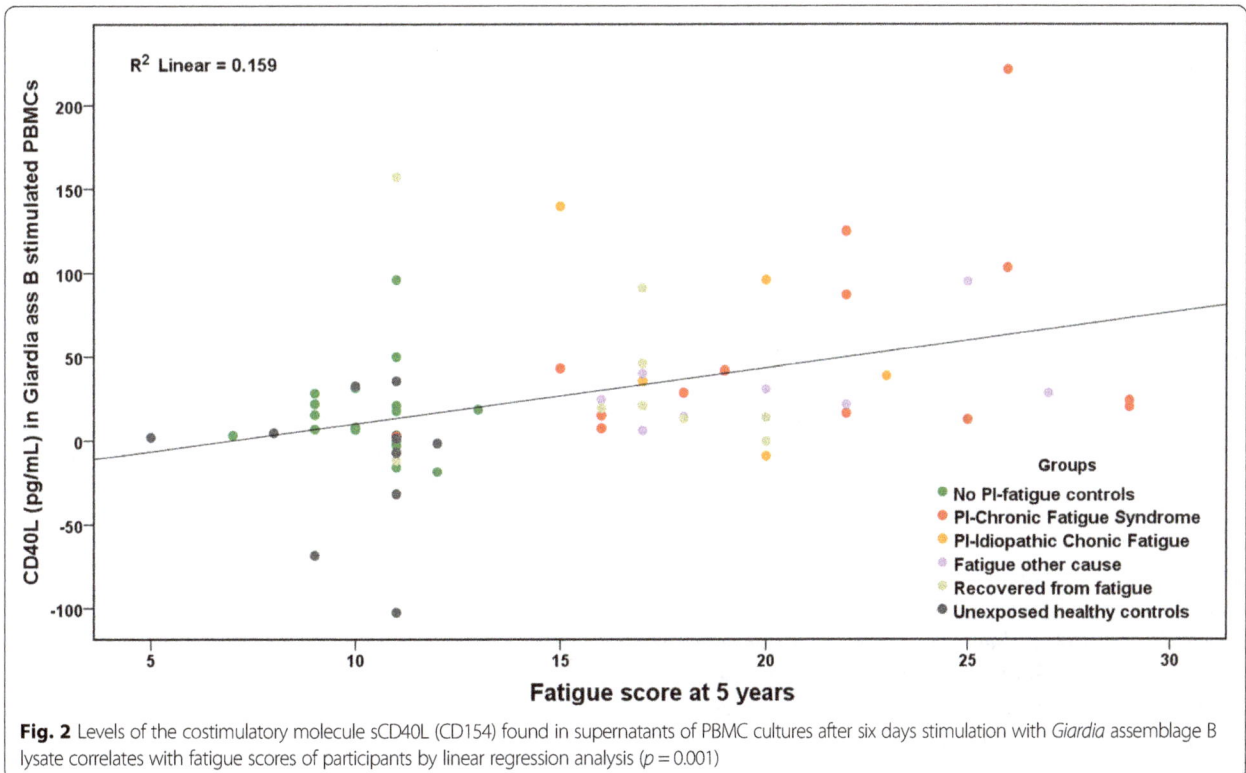

Fig. 2 Levels of the costimulatory molecule sCD40L (CD154) found in supernatants of PBMC cultures after six days stimulation with *Giardia* assemblage B lysate correlates with fatigue scores of participants by linear regression analysis ($p = 0.001$)

and this could be a mechanism deserving further research [19].

Few studies are available to compare our data with. In line with the present study an analysis of specific humoral immunity in PI-CFS after parvovirus B19 infection did not identify any pattern distinguishing this illness [20]. Epstein-Barr virus specific cellular immune responses have been investigated in a CFS patient group of uncharacterized etiology, finding lower levels of polyfunctional ebna-1 specific T cells, whereas no differences in cytomegalovirus-responses were detected [21].

Curriu et al. found general cellular proliferative responses to be decreased in PBMCs from CFS patients [22], possibly due to increased number of regulatory T cells. We did observed a weaker proliferative response to strong T cell activation with anti-CD3/anti-CD28 stimulation in the CFS/ICF group, but these results were not statistically significant. Additionally, we also observed weaker, but non-significant, proliferative responses in the other exposed groups.

Our patient cohort offered a rare chance to study cellular immune responses to the eliciting pathogen. However, participants were recruited from a group of people who had a common exposure five years previously, and were therefore limited in number. We included those who were willing to participate, and had no chance to expand recruitment. From talking to individuals who did not wish to participate we learned that many of these experienced a substantial improvement in their condition between three and five years after the outbreak.

There was a large variation observed in measurements, causing large SDs. Some of this is likely due to the multiplicative effect of even small differences after culturing cells for six days.

The cytokine IL-17 which we have shown to play a role in human memory responses against *Giardia* infections [23] had high background levels in supernatants in the present study, leaving too few values measurable, and could not be analyzed.

Examination at an earlier time point where we would have been able to recruit more individuals still fulfilling the CFS criteria into the study could have increased the statistical power, and could possibly have resulted in stronger, more distinct immune responses.

Conclusion

While these data confirm previous finding of T cell memory responses towards *Giardia* and bring new data on cytokine profiles, they did not reveal a difference in the magnitude of *Giardia*-specific T cell responses with respect to post-giardiasis CFS. Neither were differences in the quality of these responses, as measured by cytokine profiles in supernatants above *Giardia* stimulated

PBMCs, found, except for sCD40L being elevated in the PI-CFS/ICF group as well as other exposed cases who experienced fatigue after the outbreak *Giardia* assemblage B infection.

Abbreviations
ATCC: American type culture collection; CFS: Chronic fatigue syndrome; EBV: Epstein barr infection; FGID: Functional gastrointestinal disorder; HIV: Human immunodeficiency virus; ICF: Idiopathic chronic fatigue; IL: Interleukin; LPS: Lipopolysaccaride; PBMC: Peripheral blood mononuclear cells; PBS: Phosphate buffered saline; PCR: Polymerase chain reaction; PI: Post-infectious; PPD: Purified protein derivate; sCD40L: Soluble cluster of differentiation 40 ligand

Acknowledgements
We want to thank the staff at the hospital clinical routine laboratory, the study participants and also Marita Wallevik, Knut-Arne Wensaas, Guri Rørtveit, Bjarte Stubhaug, Marit Tellevik, Christel Haanshuus, Geir Egil Eide, Halvor Næss, Ann Christin Rivenes, Jørn Eilert Bødtker and Harald Inge Nyland for their cooperation, advice and assistance in this project.

Funding
This work was supported by The Western Norway Regional Health Authority project number 911571 and the University of Bergen. Data were analyzed and evaluated independently by the authors, without any interference from the funding institution.

Authors' contributions
Laboratory work, data collection and analyses were done by KH, EKK, SSø and KPR. *Giardia* antigens were prepared and supplied by SSv. Clinical evaluation and classification of patients was done by KM. OB and KPR assisted in planning and cytokine analysis. NL supervised all parts of the study. All authors assisted in preparation of, and approved, the final manuscript.

Competing interests
K.H. has been a consultant for Lupin Pharmaceuticals Inc. The other authors declare that they have no competing interests.

Author details
[1]Department of Clinical Science, Lab-building 8.floor, University of Bergen, N-5021 Bergen, Norway. [2]Center for Tropical Infectious Diseases, Haukeland University Hospital, Bergen, Norway. [3]Department of immunology and transfusion medicine, Haukeland University Hospital, Bergen, Norway. [4]Department of Cell and Molecular biology, Uppsala University, Uppsala, Sweden.

References

1. Hickie I, Davenport T, Wakefield D, Vollmer-Conna U, Cameron B, Vernon SD, Reeves WC, Lloyd A. Post-infective and chronic fatigue syndromes precipitated by viral and non-viral pathogens: prospective cohort study. BMJ. 2006;333(7568):575.

2. Gow JW, Hagan S, Herzyk P, Cannon C, Behan PO, Chaudhuri A. A gene signature for post-infectious chronic fatigue syndrome. BMC Med Genomics. 2009;2:38.

3. Masuda A, Munemoto T, Yamanaka T, Takei M, Tei C. Psychosocial characteristics and immunological functions in patients with postinfectious chronic fatigue syndrome and noninfectious chronic fatigue syndrome. J Behav Med. 2002;25(5):477–85.

4. Devanur LD, Kerr JR. Chronic fatigue syndrome. J Clin Virol. 2006;37(3):139–50.

5. Spiller R, Garsed K. Postinfectious irritable bowel syndrome. Gastroenterology. 2009;136(6):1979–88.

6. Hardcastle SL, Brenu EW, Johnston S, Nguyen T, Huth T, Ramos S, Staines D, Marshall-Gradisnik S. Longitudinal analysis of immune abnormalities in varying severities of chronic fatigue syndrome/myalgic encephalomyelitis patients. J Transl Med. 2015;13:299.

7. Nygard K, Schimmer B, Sobstad O, Walde AK, Tveit I, Langeland N, Hausken T, Aavitsland P. A large community outbreak of waterborne giardiasis-delayed detection in a non-endemic urban area. BMC Public Health. 2006;6(1):141.

8. Morch K, Hanevik K, Rortveit G, Wensaas KA, Langeland N. High rate of fatigue and abdominal symptoms 2 years after an outbreak of giardiasis. Trans R Soc Trop Med Hyg. 2009;103(5):530-2. doi: 10.1016/j.trstmh.2009.01.010.

9. Wensaas KA, Langeland N, Hanevik K, Morch K, Eide GE, Rortveit G. Irritable bowel syndrome and chronic fatigue 3 years after acute giardiasis: historic cohort study. Gut. 2012;61(2):214–9.

10. Morch K, Hanevik K, Rortveit G, Wensaas KA, Eide GE, Hausken T, Langeland N. Severity of giardia infection associated with post-infectious fatigue and abdominal symptoms two years after. BMC Infect Dis. 2009;9(1):206.

11. Morch K, Hanevik K, Rivenes AC, Bodtker JE, Naess H, Stubhaug B, Wensaas KA, Rortveit G, Eide GE, Hausken T, et al. Chronic fatigue syndrome 5 years after giardiasis: differential diagnoses, characteristics and natural course. BMC Gastroenterol. 2013;13:28.

12. Fukuda K, Straus SE, Hickie I, Sharpe MC, Dobbins JG, Komaroff A. The chronic fatigue syndrome: a comprehensive approach to its definition and study. International chronic fatigue syndrome study group. Ann Intern Med. 1994;121(12):953–9.

13. Hanevik K, Kristoffersen EK, Sornes S, Morch K, Naess H, Rivenes AC, Bodtker JE, Hausken T, Langeland N. Immunophenotyping in post-giardiasis functional gastrointestinal disease and chronic fatigue syndrome. BMC Infect Dis. 2012;12:258.

14. Verweij JJ, Blange RA, Templeton K, Schinkel J, Brienen EA, van Rooyen MA, van Lieshout L, Polderman AM. Simultaneous detection of entamoeba histolytica, giardia lamblia, and cryptosporidium parvum in fecal samples by using multiplex real-time PCR. J Clin Microbiol. 2004;42(3):1220–3.

15. Chalder T, Berelowitz G, Pawlikowska T, Watts L, Wessely S, Wright D, Wallace EP. Development of a fatigue scale. J Psychosom Res. 1993;37(2):147–53.

16. Drossman DA. The functional gastrointestinal disorders and the Rome II process. Gut. 1999;45 Suppl 2:II1–5.

17. Hanevik K, Kristoffersen E, Svard S, Bruserud O, Ringqvist E, Sornes S, Langeland N. Human cellular immune response against giardia lamblia 5 years after acute giardiasis. J Infect Dis. 2011;204(11):1779–86.

18. White AT, Light AR, Hughen RW, Bateman L, Martins TB, Hill HR, Light KC. Severity of symptom flare after moderate exercise is linked to cytokine activity in chronic fatigue syndrome. Psychophysiology. 2010;47(4):615–24.

19. Davidson DC, Hirschman MP, Sun A, Singh MV, Kasischke K, Maggirwar SB. Excess soluble CD40L contributes to blood brain barrier permeability in vivo: implications for HIV-associated neurocognitive disorders. PLoS One. 2012;7(12):e51793.

20. Kerr JR, Bracewell J, Laing I, Mattey DL, Bernstein RM, Bruce IN, Tyrrell DA. Chronic fatigue syndrome and arthralgia following parvovirus B19 infection. J Rheumatol. 2002;29(3):595–602.

21. Loebel M, Strohschein K, Giannini C, Koelsch U, Bauer S, Doebis C, Thomas S, Unterwalder N, von Baehr V, Reinke P, et al. Deficient EBV-specific B- and T-cell response in patients with chronic fatigue syndrome. PLoS One. 2014;9(1):e85387.

22. Curriu M, Carrillo J, Massanella M, Rigau J, Alegre J, Puig J, Garcia-Quintana AM, Castro-Marrero J, Negredo E, Clotet B, et al. Screening NK-B- and T-cell phenotype and function in patients suffering from chronic fatigue syndrome. J Transl Med. 2013;11:68.

23. Saghaug CS, Sornes S, Peirasmaki D, Svard S, Langeland N, Hanevik K. Human memory CD4+ T cell immune responses against giardia lamblia. Clin Vaccine Immunol. 2016;23(1):11–8.

12

Human NK cells adapt their immune response towards increasing multiplicities of infection of *Aspergillus fumigatus*

Lothar Marischen[*], Anne Englert, Anna-Lena Schmitt, Hermann Einsele and Juergen Loeffler

Abstract

Background: The saprophytic fungus *Aspergillus fumigatus* reproduces by generation of conidia, which are spread by airflow throughout nature. Since humans are inhaling certain amounts of spores every day, the (innate) immune system is constantly challenged. Even though macrophages and neutrophils carry the main burden, also NK cells are regarded to contribute to the antifungal immune response. While NK cells reveal a low frequency, expression and release of immunomodulatory molecules seem to be a natural way of their involvement.

Results: In this study we show, that NK cells secrete chemokines such as CCL3/MIP-1α, CCL4/MIP-1β and CCL5/RANTES early on after stimulation with *Aspergillus fumigatus* and, in addition, adjust the concentration of chemokines released to the multiplicity of infection of *Aspergillus fumigatus*.

Conclusions: These results further corroborate the relevance of NK cells within the antifungal immune response, which is regarded to be more and more important in the development and outcome of invasive aspergillosis in immunocompromised patients after hematopoietic stem cell transplantation. Additionally, the correlation between the multiplicity of infection and the expression and release of chemokines shown here may be useful in further studies for the quantification and/or surveillance of the NK cell involvement in antifungal immune responses.

Keywords: *Aspergillus fumigatus*, Aspergillosis, NK cells, Chemokines, CCL4, MIP-1β, Multiplicity of infection

Background

As a mold fungus, *Aspergillus (A.) fumigatus* is part of our everyday environment. Naturally living in the soil, *A. fumigatus* is capable of colonizing dead plants, rotting wood, and also wet areas often frequented by humans, as for example cellars or swimming pools. Within its reproductive cycle, *A. fumigatus* generates spores ("conidia"), that are easily distributed by air flow [1]. Therewith, humans often inhale certain amounts of spores per day [2]. Fungal pathogens are recognized by the innate immune system via pattern recognition receptors such as Toll-like receptors (TLRs), c-type lectin receptors (CLRs), complement receptor 3 and galectin family proteins, and subsequently damaged by neutrophils and/or finally phagocytosed by alveolar macrophages. Since dendritic cells may get involved, different subgroups of T cells will eventually contribute to the immune response [3]. Nevertheless, *A. fumigatus* can bring on allergies like asthma or allergic bronchopulmonary aspergillosis (ABPA) [4]. Furthermore, immunocompromised patients in general, and – increasingly encountered in clinical practice – patients after hematopoietic stem cell transplantation (HSCT), are severely endangered to develop invasive aspergillosis (IA) after *A. fumigatus* infection [5]. The recovery of the immune system after HSCT starts with the appearance of innate immune cells such as granulocytes, monocytes and dendritic cells within the first weeks. Natural killer (NK) cells are the first lymphoid cells to show up in peripheral blood, and their numbers are reciprocally correlated with the severity of IA [6, 7].

NK cells are cluster of differentiation (CD)56[+] CD3[−] lymphocytes originally characterized by their ability to arrange apoptosis of virus-infected or neoplastic cells

---

* Correspondence: Marischen_L@ukw.de
Department of Internal Medicine II, WÜ4i, University Hospital Wuerzburg, Wuerzburg, Germany

without a previous sensitization process. Up to now, NK cells or adequate subsets were found in several tissues of the human body such as lungs, liver, skin, intestine, uterus, bone marrow, spleen, lymph nodes [8], blood, decidua [9], or central nervous system [10]. In broncho-alveolar lavage fluid, macrophages account for more than 80% of total immune cells, while NK cells constitute just around 1% [11]. Even though this hardly suggests a major contribution of NK cells, several studies lay special emphasis on the fact that NK cells still account for 10% of the lymphocytes in the lung, while they additionally show a higher percentage of differentiated/matured cells than in other peripheral organs such as liver, skin and secondary lymphoid tissues. The fast recruitment of additional NK cells just hours (h) after the onset of inflammation may be supported by the regular dynamic movement of NK cells between blood and lung tissue, that leaves just a very small subpopulation of tissue-resident CD69+ NK cells as required for immune surveillance [8, 12, 13]. It is therefore tempting to speculate, that the low amount of NK cells initially present in the lung can increase very rapidly when needed, and subsequently contribute substantially to the immune response.

It is still under discussion, whether the contribution of NK cells to the immune response against pathogens is strongly dependent on accessory cells [14] or can be fully or in part explained by their expression of pattern recognition receptors like TLRs and nucleotide oligomerization domain (NOD)-like receptors [15]. In this context, Chalifour et al. showed a TLR-dependent release of α-defensin by highly purified NK cells [16]. Expression of other peptides with antimicrobial characteristics, for example X-C motif chemokine ligand 1 (XCL1)/lymphotactin, lysozyme, granulysin, α-defensin 6 [17], perforin [18] and cathelicidin/LL-37 [19], was reported.

Further studies have characterized the integration of NK cells within the cytokine network of the immune system. NK cell functions are affected by several interleukins (IL) as IL-1, IL-10, IL-12, IL-15 and IL-18 [20], and by chemokines such as CC chemokine ligand (CCL)2/monocyte chemo-attractant protein (MCP)-1, CCL3/macrophage inflammatory protein (MIP)-1α, CCL4/MIP-1β, CCL5/regulated and normal T cell expressed and secreted (RANTES), CCL10/N-gamma-inducible protein-10 (IP-10), CCL19/MIP-3β, CCL21/ secondary lymphoid tissue chemokine (SLC) and chemokine (C–X3–C motif) ligand 1 (CX3CL1)/fractalkine [21]. Recruitment of NK cells is mediated by CCL3/MIP-1α, CCL4/MIP-1β, CCL5/RANTES, CCL19/MIP-3β, CCL21/SLC, CXCL8/IL-8, CXCL10/IP-10, CXCL11, CXCL12/stromal cell-derived factor 1 and CX3CL1/fractalkine [21, 22]. By themselves, NK cells can produce tumor necrosis factor-α (TNF-α) and interferon-γ (IFN-γ) most prominently, as well as IL-5, IL-10, IL-13, granulocyte-macrophage colony-stimulating factor (GM-CSF), CCL2/MCP-1, CXCL8/IL-8, CXCL10/IP-10, XCL1/lymphotactin, CCL1 and CCL22/ macrophage-derived chemokine [20, 21]. CCL3/MIP-1α, CCL4/MIP-1β and CCL5/RANTES were found early on in the supernatant of stimulated NK cells [20].

In conclusion, NK cells are present at the typical gateway for fungal infections, are expressing pattern recognition receptors and antimicrobial peptides, and are involved in the cytokine network of the immune system. Recent reviews from Schmidt et al. [23] and Ogbomo and Mody [24] summarize current knowledge about the interaction of NK cells with fungal pathogens in general. Concerning A. fumigatus, the essential role of NK cells is underscored by animal studies in neutropenic mice [25, 26] and in vitro experiments pointing to a critical role of IFN-γ and perforin [27, 28]. CD56 [29], NKp30 [30] and NKp46 [31], which are prototypic surface molecules for NK cells, are reported as binding receptors for fungal ligands. Interestingly, the morphotype of A. fumigatus is critical for the onset of an immune response by NK cells. As published by Schmidt et al. and our study group, respectively, germlings and hyphae induce fungicidal activity, while conidia seem to pass unnoticed [27, 28]. In this respect, Aimanianda et al. have shown the rodlet/hydrophobin layer on A. fumigatus conidia to prevent immune recognition [32]. It appears to be obvious, that this rodlet/hydrophobin layer becomes fragile during the germination and growing processes of the fungus, and therefore exposes immunogenic structures below. On the other hand, A. fumigatus actively interact with lung epithelial cells, macrophages, neutrophils and components of the complement system [33]. As well, A. fumigatus impairs NK cell-derived immune functions by downregulating the levels of GM-CSF and IFN-γ in the supernatant of pre-stimulated NK cells [28, 34].

Here, we aimed to characterize the expression and release of immunomodulatory molecules by NK cells early on after stimulation with A. fumigatus, and accessed the effects of a varying multiplicity of infection (MOI). Thereby, this study contributes to the understanding of the interaction between NK cells and A. fumigatus, which is regarded to be more and more important in the progression of fungal infections in immunocompromised patients recovering from HSCT.

Results

Cytokine expression levels in NK cells after A. fumigatus stimulation

In a first approach, expression of selected cytokines was screened by quantitative polymerase chain reaction (qPCR) analysis of NK cells after stimulation with A. fumigatus. Therefore, freshly isolated NK cells were pre-incubated overnight with IL-2 and subsequently stimulated with IL-2/

IL-15 or *A. fumigatus* germ tubes for 6 h. Unstimulated controls were included. Ribonucleic acid (RNA) was isolated and used for qPCR screening analysis (Fig. 1). As shown, the expressions of the chemokines CCL3/MIP-1α, CCL4/MIP-1β, CXCL8/IL-8, XCL1/lymphotactin and the cytokines IFN-γ, TNF-α, GM-CSF and IL-1α were increased due to stimulation by *A. fumigatus* or – as for granzyme B – just by IL-2/IL-15. CCL5/RANTES and IL-16 expressions, on the other hand, were significantly downregulated.

In the qPCR analysis, relative cytokine messenger RNA (mRNA) expression was calculated by normalization to 5′-aminolevulinate synthase 1 (ALAS1) expression levels. Thereby, factors as (due to stimulation) additionally produced mRNAs or the real number of NK cells before/during/after stimulation were intentionally taken out of calculation. Now, in order to visualize the situation considering these factors, corresponding PCR fragments for CCL3/MIP-1α, CCL4/MIP-1β and XCL1/lymphotactin were analyzed by gel electrophoresis. Consistently, subsequent densitometric evaluations were performed without including ALAS1 for normalization (Fig. 2). The expression levels of all three tested chemokines were upregulated in NK cells already after 3 h stimulation, with just a marginal difference to the expression levels after 6 h. Due to the normalization mentioned above, qPCR analysis revealed a higher expression level for CCL3/MIP-1α and CCL4/MIP-1β after *A. fumigatus* versus (vs.) IL-2/IL-15 stimulation. Here, a densitometric evaluation detects the same expression level for both stimulations, or even a higher expression level for IL-2/IL-15 stimulation.

Release of CCL4/MIP-1β

In Fig. 2, expression increase of CCL4 – but not of CCL5 or XCL1 – after 6 h stimulation with *A. fumigatus* is not only significant, but also on a similar level as the expression increase after IL-15 stimulation. Additionally, CCL4/MIP-1β has already been shown to reveal higher concentrations in the supernatant of stimulated NK cells than 24 other tested cytokines – including IFN-γ, TNF-α, CCL3/MIP-1α and CCL5/RANTES [20]. Therefore, CCL4/MIP-1β was expected to be detected easier than other cytokines and was exemplarily selected for further analysis of protein release by different methods (Fig. 3). Freshly isolated NK cells were stimulated as mentioned above, the supernatant was analyzed by immunoprecipitation and subsequent Western Blot analysis for the presence of CCL4/MIP-1β. A protein band of similar size as the positive control (approximately 7.8 kDa) was detected in the immunoprecipitate of the supernatants from stimulated, but not from unstimulated, NK cells. Additionally, the Western Blots from four different experiments were densitometrically evaluated. In line with the results from Figs. 1 and 2, NK cells showed a significant higher release of CCL4/MIP-1β after stimulation with IL-2/IL-15 or *A. fumigatus*, while the CCL4/MIP-1β concentration was highest after stimulation with IL-2/IL-15 (Fig. 3a and b).

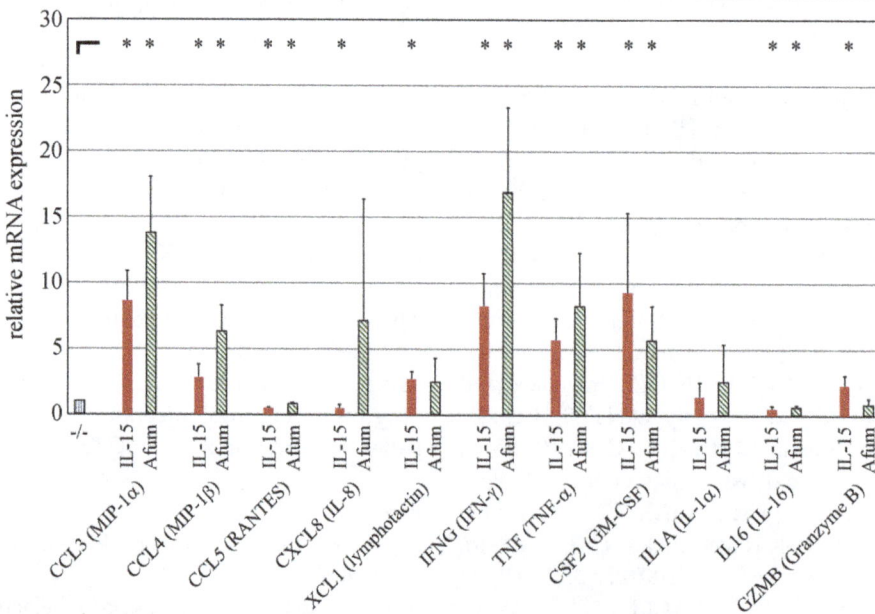

Fig. 1 Screening for cytokine mRNA expression by quantitative PCR. Freshly isolated NK cells were pre-incubated overnight with pro-leukin and stimulated with IL-2/IL-15 (IL-15) or *A. fumigatus* (Afum) germ tubes for 6 h. RNA was isolated and analyzed for the relative expression of the indicated genes by qPCR. Results were normalized for the value of unstimulated NK cells (−/−) – which was specified as "1". *n* = 5, means and standard deviations are shown. *$p < 0.05$. Please note CCL5/RANTES, which was significantly downregulated in a very small range

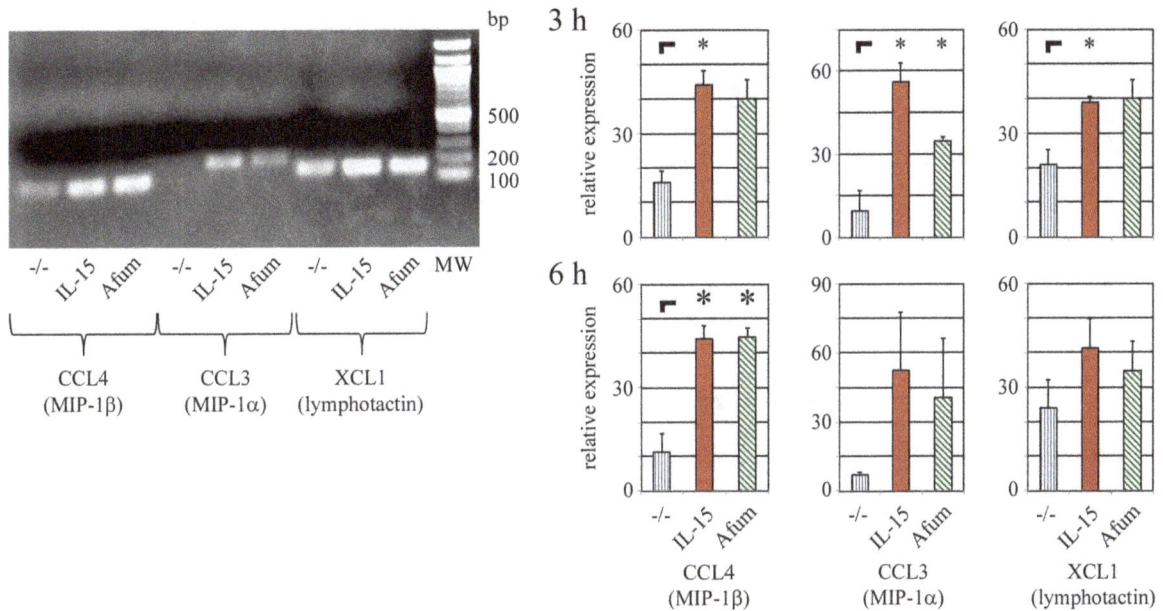

Fig. 2 Expression of cytokine mRNA after 3 and 6 h of stimulation analyzed by conventional PCR. Left side: Freshly isolated NK cells were pre-incubated overnight with pro-leukin and stimulated with IL-2 / Il-15 (IL-15) or *A. fumigatus* (Afum) germ tubes for 3 h. Unstimulated controls were included (–/–). RNA was isolated and used for RT-PCR detection of CCL4/MIP-1β, CCL3/MIP-1α, and XCL1/lymphotactin expression. PCR products were analyzed by gel electrophoresis. Right side: The experiment was performed three times in total for 3 (upper row) and 6 h (lower row) of stimulation, as indicated. Using ImageJ, the relative color intensity of each DNA band was quantified as a measure for the initial expression rate of the appropriate mRNA. Means and standard deviations were summarized in diagrams, *$p < 0.05$

In order to further corroborate the release of CCL4/MIP-1β, intracellular fluorescence-activated cell scanning (FACS) analysis was performed. Freshly isolated NK cells were stimulated as described above, but additionally had Brefeldin A added after 1 h of stimulation. After 6 h of stimulation in total, cells were collected, fixed, permeabilized and finally stained with α-CCL4/MIP-1β and a fluorochrome-conjugated second step antibody (Fig. 3c). CCL4/MIP-1β was detected to a minor extent in unstimulated, on a higher level with *A. fumigatus* stimulated, and clearly visible with IL-2/IL-15 stimulated NK cells. Three different experiments were taken into account for a statistical approach (Fig. 3d). In line with former results, expression of CCL4/MIP-1β was increased due to stimulation to a higher extent by IL-2/IL-15 vs. *A. fumigatus*.

Finally, supernatants of stimulated and unstimulated NK cells were analyzed for CCL4/MIP-1β by enzyme-linked immunosorbent assays ELISA (Fig. 3e). The release of CCL4/MIP-1β was significantly increased by stimulation with IL-2/IL-15 or *A. fumigatus*.

Cytokine production and release are adjusted to the MOI of *A. fumigatus*

In order to elucidate a potential dose dependent effect on the cytokine release, NK cells were stimulated as described above but with increasing MOIs of *A. fumigatus*.

In order to get a first impression, expression of CCL4 mRNA was found to increase dose dependently according to the MOI (Fig. 4).

Subsequently, cytokine release was analyzed by ELISA (Fig. 5). Chemokines such as CCL3/MIP-1α, CCL4/MIP-1β and CCL5/RANTES showed a significant stepwise increase up to 1000 (CCL4/MIP-1β) pg/ml referring to an increasing MOI. The cytokines TNF-α and IL-1α revealed a gradually increasing release, as well, but – presumably due to low absolute concentrations – showed significant difference to the release of unstimulated NK cells only with the highest MOIs. IFN-γ release was increased in general, but did not show a continuous rise according to the MOIs. Taken together, protein releases of all cytokines but IFN-γ were gradually amplifying due to increasing MOIs.

CD56 availability and CD69 expression on NK cells reflect the MOI of *A. fumigatus*

While this study was in preparation, our group published data revealing CD56 as a pathogen recognition receptor (not only) for *A. fumigatus*. In line with these results, we verified the gradually decrease of CD56 availability on the surface of NK cells after stimulation with the MOIs used in the present study. Additionally, CD69 and NKp30 expressions were examined (Fig. 6). As

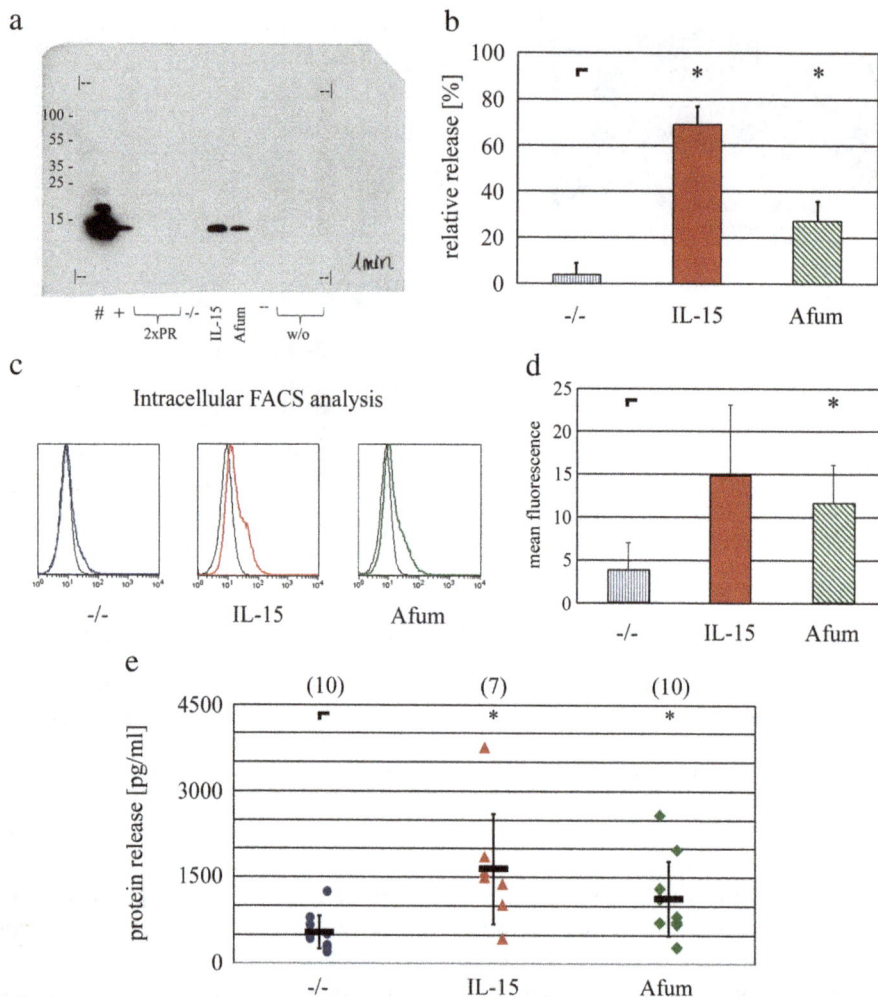

Fig. 3 Release of CCL4/MIP-1β by stimulated NK cells. NK cells were prepared and stimulated as described in methods. **a** Supernatants were incubated with αCCL4/MIP-1β and A/G sepharose beads, culture medium was included as negative control (–). Immunoprecipitated proteins were analyzed by SDS page and subsequent Western Blot for CCL4/MIP-1β protein. 100 ng (#) and 100 pg (+) rhCCL4/MIP-1β were provided as positive controls. Two lanes were used for molecular weight standards (PR), results are indicated in kDa on the very left. Another two lanes were not used (w/o). For your convenience, the whole X-ray film is shown, the size of the membrane is marked with "|--". Please note the exposition time on the right corner (1 min) and the appearance of high molecular weight aggregates within the overloaded positive control (#). **b** The experiment described in (**a**) was performed four times in total and analyzed by ImageJ. Means and standard deviations were summarized into one diagram. **c** Cytokine release was blocked by Brefeldin A. CCL4/MIP-1β expression was analyzed by intracellular FACS analysis (colored, thick lines) including isotype controls (thin, black lines) as shown here in a representative result. **d** The experiment described in (**c**) was performed three times in total. MFI values were corrected as described in the method section, means and standard deviations were summarized into one diagram. **e** Supernatants of stimulated NK cells were analyzed by ELISA for CCL4/MIP-1β. The number of samples is indicated for each stimulation condition. Individual results as well as means and standard deviations are depicted. *$p < 0.05$

expected, CD69 expression increased significantly due to higher MOIs. NKp30 expression, on the other hand, was barely influenced by the presence of *A. fumigatus*.

Discussion

In clinical practice, *A. fumigatus* infections in immunocompromised patients are an increasing problem. NK cells are more and more considered as a mandatory factor for the outcome, since they are known for the release of a wide spectrum of cytokines and thereby intended to

play a major role in the early phases of an immune response. In this study, the expression and release of cytokines by freshly isolated human NK cells after *A. fumigatus* stimulation were analyzed. Cytokine expression by (q)PCR and analysis of protein release by ELISA and – for CCL4/MIP-1β – by complimentary experiments including Western Blot and FACS analysis were evaluated. Additionally, the release of chemokines, cytokines, and the expression of surface markers by NK cells after stimulation with different MOIs of *A. fumigatus* were examined.

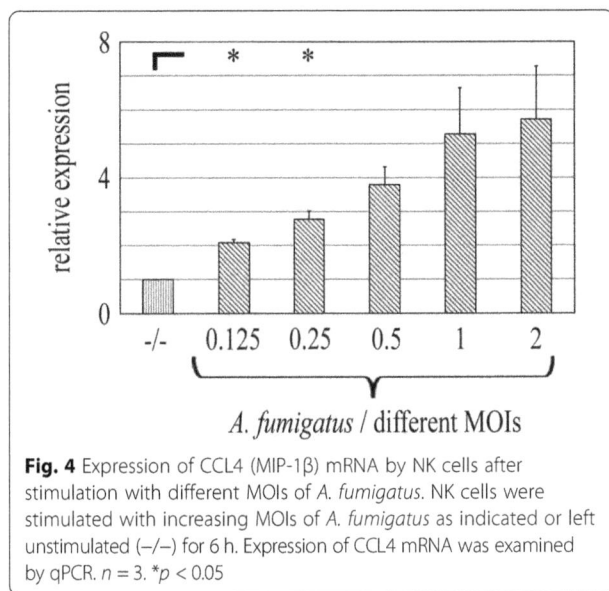

Fig. 4 Expression of CCL4 (MIP-1β) mRNA by NK cells after stimulation with different MOIs of *A. fumigatus*. NK cells were stimulated with increasing MOIs of *A. fumigatus* as indicated or left unstimulated (−/−) for 6 h. Expression of CCL4 mRNA was examined by qPCR. $n = 3$. *$p < 0.05$

Chemokines such as CCL3/MIP-1α and CCL4/MIP-1β were most prominently upregulated in stimulated NK cells, while CCL5/RANTES showed a slight downregulation on mRNA level, but a marked increase on protein release. Furthermore, the chemokine concentration was correlated with the MOI of *A. fumigatus*.

The expression and – in part – the release of cytokines by other immune cells after confrontation with *A. fumigatus* is already known. Since CCL3/MIP-1α, CCL4/MIP-1β and TNF-α mRNA expression in dendritic cells (DCs) or monocytes is upregulated after co-incubation with *A. fumigatus*, these results are in line with the present study. On the contrary, the analysis of CCL5/RANTES expression and release by further immune cells shows inconsistent results. While the mRNA is upregulated in DCs, the corresponding protein is hardly detectable after 20 h of co-cultivation with *A. fumigatus*. In monocytes, mRNA expression and the release of CCL5/RANTES is even downregulated [35–39]. Platelets, on the other hand, show an increase of CCL5/RANTES protein after *A. fumigatus* stimulation [40]. It should be noted, that CCL5/RANTES expression in T cells was intensively analyzed around 20 years ago, mainly due to its anti-HIV effect, but also due to the characteristically late expression of the CCL5 gene [41].

Beside that particular CCL5 mRNA expression characteristic, there are other possible mechanisms to explain the results of the present study. For example, resting murine NK cells contain low amounts of perforin and granzyme B proteins, while the corresponding mRNAs are abundant. Upon activation, the available mRNAs are translated, while there are just slight changes to the amount of mRNAs available [42]. It is tempting to speculate, that there may be a similar mechanism for

CCL5/RANTES. Alternatively, NK cells may simply empty their granules upon *A. fumigatus* recognition, but further focus on the expression of cytokines other than CCL5/RANTES for acute treatment of the fungal infection. It may be of interest for further studies, whether, and if so when, the expression level of CCL5/RANTES is increasing again after the stimulation has taken place.

In addition, genetic studies revealed single nucleotide polymorphisms (SNPs) in CCL3 and CCL4, which are significantly correlated to fungal infections [43]. In particular, CCL3/MIP-1α is regarded as a critical mediator of host defense against *A. fumigatus* infection due to several studies of animal infection models [44–47]. Together with CCL4/MIP-1β and CCL5/RANTES, CCL3/MIP-1α is responsible for the recruitment of various immune cells such as monocytes, T cells, all kinds of granulocytes, DCs and NK cells [48–51]. Therefore, these chemokines might play a substantial role in orchestrating an early antifungal response against *A. fumigatus*.

Cytokines such as IFN-γ, TNF-α and IL-1α revealed a vast upregulation on mRNA level and – except for IFN-γ – a slight but stepwise increase on the protein release when stimulated with different MOIs of *A. fumigatus*. Even though IFN-γ release showed a significant upregulation after stimulation with an MOI of 1 or 2, the respective gain of IFN-γ did not fully correspond to the stepwise increase of the MOI. That may be due to the combination of different characteristics of IFN-γ release by NK cells. First, cytokine vs. chemokine release by stimulated NK cells generally reveals a greater requirement for receptor cooperation and, probably therefore, occurs at later time points after stimulation [20]. Second, the release of IFN-γ by NK cells after 6 h of *A. fumigatus* stimulation is very low in general as seen in the present and in a preceding study by Bouzani et al. In the latter publication, IFN-γ release was shown to reach a peak not until 12 h of incubation [27]. Third, according to Schneider et al., *A. fumigatus* actively impairs the release of IFN-γ (and GM-CSF) by NK cells [34]. Taken together, these effects could be responsible for the inconsistent results of the MOI-dependent analysis of IFN-γ release by stimulated NK cells.

IFN-γ is a main activator of macrophages and cytotoxic T cells, and favors T helper cell type 1 immune responses. Former studies have already demonstrated beneficial effects of IFN-γ against *A. fumigatus* infection [26, 52–54]. Moreover, Bouzani et al. showed that NK cell-derived IFN-γ has a direct antifungal activity. In line with the results of the present study, IFN-γ mRNA expression was already detectable after 6 h, while IFN-γ protein was just slightly released after 6 h, but substantially present in the supernatant of NK cells after 12 h of stimulation. In contrast, TNF-α mRNA expression and protein release could be detected already after 6 h [27] – again in line with

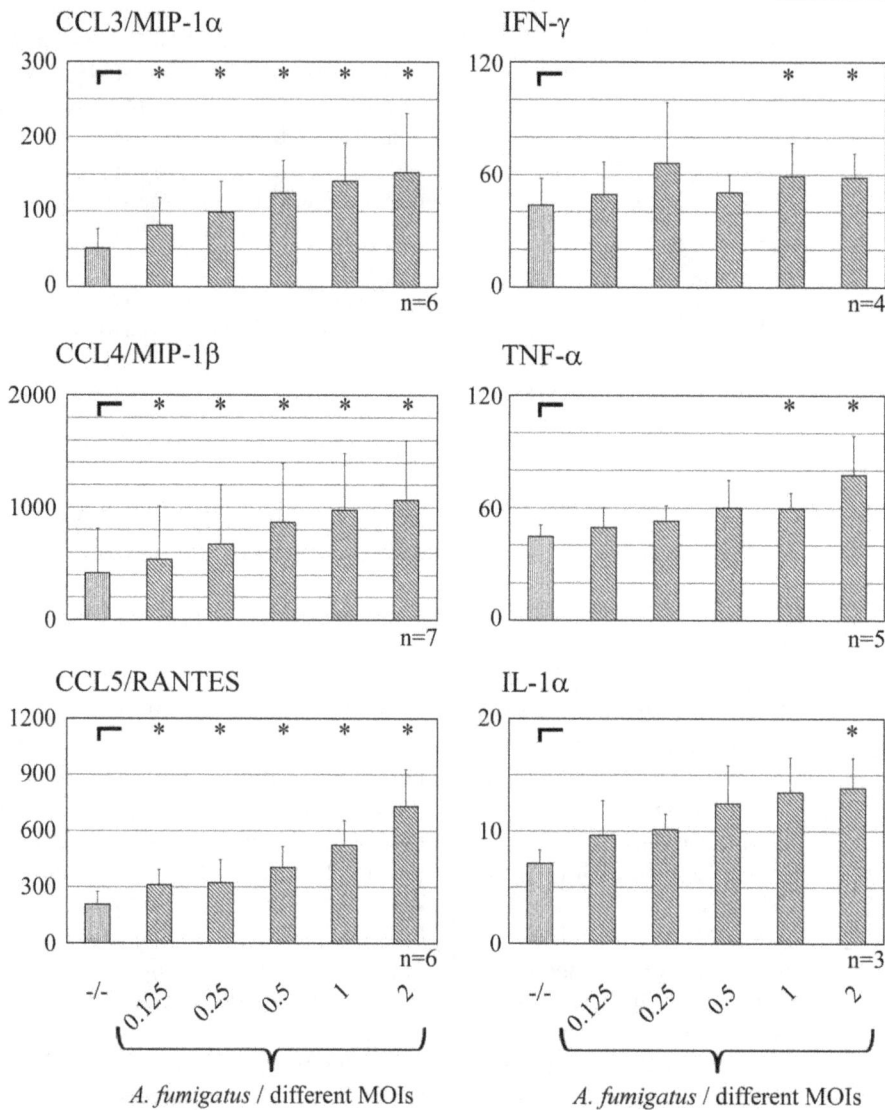

Fig. 5 Release of cytokines by NK cells after stimulation with different MOIs of *A. fumigatus*. NK cells were stimulated with increasing MOIs of *A. fumigatus* as indicated or left unstimulated (–/–) for 6 h. The release of cytokines was analyzed by ELISA. All measurements are noted in pg/ml, the number of independent experiments for every cytokine is indicated. *$p < 0.05$

results of this study. Furthermore, genetic studies show a correlation between SNPs in the genes for IFN-γ (IFNG) and tumor necrosis factor receptor 2 (TNFR2) and the risk of suffering from a disease caused by *A. fumigatus* [55].

IL-1α is a major cytokine to induce and regulate inflammation in general. With regard to antifungal effects, IL-1α was described as crucial for optimal leukocyte recruitment during a pulmonary *A. fumigatus* infection [56], identified as an inductor for antimicrobial peptide expression in epithelial cells [57] and shown to be a main coordinator in the neutrophil response to *Candida albicans* [58]. IL-1α was found to be effective already at concentrations of about 10 pg/ml [59], which is lower

than the IL-1α concentration found in this study. Taken together, the upregulation of IFN-γ mRNA expression, which – according to Bouzani et al. [27] – will likely be followed by an upregulated protein release later on, and the increase of TNF-α and IL-1α release demonstrated in this study can be regarded as substantial contribution to an immune response against *A. fumigatus*.

With regard to the comparison of chemokine (CCL3/MIP-1α, CCL4/MIP-1β) vs. cytokine (IFN-γ, TNF-α) release by stimulated NK cells, Fauriat et al. have already characterized the cytokine secretion profile of NK cells after contact with K562. While chemokines such as CCL3/MIP-1α, CCL4/MIP-1β and CCL5/RANTES were detected right after stimulation, cytokines such as

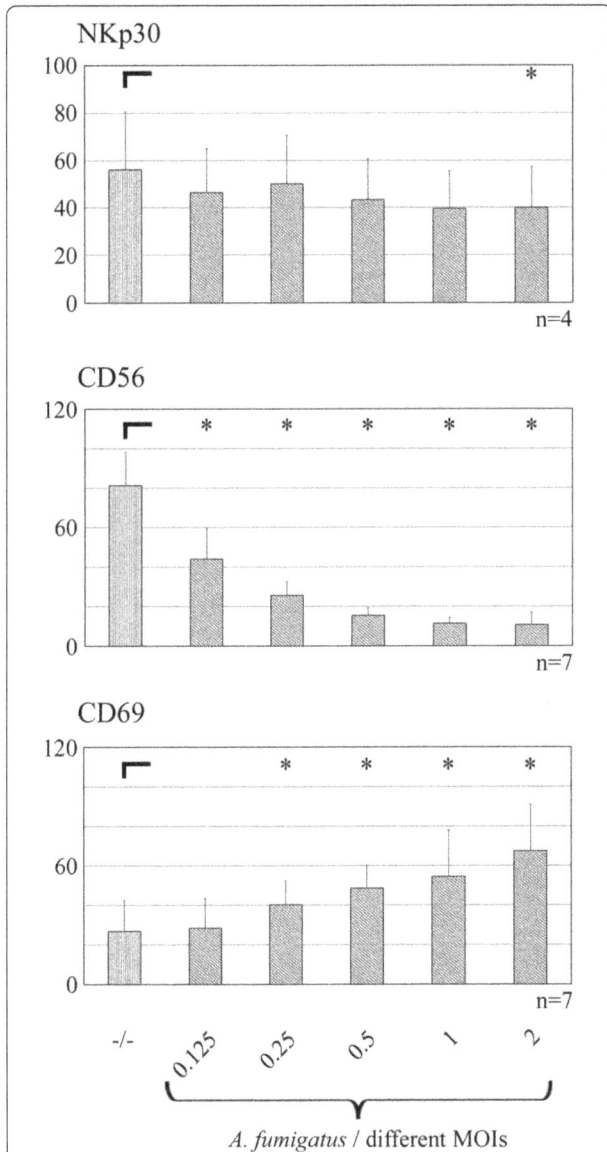

Fig. 6 Expression / availability of receptors on NK cells after stimulation with different MOIs of *A. fumigatus*. NK cells were stimulated with increasing MOIs of *A. fumigatus* as indicated or left unstimulated (−/−) for 6 h. NKp30, CD56 and CD69 were examined by FACS analysis. Mean fluorescence intensity values are shown. The number of independent experiments for every cytokine is indicated. *$p < 0.05$

increasing MOI was just recognizable in an initial stage. At this early time point after stimulation, relatively high MOIs of 1 or 2 are needed for the initiation of a significantly increased release of the cytokines. NK cells seem to stepwise counteract a fungal infection with recruitment of macrophages and neutrophils in the early phases, while adaptive immunity will be alarmed by cytokines in case the infection persists.

Very recently, Schneider et al. analyzed cytokine expression by NK cells after stimulation with *A. fumigatus*, as well [34]. In accordance with the present study, that publication reported a downregulation of GZMB (granzyme B) and an upregulation of IFNG (IFN-γ), CSF2 (GM-CSF), CCL3 (MIP-1α) and CCL4 (MIP-1β) mRNA expression, and an increase of the intracellular protein level of IFN-γ after *A. fumigatus* stimulation. In contrast to the results obtained here, subsequent analysis of the supernatant revealed a non-significant downregulation of IFN-γ, CCL3/MIP-1α or CCL4/MIP-1β release. That may be explained by the different pre-treatment of the NK cells used in both studies. Schneider et al. focused their research on a clinical background and therefore pre-stimulated NK cells over 10 days with the addition of 1000 U/ml IL-2 every three days, before the cells were co-incubated with *A. fumigatus*. The authors discuss that procedure with regard to perforin release, revealing that IL-2 pre-stimulation of NK cells alone already results in relatively high extracellular perforin levels, and that – presumably therefore – *A. fumigatus* had only a marginal additional effect on the extracellular perforin concentration. It is tempting to speculate, that this is valid not only for perforin, but also for cytokine production in general, and that IL-2 pretreatment only overnight – as in our study – just ignite NK cell activity and thereby leaves room for an increase of IFN-γ, CCL3/MIP-1α and CCL4/MIP-1β release after *A. fumigatus* stimulation.

The **surface markers** NKp30 and CD56 were reported as binding receptors for fungal ligands in former publications. Li et al. pretreated NK cells with increasing amounts of a preparation of the cryptococcal cell wall/membrane and subsequently showed a decreasing accessibility of NKp30 by an adequate antibody [30]. Here, the surface availability of NKp30 decreased just roughly according to increasing MOIs of *A. fumigatus*, but showed a significant difference in comparison of unstimulated vs. NK cells after stimulation with the highest MOI. As expected due to results by Ziegler et al. [29], the accessibility of CD56 on the cell surface decreased significantly and stepwise according to increasing MOIs. In turn, that indicated a gradually increased amount of CD56 molecules engaged in the binding process. Moreover, a correlation between CD56 binding activity and the activation status reflected by CD69 expression depending on different MOIs of *A. fumigatus* was shown.

TNF-α and IFN-γ were found only later on [20]. These results are in line with data published by Bouzani et al., showing a vast increase of IFNG and TNF expression and – only for TNF-α – a relatively moderate increase of protein release after 6 h. After 12 h, though, IFN-γ and TNF-α release showed a strong and significant increase after stimulation with *A. fumigatus*. In line with these publications, IFN-γ and TNF-α secretions after just 6 h stimulation in the present study were very low. Thereby, a fine-tuning of the release by stepwise

The **correlation of the *A. fumigatus* MOI** with the cytokine expression and release was described here – at least to our knowledge – for the first time. NK cells seem to fine-tune their immunological reactions according to the threat level, thereby not only providing information about the mere presence, but also about the relative amount of *A. fumigatus*. Future studies will analyze whether this feature of NK cells can be shown as well for the expression and release of other immunomodulatory molecules and/or toward further pathogens. Additionally, the relatively simple comparative measurement of chemokine expression by qPCR, chemokine release by ELISA or CD69 expression by FACS analysis may become an instrument to quantify the involvement of NK cells in an ongoing immune reaction.

Conclusions

In summary, we corroborate the results from Li et al. [30] and Ziegler et al. [29] with regard to the surface markers, but further provide evidence for an MOI-dependent activation status of and a cytokine release by NK cells after stimulation with *A. fumigatus*. The contribution of NK cells to the immune response against *A. fumigatus* infection may therefore be based upon their early intervention in the cytokine network. Since the dose-dependent release of CCL4/MIP-1β provides relatively high concentrations in a short period after stimulation, it may be regarded as a marker protein for NK cell activation in further studies. These results will contribute to our understanding of the interactions between NK cells and *A. fumigatus*, which may be critical in patients suffering from IA while recovering from HSCT.

Methods

NK cell purification and stimulation

Peripheral blood mononuclear cells (PBMCs) were isolated by Ficoll (Biochrom AG) density gradient centrifugation using leukoreduction system chambers obtained from healthy adult blood donors. Usage of the human blood specimens was approved by the Ethical Committee of the University Hospital Wuerzburg, and written consent was provided by all blood donors. NK cells were isolated by magnetic-activated cell separation (MACS) NK negative selection kit (Miltenyi Biotec). The purity was checked by FACS analysis using CD14-Fitc, NKp46-PE, CD56-APC (all from BD Pharmingen) and CD3-PerCP (Miltenyi Biotec) antibodies, and was always > 95% (please see Additional file 1). NK cells were cultured overnight in RPMI 1640 (Invitrogen) with 10% heat-inactivated fetal bovine serum, 120 µg/ml gentamicin (Refobacin; Merck) and supplemented with 1000 U/ml recombinant human IL-2 (Novartis) at 37 °C and 5% CO_2. *A. fumigatus* (ATCC 46645) germ tubes were prepared as described previously [37] and added to NK cells at an

MOI of 0.5 unless indicated otherwise. For comparison, NK cells were left unstimulated or – for usage as positive control – added IL-2 (500 U/ml) and IL-15 (500 U/ml = 62.5 ng/ml), which stimulate for NK cell activation [60, 61]. While preceding studies using *A. fumigatus* conidia for stimulation on macrophages or epithelial cells revealed a minimum incubation time of about 8 h to take effect [39, 62], studies using already prepared germlings provide an incubation time of around 6 h as adequate for a subsequent simultaneous analysis of mRNA and protein expression for early expressed genes [27]. Therefore, the latter method was chosen, while partially additional samples were collected after 3 h. Cells were used for RNA isolation or FACS analysis, while the supernatants were submitted to ELISA or immunoprecipitation of CCL4/MIP-1β with subsequent Western Blot analysis.

Gene expression analysis

RNA isolation was performed using RNeasy Mini Kits (Qiagen), while subsequent cDNA synthesis was done using First Strand cDNA Synthesis Kit (Thermo Fisher), each according to the manufacturer protocol. Nucleic acid concentration was determined by nanodrop quantification (Thermo Scientific). qPCR analysis was processed using primers (Table 1) from Sigma-Aldrich and SYBRGreen Master Mix from Biorad in a Step One Plus (Applied Biosystems).

Expression of every gene was normalized to the expression of the housekeeping gene ALAS1. Relative expression of the respective gene in unstimulated NK cells was converted to "1", its expression level in stimulated NK cells was calculated in correlation to that.

PCR amplicons of CCL3 (MIP-1α), CCL4 (MIP-1β) and XCL1 (lymphotactin) were submitted to agarose (Roth) gel electrophoresis, using ethidium bromide from Thermo Fisher and an electrophoresis system from Serva. The results were documented by a Multi-Image Light Cabinet (Alpha Innotech) and densitometrically analyzed by ImageJ. The intensities of bands generated by stimulated and non-stimulated NK cells of one experiment were added up und accounted for 100%. For every stimulation condition, the respective percentage was calculated.

Quantification of released CCL4/MIP-1β by immunoprecipitation and Western blot

0.5 µg monoclonal mouse anti human CCL4/MIP-1β antibody (R&D Systems) was pre-incubated with 15 µl Protein A/G Plus Agarose Beads (Santa Cruz Biotechnology) for 3 h at 4 °C, then added for overnight incubation to the NK cell supernatants generated above. After that, the beads were submitted for running on a 15% sodium dodecyl sulfate (SDS) gel, transferred to a nitrocellulose membrane and blotted with 0.1 µg/ml polyclonal biotinylated

Table 1 Primers for qPCR analysis

Gene	Forward	Reverse	Product size (bp)
ALAS1[a]	GGCAGCACAGATGAATCAGA	CCTCCATCGGTTTTCACACT	150
CCL3 (MIP-1α)	TGCAACCAGTTCTCTGCATC	TTTCTGGACCCACTCCTCAC	198
CCL4 (MIP-1β)	GCTTCCTCGCAACTTTGTGG	TCACTGGGATCAGCACAGAC	111
CCL5 (RANTES)	TCATTGCTACTGCCCTCTGC	TACTCCTTGATGTGGGCACG	115
CXCL8 (IL-8)	GGTGCAGTTTTGCCAAGGAG	TTCCTTGGGGTCCAGACAGA	183
XCL1 (lymphotactin)[b]	CTCCTTGGCATCTGCTCTCT	CCTTCCGTGATGGTGTAGGTC	137
IFNG (IFN-γ)[c]	GCATCCAAAAGAGTGTGGAG	GCAGGCAGGACAACCATTAC	255
TNF (TNF-α)	TGCTTGTTCCTCAGCCTCTT	TGGGCTACAGGCTTGTCACT	185
CSF2 (GM-CSF)	GCCCTGGGAGCATGTGAATG	CTTGTAGTGGCTGGCCATCAT	223
IL1A (IL-1α)	TGATCAGTACCTCACGGCTG	TGGTCTTCATCTTGGGCAGT	156
IL16 (IL-16)	CGAAGACTCAGCTGCAAATGG	GCAGGGAGATAACGGACTGAC	167
GZMB (granzyme B)	TGCGAATCTGACTTACGCCA	GCATGCCATTGTTTCGTCCA	160

[a]ALAS1 is well established as a housekeeping gene for the normalization of gene expression by cells confronted with different stimuli [63–67]. In general, primers were designed to include as much transcript variants of the mentioned gene as possible. Within this context, [b]primers for XCL1/lymphotactin qualify also for the amplification of XCL2, which differs just slightly with regard to the amino acids, but show the same functionality in vitro [68]. [c]Primers for IFNG were already published by Bouzani et al. [27]

anti-CCL4/MIP-1β (R&D Systems). After 2 h at 4 °C, the membrane was supplemented with Streptavidin-HRP (Biolegend) and finally developed using ECL chemiluminescence reagent. Recombinant human CCL4/MIP-1β (R&D Systems) was included as positive control. The X-ray film was scanned and densitometrically analyzed by ImageJ as described above.

Intracellular detection of CCL4/MIP-1β by FACS analysis
NK cells were isolated and initially stimulated as mentioned above, but supplemented with 10 μg/ml Brefeldin A after 1 h of incubation with *A. fumigatus*, IL-2/IL-15 or nothing. After 6 h in total, cells were permeabilized (Cytofix/Cytoperm Kit / BD Biosciences) and intracellularly stained with monoclonal mouse anti human CCL4/MIP-1β or IgG Isotype control (both R&D Systems), and subsequently treated with PE-conjugated anti mouse antibody (Jackson Immunotech). All samples were measured on a FACS Calibur flow cytometer (BD Biosciences) using the Cell Quest Pro software. The mean fluorescence intensity (MFI) obtained by the isotype control was subtracted from the respective MFI obtained by the CCL4/MIP-1β analysis in order to receive a corrected MFI for further evaluation.

Quantification of released molecules by ELISA
The concentration of immunomodulatory molecules were quantified using ELISA Kits from R&D Systems (CCL3/MIP-1α, CCL4/MIP-1β, IFN-γ) and Biolegend (CCL5/RANTES, IFN-γ, TNF-α and IL-1α) according to the manufacturer's protocol.

Expression of surface molecules by FACS analysis
αNKP30-PE (Biolegend), αCD56-Fitc (Becton Dickinson), αCD69-APC (Miltenyi) and respective isotype controls from the same companies were used for the analysis of the surface expression.

Statistical analysis
In figures, n refers to the number of independent experiments. Statistical significance was tested for results obtained from unstimulated vs. IL-2/IL-15 stimulated ("IL-15") or vs. *A. fumigatus* stimulated ("Afum") NK cells, respectively, using student's t-test. Therefore, in the presentation of the figure, results from unstimulated NK cells were marked with ⊢ for being the standard, while results from stimulated NK cells were marked with * ($p < 0.05$) or nothing ($p \geq 0.05$).

Abbreviations
(m)RNA: (messenger) ribonucleic acid; (q)PCR: (quantitative) polymerase chain reaction; *A.*: *Aspergillus*; ALAS1: 5′-aminolevulinate synthase 1; CCL: CC chemokine ligand; CD: Cluster of differentiation; CXC3L1: Chemokine (C–X3–C motif) ligand 1; DC: Dendritic cell; ELISA: Enzyme-linked immunosorbent assay; FACS: Fluorescence-activated cell scanning; GM-CSF: Granulocyte-macrophage colony-stimulating factor; h: Hours; HSCT: Hematopoietic stem cell transplantation; IA: Invasive aspergillosis; IFN: Interferon; IL: Interleukin; IP-10: N-gamma-inducible protein-10; MACS: Magnetic-activated cell separation; MCP-1: Monocyte chemoattractant protein 1; MFI: Mean fluorescence intensity; MIP: Macrophage inflammatory protein; MOI: Multiplicity of infection;

PBMC: Peripheral blood mononuclear cells; RANTES: Regulated and normal T cell expressed and secreted; SDS: Sodium dodecyl sulfate; SLC: Secondary lymphoid tissue chemokine; SNP: Single nucleotide polymorphism; TLR: Toll-like receptor; TNF: Tumor necrosis factor; vs.: Versus; XCL1: X-C motif chemokine ligand 1

Acknowledgements
We would like to thank the Collaborative Research Center CRC124 FungiNet, funded by the German Research Council (DFG), for establishing a platform to exchange ideas and protocols. Furthermore, we wish to thank all blood donors not only for supporting us, but also for providing a vital contribution to the health care system in general. This work forms part of the Ph.D. thesis of AE.

Funding
This work was supported by the Deutsche Forschungsgemeinschaft (DFG) within the Collaborative Research Center CRC124 FungiNet "Pathogenic fungi and their human host: Networks of interaction" (project A2 to HE and JL). The funders had no role in study design, data collection, analysis and interpretation, decision to publish, or preparation of the manuscript.

Authors' contributions
LM participated in the design of the study, performed analysis by intracellular FACS, ELISA and qPCR, evaluated images by ImageJ and drafted the manuscript. AE carried out experiments with varying MOIs and subsequent analysis by ELISA and FACS. ALS performed the Western Blot analysis and repeated qPCR and ELISA experiments for complementation. HE and JL participated in the design of the study, reviewing and interpreting of the results. All authors read and approved the final manuscript.

Competing interests
The authors declare that they have no competing interests.

References
1. Latge JP. Aspergillus fumigatus and aspergillosis. Clin Microbiol Rev. 1999; 12(2):310–50.
2. Hospenthal DR, Kwon-Chung KJ, Bennett JE. Concentrations of airborne aspergillus compared to the incidence of invasive aspergillosis: lack of correlation. Med Mycol. 1998;36(3):165–8.
3. Romani L. Immunity to fungal infections. Nat Rev Immunol. 2011;11(4):275–88.
4. Shah A, Panjabi C. Allergic bronchopulmonary aspergillosis: a perplexing clinical entity. Allergy Asthma Immunol Res. 2016;8(4):282–97.
5. Dagenais TR, Keller NP. Pathogenesis of aspergillus fumigatus in invasive aspergillosis. Clin Microbiol Rev. 2009;22(3):447–65.
6. Mehta RS, Rezvani K. Immune reconstitution post allogeneic transplant and the impact of immune recovery on the risk of infection. Virulence. 2016;7(8): 901–16.
7. Stuehler C, et al. Immune reconstitution after allogeneic hematopoietic stem cell transplantation and association with occurrence and outcome of invasive aspergillosis. J Infect Dis. 2015;212(6):959–67.
8. Bjorkstrom NK, Ljunggren HG, Michaelsson J. Emerging insights into natural killer cells in human peripheral tissues. Nat Rev Immunol. 2016;16(5):310–20.
9. Montaldo E, et al. Unique Eomes(+) NK cell subsets are present in uterus and decidua during early pregnancy. Front Immunol. 2015;6:646.
10. Poli A, et al. NK cells in central nervous system disorders. J Immunol. 2013; 190(11):5355–62.
11. Papakosta D, et al. Bronchoalveolar lavage fluid and blood natural killer and natural killer T-like cells in cryptogenic organizing pneumonia. Respirology. 2014;19(5):748–54.
12. Marquardt N, et al. Human lung natural killer cells are predominantly comprised of highly differentiated hypofunctional CD69(–)CD56(dim) cells. J Allergy Clin Immunol. 2017;139(4):1321–30 e4.
13. Hesker PR, Krupnick AS, The role of natural killer cells in pulmonary immunosurveillance. Front Biosci (Schol Ed). 2013;5:575–87.
14. Zanoni I, et al. IL-15 cis presentation is required for optimal NK cell activation in lipopolysaccharide-mediated inflammatory conditions. Cell Rep. 2013;4(6):1235–49.
15. Souza-Fonseca-Guimaraes F, Adib-Conquy M, Cavaillon JM. Natural killer (NK) cells in antibacterial innate immunity: angels or devils? Mol Med. 2012; 18:270–85.
16. Chalifour A, et al. Direct bacterial protein PAMP recognition by human NK cells involves TLRs and triggers alpha-defensin production. Blood. 2004; 104(6):1778–83.
17. Hanna J, et al. Novel insights on human NK cells' immunological modalities revealed by gene expression profiling. J Immunol. 2004;173(11):6547–63.
18. Marr KJ, et al. Cryptococcus neoformans directly stimulates perforin production and rearms NK cells for enhanced anticryptococcal microbicidal activity. Infect Immun. 2009;77(6):2436–46.
19. Agerberth B, et al. The human antimicrobial and chemotactic peptides LL-37 and alpha-defensins are expressed by specific lymphocyte and monocyte populations. Blood. 2000;96(9):3086–93.
20. Fauriat C, et al. Regulation of human NK-cell cytokine and chemokine production by target cell recognition. Blood. 2010;115(11):2167–76.
21. Robertson MJ. Role of chemokines in the biology of natural killer cells. J Leukoc Biol. 2002;71(2):173–83.
22. Maghazachi AA. Role of chemokines in the biology of natural killer cells. Curr Top Microbiol Immunol. 2010;341:37–58.
23. Schmidt S, et al. Natural killer cells and antifungal host response. Clin Vaccine Immunol. 2013;20(4):452–8.
24. Ogbomo H, Mody CH. Granule-dependent natural killer cell cytotoxicity to fungal pathogens. Front Immunol. 2016;7:692.
25. Morrison BE, et al. Chemokine-mediated recruitment of NK cells is a critical host defense mechanism in invasive aspergillosis. J Clin Invest. 2003;112(12): 1862–70.
26. Park SJ, et al. Early NK cell-derived IFN-{gamma} is essential to host defense in neutropenic invasive aspergillosis. J Immunol. 2009;182(7):4306–12.
27. Bouzani M, et al. Human NK cells display important antifungal activity against aspergillus fumigatus, which is directly mediated by IFN-gamma release. J Immunol. 2011;187(3):1369–76.
28. Schmidt S, et al. Human natural killer cells exhibit direct activity against aspergillus fumigatus hyphae, but not against resting conidia. J Infect Dis. 2011;203(3):430–5.
29. Ziegler S, et al. CD56 is a pathogen recognition receptor on human natural killer cells. Sci Rep. 2017;7(1):6138.
30. Li SS, et al. The NK receptor NKp30 mediates direct fungal recognition and killing and is diminished in NK cells from HIV-infected patients. Cell Host Microbe. 2013;14(4):387–97.
31. Vitenshtein A, et al. NK cell recognition of Candida glabrata through binding of NKp46 and NCR1 to fungal ligands Epa1, Epa6, and Epa7. Cell Host Microbe. 2016;20(4):527–34.
32. Aimanianda V, et al. Surface hydrophobin prevents immune recognition of airborne fungal spores. Nature. 2009;460(7259):1117–21.
33. Heinekamp T, et al. Interference of aspergillus fumigatus with the immune response. Semin Immunopathol. 2015;37(2):141–52.
34. Schneider A, et al. Aspergillus fumigatus responds to natural killer (NK) cells with upregulation of stress related genes and inhibits the immunoregulatory function of NK cells. Oncotarget. 2016;7(44):71062–71.
35. Cortez KJ, et al. Functional genomics of innate host defense molecules in normal human monocytes in response to aspergillus fumigatus. Infect Immun. 2006;74(4):2353–65.
36. Gafa V, et al. In vitro infection of human dendritic cells by aspergillus fumigatus conidia triggers the secretion of chemokines for neutrophil and Th1 lymphocyte recruitment. Microbes Infect. 2007;9(8):971–80.

37. Morton CO, et al. Gene expression profiles of human dendritic cells interacting with aspergillus fumigatus in a bilayer model of the alveolar epithelium/endothelium interface. PLoS One. 2014;9(5):e98279.

38. Morton CO, et al. The temporal dynamics of differential gene expression in aspergillus fumigatus interacting with human immature dendritic cells in vitro. PLoS One. 2011;6(1):e16016.

39. Steele C, et al. The beta-glucan receptor dectin-1 recognizes specific morphologies of aspergillus fumigatus. PLoS Pathog. 2005;1(4):e42.

40. Rodland EK, et al. Activation of platelets by aspergillus fumigatus and potential role of platelets in the immunopathogenesis of aspergillosis. Infect Immun. 2010;78(3):1269–75.

41. Song A, Nikolcheva T, Krensky AM. Transcriptional regulation of RANTES expression in T lymphocytes. Immunol Rev. 2000;177:236–45.

42. Fehniger TA, et al. Acquisition of murine NK cell cytotoxicity requires the translation of a pre-existing pool of granzyme B and perforin mRNAs. Immunity. 2007;26(6):798–811.

43. Loeffler J, et al. Genetic polymorphisms in the cytokine and chemokine system: their possible importance in allogeneic stem cell transplantation. Curr Top Microbiol Immunol. 2010;341:83–96.

44. Mehrad B, Moore TA, Standiford TJ. Macrophage inflammatory protein-1 alpha is a critical mediator of host defense against invasive pulmonary aspergillosis in neutropenic hosts. J Immunol. 2000;165(2):962–8.

45. Schelenz S, Smith DA, Bancroft GJ. Cytokine and chemokine responses following pulmonary challenge with aspergillus fumigatus: obligatory role of TNF-alpha and GM-CSF in neutrophil recruitment. Med Mycol. 1999;37(3):183–94.

46. Shahan TA, et al. Concentration- and time-dependent upregulation and release of the cytokines MIP-2, KC, TNF, and MIP-1alpha in rat alveolar macrophages by fungal spores implicated in airway inflammation. Am J Respir Cell Mol Biol. 1998;18(3):435–40.

47. Gao JL, et al. Impaired host defense, hematopoiesis, granulomatous inflammation and type 1-type 2 cytokine balance in mice lacking CC chemokine. Receptor 1. J Exp Med. 1997;185(11):1959–68.

48. Menten P, Wuyts A, Van Damme J. Macrophage inflammatory protein-1. Cytokine Growth Factor Rev. 2002;13(6):455–81.

49. Lukacs NW, et al. C-C chemokine-induced eosinophil chemotaxis during allergic airway inflammation. J Leukoc Biol. 1996;60(5):573–8.

50. Schall TJ, et al. Selective attraction of monocytes and T lymphocytes of the memory phenotype by cytokine RANTES. Nature. 1990;347(6294):669–71.

51. Le Y, et al. Chemokines and chemokine receptors: their manifold roles in homeostasis and disease. Cell Mol Immunol. 2004;1(2):95–104.

52. Bandera A, et al. Interferon-gamma and granulocyte-macrophage colony stimulating factor therapy in three patients with pulmonary aspergillosis. Infection. 2008;36(4):368–73.

53. Maheshwari RK, et al. Interferon inhibits aspergillus fumigatus growth in mice: an activity against an extracellular infection. J Interf Res. 1988;8(1):35–44.

54. Shao C, et al. Transient overexpression of gamma interferon promotes aspergillus clearance in invasive pulmonary aspergillosis. Clin Exp Immunol. 2005;142(2):233–41.

55. Ok M, Einsele H, Loeffler J. Genetic susceptibility to aspergillus fumigatus infections. Int J Med Microbiol. 2011;301(5):445–52.

56. Mayer-Barber KD, Yan B. Clash of the cytokine titans: counter-regulation of interleukin-1 and type I interferon-mediated inflammatory responses. Cell Mol Immunol. 2017;14(1):22–35.

57. Bando M, et al. Interleukin-1alpha regulates antimicrobial peptide expression in human keratinocytes. Immunol Cell Biol. 2007;85(7):532–7.

58. Altmeier S, et al. IL-1 Coordinates the Neutrophil Response to C. albicans in the Oral Mucosa. PLoS Pathog. 2016;12(9):e1005882.

59. Eigenbrod T, et al. Cutting edge: critical role for mesothelial cells in necrosis-induced inflammation through the recognition of IL-1 alpha released from dying cells. J Immunol. 2008;181(12):8194–8.

60. Brehm C, et al. IL-2 stimulated but not unstimulated NK cells induce selective disappearance of peripheral blood cells: concomitant results to a phase I/II study. PLoS One. 2011;6(11):e27351.

61. Liu CC, Perussia B, Young JD. The emerging role of IL-15 in NK-cell development. Immunol Today. 2000;21(3):113–6.

62. Balloy V, et al. Aspergillus fumigatus-induced interleukin-8 synthesis by respiratory epithelial cells is controlled by the phosphatidylinositol 3-kinase, p38 MAPK, and ERK1/2 pathways and not by the toll-like receptor-MyD88 pathway. J Biol Chem. 2008;283(45):30513–21.

63. Song W, et al. Validation of housekeeping genes for the normalization of RT-qPCR expression studies in oral squamous cell carcinoma cell line treated by 5 kinds of chemotherapy drugs. Cell Mol Biol (Noisy-le-grand). 2016;62(13):29–34.

64. Xie J, et al. Validation of RT-qPCR reference genes and determination of Robo4 expression levels in human retinal endothelial cells under hypoxia and/or hyperglycemia. Gene. 2016;585(1):135–42.

65. Taihi I, et al. Validation of housekeeping genes to study human gingival stem cells and their in vitro osteogenic differentiation using real-time RT-qPCR. Stem Cells Int. 2016;2016:6261490.

66. Almeida TA, et al. A high-throughput open-array qPCR gene panel to identify housekeeping genes suitable for myometrium and leiomyoma expression analysis. Gynecol Oncol. 2014;134(1):138–43.

67. Ohl F, et al. Gene expression studies in prostate cancer tissue: which reference gene should be selected for normalization? J Mol Med (Berl). 2005;83(12):1014–24.

68. Fox JC, et al. Structural and agonist properties of XCL2, the other member of the C-chemokine subfamily. Cytokine. 2015;71(2):302–11.

13

In silico prediction of cancer immunogens: current state of the art

Irini A. Doytchinova[1] and Darren R. Flower[2*]

Abstract

Cancer kills 8 million annually worldwide. Although survival rates in prevalent cancers continue to increase, many cancers have no effective treatment, prompting the search for new and improved protocols. Immunotherapy is a new and exciting addition to the anti-cancer arsenal. The successful and accurate identification of aberrant host proteins acting as antigens for vaccination and immunotherapy is a key aspiration for both experimental and computational research. Here we describe key elements of *in silico* prediction, including databases of cancer antigens and bleeding-edge methodology for their prediction. We also highlight the role dendritic cell vaccines can play and how they can act as delivery mechanisms for epitope ensemble vaccines. Immunoinformatics can help streamline the discovery and utility of Cancer Immunogens.

Keywords: Cancer immunogens, Databases of cancer immunogens, Prediction of cancer immunogens, Dendritic cell-based vaccines, Multi-epitope vaccines

Background

Cancer is a catch-all term for a constellation of diseases typically characterised by abnormal cell division. The term cancer can be traced to the Greek physician Hippocrates (460-370 BC), who used the terms *carcinoma* and *carcinos* to refer to ulcer-forming tumours and non-ulcer forming tumours. In Greek, these words refer to a crab. The Roman physician, Celsus (28-50 BC), translated this to cancer, the Latin for crab. Galen (130-200 AD) used the Greek word *oncos*, meaning swelling to describe tumours. Almost all cells and tissues can become cancerous, but fortunately most cancers are very rare. Yet cancer remains one of the prime health issues of our time [1].

In 2012, there were about 14 million new cancer cases worldwide and 8.2 million deaths. Deaths caused by cancer is very high in developed countries [1]. In 2014, the US recorded 591,700 deaths from cancer, with approximately 197,233 deaths in women and 394,466 deaths in men; about 22% of all deaths. The equivalent UK figures were 163,000 deaths, or 450 deaths per day; with approximately 86,500 cancer deaths in men and 76,900

deaths in women; about 25% of all deaths. Yet over half of the global cancer burden occurs in less well developed countries. Lung, bowel, liver, and stomach, are the commonest cancers globally, equating to 4 in 10 deaths worldwide. At about 1 in 10 cases, smoking-related lung cancer is the commonest male cancer.

A cancer can be classed as either "common" or "rare" based on relative prevalence. The precise threshold between classes remains open. The US National Cancer Institute (NCI) identifies "rare" as those cancers with a prevalence below 15 in 100,000 [2]. This means only 11 adult cancers are defined as common in the US: prostate, breast, lung, bowl, cervical, bladder, rectum, ovary, kidney, melanoma, and non-Hodgkin lymphoma [3]. Other adult cancers - about 25% of all adult cancers - are, by this definition, "rare" [3].

Driven by the financial exigencies governing drug discovery and development, effective cancer treatment is significantly skewed towards common cancers. As an example, there are over 20 Category 1 intervention - uniform consensus that intervention is appropriate and based on significant evidence - for prostate and breast cancer, the commonest cancers in men and women [4–6]. Yet none exist for say the bone cancers, chondrosarcoma or chordoma, which affect under 1000 individuals annually in the US [7–9].

* Correspondence: d.r.flower@aston.ac.uk
[2]School of Life and Health Sciences, Aston University, Aston Triangle, Birmingham B4 7ET, UK
Full list of author information is available at the end of the article

Survival varies considerably between different cancers. It ranges from 98% for testicular cancer to about 1% for pancreatic cancer. Most common cancers have a 10-year survival above 50%. Over 80% of those with cancers which are easy to treat and/or diagnose survive for 10+ years, yet less than 1 in 5 people with hard-to-treat or hard-to-diagnose cancers survive for 10 years or more [10]. Thus cancer remains a pivotal unmet medical need, driving both technical innovations and improved clinical practice, resulting in dramatic improvement in cancer treatment. In the UK, mortality rates peaked in the 1980s, with overall cancer mortality falling by 14% since the early 1970s, with a 22% decrease in men and an 8% decrease in women. In the UK, mortality for all cancers is predicted to decrease by 15% in the period 2014-2035, reaching less than 280 deaths per 1 hundred thousand by the year 2035 [10].

According to somatic mutation theory, mutations in DNA and epi-mutations disrupt the programmed regulation of cell division, upsetting the balance between proliferation and apoptotic cell death, resulting in excessive and uncontrolled division. Many mutations lead to cancer, but most do not. The treatment of solid tumours in particular has changed dramatically in recent years due to enhanced molecular diagnostics helping to identify a burdening number of addressable oncogenic abnormalities including in-frame insertions/deletions and amplification or rearrangements and gene activating point mutations.

Historically, cancer has been treated by small molecule drugs. A number of anti-cancer drugs are classed as agents of so-called chemotherapy. These are typically characterised by significant side-effects, as many affect cells indiscriminately. The main types of chemotherapy include DNA-damaging alkylating agents, including structurally-simple reactive molecules such as Busulfan; Antimetabolites, which compete with natural nucleotides for incorporation into DNA or RNA, impairing DNA replication, such as 5-fluorouracil; Anti-tumour antibiotics, such as complex natural product Epirubicin; Topoisomerase inhibitors, which interfere with DNA unzipping prior to replication, such as Topotecan; Mitotic inhibitors, such as plant-derived natural product Paclitaxel; and Corticosteroids, such as Prednisone [11]. Other, more targeted therapies are now appearing. Precision medicine can be defined as therapy individualised to each tumour, achieving this by exploiting quantifiable genetic alterations as de fact predictive biomarkers and/or as therapeutic or prophylactic targets for the next generation of cancer treatments.

Most recently, immune based approaches have gained significant saliency. Immunotherapy directed against cancer, include a triumvirate of main approaches: monoclonal antibodies, immune checkpoint inhibitors, and vaccines. The immune response has two arms: the humoral, or antibody-mediated, arm and the cellular arm, mediated primarily by T cells. Historically, almost all vaccine prophylactic responses have been mediated by Antibodies. Each human has billions of potential antibodies capable of recognizing proteins and tagging them for elimination. The individual 'baseline' for addressing antigen challenge is the primary naïve antibody repertoire. The structural and sequence diversity of this baseline enables the immune system to recognize, at least weakly, a very large set of antigens. Unfortunately, only a subset of Tumour Associated Antigens (TAAs) are amendable to the antibody mediated responses necessitating the exploration of cellular immune mechanisms as a replacement or adjunct therapy.

The effectiveness of potential therapeutic cancer vaccines is often reduced by mechanisms in cancer patients that suppress T-cells and antigen presenting cells (APCs). Most cancer vaccines induce anti-tumour immune responses when formulated with strong adjuvants, due to the general lack of immunogenicity exhibited by vaccines not derived from whole pathogens. Vaccination against cancer takes several forms: DNA-based vaccines, RNA-based vaccines, and DC-based vaccines.

DNA vaccines: trials to evaluate the efficacy of Inovio Pharmaceuticals combination vaccine INO-3112 are planned against cervical, head, and neck cancers (NCT02172911, NCT02163057) "http://ir.inovio.com/news-and-media/news/press-release-details/2017/Inovio-Begins-Phase-3-Clinical-Trial-of-VGX-3100-for-the-Treatment-of-HPV-Related-Cervical-Pre-Cancer/default.aspx". INO-3112 contains plasmids encoding E6 and E7 (VGX-3100) [12] combined with DNA-based IL12 delivery (INO-9012). Inovio's preventive anti-HIV DNA vaccine, PENNVAX-G, used in a prime-boost protocol with altered pox virus vector, has a satisfactory safety and immunogenicity profile [13]. This study should foment design of anti-cancer therapeutic vaccines by exploring prime-boost regimens using DNA vaccines and viral boosts. The Vaccibody-developed DNA-based vaccine VB10.16 targets HPV16 "http://www.vaccibody.com/vb10-16/". A trial (NCT02529930) is set to launch; if successful it should provide an innovative and much needed non-invasive way to treat HPV-induced cervical cancers.

RNA vaccines: Sahin's group pioneered use of lipid-based positively-charged nanoparticles delivering RNA encoding TAAs, to target DCs in vivo and thus simulate an anti-viral response [14]. This is currently undergoing a phase I trial in melanoma patients (NCT02410733). A two component RNA vaccine platforms launched by Curevac has also yielded promising results in early trials (NCT00923312) [15].

DC-based vaccines: multiple platforms are being developed to harness ex vivo activated DC vaccines for cancer immunotherapy. These platforms include the with-antigen loading vaccine DCVax-Direct "https://

www.nwbio.com/dcvax-direct/" and the without-loading vaccine DCVaxL "https://www.nwbio.com/dcvax-technology/". Similarly, the Individualized Vaccines Against Cancer (IVAC) platform uses autologous DCs loaded with individually sequenced neo-antigens (NCT02035956, NCT02316457). The potential of DC vaccines is only beginning to be explored.

Protein-based vaccines: As TAA are poorly immunogenic, an adjuvant able to generate effective immune response should be added in the protein-based vaccines [16, 17]. Aluminum salts (alum) are used as adjuvants promoting protective humoral immunity, while for the activation of cell-mediated immunity are used conserved moieties associated with pathogen or endogenous alarmins like head shock proteins (HSPs). HSPs are able to induce both innate and addaptive immune responses. The first autologous HPS vaccine, Oncophage, failed to demonstrate survival benefits in Stage IV melanoma patients although stage I and II patients seemed to benefit from vaccination [18]. Wang et al. [19] have developed a platform for generating of chaperone complexes between HSPs and clinically relevant TAA.

Computational prediction can give important insight into both antibody and cellular immune responses. Here we examine non-experimental approaches to the cataloguing and prediction of TAAs. We describe the classification of TAAs into separate categories, databases that curate and classify TAAs, servers that facilitate the accurate and robust prediction of TAAs, and the role of DC vaccines to fight cancer and deliver pre-loaded epitope ensemble vaccines.

Classification of tumour antigens

Tumour Antigens are expressed largely, but not solely, by tumour cells. Utilisation of defined tumour antigens represents perhaps the most likely current approach accurately to directing immunotherapies towards differentiating cancer from neoplastic cells. As such, tumour antigens form the underpinning bedrock of modern tumour immunotherapy.

Tumour Antigens can be effectively classified using a scheme based primarily on their origin and distribution. Although there is no officially sanctioned classification system for tumour antigens, most experts in the field [20] broadly accept a classification protocol that makes use of the broadness of expression of individual antigens and how specific they are to a particular form of tumour. According to such a classification, tumour-associated antigens can be broadly divided into the following thematic categories:

1) Unique tumour-specific antigens (TSA). They occur within a single type of tumour in one patient. Such antigens can form excellent targets for personalized cancer immunotherapy. Examples include MAGE melanoma-associated genes.

2) Shared lineage-specific differentiated antigens. They are expressed in both tumor and healthy tissue and typically viewed as poorer or secondary targets for immunotherapy. However, CD19, a B cell marker, is one of the most successful cancer targets [21].

3) Shared tumour-specific antigens or cancer neo-antigens. They are expressed in different tumour but not in healthy tissues and can form the basis of 'off-the-shelf' vaccines applicable in a broad array of cancers and patient populations. These are unique MHC restricted antigens created by mutations in tumour cells. Vaccines designed to target these antigens should theoretically be able to target tumour cells specifically while obviating the induction of general autoimmunity or tolerance. However, not all tumours express immunogenic neo-antigens. Moreover, tumours and patients have unique neo-antigen repertoires necessitating personalized neo-antigen discovery programs that facilitate the development of personalized vaccines against predicted neo-antigen epitopes.

4) Shared over-expressed antigens. They are not tumour-specific but have a much greater expression in tumours compared to neoplastic cells. This category covers antigens that are present in both normal and tumour cells but which are substantially over-expressed by tumour cells. Example antigens falling into this category include Her2/Neu [22], mesothelin [23], lineage and tissue restricted differentiation antigens such as melanoma differentiation antigens (Tyrosinase Related Protein-2 and Melan-A (MART-1)) and Oncofetal antigens (Carcinoembryonic antigen) [24].

5) Oncoviral Antigens: These are antigens expressed by viruses, like human papilloma virus (HPV) and Merkel cell polyomavirus that cause tumorigenic transformation in cells. As these antigens are typically only found expressed on infected cells, they are able to be recognized by the immune system as 'non-self' distinct from the "self" or host protein [25].

As is made evident by the above classification, not all TAA are suitable for cancer immunotherapy. According to Kessler and Melief [20], a TAA could be considered as a potential cancer immunogen, if it responds to the following criteria: to be tumour-specific and widely shared, to play a role in the oncogenic process, or to promote cancer cell survival and thus provoke an immune response. It is possible, at least theoretically, to target TAAs using either an antibody or a cellular approach, although in practice this depends on the level and time-course of antigen expression. Antigens selectively expressed on the cell surface either constitutively or for periods of long duration are potent targets for antibodies, but antigens that only appear on the surface as epitopes bound to MHCs are clearly only amenable to surveillance by cellular immunity.

Databases of cancer immunogens

Due to the very extensive and intensive research efforts focussing on cancer aetiology and therapy seen during the last few decades, a plethora of cancer-associated data has accumulated and has subsequently been archived in a wide variety of different databases and repositories [26]. Here, we review only the most relevant databases for cancer immunogens available free on the web:

1) The Peptide Database of the Cancer Research Institute [27] has been established in 2001 and today it comprises more than 400 fully validated tumour antigenic peptides (URL: https://www.cancerresearch.org/scientists/events-and-resources/peptide-database). They are classified as mutated, tumour-specific, differentiated, and overexpressed. Other antigens are classed as potential, as a catch-all for those antigens whose comprehensive characterization is not yet reported.

2) The database of differentially expressed proteins (or dbDEPC) contains 4029 differentially expressed proteins, collected from 331 mass spectrometry experiments across 20 types of human cancer [28, 29]. This database allows one o search for proteins undergoing changes in certain cancers, shows protein expression heat-maps across various cancers, and relates protein expression changes to changes at the genetic level. Moreover, it also includes information on experimental methodology used, sophisticated tools for filtering user-specified analysis, and a tool for ana-lysing networks.

3) The Cancer-Testis database (CTdatabase; URL: http://www.cta.lncc.br/) contains known cancer testis antigens, typically proteins of known immunogenicity differentially expressed by different forms of cancer versus normal tissue [30]. The database contains links to relevant CT antigen articles plus basic information such as gene names, their aliases, genomic location and corresponding RefSeq accession numbers, known splice variants, reported gene duplications, mRNA levels in cancer and normal tissues, as well as antigen-specific immunological responses in cancer patients.

4) TANTIGEN (URL: http://cvc.dfci.harvard.edu/tadb/) is a database housing a comprehensive collection of cancer antigens, with over 1000 measured tumour peptides from 368 proteins [31]. TANTIGEN is thus a rich data source for those working to discover tumour-associated epitopes and neo-epitopes. Archived peptides are classified in a set of categories:

A. Peptides which bind in vitro to HLA but are not reported to engender in vivo or in vitro cell responses.

B. Peptides found to bind HLA and to engender an in vitro T cell response.

C. Peptides shown to mediate in vivo tumour rejection.

D. Peptides naturally processed and presented, as identified by physical techniques.

Servers for prediction of cancer immunogens

As both CD8+ and CD4+ T cells play a significant role in tumour rejection, most of the in silico methods for cancer immunogens prediction utilize servers for T-cell epitope prediction. Cancer immunogens are processed mainly in the dendritic cells by a cascade of enzymatic digestion in proteasomes or endosomes followed by assembling with HLA class I or class II proteins in the endoplasmic reticulum and presentation of the complexes on the cell surface where they are recognized by the CD8+ and CD4+ T cells, respectively [21]. The servers for T cell prediction utilize a wide range of different algorithms for prediction of peptide binding to HLA class I and class II proteins [32–34]. Servers trained to recognize whole cancer immunogens include:

1) VaxiJen was the first server for prediction of cancer immunogens applying a unique alignment-free algorithm [35]. The hydrophobicity, molecular size and polarity of amino acid residues were presented by z-scores [36]. The strings were converted into uniform vectors by auto- and cross covariance (ACC) transformation [37]. The algorithm was trained on a set of 75 known tumour antigens and 75 randomly chosen human proteins and tested on a set of 25 known tumour antigens and 25 human proteins. VaxiJen identified 96% of the test tumour antigens and 76% of the test human proteins with overall accuracy of 86% at threshold of 0.5.

2) TIminer (Tumor Immunology miner) is a pipeline for mining tumour-immune cell interactions from next-generation sequencing data [38]. It provides HLA class I typing by RNA-seq, characterization of immune infiltrates and quantification of tumour immunogenicity through immunophenogram and immunophenoscore, and neoantigen prediction from mutated proteins binding to patient-specific HLA class I proteins.

3) MuPeXI (mutant peptide extractor and informer) identifies tumour-specific peptides and assess their potential to be neo-epitopes [39]. It consists of several steps: identifies protein sequence changes that result from a genomic alteration, retains the alteration-containing peptides as potential neo-

peptides, compares them to the human proteome and penalizes the identical as non-immunogenic, predicts the binding affinities of neo-peptides to patient-specific HLA types, and prioritize the neo-peptides which are likely to be abundantly presented by patient's HLA and recognized by the T cells.

To improve these servers, we need both an improvement to the underlying data – in terms of quantity and quality - and to the breadth and robustness of algorithms. What is also very much required is a much better and much more carefully constructed tranche of negative training sets and algorithmic learning protocols over and above just simple improvements in reported accuracy. We should balance the selection of negative test sets so that any signal present reflects antigenicity and no other quality, selecting similar origin species, similar subcellular locations, similar protein lengths, and similar functions. Robustness in particular is seldom addressed by method developers. An over-specified algorithm which works well interpolating within a poorly-defined multidimensional subset of the overall chemical space is seldom likely to extrapolate well to unseen data that clearly lies outside such a space.

Antigen selection for cell-based cancer treatment: subunit and epitope ensemble vaccines delivered by dendritic cell and antigen selection for CAR T-cell therapy

Several decades ago, the advent of biologics revolutionized the pharmaceutical industry. Today, biomedicine is on the cusp of another revolution: cells as therapies. The potential of such novel therapies is enormous but significant challenges remain. Natural in origin or designed, such cells will present problems scientific, regulatory, and economic in nature. Cellular medicines will necessitate the development of a foundational cellular engineering science providing a systematic framework for the safe and predictable modulation of cell behaviour. In the vanguard of cellular medicine is the development of DC-based vaccines and the advent of CAR T-cell therapy. It should be noted that the immunoinformatic prediction of cancer antigens, as adumbrated in preceding sections, potentially underpins several important therapeutic strategies - CAR T-cell therapy and DC vaccines – as well as epitope ensemble vaccines. We explore these exciting strategies here.

Amongst all APCs, so-called dendritic cells (DCs), have the greatest perceived capacity to initiate innate and adaptive immune responses. DC based vaccines offer the potential therapeutic benefits of suppressive therapies against pathogens, tumours, and/or auto-immune diseases [40]. Consequently, there has been a maelstrom of activity in creating and testing DC cancer immunotherapy. DC vaccines are primarily used to treat

cancer. For example, sipuleucel-T is a US approved DC-based vaccine for treatment of hormone-insensitive prostate cancer.

In the 1970's, Ralph Steinman discovered DCs in the spleen. Post 1970's, it was revealed that DCs exist in non-lymphoid and lymphoid tissues as antigen presenting cells. The theoretical framework was based on Daniel Hawiger's experiment which utilised antigens specific for diseases such as: tuberculosis, diabetes, HIV, allergy or cancer. The specific antibody was used as a delivery vehicle and carried these antigens to DCs. This notion was applied by Steinman, exploiting varying receptors to trigger an immune response by targeting DCs [41].

DCs are present in an immature state in the blood, upon activation they migrate to the lymph tissue where they network with B cells and T cells. Immature DCs migrate through the blood stream from the bone marrow to enter tissues, ingesting particulate matter by phagocytosis and persistently absorb large amounts of extracellular fluid by micropinocytosis. Also presenting where there is contact with the external environment as they are portals of entry for infectious organisms, including the lining of the nose, lungs, intestine and stomach. DCs take up and process antigens and migrate to regional lymph nodes.

Manipulation of the immune system to eliminate cancer cells has long been a clinical and preclinical focus. Although achieving some success with cytokines such as IFN-γ and IL-2, an immunotherapy with proven clinical outcomes remain elusive. As previously, peptide-based approaches were discouraging, isolating stem cells from cultured blood resulted in sipuleucel-T (Provenge). Stem cells were loaded with cancer antigens and became sensitised. Sensitised DCs are injected into the skin and travel to the lymph node where they seek out specific lymphocytes. The DCs then initiate specific lymphocytes to multiply and attack cancer cells [42].

Thus the secret to future effective DC-based vaccines capable of combatting cancer is the identification of potent cancer antigens. A key alternative to whole protein immunogens is the idea of loading DCs with an epitope ensemble vaccine as a prelude to creating an anti-cancer vaccine. Here immunoinformatics can help.

Efforts supporting the development of a T-cell poly-epitope or epitope ensemble vaccine fall into two camps: un-validated prediction-only methods that predict supposedly high-binding epitopes [43] and more modern approaches that use immunoinformatics to select rather than predict the best epitopes suitable for forming a vaccine [44, 45]. Both rely on the development of accurate, reliable, and robust algorithms for the prediction of epitope affinity [46] and processing [47]. Here accurate refers to the nearness of results to reality, reliable – to the broadness of this accuracy in terms of distinct epitopes and MHC alleles, and robust – to the ability to deal with new data radically different from that it has seen before. Most algorithms, show variable performance in regard to these different criteria.

Prior to DC-based vaccines, small-molecule based chemotherapy and other toxic therapies were used to prevent or slow the progression of tumours. DC-based vaccines have the ability to initiate an immunological response that will hinder the development of malignancies even whilst the cancer cells mutate, and thus represent a potential step-change in cancer treatment. DC vaccine studies have shown that stimulating antigen specific cytotoxicity in vivo and in vitro exhibit a lack of toxicity and increase survival rates. In 16 different clinical trials, over 200 patients were treated for brain tumours, and have proven to treat metastasis although the clinical response is seemingly dependent on when immunotherapy is administered. Patients who benefit most are patients in early stage metastasis with a lower tumour burden. Multiple vaccines rather than a single vaccine stimulate a more multivalent response.

Currently, most DC therapies are rather limited in their scope, since they are typically used as part of a complex combination treatment rather than a monotherapy. Nonetheless, current state-of-the-art DC-based therapies is the cause for much optimism since they are clearly a prime candidate for future elaboration, leading to a wealth of promising future treatments.

Recently, immunotherapy, rather than vaccination per se, has the potential "fifth pillar" of cancer treatment. So-called Adoptive Cell Transfer, or ACT, collects patients' immune cells to treat cancer; of the various types of ACT, Chimeric antigen receptors (CARs) T-cells seems the most promising. When a CAR is derived from an antibody, the resulting T-cell will combine its own effector functions with an antibody's ability to recognize non-protein antigens and be freed from obligatory major histocompatibility complex restriction.

Hitherto, CAR T-cell therapy has been limited to small-scale clinical trials, mostly in blood cancer patients. In 2017, two CAR T-cell therapies gained approval by the Food and Drug Administration (FDA): one for patients with advanced lymphomas, the other for acute paediatric lymphoblastic leukemia. Yet this is still an early phase for CAR T-cell therapy, with questions over their potential effectiveness against solid tumours. In particular, technical questions about the identification and selection of appropriate antigens for incorporation into CARs remain.

To a crude, first approximation, a CAR is composed of an extracellular targeting domain (ectodomain), and transmembrane region, and an intracellular T-cell signalling domain (endodomain) [48]. The ectodomain can constructed from a limited repertoire of signalling domains, such as ZAP70 or CD28. The ectodomain is a more challenging design puzzle, as it is exquisitely linked to the form of cancer being targeted. While immunoglobulin domains in their antibody and TCR guises are perhaps the most obvious candidates, a plethora of ever-increasing number and diversity continue to emerge [49, 50]. These include, inter alia, adnectins, Affibodies, Avimers, DARPIns, Fynomers, Kunitz domains, knottins, and Nanobodies. The challenge here is twofold: one predicting using VaxiJen or equivalent approach the appropriate target.

However, perhaps the most interesting, intriguing, and exciting alternative is the possibility of including anticalins [51, 52] as antibody surrogates. Anticalins are non-natural engineered lipocalins able to bind small molecules in a hapten-dependent but conjugate antigen-independent manner. This would open up metabolites secreted in a cancer-dependent fashion by tumours as putative targets for anti-cancer CAR T-cells. Moreover, lipocalins as well as binding small molecule ligands of all kinds, also have the capacity to bind macromolecules with high specificity [51]. This could open the way to dual specificity anticalin CAR T-cells able to bind both cancer-specific metabolites and cell surface receptors, enlarging the homing capacity and cell-targeting abilities native to T cells.

Discussion

The worth, value, and utility of vaccines, though clear for all to see, is not yet unchallenged; yet most reasonable people are likely to agree that they are, qualifications apart, a thing of inestimable value and utility. Existing vaccines are not perfect. One might argue that their intrinsic complexity, and the highly empirical nature of their discovery over decades, and the fraught nature of their manufacture, is a root of current mistrust. In some senses this also hampered the progress of cancer vaccines and immunotherapy. Finally, these are beginning to make some headway.

Computational prediction has a part to play, one of the strongest messages to emerge from this review is that immunogenicity is a multi-factorial property: some protein antigens are immunogenic for one reason, or set of reasons, while another protein will be immunogenic for another possibly-tangential reason or set of reasons. Each such a causal manifold seems dauntingly complex and confusing. The prediction of immunogenicity for cancer antigens is a greater problems still in multi-factorial prediction since we must factor in the high degree of antigenic similarity to other host proteins. Thus the search for new antigens is a search through a multi-factorial landscape of contingent causes. As noted above, the immunoinformatic prediction of cancer antigens potentially underpins several important therapeutic strategies, including epitope ensemble vaccines, CAR T-cell therapy, and DC vaccines.

To develop proper predictive approaches to the prediction of cancer and other immunogenic antigens we need to address several issues. We require more "positive" and carefully curated, validated data focussed on cancer. While there are databases of vaccine antigens - AntigenDB [53] is a dedicated resource directly addressing this, as well as IEDB [54] - similar yet better data resources are still required, suggesting the need to enlarge, deepen, and broaden available data collections. We also require much better and much deeper representations of the sequence data. Single descriptors characterising the whole sequence [55], and other multivariate descriptors of sequences. One could envisage a phase space of disjoint descriptor variables from which variable selection protocols could extract a compact, near-optimal choice of indicative variables. Also, better algorithms are needed. Powerful machine learning toolkits, such as Weka, are already available, and these are more than capable of delivering robust and extensible methods provided the data and the data representation are adequate. Yet, as new algorithms appear we must not be complacent but open, embracing proven innovations.

Better protocols for establishing the immunogenicity of identified potential vaccines are desperately needed. This work is that of the experimentalist. Here a fast, straightforward methodology is required which projects a more consistent, clearer, and much more accurate picture of the immunogenicity of individual proteins. As with many computational studies of real world problems, there is also general need for experiments able to validate predictions. The *in silico* analyses of pathogen genomes and virtual proteomes, has led to the publication of innumerable papers reporting potential but unverified vaccine candidates [56–58]. Such papers typically use methodology largely embodied in web-servers: operating such systems is facile, and the resulting analysis straightforward. Publishing unverified papers ultimately becomes counterproductive. Science progresses through independent corroboration by verification by peers. Science progresses faster when people do not waste time on fruitless research. Many are rightly alarmed by the increasing perception that the complex results of present day science cannot be reproduced and validated. Explanations are legion, including increased levels of scrutiny and institutional pressure on research and individual researchers. Arguably, the greatest issues are the increasing complexity and instrumentality of modern experimentation, in the opaqueness of many systems being studied, and the daunting technicality of analysing and teasing out the nature of many experiments. Computational experiments may be reproducible in themselves but without robust and reproducible experimental validation mean little. Other vaccine prediction studies give credibility to their results [59, 60] by linking vaccine design to experimental validation. Even in the current atmosphere of hysteria and hyperbole over AI, prediction lacking validation exerts slight influence and convinces few.

Conclusions

The utility of vaccines, though clear to most of us, is not yet unchallenged. Existing vaccines are not perfect. This also hampered cancer vaccines and immunotherapy. Finally, these are beginning to make some headway. Computational prediction has a part to play, one of the strongest messages to emerge from this review is that immunogenicity is a multi-factorial property. The prediction of immunogenicity for cancer antigens is a greater problems still in multi-factorial prediction since we must factor in the high degree of antigenic similarity to other host proteins. Immunoinformatics is poised to deliver on its potential and open up a whole new era in Cancer immunotherapy.

Abbreviations

AI: Artificial intelligence; APC: Antigen presenting cell; DC: Dendritic Cell; DNA: Deoxyribose nucleic acid; IEDB: Immune epitope database; RNA: Ribonucleic acid; TAA: Tumour associated antigen; TSA: Tumour specific antigen

Acknowledgements

Not applicable.

Funding

The authors' research was funded by Aston University, the National Science Fund, Bulgaria, and the Medical Research Council of the Medical University of Sofia, Bulgaria.

Authors' contributions

ID and DRF were PIs of certain research projects covered in this review. Both authors drafted, reviewed and approved the final manuscript.

Competing interests

The authors declare that they have no competing interests.

Author details

[1]Faculty of Pharmacy, Medical University of Sofia, 2 Dunav st, 1000 Sofia, Bulgaria. [2]School of Life and Health Sciences, Aston University, Aston Triangle, Birmingham B4 7ET, UK.

References

1. Siegel RL, Ma J, Zou Z, Jemal A. Cancer statistics, 2014. CA Cancer J Clin. 2014;64:9–29.
2. National Cancer Institute. (2007). Synergizing epidemiologic research on rare cancers. https://epi.grants.cancer.gov/events/rare-cancers/
3. Greenlee RT, Goodman MT, Lynch CF, Platz CE, Havener LA, Howe HL. The occurrence of rare cancers in United States adults, 1995-2004. Public Health Rep. 2010;125(1):28–43.
4. Gradishar WJ, Anderson BO, Balassanian R, Blair SL, Burstein HJ, Cyr A, Elias AD, Farrar WB, Forero A, Giordano SH, Goetz MP, Goldstein LJ, Isakoff SJ, Lyons J, Marcom PK, Mayer IA, McCormick B, Moran MS, O'Regan RM, Patel SA, Pierce LJ, Reed EC, Salerno KE, Schwartzberg LS, Sitapati A, Smith KL, Smith ML, Soliman H, Somlo G, Telli M, Ward JH, Shead DA, Kumar R. NCCN Guidelines Insights: Breast Cancer, Version 1.2017. J Natl Compr Canc Netw. 2017;15(4):433-51.
5. Carroll PR, Parsons JK, Andriole G, Bahnson RR, Castle EP, Catalona WJ, Dahl DM, Davis JW, Epstein JI, Etzioni RB, Farrington T, Hemstreet GP 3rd, Kawachi MH, Kim S, Lange PH, Loughlin KR, Lowrance W, Maroni P, Mohler J, Morgan TM, Moses KA, Nadler RB, Poch M, Scales C, Shaneyfelt TM, Smaldone MC, Sonn G, Sprenkle P, Vickers AJ, Wake R, Shead DA, Freedman-Cass DA. NCCN Guidelines Insights: Prostate Cancer Early Detection, Version 2.2016. J Natl Compr Canc Netw. 2016;14(5):509-19.
6. Siegel RL, Miller KD, Jemal A. Colorectal Cancer mortality rates in adults aged 20 to 54 years in the United States, 1970-2014. JAMA. 2017;318(6):572–4.
7. Biermann JS, Chow W, Reed DR, Lucas D, Adkins DR, Agulnik M, Benjamin RS, Brigman B, Budd GT, Curry WT, Didwania A, Fabbri N, Hornicek FJ, Kuechle JB, Lindskog D, Mayerson J, McGarry SV, Million L, Morris CD, Movva S, O'Donnell RJ, Randall RL, Rose P, Santana VM, Satcher RL, Schwartz H, Siegel HJ, Thornton K, Villalobos V, Bergman MA, Scavone JL. NCCN Guidelines Insights: Bone Cancer, Version 2.2017. J Natl Compr Canc Netw. 2017;15(2):155-67.
8. McMaster ML, Goldstein AM, Bromley CM, Ishibe N, Parry DM. Chordoma: incidence and survival patterns in the United States, 1973-1995. Cancer Causes Control. 2001;12:1–11.
9. Orphanet. Prevalence and incidence of rare diseases: bibliographic data. 2016. http://www.orpha.net/orphacom/cahiers/docs/GB/Prevalence_of_rare_diseases_by_alphabetical_list.pdf.
10. http://www.cancerresearchuk.org/health-professional/cancer-statistics-for-the-uk.
11. Isoldi MC, Visconti MA, Castrucci AM. Anti-cancer drugs: molecular mechanisms of action. Mini Rev Med Chem. 2005;5(7):685–95.
12. Morrow MP, Kraynyak KA, Sylvester AJ, Shen X, Amante D, Sakata L, Parker L, Yan J, Boyer J, Roh C, et al. Augmentation of cellular and humoral immune responses to HPV16 and HPV18 E6 and E7 antigens by VGX-3100. Mol Ther Oncolytics. 2016;3:16025.
13. Nilsson C, Hejdeman B, Godoy-Ramirez K, Tecleab T, Scarlatti G, Brave A, Earl PL, Stout RR, Robb ML, Shattock RJ, et al. HIV-DNA given with or without intradermal electroporation is safe and highly immunogenic in healthy Swedish HIV-1 DNA/MVA vaccinees: a phase I randomized trial. PLoS One. 2015;10:e0131748.
14. Vormehr M, Schrörs B, Boegel S, Löwer M, Türeci Ö, Sahin U. Mutanome engineered RNA immunotherapy: towards patient-centered tumor vaccination. J Immunol Res. 2015;2015:595363.
15. Rauch S, Lutz J, Kowalczyk A, Schlake T, Heidenreich R. RNActive (R) technology: generation and testing of stable and immunogenic mRNA vaccines. Methods Mol Biol. 2017;1499:89–107.
16. Guo C, Manjili MH, Subjeck JR, Sarkar D, Fisher PB, Xiang-Yang Wang XY. Therapeutic Cancer vaccines: past, present and future. Adv Cancer Res. 2013;119:421–75.
17. Flower DR. Towards the systematic discovery of immunomodulatory adjuvants. In: Flower DR, Perrie Y, editors. Immunomic discovery of adjuvants and candidate subunit vaccines: Springer; 2013. p. 155–80.
18. Wood C, Srivastava P, Bukowski R, Lacombe L, Gorelov A, Gorelov S, et al. An adjuvant autologous therapeutic vaccine (HSPPC-96; vitespen) versus observation alone for patients at high risk of recurrence after nephrectomy for renal cell carcinoma: a multicentre, open-label, randomised phase III trial. Lancet. 2008;372:145–54.
19. Wang XY, Sun X, Chen X, Facciponte J, Repasky EA, Kane J, et al. Superior antitumor response induced by large stress protein chaperoned protein antigen compared with peptide antigen. J Immunol. 2010;184:6309–19.
20. Kessler JH, Melief CJM. Identification of T-cell epitopes for cancer immunotherapy. Leukemia. 2007;21:1859–74.
21. Tonecka K, Plich Z, Ramji K, Taclak B, Kiraga L, Krol M, et al. Immune cells as targets and tools for cancer therapy. Immunotherapy. 2017;3:143.
22. Clifton GT, Mittendorf EA, Peoples GE. Adjuvant HER2/neu peptide cancer vaccines in breast cancer. Immunotherapy. 2015;7:1159–68.
23. Morello A, Sadelain M, Adusumilli PS. Mesothelin-targeted CARs: driving T cells to solid tumors. Cancer Discov. 2016;6:133–46.
24. Butterfield LH. Lessons learned from cancer vaccine trials and target antigen choice. Cancer Immunol Immunother. 2016;65:805–12.
25. Kenter GG, Welters MJ, Valentijn AR, Lowik MJ, Berends-van der Meer DM, Vloon AP, Essahsah F, Fathers LM, Offringa R, Drijfhout JW, et al. Vaccination against HPV-16 oncoproteins for vulvar intraepithelial neoplasia. N Engl J Med. 2009;361:1838–47.
26. Pavlopoulou A, Spandidos DA, Michalopoulos I. Human cancer databases. Oncol Rep. 2015;33:3–18.
27. Jongeneel V. Towards a cancer immunome database. Cancer Immun. 2001;1:3.
28. Li H, He Y, Ding G, Wang C, Xie L, Li Y. dbDEPC: a database of differentially expressed proteins in human cancers. Nucleic Acids Res. 2010;38:D658–64.
29. He Y, Zhang M, Ju Y, Yu Z, Lv D, Sun H, et al. dbDEPC 2.0: updated database of differentially expressed proteins in human cancers. Nucleic Acids Res. 2012;40:D964–71.
30. Almeida LG, Sakabe NJ, deOliveira AR, Silva MC, Mundstein AS, Cohen T, et al. CTdatabase: a knowledge-base of high-throughput and curated data on cancer-testis antigens. Nucleic Acids Res. 2009;37:D816–9.
31. Olsen LR, Tongchusak S, Lin H, Reinherz EL, Brusic V, Zhang GL. TANTIGEN: a comprehensive database of tumor T cell antigens. Cancer Immunol Immunother. 2017;66:731–5.
32. Flower DR. Designing immunogenic peptides. Nat Chem Biol. 2013;9:749–53.
33. Patronov A, Doytchinova I. T-cell epitope vaccine design by immunoinformatics. Open Biol. 2013;3:120139.
34. Flower DR, Macdonald IK, Ramakrishnan K, Davies MN, Doytchinova IA. Computer aided selection of candidate vaccine antigens. Immunome Res. 2010;6(Suppl 2):S1.
35. Doytchinova IA, Flower DR. VaxiJen: a server for prediction of protective antigens, tumour antigens and subunit vaccines. BMC Bioinformatics. 2007;8:4.
36. Hellberg S, Sjöström M, Skagerberg B, Wold S. Peptide quantitative structure-activity relationships, a multivariate approach. J Med Chem. 1987;30:1126–35.
37. Nyström Å, Andersson PM, Lundstedt T. Multivariate data analysis of topographically modified á-melanotropin analogues using auto and cross auto covariances (ACC). Quant Struct Act Relat. 2000;19:264–9.
38. Tappeiner E, Finotello F, Charoentong P, Mayer C, Rieder D, Trajanoski Z. TIminer: NGS data mining pipeline for cancer immunology and immunotherapy. Bioinformatics. 2017;33:3140–1.
39. Bjerregaard AM, Nielsen M, Hadrup SR, Szallasi Z, Eklund AC. MuPeXI: prediction of neo-epitopes from tumor sequencing data. Cancer Immunol Immunother. 2017;66:1123–30.
40. Merad M, Sathe P, Helft J, Miller J, Mortha A. The dendritic cell lineage: ontogeny and function of dendritic cells and their subsets in the steady state and the inflamed setting. Annu Rev Immunol. 2013;31:563–604.
41. Tesfatsion DA. Dendritic cell vaccine against leukemia: advances and perspectives. Immunotherapy. 2014;6(4):485–96.
42. Datta J, Berk E, Cintolo J, Xu S, Roses R, Czerniecki B. Rationale for a multimodality strategy to enhance the efficacy of dendritic cell-based Cancer immunotherapy. Front Immunol. 2015;6:271.
43. Rai J, Lok KI, Mok CY, Mann H, Noor M, Patel P, Flower DR. Immunoinformatic evaluation of multiple epitope ensembles as vaccine candidates: E coli 536. Bioinformation. 2012;8(6):272–5.
44. Molero-Abraham M, Lafuente EM, Flower DR, Reche PA. Selection of conserved epitopes from hepatitis C virus for pan-populational stimulation of T-cell responses. Clin Dev Immunol. 2013;2013:601943.
45. Sheikh QM, Gatherer D, Reche PA, Flower DR. Towards the knowledge-based design of universal influenza epitope ensemble vaccines. Bioinformatics. 2016;32(21):3233–9.
46. Dimitrov I, Atanasova M, Patronov A, Flower DR, Doytchinova I. A cohesive and integrated platform for immunogenicity prediction. Methods Mol Biol. 2016;1404:761–70.

47. Doytchinova IA, Guan P, Flower DR. EpiJen: a server for multistep T cell epitope prediction. BMC Bioinformatics. 2006;7:131.

48. Dotti G, Gottschalk S, Savoldo B, Brenner MK. Design and development of therapies using chimeric antigen receptor-expressing T cells. Immunol Rev. 2014;257:107–26.

49. Wurch T, Pierré A, Depil S. Novel protein scaffolds as emerging therapeutic proteins: from discovery to clinical proof-of-concept. Trends Biotechnol. 2012;30:575–82.

50. Simeon R, Chen Z. In vitro-engineered non-antibody protein therapeutics. Protein Cell. 2018;9:3–14.

51. Flower DR. The lipocalin protein family: structure and function. Biochem J. 1996;318:1–14.

52. Gebauer M, Skerra A. Engineered protein scaffolds as next-generation antibody therapeutics. Curr Opin Chem Biol. 2009;13:245–55.

53. Ansari HR, Flower DR, Raghava GP. AntigenDB: an immunoinformatics database of pathogen antigens. Nucleic Acids Res. 2010;38(Database issue):D847–53.

54. Vita R, Overton JA, Greenbaum JA, Ponomarenko J, Clark JD, Cantrell JR, Wheeler DK, Gabbard JL, Hix D, Sette A, Peters B. The immune epitope database (IEDB) 3.0. Nucleic Acids Res. 2015;43(Database issue):D405–12.

55. Chattopadhyay AK, Nasiev D, Flower DR. A statistical physics perspective on alignment-independent protein sequence comparison. Bioinformatics. 2015; 31(15):2469–74.

56. Akhoon BA, Slathia PS, Sharma P, Gupta SK, Verma V. In silico identification of novel protective VSG antigens expressed by Trypanosoma brucei and an effort for designing a highly immunogenic DNA vaccine using IL-12 as adjuvant. Microb Pathog. 2011;51(1-2):77–87.

57. Gupta A, Chaukiker D, Singh TR. Comparative analysis of epitope predictions: proposed library of putative vaccine candidates for HIV. Bioinformation. 2011;5(9):386–9.

58. Barh D, Misra AN, Kumar A, Vasco A. A novel strategy of epitope design in Neisseria gonorrhoeae. Bioinformation. 2010;5(2):77–85.

59. Seyed N, Zahedifard F, Safaiyan S, Gholami E, Doustdari F, Azadmanesh K, Mirzaei M, Saeedi Eslami N, Khadem Sadegh A, Eslami Far A, Sharifi I, Rafati S. In silico analysis of six known Leishmania major antigens and in vitro evaluation of specific epitopes eliciting HLA-A2 restricted CD8 T cell response. PLoS Negl Trop Dis. 2011;5(9):e1295.

60. Wieser A, Romann E, Magistro G, Hoffmann C, Nörenberg D, Weinert K, Schubert S. A multiepitope subunit vaccine conveys protection against extraintestinal pathogenic Escherichia coli in mice. Infect Immun. 2010; 78(8):3432–42.

Validation of T-Track® CMV to assess the functionality of cytomegalovirus-reactive cell-mediated immunity in hemodialysis patients

Bernhard Banas[1*], Carsten A. Böger[1], Gerhard Lückhoff[2], Bernd Krüger[3], Sascha Barabas[4], Julia Batzilla[4], Mathias Schemmerer[4,5], Josef Köstler[5], Hanna Bendfeldt[4], Anne Rascle[4], Ralf Wagner[5], Ludwig Deml[4], Joachim Leicht[6] and Bernhard K. Krämer[3]

Abstract

Background: Uncontrolled cytomegalovirus (CMV) replication in immunocompromised solid-organ transplant recipients is a clinically relevant issue and an indication of impaired CMV-specific cell-mediated immunity (CMI). Primary aim of this study was to assess the suitability of the immune monitoring tool T-Track® CMV to determine CMV-reactive CMI in a cohort of hemodialysis patients representative of patients eligible for renal transplantation. Positive and negative agreement of T-Track® CMV with CMV serology was examined in 124 hemodialysis patients, of whom 67 (54%) revealed a positive CMV serostatus. Secondary aim of the study was to evaluate T-Track® CMV performance against two unrelated CMV-specific CMI monitoring assays, QuantiFERON®-CMV and a cocktail of six class I iTAg™ MHC Tetramers.

Results: Positive T-Track® CMV results were obtained in 90% (60/67) of CMV-seropositive hemodialysis patients. In comparison, 73% (45/62) and 77% (40/52) positive agreement with CMV serology was achieved using QuantiFERON®-CMV and iTAg™ MHC Tetramer. Positive T-Track® CMV responses in CMV-seropositive patients were dominated by pp65-reactive cells (58/67 [87%]), while IE-1-responsive cells contributed to an improved (87% to 90%) positive agreement of T-Track® CMV with CMV serology. Interestingly, T-Track® CMV, QuantiFERON®-CMV and iTAg™ MHC Tetramers showed 79% (45/57), 87% (48/55) and 93% (42/45) negative agreement with serology, respectively, and a strong inter-assay variability. Notably, T-Track® CMV was able to detect IE-1-reactive cells in blood samples of patients with a negative CMV serology, suggesting either a previous exposure to CMV that yielded a cellular but no humoral immune response, or TCR cross-reactivity with foreign antigens, both suggesting a possible protective immunity against CMV in these patients.

Conclusion: T-Track® CMV is a highly sensitive assay, enabling the functional assessment of CMV-responsive cells in hemodialysis patients prior to renal transplantation. T-Track® CMV thus represents a valuable immune monitoring tool to identify candidate transplant recipients potentially at increased risk for CMV-related clinical complications.

Keywords: Cytomegalovirus, CMV, IE-1, pp65, Cell-mediated immunity, IFN-γ ELISpot, T-Track® CMV, QuantiFERON®-CMV, iTAg™ MHC Tetramers, Hemodialysis

* Correspondence: Bernhard.Banas@ukr.de
[1]Department of Nephrology, University Medical Center Regensburg, Regensburg, Germany
Full list of author information is available at the end of the article

Background

Cytomegalovirus (CMV) is a major cause of infectious complications in immunocompromised individuals. Protection against CMV infection or reactivation is normally assured by both the innate and adaptive arms of the immune system [1, 2]. While the humoral and innate responses are essential for the early response to infection [1, 3, 4], cellular immunity is required to control latency and prevent CMV reactivation in latently infected individuals [1]. CD8$^+$ cytotoxic T cells (CTL) and CD4$^+$ T helper (Th) cells are both required to assure efficient immune protection against CMV reactivation [1, 5–8]. Primary infection is dominated by CD8$^+$ T cell response, preferentially targeting CMV immediate early-1 (IE-1) antigen, while long-term recovery is dominated by CD4$^+$ T cell response and a switch of reactivity toward CMV lower matrix phosphoprotein 65 (pp65) [6, 8–11]. The frequency of CMV-specific CD8$^+$ and CD4$^+$ T cells is highly variable, both between healthy CMV-seropositive individuals and during the course of CMV reactivation, and correlates with varying levels of protection [6, 9, 11–13]. Beside changes in T cell frequency, alterations in T cell functionality are associated with impaired response to chronic viral infection [14–17].

Functional impairment of cell-mediated immunity (CMI) in the course of immunosuppression, such as in solid-organ transplant recipients, is a major cause of uncontrolled CMV replication and related clinical complications [18–21]. Treatment regimens with antivirals are costly and associated with harmful side effects. Assessment of CMV-specific immunity may be beneficial to identify patients at increased risk of viral complications, possibly allowing personalized adjustment of antiviral and immunosuppressive therapies.

Various experimental approaches exist to measure CMV-specific CMI. Direct T cell staining with for instance class I iTAg™ MHC Tetramers (Beckman Coulter) allows the quantification of epitope-specific CD8$^+$ cells by flow cytometry [18, 22–24]. The sensitivity of tetramer-based assays strictly depends on the coverage of the patient population by the selected HLA types, and this method cannot assess the functionality of CD8$^+$ cells. Several assays assessing CMV-specific T cell function have been described. Principally, they measure the production of activation markers (e.g. cytokines such as IFN-γ) in response to antigen stimulation, using intracellular cytokine staining followed by flow cytometry [6, 7, 12, 13, 25, 26], ELISA [21, 27–30], or ELISpot [31–33] assays. These approaches differ not only in their read-out format but also in the antigen (peptide vs. protein) used for the *ex vivo* stimulation. Peptide-based immune monitoring tests such as QuantiFERON®-CMV (Qiagen) allow the quantification of IFN-γ produced by epitope-specific CD8$^+$ T cells. Whole blood samples are stimulated with a pool of 22 immunogenic peptides (mapping at IE-1, IE-2, pp28, pp50, pp65 and gB CMV antigens) and covering > 98% of HLA class-I haplotypes. Reactive CD8$^+$ T cells are monitored by quantifying secreted IFN-γ by ELISA [34]. QuantiFERON®-CMV was used in a number of studies to assess the risk of CMV reactivation and related disease following solid-organ transplantation [21, 27–30]. A disadvantage of QuantiFERON®-CMV is that it does not assess CMV-specific CD4$^+$ T cell function and that it often yields indeterminate results that cannot be interpreted [28, 35, 36]. T-Track® CMV is based on the stimulation of freshly isolated peripheral blood mononuclear cells (PBMC) with recombinant urea-formulated (T-activated®) immunodominant CMV IE-1 and pp65 proteins, and the subsequent quantification of antigen-reactive effector cells using an IFN-γ ELISpot assay. T-activated® proteins (aproteins) are processed via the exogenous and endogenous antigen processing pathways, resulting in the presentation of naturally-generated peptides by MHC class I and class II molecules, thus enabling the stimulation of a broad spectrum of CMV-protective cells including CD8$^+$ and CD4$^+$ T cells, as well as the bystander activation of NK and NKT-like cells [37, 38]. As such, T-Track® CMV is not restricted to particular HLA types. Performance of T-Track® CMV has been recently characterized [38]. A recent study demonstrated its high sensitivity in evaluating changes in CMV-specific CMI during and after pregnancy [39].

Primary aim of this cross-sectional prospective multicenter study was to evaluate the suitability of T-Track® CMV to assess the functionality of CMV-specific CMI in a cohort of patients on hemodialysis due to end-stage renal failure, and thus being representative of patients prior to renal transplantation. Secondary aim of the study was to compare the performance of T-Track® CMV to that of QuantiFERON®-CMV and iTAg™ MHC Tetramers in terms of positive and negative agreement with CMV serology (gold standard reference).

Methods

Study design and participants

Hemodialysis patients of any gender and race aged at least 18 years were recruited in the study. Patients requiring systemic immunosuppressive treatment within the last 3 months before study inclusion or suffering from chronic or uncontrolled infections (e.g. HIV or chronic hepatitis) were ineligible for study participation. All subjects gave written informed consent. The study was registered and approved according to the rules, at the German Institute of Medical Documentation and Information (DIMDI). Patient enrolment was started only after receiving the exemption of the permit requirement by the BfArM (Federal Institute for Drugs and Medical Devices) and approval by the ethics committee of the University of Regensburg (approval number 11-122-0205). For reasons of transparency and completeness, the study was prospectively registered at clinicaltrials.gov. The authors confirm that all ongoing and related trials for this intervention are registered at clinicaltrials.gov.

Blood collection

Lithium heparinized whole blood was collected during routine withdrawal, prior to the start of the dialysis session. For T-Track® CMV and iTAg™ MHC Tetramer staining, 15 ml blood was collected for further PBMC isolation. For QuantiFERON®-CMV, 0.8 to 1.2 ml whole blood was collected into each of the three assay tubes. CMV serology was performed from 2.6 ml whole blood.

CMV serology

Anti-CMV serological testing was performed using fully automated anti-CMV IgM and IgG tests on the BEP III system (Siemens Healthcare, Eschborn, Germany). CMV IgG-serology was used as primary reference measurement procedure (gold standard method).

CMV-specific cellular immunity assays

T-Track® CMV (Lophius Biosciences GmbH, Regensburg, Germany) was performed according to manufacturer's instructions. Briefly, PBMC were isolated and stimulated individually with T-activated® CMV-specific immediate-early 1 (aIE-1) and phosphoprotein pp65 ($a$pp65) proteins for 19 h at 37°C. Staphylococcus enterotoxin B (SEB) and medium served as positive and negative controls for the stimulation, respectively. IFN-γ ELISpot assays were performed following manufacturer's recommendations. IFN-γ-specific spot-forming cells (SFC) were enumerated on a Bioreader® 5000 Pro-Eα (BIO-SYS GmbH, Karben, Germany). Test results were considered positive if the geometric mean of the spots resulting from at least one of the $a$pp65 and aIE1 stimulations was ≥ 10 SFC/200,000 PBMC and when the ratio of the geometric means of stimulated and non-stimulated conditions was ≥ 2.5. Positivity rules were calculated as described in the Statistics section.

The QuantiFERON®-CMV assay (Qiagen, Hilden, Germany) was performed according to manufacturer's instructions. Briefly, QuantiFERON®-CMV collection tubes (Nil Control, CMV Antigen and Mitogen Control) were incubated for 16–24 h at 37°C. IFN-γ levels were determined by enzyme-linked immunosorbent assay (ELISA). Calculation of results was achieved using QuantiFERON®-CMV Analysis Software. QuantiFERON®-CMV test results were considered positive when IFN-γ level (IU/mL) in the CMV Antigen-specific assay minus that in the Nil Control was ≥ 0.2, as recommended by the manufacturer. ELISA

measurements are accurate up to 10 IU/mL. Values ≥ 10 IU/mL cannot be quantitatively evaluated.

For the CMV-specific tetramer assay, CMV peptide-specific CD8+ T cells were quantified by flow cytometry using a mixture of six class I iTAg™ MHC Tetramers (Beckman Coulter), including: MHC A*0101 Class I Tetramer CMV pp50 (VTEHDTLLY), MHC A*0201 Class I Tetramer CMV pp65 (NLVPMVATV), MHC A*2402 Class I Tetramer CMV pp65 (QYDPVAALF), MHC B*0702 Class I Tetramer CMV pp65 (TPRVTGGGAM), MHC B*0801 Class I Tetramer CMV IE-1 (ELRRKMMYM) and MHC B*3501 Class I Tetramer CMV pp65 (IPSINVHHY). iTAg™ MHC Negative Tetramer PN T01044 (Beckman Coulter) served as negative control. Preselected HLA types are predicted to cover at least 80% of the Caucasian population [40]. Each 1×10^6 PBMC were stained with 10 μl tetramer mix, 10 μl anti-CD8-FITC (T8-FITC, Beckman Coulter) and 5 μl human CD3 APC-Alexa Fluor® 750 conjugate (Invitrogen/Thermo Fisher Scientific) for 30 min at room temperature protected from light. Cells were washed once in PBS and incubated 45 min at 4 °C protected from light. Dead cells were further stained with SYTOX® RED dead cell stain (Invitrogen/Thermo Fisher Scientific) for 15 min at 4 °C protected from light, prior to flow cytometry analysis. Measurements were performed using a Cytomics FC 500 MPL cytometer (Beckmann Coulter), gating on living and CD3-positive cells. Cell count from the iTAg™ MHC Tetramer Negative staining was subtracted from that of the iTAg™ MHC Tetramer CMV-specific cocktail staining. Data were expressed as the % of CMV-specific tetramer-positive CD8+ T cells relative to total CD8+ T cells. Test results were considered positive, when the proportion of tetramer-positive CD8+ cells was ≥ 0.1% of total CD8+ T cells.

Statistics

Calculations were performed with SAS 9.2 Software and VFP (Variance Function Program) 10.0. Figures were generated using GraphPad Prism. In case of categorically scaled data, absolute and relative frequencies were reported. For continuously scaled data, mean, median, geometric mean, standard deviation, minimum and maximum have been reported. Diagnostic accuracies (sensitivity and specificity) were analyzed from 2 × 2 contingency tables referring bivariate test results to CMV serostatus (reference method). Since the reference standard was not disease but a comparative method, the terms "percent positive agreement" and "percent negative agreement" were used instead of "sensitivity" and "specificity" respectively. The measures are reported with their exact Pearson-Clopper confidence intervals. Kappa (κ) according to Altman and McNemar's test were used to indicate overall agreement and consistency of pairs of methods respectively. Significance was accepted at $p < 0.05$.

The cut-off of T-Track® CMV positivity was determined using z-statistics (α-level = 0.05) on log10-transformed geometric mean values. Values = 0 were replaced by values near detection limit, which was assumed to be 0.5. Intra-assay standard deviation (SD) of ELISpot measurements from the hemodialysis patient cohort ($n = 124$) and from a cohort of healthy donors ($n = 45$; [38]) was calculated. SD was for the unstimulated control, IE-1 stimulation and pp65 stimulation 0.199, 0.240 and 0.220 (hemodialysis patients), and 0.234, 0.192 and 0.136 (healthy donors), respectively. Considering an intra-assay SD of 0.2 and assuming that 4 replicates are measured for each negative control and test samples, a criterion that the ratio of geometric means of stimulated to unstimulated values is at least 2.5 was obtained. In addition, precision profiles were generated from both IE-1- and pp65-specific test results, whereby a coefficient of variation (CV) no higher than 40% was used as a limit of acceptance of assay validity to determine the respective limit of quantitation (LoQ). Precision profiles for IE-1- and pp65-specific T-Track® CMV yielded LoQ values of 7.8 and 8.3 respectively (see Additional file 1). Comparable limits of quantitation were obtained from precision profiles generated from T-Track® CMV assays performed on PBMC from healthy donors [38]. Based on these analyses, a technical cut-off of 10 SFC/200,000 PBMC was chosen. Altogether, T-Track® CMV test results were considered positive if the geometric mean of the spots resulting from at least one of app65 and aIE1 stimulations was ≥ 10 SFC/200,000 PBMC and if the ratio of the geometric means of stimulated to non-stimulated conditions was ≥ 2.5.

Results

Patient characteristics

One hunderd twenty-four hemodialysis patients (68 men, 56 women, mean age 65 ± 13 years) were enrolled in this study. The mean duration of dialysis was 1,913 days (range 21 to 11,640 days). A positive CMV-IgG serostatus was measured in 67/124 (54%) of hemodialysis patients (Table 1). Blood was collected before the start of the dialysis session. Routine blood parameters and inflammation markers are depicted in Table 1.

One hunderd twenty-four T-Track® CMV, 123 QuantiFERON®-CMV and 97 iTAg™ MHC Tetramer measurements were carried out from whole-blood (QuantiFERON®-CMV) or from freshly isolated PBMC (T-Track® CMV, iTAg™ MHC Tetramers). Insufficient amount of blood and/ or PBMC did not allow the performance evaluation of all tests for all 124 patients. CMV serology served as a primary reference measurement procedure (gold standard reference) in the performance study.

Table 1 Demographic and blood parameters of hemodialysis patients

Age (years), mean ± SD (range)	65 ± 13 (26; 88)
Gender, N (%)	
Male	68 (54.8%)
Female	56 (45.2%)
CMV serostatus, N (%)	
Positive	67 (54%)
Negative	57 (46%)
Duration of dialysis (days), mean ± SD (range)	1,913 ± 2,079 (21; 11,640)
Blood count, mean ± SD (range)	
Hemoglobin (g/dl)	11.3 ± 1.2 (7.8; 16.1)
Erythrocytes (Tpt/l)	3.7 ± 0.44 (2.5; 5.2)
Leukocytes (pt/nl)	7.5 ± 2.4 (3.0; 17.8)
Thrombocytes (Tsd/μl)	234 ± 65 (84; 426)
Inflammation marker, mean ± SD (range)	
CRP (mg/l)[a]	9.7 ± 17.6 (1.0; 143.0)
Absolute number of PBMC x 10^6 / 15 ml whole blood (mean ± SD (range)	13.5 ± 9.8 (3.2; 87.3)

[a]CRP values were available for 80 out of 124 patients

Performance of T-Track® CMV

Positive and negative agreement of T-Track® CMV with CMV serology was investigated using PBMC samples from 124 hemodialysis patients. 58 of the 67 CMV-seropositive patients showed a positive response to app65 (Table 2) with a median of 165 spot-forming cells (SFC)/200,000 PBMC and a maximum of 1,040 SFC/200,000 PBMC (Fig. 1a). 33 of the 67 CMV-seropositive patients demonstrated an aIE-1-specific response in the T-Track® CMV ELISpot assay, with a median of 9.7 SFC/200,000 PBMC and a maximum of 696 SFC/200,000 PBMC (Table 2 and Fig. 1a). By taking into account the outcome of both aIE-1 and app65 stimulations, T-Track® CMV results were positive in 60 out of 67 CMV-seropositive patients, corresponding to an overall positive agreement with CMV serology of 89.6% (Table 2).

Interestingly, 12 out of 57 (21.1%) study participants who scored negative in a conventional serological assay presented with CMV-reactive effector cells in T-Track® CMV, equivalent to a negative agreement with CMV serology of 78.9% (Table 3). With one exception, positive T-Track® CMV results in CMV-seronegative patients were observed in aIE-1-stimulated PBMC samples, and were mostly associated with low spot counts (10.3–23.6 SFC/200,000 PBMC in 9 out 12 patients; Fig. 1a). Three patients however exhibited higher spot counts (93.6–116.5 SFC/200,000 PBMC). In contrast, one app65-positive test result with a spot count of 94 SFC/200,000 PBMC was observed among the 57 CMV-seronegative patients (Fig. 1a). Of note, this patient also showed a positive test result for aIE-1, with 109.2 SFC/200,000 PBMC (Fig. 1a).

Table 2 Positive agreement of T-Track® CMV, QuantiFERON®-CMV and iTAg™ MHC Tetramers with CMV serology in hemodialysis patients

Test	CMV positive serology[a]	CMI+	CMI-	Positive agreement	95% CI
T-Track® CMV	67	60	7	0.896	0.797–0.957
CMV aIE-1	67	33	34	0.493	0.368–0.618
CMV app65	67	58	9	0.866	0.760–0.937
QuantiFERON®-CMV[b]	62	45	17	0.726	0.598–0.831
iTAg™ MHC Tetramers	52	40	12	0.769	0.632–0.875

[a]CMV-serology served as primary reference measurement procedure; [b]calculation of the positive agreement and associated 95% CI do not take into account the 4 indeterminate QuantiFERON®-CMV results out of the 66 CMV-seropositive patients; *CMI+* positive test result, *CMI-* negative test result, *CI* confidence interval

These observations suggest that T-Track® CMV might have the capacity to detect CMV-reactive cells resulting from a previous CMV infection that was however not sufficient to yield an antibody response.

Performance of QuantiFERON®-CMV and iTAg™ MHC Tetramers

The QuantiFERON®-CMV assay was performed on blood samples from 66 CMV-seropositive and 57 CMV-seronegative hemodialysis patients. QuantiFERON®-CMV was positive (reactive) in 45/66, negative (non-reactive) in 17/66 and indeterminate in 4/66 of CMV-seropositive patients. Conversely, 7/57, 48/57 and 2/57 of CMV-seronegative patients showed positive, negative and indeterminate test results, respectively. Indeterminate results

were excluded from subsequent analyses, as a repetition of the QuantiFERON®-CMV assay from fresh blood samples was not possible. Thus, the results of the QuantiFERON®-CMV assay revealed a positive and negative agreement with CMV serology of 72.6% (45/62) and 87.3% (48/55) respectively (Tables 2 and 3; Fig. 1b).

A mixture of six preselected CMV-specific class I iTAg™ MHC Tetramers based on IE-1, pp65 and pp50 epitopes and predicted to cover at least 80% of the Caucasian population was used to quantify the proportion of CMV-specific CTL in freshly isolated PBMC of 52 CMV-seropositive and 45 CMV-seronegative hemodialysis patients. In these experiments, 40/52 (76.9%) of CMV-seropositive patients were test-positive with a median proportion of 0.98% CMV-specific CD8$^+$ T cells / total CD8$^+$ T

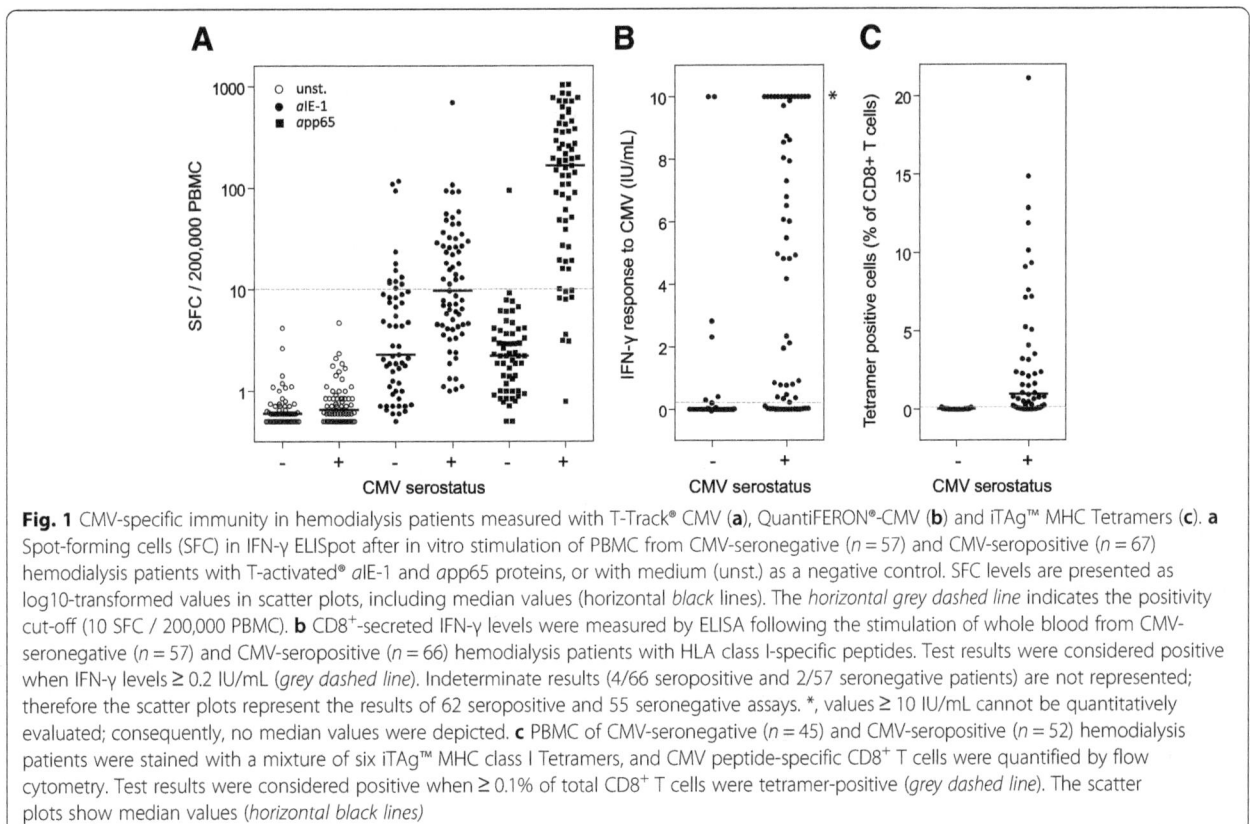

Fig. 1 CMV-specific immunity in hemodialysis patients measured with T-Track® CMV (**a**), QuantiFERON®-CMV (**b**) and iTAg™ MHC Tetramers (**c**). **a** Spot-forming cells (SFC) in IFN-γ ELISpot after in vitro stimulation of PBMC from CMV-seronegative ($n = 57$) and CMV-seropositive ($n = 67$) hemodialysis patients with T-activated® aIE-1 and app65 proteins, or with medium (unst.) as a negative control. SFC levels are presented as log10-transformed values in scatter plots, including median values (horizontal *black* lines). The *horizontal grey dashed line* indicates the positivity cut-off (10 SFC / 200,000 PBMC). **b** CD8$^+$-secreted IFN-γ levels were measured by ELISA following the stimulation of whole blood from CMV-seronegative ($n = 57$) and CMV-seropositive ($n = 66$) hemodialysis patients with HLA class I-specific peptides. Test results were considered positive when IFN-γ levels ≥ 0.2 IU/mL (*grey dashed line*). Indeterminate results (4/66 seropositive and 2/57 seronegative patients) are not represented; therefore the scatter plots represent the results of 62 seropositive and 55 seronegative assays. *, values ≥ 10 IU/mL cannot be quantitatively evaluated; consequently, no median values were depicted. **c** PBMC of CMV-seronegative ($n = 45$) and CMV-seropositive ($n = 52$) hemodialysis patients were stained with a mixture of six iTAg™ MHC class I Tetramers, and CMV peptide-specific CD8$^+$ T cells were quantified by flow cytometry. Test results were considered positive when ≥ 0.1% of total CD8$^+$ T cells were tetramer-positive (*grey dashed line*). The scatter plots show median values (*horizontal black lines*)

Table 3 Negative agreement of T-Track® CMV, QuantiFERON®-CMV and iTAg™ MHC Tetramers with CMV serology in hemodialysis patients

Test	CMV negative serology[a]	CMI-	CMI+	negative agreement	95% CI
T-Track® CMV	57	45	12	0.789	0.661–0.886
CMV aIE-1	57	45	12	0.789	0.661–0.886
CMV app65	57	56	1	0.982	0.906–1.000
QuantiFERON®-CMV[b]	55	48	7	0.873	0.755–0.947
iTAg™ MHC Tetramers	45	42	3	0.933	0.817–0.986

[a]CMV-serology served as primary reference measurement procedure; [b]calculation of the negative agreement and associated 95% CI do not take into account the 2 indeterminate QuantiFERON®-CMV results out of the 57 CMV-seronegative patients; *CMI-* negative test result, *CMI+* positive test result, *CI* confidence interval

cells and a maximum of 21.1% tetramer-positive CD8[+] T cells (Table 2 and Fig. 1c). Among 45 CMV-seronegative patients 3 were assay-positive, corresponding to a negative agreement with CMV-serology of 93.3% (Table 3 and Fig. 1c).

Assessment of agreement between the different assays

The results of T-Track® CMV, QuantiFERON®-CMV and iTAg™ MHC Tetramers were compared to assess their level of agreement. Results of T-Track® CMV moderately agreed with that of QuantiFERON®-CMV (κ = 0.445) and of the CMV iTAg™ MHC Tetramers (κ = 0.434) (Table 4). Statistical analysis of the number of discordant results between T-Track® CMV, QuantiFERON®-CMV and iTAg™ MHC Tetramers using the McNemar's test revealed that the consistency in the pairs of methods was statistically different between T-Track® CMV and both QuantiFERON®-CMV ($p = 0.0090$) and iTAg™ MHC Tetramers ($p = 0.0082$) (Table 4).

Notably, 14/17 and 12/12 CMV-seropositive patients with negative results in QuantiFERON®-CMV and iTAg™ MHC Tetramer respectively, were assay-positive in T-Track® CMV. Moreover, 5/5 CMV-seropositive patients with negative results for both QuantiFERON®-CMV and iTAg™ MHC Tetramers showed positive T-Track® CMV results. Conversely, the 7 CMV-seropositive patients with a negative T-Track® CMV result showed either positive or negative results by QuantiFERON®-CMV and iTAg™ MHC Tetramers, revealing inter-assay discordance. Interestingly, 3/4 CMV-seropositive patients with indeterminate QuantiFERON®-CMV results showed a positive T-

Table 4 Assessment of strength (κ) and consistency (McNemar's Test) of agreement of T-Track® CMV results with QuantiFERON®-CMV and iTAg™ MHC Tetramers results

Test 1	Test 2	κ	95% CI	McNemar
T-Track® CMV	QuantiFERON®-CMV	0.445	0.289–0.601	0.009
T-Track® CMV	iTAg™ MHC Tetramers	0.434	0.264–0.604	0.008

According to Altman, kappa (κ) values between 0.4 and 0.6 refer to moderate agreement. Consistency was evaluated by comparing the number of discordant results using the McNemar's Test ($p < 0.05$ was considered statistically significant). Of note, assessment does not take into consideration indeterminate results of the QuantiFERON®-CMV assay. *CI* confidence interval

Track® CMV result, of which 2 were also CMV-Tetramer positive. Finally, among the CMV-seronegative patients, only 1 out of 12 positive T-Track® CMV assays was also positive in QuantiFERON®-CMV while 6/7 and 3/3 positive results in QuantiFERON®-CMV and iTAg™ MHC Tetramers respectively were negative in T-Track® CMV.

Discussion

T-Track® CMV represents a novel assay format, which relies on the functional assessment of various CMV protein-reactive effector cells, including CD4[+] (Th) cells, CD8[+] (CTL), NK and NKT-like cells [37, 38], all of which being described to contribute to the clearance of CMV replication [1, 6–8, 41–44]. In this study, the suitability of T-Track® CMV to measure CMV-specific CMI in a cohort of dialysis patients and its performance against QuantiFERON®-CMV [34] and iTAg™ MHC Tetramer assays [24] were evaluated.

T-Track® CMV revealed a positive agreement with CMV-serology of 90% in hemodialysis patients, higher than that measured with QuantiFERON®-CMV (73%) and a mixture of 6 preselected CMV-specific iTAg™ MHC Tetramers (77%), indicating a higher sensitivity of T-Track® CMV compared to QuantiFERON®-CMV and iTAg™ MHC Tetramers. This difference in positive agreement with CMV-serology is likely due to the difference in format of the three assays. Beside the detection of a broad repertoire of CD8[+] T cells as a result of antigen cross-presentation [37], T-Track® CMV is indeed able to assess the functionality of CMV-reactive CD4[+] cells but also the bystander activation of IFN-γ-producing NK and NKT-like cells [41, 43–46]. In contrast, QuantiFERON®-CMV and iTAg™ MHC Tetramers are restricted to the detection of selected CMV-specific CD8[+] cells. In addition to the assay format, the combination of results of the separate measurement of pp65- and IE-1-responsive effector cells by T-Track® CMV contributes to the increased positive agreement with CMV serology, from 87% with pp65-specific CMI alone to 90% with both pp65- and IE-1-specific CMI. This positive contribution of IE-1 to the sensitivity of T-Track® CMV is in agreement with the demonstration that CMV-seropositive healthy donors do not always exhibit a pp65-specific CD8$^+$ T cell response and that a non-negligible proportion of individuals only show a CD8$^+$ T cell response to IE-1 [47]. Other factors potentially enhancing the sensitivity of T-Track® CMV are the standardization of the assay, which uses a constant number of PBMC (as opposed to whole blood in QuantiFERON®-CMV, possibly resulting in high inter-individual variability), its HLA-type-independence (as opposed especially to the iTAg™ MHC Tetramer assay) and the absence of indeterminate results (as opposed to QuantiFERON®-CMV). In that regard, 4/66 CMV-seropositive and 2/57 CMV-seronegative hemodialysis patients yielded indeterminate results with QuantiFERON®-CMV, which - with a rate of 5% - is lower than what was reported in transplant recipients [28, 35, 36].

Interestingly, the positive agreement of T-Track® CMV with CMV-serology of 90% measured in this cohort of hemodialysis patients was lower than that obtained in CMV-seropositive healthy individuals (97%; [38]). Similarly, the positive agreement of QuantiFERON®-CMV results with CMV-serology in hemodialysis patients (73%) is below the positive agreement of 88% to 97% previously reported in healthy adults [27, 34]. This difference might be explained by a functional impairment of Th cells, CTL, Antigen-presenting cells (APC), NK and NKT cells in patients with end-stage renal failure undergoing hemodialysis [48–52]. A reduced CMV-CMI prior to renal transplantation might be associated with an increased risk of CMV reactivation following transplantation. In support to this proposition, several studies reported an association between impaired CMV-specific CMI pre-transplantation and increased risk for CMV viremia post-transplantation [29, 31, 53]. The high positive agreement of T-Track® CMV with CMV serology observed in this cohort of hemodialysis patients therefore emphasizes the suitability and clinical relevance of T-Track® CMV for patients eligible for renal transplantation.

Although both CMV pp65 and IE-1 antigens contain multiple CD4$^+$ and CD8$^+$ T cell epitopes presented by different HLA alleles [40], the number of reactive effector cells responding to stimulation with $a$pp65 was substantially higher than that responding to aIE-1. This difference might result in part from the dynamics of pp65- and IE-1-reactive CD4$^+$ and CD8$^+$ T cells in the course of the immune response to CMV infection, long-term seroconversion being dominated by pp65- over IE-1-reactive T cells [8–11, 53, 54]. Moreover, mechanisms of immune evasion involving CMV-encoded unique short (US) proteins and resulting in the inhibition of the MHC-I-dependent antigen presentation pathway appear to be responsible for impaired IE-1 antigen processing and presentation, and thus in the low frequency of IE-1-reactive CD8$^+$ T cells [55–57]. On the other hand,

differential antigen uptake, processing and presentation by APC, possibly influenced by pp65 and IE-1 intrinsic properties [54, 58, 59], might explain inter-individual differences in the frequency of CMV antigen-specific T cells. Accordingly, comparable CD8$^+$ T cell response to IE-1 and pp65 has also been described in some CMV-seropositive healthy donors [47, 60]. The clinical significance of the differential responses to different antigens using T-Track® CMV needs to be elucidated in future studies.

12/57 CMV-seronegative patients revealed positive T-Track® CMV results, corresponding to a negative agreement of T-Track® CMV with CMV serology of 79%. Positive test results were mainly attributed to aIE-1 stimulation, and negative agreement raised to 98% when considering the results of $a$pp65 stimulation alone. IE-1-induced spot counts were close to T-Track® CMV positivity threshold in 9/12 patients and only 3 CMV-seronegative patients showed higher IE-1-induced spot counts. We can reasonably rule out false negative CMV serology test results in these patients, as repetition of CMV serology 6 months upon completion of the study in 9 patients who were still available, confirmed their negative serostatus for IgG and IgM (data not shown). Comparatively, 7/55 QuantiFERON®-CMV and 3/45 CMV iTAg™ MHC Tetramer measurements also revealed positive test results in seronegative dialysis patients. Interestingly, with one exception, the 12, 7 and 3 CMV seronegative patients with positive test results in T-Track® CMV, QuantiFERON®-CMV and CMV iTAg™ MHC Tetramers, respectively, were different. This inter-assay variability contributes to the moderate agreement (κ = ~0.4) observed between T-Track® CMV and the 2 alternative assays, and is in agreement with previous studies reporting discordant results between IFN-γ ELISpot and QuantiFERON®-CMV [61, 62]. This inter-assay variability likely reflects differences in the ability of antigen stimulants in each assay to activate distinct subsets of CMV-reactive T cells. Urea formulation of T-activated® CMV antigens increases protein uptake and promotes antigen processing and presentation in the context of both MHC-I (cross-presentation) and MHC-II [37]. T-Track® CMV is thus able to activate a broad range of CD8$^+$ and CD4$^+$ T cells, encompassing a larger T cell repertoire than QuantiFERON®-CMV or iTAg™ MHC-I Tetramers, and possibly explaining the higher number of CMV-seronegative patients with positive T-Track® CMV test results.

Interestingly, detection of CMV-reactive effector T cells within CMV-seronegative individuals has been described by others, both in healthy individuals and in transplant recipients, at frequencies of 2–11% among healthy donors and up to 30% in renal transplant recipients [13, 63–65]. With 21% CMV-seronegative hemodialysis patients with positive T-Track® CMV results, our data are in concordance with these published studies. Although Sester et al.

questioned the accuracy of serologic testing, in particular in case of borderline immunoglobulin titers [65], Loeth et al. elegantly demonstrated in their study on healthy individuals, that the frequency of 11% seronegative donors with pp65-specific $CD4^+$ and $CD8^+$ response was neither due to wrong serological assignment, nor to immune cross-reactivity with the closely related herpes virus HHV6, nor to *in vitro* priming. Instead, their demonstration that a large proportion of seronegative donors could mount a strong pp65-specific $CD4^+$ (and to a lesser extent $CD8^+$) response upon *in vitro* stimulation, led the authors to suggest that these individuals were previously exposed to CMV but failed to mount a humoral immune response [63]. We cannot exclude at this point this possibility nor that TCR cross-reactivity with closely related herpes viruses [66, 67] or with environmental antigens [68, 69] is responsible for the detection of CMV-reactive cells in CMV-seronegative hemodialysis patients. On the other hand, we can reasonably exclude the possibility that signals detected by IFN-γ ELISpot following 19 h of antigen stimulation originate from CMV-specific naïve T cells present in the PBMC population [70–72]. Indeed, although antigen-specific naïve T cells can be primed and expanded in vitro and in vivo [69, 72–78], the vast majority of antigen-stimulated naïve T cells produce no IFN-γ and do not divide for the first ~3 days of stimulation [69, 76, 79–82]. The higher proportion of CMV-reactive cells in seronegative dialysis patients in T-Track® CMV compared to QuantiFERON®-CMV and iTAg™ MHC Tetramers supports the hypothesis that IE-1-specific $CD4^+$ T cells (and possibly $CD8^+$ T cells through cross-presentation) contribute to the detected signals. On the other hand, the increased proportion of IE-1-reactive cells over pp65-reactive cells in CMV-seronegative patients supports the idea of a recent exposure to CMV, as response to primary infection is usually dominated by IE-1-reactive (predominantly $CD8^+$) effector cells [6, 8–11]. Additional experiments will be necessary to address these propositions. Whatever the mechanism involved in the generation of CMV-reactive effector cells in CMV-seronegative patients, these observations raise the attractive possibility that these individuals might have a protective immunity against CMV infection. Clearly, further investigations are needed to address this possibility. Altogether, our data suggest that T-Track® CMV exhibits a performance superior to that of QuantiFERON®-CMV and of iTAg™ MHC Tetramers, and possibly also superior to that of CMV-IgG serology, for the detection of possible immunity against CMV.

Conclusions

T-Track® CMV represents a highly standardized and sensitive assay suitable for the monitoring of CMV-specific cell-mediated immunity in end-stage renal failure patients, representative of patients prior to renal transplantation. Further validation of T-Track® CMV in multi-center clinical studies on kidney and allogeneic stem cell transplant patients is currently on-going, to evaluate its use for the risk assessment and prediction of CMV-related clinical complications in transplant recipients. In these situations, monitoring of CMV-specific CMI could help physicians better define patient populations that would benefit from prophylactic antiviral therapy, and assist the decision as to when to withdraw prophylaxis safely. Reducing prophylactic antiviral treatment would be beneficial in limiting both treatment-related nephrotoxic side effects and costs.

Abbreviations

APC: Antigen-presenting cell; αprotein: T-activated® protein; CMI: Cell-mediated immunity; CMV: Cytomegalovirus; CTL: Cytotoxic T lymphocyte; CV: Coefficient of variation; ELISA: Enzyme-linked immunosorbent assay; ELISpot: Enzyme-linked immunospot; HIV: Human immunodeficiency virus; HLA: Human leukocyte antigen; IE-1: Immediate early-1 protein; IFN-γ: Interferon gamma; LoQ: Limit of quantitation; NK: Natural killer cell; NKT: Natural killer T cell; PBMC: Peripheral blood mononuclear cell; pp65: 65 kDa lower matrix phosphoprotein; SD: Standard deviation; SFC: Spot-forming cell; Th: T helper cell

Acknowledgements

The authors are grateful to Theresa Spindler, Tamara Lugner, Charlotte Tonar and Astrid Starke for their expertise and technical assistance in laboratory testing as well as in data collection and analysis. We thank Dr. Thomas Keller (ACOMED Statistik) for statistical evaluation. T-Track® CMV tests were provided by Lophius Biosciences GmbH, Regensburg.

Funding

This project was funded in part by the Bayerische Forschungsstiftung Grants AZ 924-10 (to L.D.) and AZ 1070-13 (ForBiMed project D5 to R.W.) and by institutional funds of the University of Regensburg (ReForM C Project 03-082 to B.K.K., later transferred to B.B.). The funding body had no role in the design of the study and in collection, analysis and interpretation of data and in writing the manuscript.

Authors' contributions

LD, BB and BKK designed the study. JB supervised the study. BB, BKK, CB, GL, BK and JL obtained patient samples and collected the data. SB, MS and JK performed the assays and analyzed the data. RW supervised the interpretation and representation of data. AR and HB drafted the manuscript and figures. All authors edited and/or approved the final version.

Competing interests

SB, JB, HB, LD, AR and MS are or were employees of Lophius Biosciences GmbH at the time of the study. LD is co-founder and Chief Scientific Officer of Lophius Biosciences GmbH. RW is Chairman of the Board of Lophius Biosciences GmbH. RW, SB and LD are shareholders of Lophius Biosciences GmbH. The participating clinical and dialysis centers have received research funding from Lophius Biosciences GmbH for this study.

Author details

[1]Department of Nephrology, University Medical Center Regensburg, Regensburg, Germany. [2]Dialysis Center Landshut, Landshut, Germany. [3]5th Department of Medicine, University Medical Center Mannheim, Medical Faculty Mannheim of the University Heidelberg, Mannheim, Germany. [4]Lophius Biosciences GmbH, Regensburg, Germany. [5]Institute of Clinical Microbiology and Hygiene, University of Regensburg, Regensburg, Germany. [6]Dialysis Center Schwandorf, Schwandorf, Germany.

References

1. Hanley PJ, Bollard CM. Controlling cytomegalovirus: helping the immune system take the lead. Viruses. 2014;6:2242–58.
2. Crough T, Khanna R. Immunobiology of human cytomegalovirus: from bench to bedside. Clin Microbiol Rev. 2009;22:76–98.
3. Schleiss MR. Cytomegalovirus in the neonate: immune correlates of infection and protection. Clin Dev Immunol. 2013;2013:501801.
4. Rossini G, Cerboni C, Santoni A, Landini MP, Landolfo S, Gatti D, et al. Interplay between human cytomegalovirus and intrinsic/innate host responses: a complex bidirectional relationship. Mediators Inflamm. 2012; 2012:607276.
5. Jeitziner SM, Walton SM, Torti N, Oxenius A. Adoptive transfer of cytomegalovirus-specific effector CD4+ T cells provides antiviral protection from murine CMV infection. Eur J Immunol. 2013;43:2886–95.
6. Sester M, Sester U, Gärtner B, Heine G, Girndt M, Mueller-Lantzsch N, et al. Levels of virus-specific CD4 T cells correlate with cytomegalovirus control and predict virus-induced disease after renal transplantation. Transplantation. 2001;71:1287–94.
7. Gamadia LE, Remmerswaal EBM, Weel JF, Bemelman F, van Lier RAW, Ten Berge IJM. Primary immune responses to human CMV: a critical role for IFN-gamma-producing CD4+ T cells in protection against CMV disease. Blood. 2003;101:2686–92.
8. Sester M, Sester U, Gärtner BC, Girndt M, Meyerhans A, Köhler H. Dominance of virus-specific CD8 T cells in human primary cytomegalovirus infection. J Am Soc Nephrol JASN. 2002;13:2577–84.
9. Widmann T, Sester U, Gärtner BC, Schubert J, Pfreundschuh M, Köhler H, et al. Levels of CMV specific CD4 T cells are dynamic and correlate with CMV viremia after allogeneic stem cell transplantation. PLoS One. 2008;3:e3634.
10. Sacre K, Carcelain G, Cassoux N, Fillet A-M, Costagliola D, Vittecoq D, et al. Repertoire, diversity, and differentiation of specific CD8 T cells are associated with immune protection against human cytomegalovirus disease. J Exp Med. 2005;201:1999–2010.
11. Sester M, Sester U, Gärtner B, Kubuschok B, Girndt M, Meyerhans A, et al. Sustained high frequencies of specific CD4 T cells restricted to a single persistent virus. J Virol. 2002;76:3748–55.

12. Dunn HS, Haney DJ, Ghanekar SA, Stepick-Biek P, Lewis DB, Maecker HT. Dynamics of CD4 and CD8 T Cell Responses to Cytomegalovirus in Healthy Human Donors. J Infect Dis. 2002;186:15–22.
13. Sinclair E, Black D, Epling CL, Carvidi A, Josefowicz SZ, Bredt BM, et al. CMV antigen-specific CD4+ and CD8+ T cell IFNgamma expression and proliferation responses in healthy CMV-seropositive individuals. Viral Immunol. 2004;17:445–54.
14. Sester U, Presser D, Dirks J, Gärtner BC, Köhler H, Sester M. PD-1 expression and IL-2 loss of cytomegalovirus- specific T cells correlates with viremia and reversible functional anergy. Am J Transplant Off J Am Soc Transplant Am Soc Transpl Surg. 2008;8:1486–97.
15. Dirks J, Tas H, Schmidt T, Kirsch S, Gärtner BC, Sester U, et al. PD-1 analysis on CD28(-) CD27(-) CD4 T cells allows stimulation-independent assessment of CMV viremic episodes in transplant recipients. Off J Am Soc Transplant Am Soc Transpl Surg. 2013;13:3132–41.
16. Engstrand M, Lidehall AK, Totterman TH, Herrman B, Eriksson B-M, Korsgren O. Cellular responses to cytomegalovirus in immunosuppressed patients: circulating CD8+ T cells recognizing CMVpp65 are present but display functional impairment. Clin Exp Immunol. 2003;132:96–104.
17. Huster KM, Stemberger C, Gasteiger G, Kastenmüller W, Drexler I, Busch DH. Cutting edge: memory CD8 T cell compartment grows in size with immunological experience but nevertheless can lose function. J Immunol. 2009;183:6898–902.
18. Sund F, Lidehäll A-K, Claesson K, Foss A, Tötterman TH, Korsgren O, et al. CMV-specific T-cell immunity, viral load, and clinical outcome in seropositive renal transplant recipients: a pilot study. Clin Transplant. 2010;24:401–9.
19. Fernández-Ruiz M, Kumar D, Humar A. Clinical immune-monitoring strategies for predicting infection risk in solid organ transplantation. Clin Transl Immunol. 2014;3:e12.
20. Kotton CN. Management of cytomegalovirus infection in solid organ transplantation. Nat Rev Nephrol. 2010;6:711–21.
21. Lisboa LF, Kumar D, Wilson LE, Humar A. Clinical utility of cytomegalovirus cell-mediated immunity in transplant recipients with cytomegalovirus viremia. Transplantation. 2012;93:195–200.
22. Koehl U, Dirkwinkel E, Koenig M, Erben S, Soerensen J, Bader P, et al. Reconstitution of cytomegalovirus specific T cells after pediatric allogeneic stem cell transplantation: results from a pilot study using a multi-allele CMV tetramer group. Klin Padiatr. 2008;220:348–52.
23. Gratama JW, Boeckh M, Nakamura R, Cornelissen JJ, Brooimans RA, Zaia JA, et al. Immune monitoring with iTAg MHC Tetramers for prediction of recurrent or persistent cytomegalovirus infection or disease in allogeneic hematopoietic stem cell transplant recipients: a prospective multicenter study. Blood. 2010;116:1655–62.
24. Klenerman P, Cerundolo V, Dunbar PR. Tracking T cells with tetramers: new tales from new tools. Nat Rev Immunol. 2002;2:263–72.
25. Bunde T, Kirchner A, Hoffmeister B, Habedank D, Hetzer R, Cherepnev G, et al. Protection from cytomegalovirus after transplantation is correlated with immediate early 1-specific CD8 T cells. J Exp Med. 2005;201:1031–6.
26. Egli A, Binet I, Binggeli S, Jäger C, Dumoulin A, Schaub S, et al. Cytomegalovirus-specific T-cell responses and viral replication in kidney transplant recipients. J Transl Med. 2008;6:29.
27. Abate D, Saldan A, Mengoli C, Fiscon M, Silvestre C, Fallico L, et al. Comparison of cytomegalovirus (CMV) enzyme-linked immunosorbent spot and CMV quantiferon gamma interferon-releasing assays in assessing risk of CMV infection in kidney transplant recipients. J Clin Microbiol. 2013;51:2501–7.
28. Manuel O, Husain S, Kumar D, Zayas C, Mawhorter S, Levi ME, et al. Assessment of cytomegalovirus-specific cell-mediated immunity for the prediction of cytomegalovirus disease in high-risk solid-organ transplant recipients: a multicenter cohort study. Clin Infect Dis Off Publ Infect Dis Soc Am. 2013;56:817–24.
29. Cantisán S, Lara R, Montejo M, Redel J, Rodríguez-Benot A, Gutiérrez-Aroca J, et al. Pretransplant interferon-γ secretion by CMV-specific CD8+ T cells informs the risk of CMV replication after transplantation. Am J Transplant Off J Am Soc Transplant Am Soc Transpl Surg. 2013;13:738–45.
30. Kumar D, Chernenko S, Moussa G, Cobos I, Manuel O, Preiksaitis J, et al. Cell-mediated immunity to predict cytomegalovirus disease in high-risk solid organ transplant recipients. Am J Transplant Off J Am Soc Transplant Am Soc Transpl Surg. 2009;9:1214–22.
31. Bestard O, Lucia M, Crespo E, Van Liempt B, Palacio D, Melilli E, et al. Pretransplant immediately early-1-specific T cell responses provide

protection for CMV infection after kidney transplantation. Am J Transplant Off J Am Soc Transplant Am Soc Transpl Surg. 2013;13:1793–805.

32. Godard B, Gazagne A, Gey A, Baptiste M, Vingert B, Pegaz-Fiornet B, et al. Optimization of an elispot assay to detect cytomegalovirus-specific CD8+ T lymphocytes. Hum Immunol. 2004;65:1307–18.

33. Schmittel A, Keilholz U, Scheibenbogen C. Evaluation of the interferon-gamma ELISPOT-assay for quantification of peptide specific T lymphocytes from peripheral blood. J Immunol Methods. 1997;210:167–74.

34. Walker S, Fazou C, Crough T, Holdsworth R, Kiely P, Veale M, et al. Ex vivo monitoring of human cytomegalovirus-specific CD8+ T-cell responses using QuantiFERON-CMV. Transpl Infect Dis Off J Transplant Soc. 2007;9:165–70.

35. Clari MÁ, Muñoz-Cobo B, Solano C, Benet I, Costa E, Remigia MJ, et al. Performance of the QuantiFERON-cytomegalovirus (CMV) assay for detection and estimation of the magnitude and functionality of the CMV-specific gamma interferon-producing CD8(+) T-cell response in allogeneic stem cell transplant recipients. Clin Vaccine Immunol CVI. 2012;19:791–6.

36. Fleming T, Dunne J, Crowley B. Ex vivo monitoring of human cytomegalovirus-specific CD8(+) T-Cell responses using the QuantiFERON-CMV assay in allogeneic hematopoietic stem cell transplant recipients attending an Irish hospital. J Med Virol. 2010;82:433–40.

37. Barabas S, Gary R, Bauer T, Lindner J, Lindner P, Weinberger B, et al. Urea-mediated cross-presentation of soluble Epstein-Barr virus BZLF1 protein. PLoS Pathog. 2008;4:e1000198.

38. Barabas S, Spindler T, Kiener R, Tonar C, Lugner T, Batzilla J, Bendfeldt H, Rascle A, Asbach B, Wagner R, Deml L. An optimized IFN-γ ELISpot assay for the sensitive and standardized monitoring of CMV protein-reactive effector cells of cell-mediated immunity. BMC Immunol. 2017. doi:10.1186/s12865-017-0195-y.

39. Reuschel E, Barabas S, Zeman F, Bendfeldt H, Rascle A, Deml L, et al. Functional impairment of CMV-reactive cellular immunity during pregnancy. J Med Virol. 2017;89:324–31.

40. Bui H-H, Sidney J, Dinh K, Southwood S, Newman MJ, Sette A. Predicting population coverage of T-cell epitope-based diagnostics and vaccines. BMC Bioinformatics. 2006;7:153.

41. van Dommelen SLH, Tabarias HA, Smyth MJ, Degli-Esposti MA. Activation of Natural Killer (NK) T Cells during Murine Cytomegalovirus Infection Enhances the Antiviral Response Mediated by NK Cells. J Virol. 2003;77:1877–84.

42. Sylwester AW, Mitchell BL, Edgar JB, Taormina C, Pelte C, Ruchti F, et al. Broadly targeted human cytomegalovirus-specific CD4+ and CD8+ T cells dominate the memory compartments of exposed subjects. J Exp Med. 2005;202:673–85.

43. Kamath AT, Sheasby CE, Tough DF. Dendritic cells and NK cells stimulate bystander T cell activation in response to TLR agonists through secretion of IFN-alpha beta and IFN-gamma. J Immunol. 2005;174:767–76.

44. Min-Oo G, Lanier LL. Cytomegalovirus generates long-lived antigen-specific NK cells with diminished bystander activation to heterologous infection. J Exp Med. 2014;211:2669–80.

45. Reschner A, Hubert P, Delvenne P, Boniver J, Jacobs N. Innate lymphocyte and dendritic cell cross-talk: a key factor in the regulation of the immune response. Clin Exp Immunol. 2008;152:219–26.

46. Ferlazzo G, Morandi B. Cross-Talks between Natural Killer Cells and Distinct Subsets of Dendritic Cells. Front Immunol. 2014;5:159.

47. Kern F, Surel IP, Faulhaber N, Frömmel C, Schneider-Mergener J, Schönemann C, et al. Target structures of the CD8(+)-T-cell response to human cytomegalovirus: the 72-kilodalton major immediate-early protein revisited. J Virol. 1999;73:8179–84.

48. Litjens NHR, Huisman M, van den Dorpel M, Betjes MGH. Impaired immune responses and antigen-specific memory CD4+ T cells in hemodialysis patients. J Am Soc Nephrol JASN. 2008;19:1483–90.

49. Girndt M, Sester U, Sester M, Kaul H, Köhler H. Impaired cellular immune function in patients with end-stage renal failure. Nephrol Dial Transplant Off Publ Eur Dial Transpl Assoc - Eur Ren Assoc. 1999;14:2807–10.

50. Girndt M, Sester M, Sester U, Kaul H, Köhler H. Defective expression of B7-2 (CD86) on monocytes of dialysis patients correlates to the uremia-associated immune defect. Kidney Int. 2001;59:1382–9.

51. Lonnemann G. Impaired NK, cell function in ESRD patients. Blood Purif. 2008;26:315–6.

52. Mattes FM, Vargas A, Kopycinski J, Hainsworth EG, Sweny P, Nebbia G, et al. Functional impairment of cytomegalovirus specific CD8 T cells predicts high-level replication after renal transplantation. Am J Transplant Off J Am Soc Transplant Am Soc Transpl Surg. 2008;8:990–9.

53. Gerna G, Lilleri D, Fornara C, Comolli G, Lozza L, Campana C, et al. Monitoring of human cytomegalovirus-specific CD4 and CD8 T-cell immunity in patients receiving solid organ transplantation. Am J Transplant Off J Am Soc Transplant Am Soc Transpl Surg. 2006;6:2356–64.

54. Tabi Z, Moutaftsi M, Borysiewicz LK. Human cytomegalovirus pp 65- and immediate early 1 antigen-specific HLA class I-restricted cytotoxic T cell responses induced by cross-presentation of viral antigens. J Immunol. 2001;166:5695–703.

55. Khan N, Bruton R, Taylor GS, Cobbold M, Jones TR, Rickinson AB, et al. Identification of cytomegalovirus-specific cytotoxic T lymphocytes in vitro is greatly enhanced by the use of recombinant virus lacking the US2 to US11 region or modified vaccinia virus Ankara expressing individual viral genes. J Virol. 2005;79:2869–79.

56. Manley TJ, Luy L, Jones T, Boeckh M, Mutimer H, Riddell SR. Immune evasion proteins of human cytomegalovirus do not prevent a diverse CD8+ cytotoxic T-cell response in natural infection. Blood. 2004;104:1075–82.

57. Gilbert MJ, Riddell SR, Li CR, Greenberg PD. Selective interference with class I major histocompatibility complex presentation of the major immediate-early protein following infection with human cytomegalovirus. J Virol. 1993;67:3461–9.

58. Scheller N, Furtwängler R, Sester U, Maier R, Breinig T, Meyerhans A. Human cytomegalovirus protein pp 65: an efficient protein carrier system into human dendritic cells. Gene Ther. 2008;15:318–25.

59. Delmas S, Martin L, Baron M, Nelson JA, Streblow DN, Davignon J-L. Optimization of CD4+ T lymphocyte response to human cytomegalovirus nuclear IE1 protein through modifications of both size and cellular localization. J Immunol. 2005;175:6812–9.

60. Khan N, Cobbold M, Keenan R, Moss PAH. Comparative analysis of CD8+ T cell responses against human cytomegalovirus proteins pp65 and immediate early 1 shows similarities in precursor frequency, oligoclonality, and phenotype. J Infect Dis. 2002;185:1025–34.

61. Forner G, Saldan A, Mengoli C, Gussetti N, Palù G, Abate D. CMV-ELISPOT but not CMV-QuantiFERON assay is a novel biomarker to determine risk of congenital CMV infection in pregnant women. J Clin Microbiol. 2016;54(8):2149–54.

62. Saldan A, Forner G, Mengoli C, Tinto D, Fallico L, Peracchi M, et al. Comparison of cell-mediated immune assays CMV-ELISPOT and CMV-QuantiFERON in CMV seropositive and seronegative pregnant and non-pregnant women. J Clin Microbiol. 2016;54(5):1352–6.

63. Loeth N, Assing K, Madsen HO, Vindeløv L, Buus S, Stryhn A. Humoral and cellular CMV responses in healthy donors; identification of a frequent population of CMV-specific, CD4+ T cells in seronegative donors. PLoS One. 2012;7:e31420.

64. Lúcia M, Crespo E, Melilli E, Cruzado JM, Luque S, Llaudó I, et al. Preformed frequencies of cytomegalovirus (CMV)-specific memory T and B cells identify protected CMV-sensitized individuals among seronegative kidney transplant recipients. Clin Infect Dis Off Publ Infect Dis Soc Am. 2014;59:1537–45.

65. Sester M, Gärtner BC, Sester U, Girndt M, Mueller-Lantzsch N, Köhler H. Is the cytomegalovirus serologic status always accurate? A comparative analysis of humoral and cellular immunity. Transplantation. 2003;76:1229–30.

66. Edson CM, Hosler BA, Respess RA, Waters DJ, Thorley-Lawson DA. Cross-reactivity between herpes simplex virus glycoprotein B and a 63,000-dalton varicella-zoster virus envelope glycoprotein. J Virol. 1985;56:333–6.

67. Vafai A, Wroblewska Z, Graf L. Antigenic cross-reaction between a varicella-zoster virus nucleocapsid protein encoded by gene 40 and a herpes simplex virus nucleocapsid protein. Virus Res. 1990;15:163–74.

68. Su LF, Kidd BA, Han A, Kotzin JJ, Davis MM. Virus-specific CD4(+) memory-phenotype T cells are abundant in unexposed adults. Immunity. 2013;38:373–83.

69. Kieper WC, Troy A, Burghardt JT, Ramsey C, Lee JY, Jiang H-Q, et al. Recent immune status determines the source of antigens that drive homeostatic T cell expansion. J Immunol. 2005;174:3158–63.

70. Yukl SA, Shergill AK, Girling V, Li Q, Killian M, Epling L, et al. Site-specific differences in T cell frequencies and phenotypes in the blood and gut of HIV-uninfected and ART-treated HIV+ adults. PLoS One. 2015;10:e0121290.

71. Dubois E, Ruschil C, Bischof F. Low frequencies of central memory CD4 T cells in progressive multifocal leukoencephalopathy. Neurol Neuroimmunol Neuroinflammation [Internet]. 2015. [cited Oct 24 2016];2. Available from: http://www.ncbi.nlm.nih.gov/pmc/articles/PMC4630684/.

72. Alanio C, Lemaitre F, Law HKW, Hasan M, Albert ML. Enumeration of human antigen–specific naive CD8+ T cells reveals conserved precursor frequencies. Blood. 2010;115:3718–25.

73. Sprent J, Surh CD. Normal T cell homeostasis: the conversion of naive cells into memory-phenotype cells. Nat Immunol. 2011;12:478–84.

74. Hanley PJ, Melenhorst JJ, Nikiforow S, Scheinberg P, Blaney JW, Demmler-Harrison G, et al. CMV-specific T cells generated from naïve T cells recognize atypical epitopes and may be protective in vivo. Sci Transl Med. 2015;7:285ra63.

75. Hanley PJ, Shaffer DR, Cruz CRY, Ku S, Tzou B, Liu H, et al. Expansion of T cells targeting multiple antigens of cytomegalovirus, Epstein-Barr virus and adenovirus to provide broad antiviral specificity after stem cell transplantation. Cytotherapy. 2011;13:976–86.

76. Brenchley JM, Douek DC, Ambrozak DR, Chatterji M, Betts MR, Davis LS, et al. Expansion of activated human naïve T-cells precedes effector function. Clin Exp Immunol. 2002;130:432–40.

77. Maroof A, Beattie L, Kirby A, Coles M, Kaye PM. Dendritic cells matured by inflammation induce CD86-dependent priming of naive CD8+ T cells in the absence of their cognate peptide antigen. J Immunol. 2009;183:7095–103.

78. Zippelius A, Pittet MJ, Batard P, Rufer N, de Smedt M, Guillaume P, et al. Thymic selection generates a large T cell pool recognizing a self-peptide in humans. J Exp Med. 2002;195:485–94.

79. Whitmire JK, Eam B, Whitton JL. Tentative T cells: memory cells are quick to respond, but slow to divide. PLoS Pathog. 2008;4:e1000041.

80. Veiga-Fernandes H, Walter U, Bourgeois C, McLean A, Rocha B. Response of naïve and memory CD8+ T cells to antigen stimulation in vivo. Nat Immunol. 2000;1:47–53.

81. Brehm MA, Mangada J, Markees TG, Pearson T, Daniels KA, Thornley TB, et al. Rapid quantification of naive alloreactive T cells by TNF-alpha production and correlation with allograft rejection in mice. Blood. 2007;109:819–26.

82. Ben-Sasson SZ, Gerstel R, Hu-Li J, Paul WE. Cell division is not a "clock" measuring acquisition of competence to produce IFN-gamma or IL-4. J Immunol. 2001;166:112–20.

15

The differences in immunoadjuvant mechanisms of TLR3 and TLR4 agonists on the level of antigen-presenting cells during immunization with recombinant adenovirus vector

Ekaterina Lebedeva[1][*] ⓘ, Alexander Bagaev[1], Alexey Pichugin[1], Marina Chulkina[1], Andrei Lysenko[2], Irina Tutykhina[2], Maxim Shmarov[2], Denis Logunov[2], Boris Naroditsky[2] and Ravshan Ataullakhanov[1][*]

Abstract

Background: Agonists of TLR3 and TLR4 are effective immunoadjuvants for different types of vaccines. The mechanisms of their immunostimulatory action differ significantly; these differences are particularly critical for immunization with non-replicating adenovirus vectors (rAds) based vaccines. Unlike traditional vaccines, rAd based vaccines are not designed to capture vaccine antigens from the external environment by antigen presenting cells (APCs), but rather they are targeted to the de novo synthesis of vaccine antigens in APCs transfected with rAd. To date, there is no clear understanding about approaches to improve the efficacy of rAd vaccinations with immunoadjuvants. In this study, we investigated the immunoadjuvant effect of TLR3 and TLR4 agonists on the level of activation of APCs during vaccination with rAds.

Results: We demonstrated that TLR3 and TLR4 agonists confer different effects on the molecular processes in APCs that determine the efficacy of antigen delivery and activation of antigen-specific CD4$^+$ and CD8$^+$ T cells. APCs activated with agonists of TLR4 were characterized by up-regulated production of target antigen mRNA and protein encoded in rAd, as well as enhanced expression of the co-activation receptors CD80, CD86 and CD40, and pro-inflammatory cytokines TNF-α, IL6 and IL12. These effects of TLR4 agonists have provided a significant increase in the number of antigen-specific CD4$^+$ and CD8$^+$ T cells. TLR3 agonist, on the contrary, inhibited transcription and synthesis of rAd-encoded antigens, but improved expression of CD40 and IFN-β in APCs. The cumulative effect of TLR3 agonist have resulted in only a slight improvement in the activation of antigen-specific T cells. Also, we demonstrated that IFN-β and TNF-α, secreted by APCs in response to TLR3 and TLR4 agonists, respectively, have an opposite effect on the transcription of the targeted gene encoded in rAd. Specifically, IFN-β inhibited, and TNF-α stimulated the expression of target vaccine antigens in APCs.

Conclusions: Our data demonstrate that agonists of TLR4 but not TLR3 merit further study as adjuvants for development of vaccines based on recombinant adenoviral vectors.

Keywords: Toll-like receptors, Agonists, Adjuvants, Immunization, Recombinant non-replicating adenoviral vector, Expression of transgenes, Antigen-presenting cells, Dendritic cells

* Correspondence: ekaterinalebedeva2612@mail.ru;
ravshan.ataullakhanov@gmail.com
[1]National Research Center Institute of Immunology, Federal
Medical-Biological Agency of Russia, Moscow, Russia
Full list of author information is available at the end of the article

Background

Activation of antigen-specific T-cell responses is the basis of the most effective approaches in vaccination and immunotherapy [1–3]. Combination of vaccines with adjuvants significantly improves antigen-specific responses of T cells.

Agonists of Toll-like receptors 3 and 4 (TLR3 and TLR4) are effective adjuvants for various vaccines [4–7]. The mechanism of adjuvant action of TLR3 and TLR4 agonists is largely associated with their ability to activate APCs [8–13]. Particularly, TLR agonists enhance uptake and presentation of vaccine antigens by APCs (up-regulation of MHC class II and class I expression, inflammasome activation); induce maturation (increase expression of co-stimulating receptors and immunostimulatory cytokines), and migration of APCs to draining lymph nodes [8]. These events, induced in APCs by TLR agonists, determine the efficacy of antigen-specific CD8$^+$ and CD4$^+$ T cell responses after vaccination.

Vaccines based on recombinant adenoviral vectors (rAds) demonstrate high efficiency in activation of antigen-specific CD8$^+$ and CD4$^+$ T cells, which allows for the successful protection of animals against malaria, tuberculosis, Ebola, and other infectious diseases [14–17]. Theoretically, combination of adenoviruses with adjuvants could be a strategy to enhance the potential of rAd vaccines. However, there is no clear understanding of benefits resulting from the inclusion of adjuvants to the rAd vaccine composition. Despite the known examples of combinations of TLR3 and TLR4 agonists with rAds [18–24], the mechanisms of their adjuvant action is not well understood. It has been shown that signals from different TLRs are necessary to induce effective responses of antigen-specific T-cells upon immunization with rAd [25]. However, responses of CD8$^+$ T cells in TLR-deficient mice (TLR2, 4, 5, 6, 7, 9) were not critically affected compared with wild-type mice. The effectiveness of vaccination was significantly decreased when the molecule MyD88 was knocked out. Therefore, an integrative action of individual TLRs in activation of MyD88 and induction of reliable responses to rAd immunization was proposed.

There is sufficient evidences that TLR3 and TLR4 agonists have an opposite effect on immunogenicity of rAd vaccines. Immunization with the rAd26-Gag vector in the presence of Poly I:C (TLR3 agonist) resulted in a decrease of Gag-specific responses of CD8$^+$ T cells, whereas TLR4 agonists significantly improved ones [26]. Moreover, mice deficient in TLR3 and its adaptor molecule TRIF demonstrated an increase in antigen-specific T-cell responses compared with wild-type mice [25].

In contrast to protein and peptide vaccines that are designed to deliver vaccine antigens to APCs from outside, rAd-based vaccines require effective expression (de novo synthesis) of target antigens within APCs.

Thus, the presentation of antigenic peptides in MHC-I and subsequent activation of CD8$^+$ T cells is significantly dependent on the expression of adenoviral vector transgenes in APCs. Quinn et al. [27] had previously investigated the expression efficacy of target antigens in DCs isolated from lymph nodes of mice immunized with rAd. An opposing relationship between the expression of target antigens and the genes involved in interferon responses in APCs was observed. The external induction of the interferon genes by TLR3 agonist Poly I:C resulted in a reduction in both the total number of DCs in lymph nodes and the expression of target antigen of rAd. TBK1 (TANK-binding kinase 1) have been shown to be involved in the suppression of adenovirus vector expression through induction of an interferon response in splenocytes of immunized mice [28].

In a previous study, we have shown that the efficacy of rAd expression in APCs could be regulated with TLR agonists. In particular, we demonstrated that TLR4 agonists enhances the production of proteins encoded in rAd, while TLR3 agonist inhibits their production [29].

In the present study, we investigated the mechanisms of immunoadjuvant action of TLR3 and TLR4 agonists upon immunization with rAd (rAdTet-off H1) encoding haemagglutinin of influenza virus (H1). We demonstrated that TLR3 and TLR4 agonists equally enhance the generation of antigen-reactive CD4$^+$ T cells in spleen of mice immunized with rAdTet-off H1. However, TLR3 and TLR4 agonists have shown different potential for activation of CD8$^+$ T cell responses. The number of CD8$^+$ T cells recognizing H1 was significantly improved in mice immunized with rAdTet-off H1 in combination with TLR4 compared to mice immunized with rAdTet-off H1 alone. TLR3 agonist did not improve responses of H1-reactive CD8$^+$ T cells.

We carried out detailed experiments to study the efficiency of target adenovirus antigens presentation in DCs activated with TLR3 and TLR4 agonists. We investigated the effect of TLR3 and TLR4 agonists on the three types of processes in APCs that can provide the final adjuvant effect of each agonist: (1) the intensity of production of target H1 antigen; (2) the expression of co-activation receptors CD80, CD86 and CD40; and (3) the production of immunostimulatory cytokines.

Results

The immunoadjuvant effect of TLR3 and TLR4 agonists

BALB/c mice were vaccinated intramuscularly with rAdTet-off H1 (10^7 PFU/mouse) alone (PBS) or in combination with TLR3 or TLR4 agonists. PBS or TLR agonists Poly I:C (5 μg), LPS (10 μg) or IMM (10 μg) were administered simultaneously (in one syringe) with rAdTet-off H1. Forty days after immunization mice were euthanized, and the number of antigen-reactive CD4$^+$ and CD8$^+$ T cells in the spleen of immunized mice were estimated with ELISPOT. The antigen-reactive populations of CD4$^+$ and CD8$^+$ cells were isolated from spleen of the mice by sorting on the FACS. Sorted CD4$^+$ (Fig. 1d) and CD8$^+$ (Fig. 1c) T cells were co-cultured with antigen loaded DCs.

The combination of rAdTet-off H1 with TLR4 agonist had significantly improved the magnitude of H1-specific T cell responses (Fig. 1). Up to 2–3 times more H1-specific CD8$^+$ (Fig. 1a) and CD4$^+$ (Fig. 1b) T cells had accumulated in the spleen of mice immunized with rAdTet-off H1 in combination with one of TLR4 agonists (LPS, IMM) compared to mice immunized with rAdTet-off H1 alone (PBS). TLR3 agonist induced an enhanced response of CD4$^+$ T cells (Fig. 1b), however, it did not exert an adjuvant effect on H1-specific CD8$^+$ T cells (Fig. 1a).

We concluded that TLR3 and TLR4 agonists enhance immune responses upon immunization with rAd based vaccines. An adjuvant effect of TLR agonists was primarily thought to affect APCs maturation which subsequently improves activation of antigen-specific T-cells [8–13]. Therefore, we further investigated the T-cells activation potential of APCs loaded with rAd and stimulated with agonists of TLR3 and TLR4.

Activation of antigen-presenting dendritic cells with TLR3 and TLR4 agonists enhances the efficiency of responses of H1-specific T cells

Bone marrow derived dendritic cells (DCs) were activated with different concentrations of TLR3 or TLR4 agonists (0–10 µg/ml) and loaded with rAdTet-off H1 (3.5–350 PFU per cell) in vitro. Next, they were co-cultured with sorted CD4$^+$ (Fig. 1d) and CD8$^+$ (Fig. 1c) T cells from the spleen of the mice immunized with rAdTet-off H1. T cell responses were evaluated according to the number of T cells secreting interferon-γ (IFN- γ) using the ELISPOT.

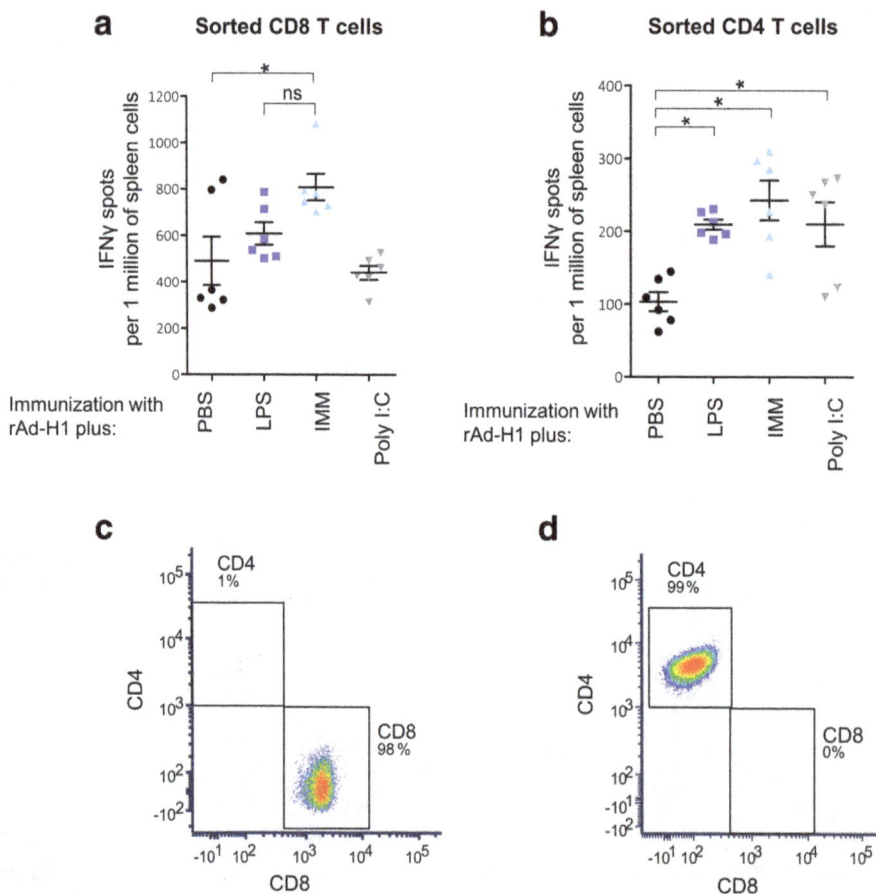

Fig. 1 Immunoadjuvant effect of TLR3 and TLR4 agonists upon immunization with rAdTet-off H1 vaccine. Balb/c mice were immunized with 10^7 PFU rAdTet-off H1 alone or in combination with 10 µg LPS, 10 µg IMM or 5 µg Poly I:C. Forty days after immunization mice were euthanized, sorted populations of CD8$^+$ (c) and CD4$^+$ (d) T cells from spleens of immune mice were co-cultured with bone marrow DCs loaded with rAdTet-off H1 (35 PFU/cell) (a) or with recombinant protein H1 (2 µg/ml) (b), respectively. Reactivated IFNγ-producing T cells were detected using ELISPOT method. The number of IFNγ-positive spots is shown as M + SD (per 1 million spleen cells). Significant differences (p < 0.05) between the control group of mice immunized with rAdTet-off H1 (PBS) alone and groups of mice immunized with rAdTet-off H1 in combination with TLR agonists (LPS, IMM or Poly I:C) are indicated by asterisks

The number of IFN-γ-secreting T cells was dependent on the concentration of rAd loaded into the DCs (Fig. 2). As the viral dose increased from 3.5 (Fig. 2a, d) to 350 (Fig. 2c, f) PFU per cell, the number of IFN-γ-secreting $CD8^+$ (Fig. 2a-c) and $CD4^+$ T cells (Fig. 2d-f) increased from 100 (Fig. 2a) to 1500 (Fig. 2c), and from 80 (Fig. 2d) to 500 cells (Fig. 2f) (per 1 million spleen cells), respectively.

Activation of rAd-loaded DCs with TLR3 and TLR4 agonists resulted in an increase in the number of antigen-activated T cells. When APCs were loaded with a minimal viral dose, the minimal responses of antigen-reactive CD8 + T cells were observed (Fig. 2a). Activation of DC with TLR3 and TLR4 agonists allowed an increase of the minimal responses of antigen-reactive $CD8^+$ T cells 4-fold ($p = 0.0005$) and 7-fold ($p = 0.0008$), respectively (Fig. 2a). At the medium rAd concentration only 1.5-fold ($p = 0.0028$) and 2.5-fold ($p = 0.0004$) improvement of responses of $CD8^+$ T cells (Fig. 2b) by

TLR3 and TLR4 agonists, respectively, were observed. At the maximum load of rAd, TLR3 agonist suppressed $CD8^+$ T cell responses, while agonists of TLR4 did not affected responses of $CD8^+$ T cells (Fig. 2c).

TLR3 or TLR4 agonists similarly affected $CD4^+$ population of T cells. TLR3 agonist doubled $CD4^+$ responses upon low virus load (Fig. 2d) and had no influence at the medium (Fig. 2e) or maximum (Fig. 2f) concentrations of rAd. TLR4 agonists increased the number of reactivated $CD4^+$ T cells at low, medium and maximum concentrations of the rAd in 5, 3 and 1.5-times, respectively (Fig. 2d-f).

T-cell responses were dependent on the expression level of the target H1 antigen in DCs (Fig. 3e). Stimulation of DCs with TLR4 agonists increased the production of the target antigen H1 (Fig. 3a-d, Additional file 1: Figure S1) in APCs. There was a direct association between the level of expression of H1 and the reactivation efficiency of $CD4^+$ or $CD8^+$ T cells (Fig. 3f, g) upon activation of DC with TLR4 agonists. Production of the H1 in DCs was

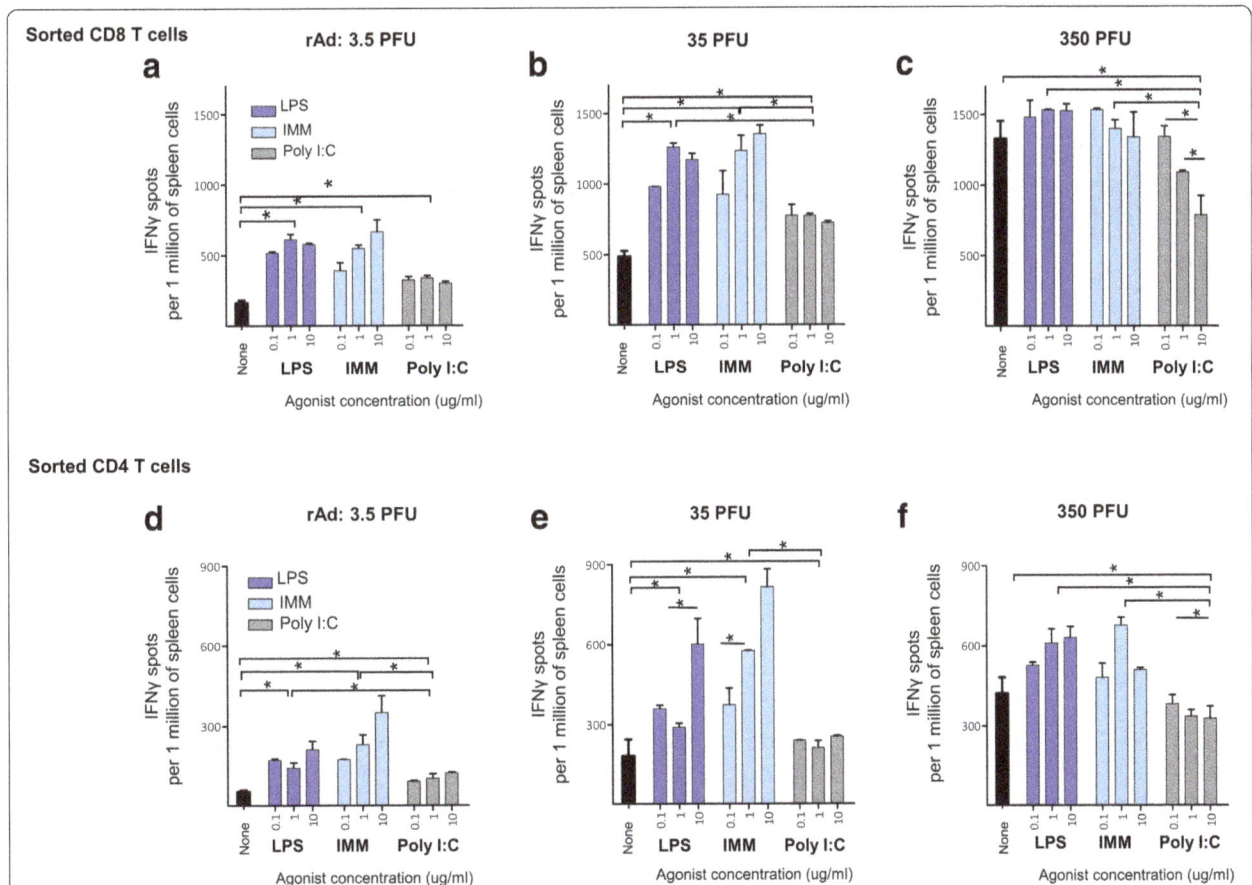

Fig. 2 The effect of TLR3 and TLR4 agonists on the efficacy of reactivation of H1-specific T cells. **a-f** balb/c mice were immunized (i.m.) with 10^8 PFU rAdTet-off H1. Forty days after immunization mice were euthanized, the pool of $CD8^+$ (**a-c**) and $CD4^+$ (**d-f**) T cells from the spleen of two immune mice was re-activated in vitro. Sorted $CD8^+$ and $CD4^+$ T cells were co-cultured with bone marrow derived DCs preloaded with 3.5 (**a, d**), 35 (**b, e**), or 350 (**c, f**) PFU/cell rAdTet-off H1 in the presence of 0–10 µg/ml agonists of TLR3 (Poly I:C) or TLR4 (LPS, IMM). The number of reactivated IFNγ-producing T-cells were detected by ELISPOT and calculated for 1 million spleen cells. Shown are M ± SD, statistically significant differences ($p < 0.05$) are indicated by asterisks

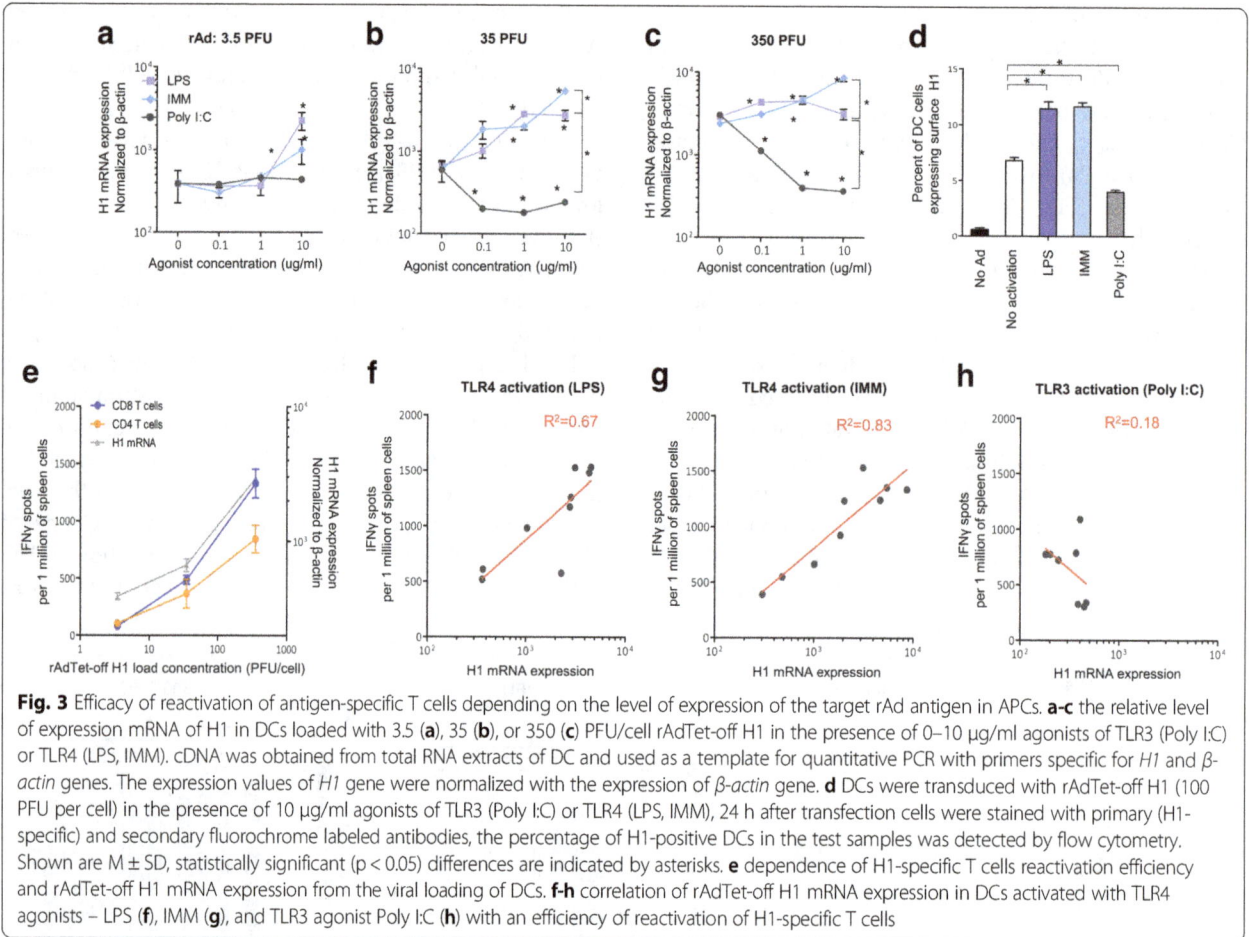

Fig. 3 Efficacy of reactivation of antigen-specific T cells depending on the level of expression of the target rAd antigen in APCs. **a-c** the relative level of expression mRNA of H1 in DCs loaded with 3.5 (**a**), 35 (**b**), or 350 (**c**) PFU/cell rAdTet-off H1 in the presence of 0–10 μg/ml agonists of TLR3 (Poly I:C) or TLR4 (LPS, IMM). cDNA was obtained from total RNA extracts of DC and used as a template for quantitative PCR with primers specific for *H1* and *β-actin* genes. The expression values of *H1* gene were normalized with the expression of *β-actin* gene. **d** DCs were transduced with rAdTet-off H1 (100 PFU per cell) in the presence of 10 μg/ml agonists of TLR3 (Poly I:C) or TLR4 (LPS, IMM), 24 h after transfection cells were stained with primary (H1-specific) and secondary fluorochrome labeled antibodies, the percentage of H1-positive DCs in the test samples was detected by flow cytometry. Shown are M ± SD, statistically significant (p < 0.05) differences are indicated by asterisks. **e** dependence of H1-specific T cells reactivation efficiency and rAdTet-off H1 mRNA expression from the viral loading of DCs. **f-h** correlation of rAdTet-off H1 mRNA expression in DCs activated with TLR4 agonists – LPS (**f**), IMM (**g**), and TLR3 agonist Poly I:C (**h**) with an efficiency of reactivation of H1-specific T cells

suppressed when antigen-presenting DCs were exposed to TLR3 agonist (Fig. 3a-d, Additional file 1: Figure S1) and no correlations between the expression of the target antigen and the responses of the T cells were observed (Fig. 2h). TLR3 agonist stimulated T cell responses at medium rAd load (Fig. 2a, b, d, e), but TLR3 agonist inhibited T cell responses at a higher concentration of rAds (Fig. 2c, f). This denotes that the production of the target antigen in the DCs activated with TLR4 agonists positively contributes to the effectiveness of T cell activation, but this does not occur when the DCs are activated with TLR3 agonist.

TLR3 and TLR4 agonists influenced the activation of T cells, regardless of the type of APCs (DCs and macrophages) used to present the rAd antigens (Additional file 1: Figure S2).

The stimulation of co-activation molecules and pro-inflammatory cytokines in antigen-presenting cells necessary for effective activation of antigen-reactive T cells

The effective stimulation of T cells in addition to the successful presentation of the target antigen in MHCI or MHCII complexes (signal 1 activating the T cell via TCR/CD3) requires at least two additional activation signals. The T cell receives the second signal through the CD28 and CD40L, which arises from binding the co-stimulating molecules CD80, CD86, CD40 on the surface of the APCs and ensures signals for T-cell stimulation and secretion of pro-inflammatory cytokines in APCs [30]. The source of the third signal are pro-inflammatory cytokines and type 1 interferons [31–36]. They maintain survival of antigen-specific T cells and development of productive antigen-specific reactions.

We measured the expression of key co-stimulatory molecules (CD80, CD86 and CD40) and pro-inflammatory cytokines (IL12, TNF-α, IL6 and IFN-β) in DCs activated with TLR3 and TLR4 agonists (Fig. 4).

TLR4 agonists significantly enhanced the expression of co-activation receptors CD40, CD80 and CD86 on the surface of DCs (Fig. 4a-c). TLR3 agonist induced increased expression of CD40 (Fig. 4a) but had not affected expression of CD80 and CD86 (Fig. 4b, c).

DCs activated with TLR3 and TLR4 agonists also differed in the level of induced expression of the genes of pro-inflammatory cytokines. TLR4 agonists significantly

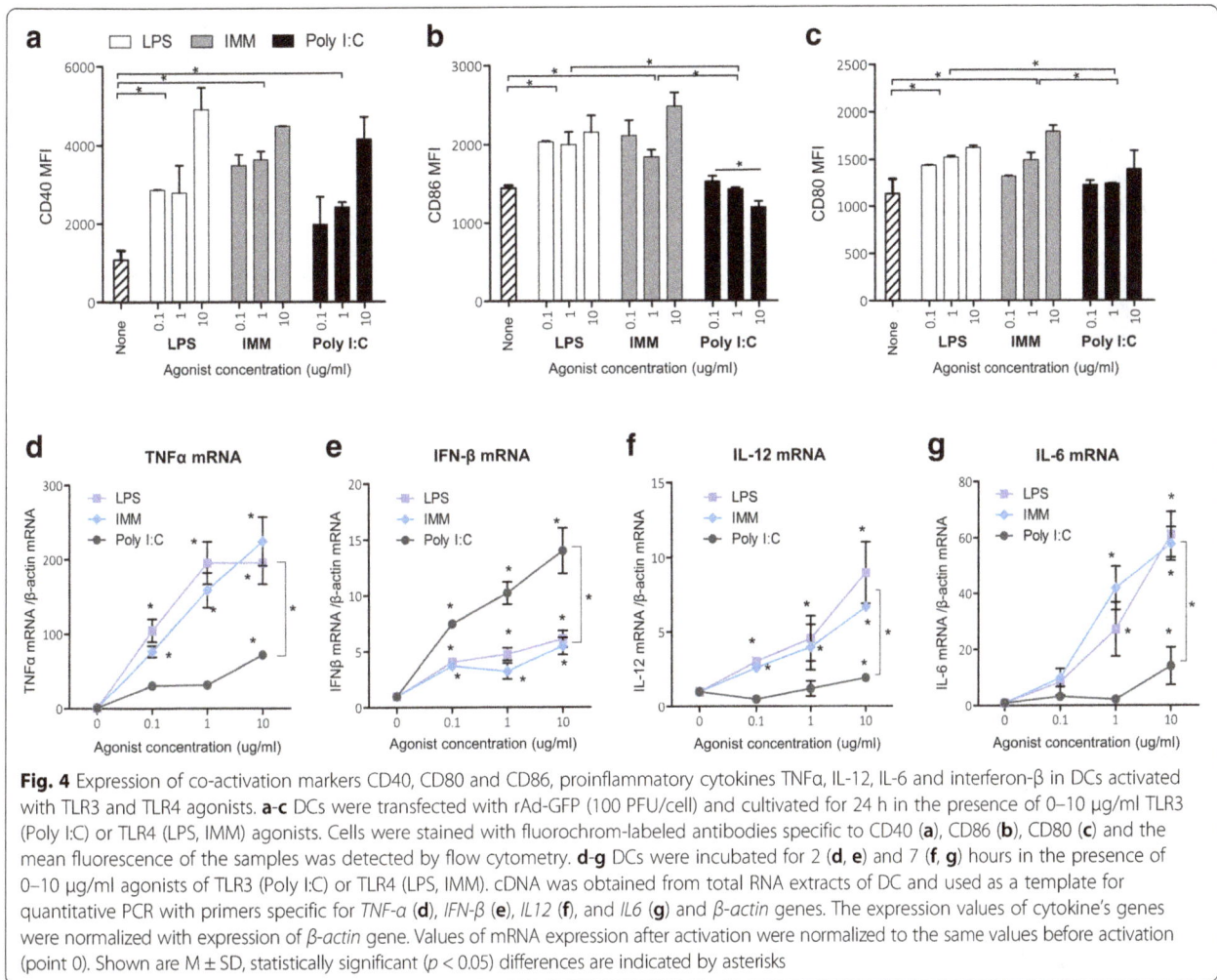

Fig. 4 Expression of co-activation markers CD40, CD80 and CD86, proinflammatory cytokines TNFα, IL-12, IL-6 and interferon-β in DCs activated with TLR3 and TLR4 agonists. **a-c** DCs were transfected with rAd-GFP (100 PFU/cell) and cultivated for 24 h in the presence of 0–10 μg/ml TLR3 (Poly I:C) or TLR4 (LPS, IMM) agonists. Cells were stained with fluorochrom-labeled antibodies specific to CD40 (**a**), CD86 (**b**), CD80 (**c**) and the mean fluorescence of the samples was detected by flow cytometry. **d-g** DCs were incubated for 2 (**d**, **e**) and 7 (**f**, **g**) hours in the presence of 0–10 μg/ml agonists of TLR3 (Poly I:C) or TLR4 (LPS, IMM). cDNA was obtained from total RNA extracts of DC and used as a template for quantitative PCR with primers specific for *TNF-a* (**d**), *IFN-β* (**e**), *IL12* (**f**), and *IL6* (**g**) and *β-actin* genes. The expression values of cytokine's genes were normalized with expression of *β-actin* gene. Values of mRNA expression after activation were normalized to the same values before activation (point 0). Shown are M ± SD, statistically significant ($p < 0.05$) differences are indicated by asterisks

stimulated transcription of *TNF-a*, *IL12* and *IL6* genes in DCs (Fig. 4d, f, g). TLR3 agonist activated *TNF-a*, *IL12* and *IL6* genes only at very low levels compared to the TLR4 agonist. However, TLR3 agonist stimulated production of IFN-β mRNA to a greater extent, than TLR4 agonists (Fig. 4e).

Enhancement and suppression of the adenoviral vector expression in antigen-presenting cells by TLR4 and TLR3 agonists can be transmitted through the secretion of cytokines in a paracrine manner

In response to activation with TLR agonists, antigen-presenting cells (dendritic cells and macrophages) secrete pro-inflammatory cytokines, chemokines, interferons and other biologically active substances capable of paracrine influence on the neighboring cells. We demonstrated that TLR4 agonists preferentially stimulate the production of pro-inflammatory cytokines, such as TNF-α, IL-6, IL-12, but TLR3 agonist activated type 1 interferons (Fig. 4). We hypothesized that differences in the spectrum of activated cytokines could determine the different effects

of TLR4 and TLR3 agonists on the expression of the adenovirus vector in antigen-presenting cells. To test this, we investigated the possibility of paracrine transfer of TLR-agonist induced regulation of the target protein expression from activated APCs to non-activated ones.

APCs were pre-activated with TLR agonists, washed from the agonists and cultured together with non-activated APCs. The combined culture of activated and non-activated APCs was transduced with rAd-GFP. Non-activated APCs were pre-labeled with the fluorescent dye Celltrace™ Violet, which further allowed us to distinguish two cell populations by flow cytometry. Intensity of production of the rAd-coded GFP protein was analysed in each of the two populations of cells (Fig. 5a). Enhanced expression of GFP was observed in APCs, which were pre-activated by TLR4 agonist. TLR4 agonist induced a 2-fold enhancement of the percentage and almost 2-fold increased mean fluorescence intensity of GFP-positive APCs (Fig. 5b, $p = 0.011$–0.041). Cells pre-activated with TLR3 had a lower GFP expression than cells transduced with rAd-GFP without TLR agonist activation. TLR3

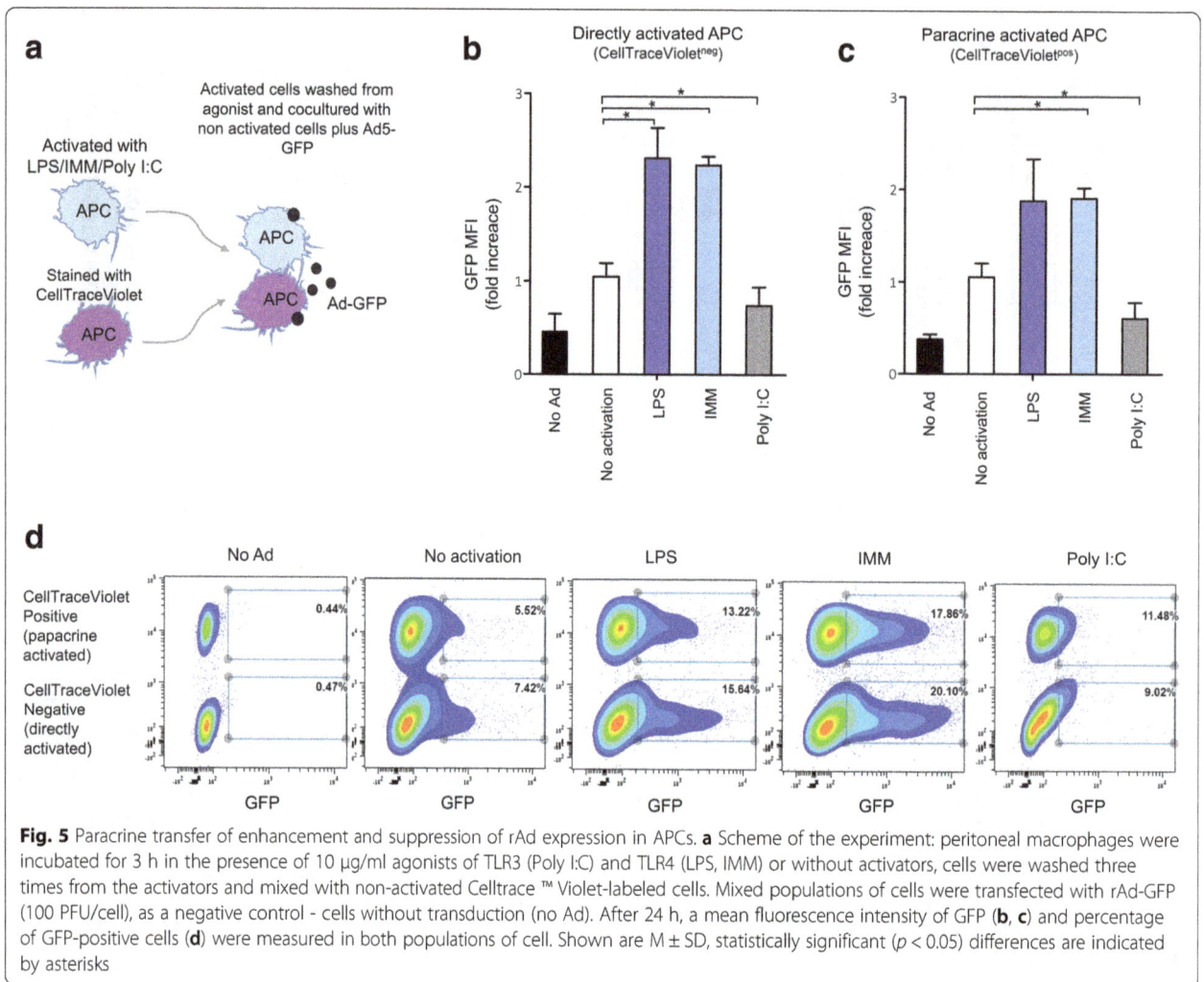

Fig. 5 Paracrine transfer of enhancement and suppression of rAd expression in APCs. **a** Scheme of the experiment: peritoneal macrophages were incubated for 3 h in the presence of 10 µg/ml agonists of TLR3 (Poly I:C) and TLR4 (LPS, IMM) or without activators, cells were washed three times from the activators and mixed with non-activated Celltrace ™ Violet-labeled cells. Mixed populations of cells were transfected with rAd-GFP (100 PFU/cell), as a negative control - cells without transduction (no Ad). After 24 h, a mean fluorescence intensity of GFP (**b**, **c**) and percentage of GFP-positive cells (**d**) were measured in both populations of cell. Shown are M ± SD, statistically significant ($p < 0.05$) differences are indicated by asterisks

agonist induced a decrease of mean fluorescence intensity of cells in the GFP channel (Fig. 5b, $p = 0.015$), while the percentage of cells producing GFP did not change significantly (Fig. 5d, $p > 0.05$).

Non-activated APCs following co-culturing with APCs pre-activated with TLR4 agonist expressed enhanced levels of GFP (Fig. 5c, $p = 0.037$) in the same manner to APCs directly activated with TLR4 agonist (Fig. 5b, $p = 0.011$–0.041). GFP synthesis was suppressed in non-activated APCs following co-culturing with APCs pre-activated with TLR3 agonist (Fig. 5c, $p = 0.01$), as well as in APCs directly activated by with TLR3 agonist (Fig. 5b, $p = 0.015$).

As can be seen from the data presented (Fig. 5), the effects of enhancement and suppression of GFP expression appeared both in cells directly activated with TLR4 or TLR3 agonists (Fig. 5b) and in non-activated cells neighboring with TLR3- or TLR4-activated APCs (Fig. 5c). Therefore, APCs activated with TLR4 or TLR3 agonists secrete signals that determine the enhancement or suppression of the production of the target rAd protein. Such signal molecules paracrinally affect non-activated

APCs and provide an enhancement/suppression of rAd expression in APCs without TLR3 and TLR4 agonists' activation.

The nature of paracrine signals determining enhancement or suppression of rAd expression in antigen-presenting cells

As indicated above, the enhancement (TLR4 agonists) and suppression (TLR3 agonist) of rAd expression in APCs occurs at the transcription level of the target gene (Fig. 3a-c) and can be paracrinally transmitted (Fig. 5). We suggested that cytokines and interferons are capable of playing the role of mediators of paracrine action of TLR-activated APCs on non-activated APCs.

The rAds used in this study encoded target genes (H1 or GFP) under the control of the NF-kB-dependent CMV promoter. TLR4 agonists have stimulated production of TNF-α (Fig. 4d), which is an effective activator of NF-kB in APCs [37]. Therefore, we proposed TNF-α mediated activation of transcription of the target gene under the NF-kB-sensitive promoter providing an enhanced expression of the target gene of rAd in APCs. In our experiments, TLR3 agonist caused enhanced production of IFN-β (Fig. 4e) and inhibited the expression of the target rAd gene in the APCs (Fig. 3a-d). Type 1 interferons are well known antiviral effectors providing destruction of viral RNA [38]. We assumed that IFN-β, secreted by TLR3-stimulated APCs, could suppress the expression of the viral vector accelerating the degradation of mRNA of the target antigen in APCs. To prove our assumptions, we used recombinant TNF-α and IFN-β proteins.

Antigen-presenting cells were transfected with rAd-GFP in the presence of recombinant TNF-α (0–30 ng/ml) (Fig. 6c) or IFN-β (0–100 ng/ml) (Fig. 6a). IFN-β suppressed (Fig. 6a), and TNF-α enhanced (Fig. 6c) the production of GFP in APCs in a dose-dependent manner. The combined effect of cytokines TNF-α + IFN-β (Fig. 6b, d) resulted in a decrease in the effects of each cytokine alone (Fig. 6a, c). In particular, the enhanced expression of GFP induced by TNF-α decreased when IFN-β was added (Fig. 6d), and conversely, the inhibited expression of GFP in the presence of IFN-β enhanced following addition of

TNF-α (Fig. 6b). The observed effects indicate that the regulation of mRNA transcription of rAd-GFP in APC could be mediated by IFN-β and TNF-α (Fig. 6e). TNF-α increases, and IFN-β inhibits (Fig. 6e) expression of target GFP mRNA in adenovirus infected APCs. The studied cytokines had no effect on the content of viral DNA in transfected cells (Fig. 6f) and, therefore, did not affect the efficiency of virus entry into APCs. Therefore, the observed effects were solely dependent on the transcription of the target antigens.

Discussion

Non-replicating recombinant adenoviral vectors (rAd) are an effective platform for the development of vaccines against a wide range of pathogens and diseases [14–17]. Combinations of rAd vaccines with adjuvant substances are capable of increasing the intensity of responses of antigen specific CD4⁺ and CD8⁺ T cells and enhancing the protective effect followingimmunization. TLR agonists demonstrated a high adjuvant potential when administered together with various adenoviral vectors [7, 18, 19, 21–23,

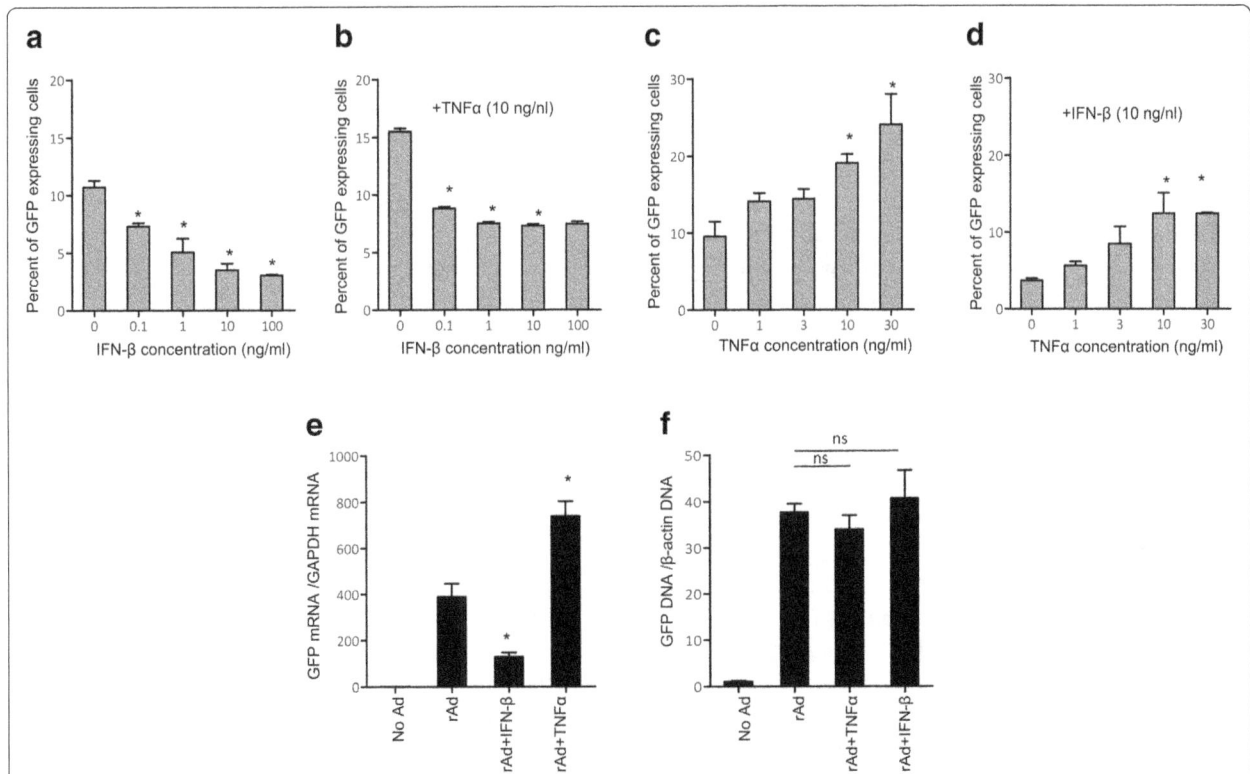

Fig. 6 Effect of TNFα and IFNβ on the expression of rAd in APCs. Peritoneal macrophages were transfected with rAd-GFP in the presence of 0–30 ng/ml of TNF-α (c, e, f), 0–100 ng/ml IFN-β (a, e, f), or in the presence of combinations of 0–100 ng/ ml IFN-β and 10 ng/ml TNF-α (b), 0–30 ng/ml TNF-α and 10 ng/ml IFN-β (d). After 24 h, the efficacy of GFP protein synthesis (a-d), the level of transcription of the GFP (e) gene mRNA and the amount of viral DNA penetrated into the cells upon transfection (f) were analyzed. a-d GFP fluorescence in cells was detected by cytometry, mRNA (e) and DNA (f) from the lysates of DCs were extracted, RNA was subjected to a reverse transcription reaction; the obtained cDNA (e) and total cellular DNA (f) were used as a template for quantitative PCR with primers specific for GFP, GAPDH and β-actin genes. The expression values of GFP gene were normalized with the expression of β–actin or GAPDH genes. Values of GFP mRNA and DNA were normalized to the control values (No rAd). Shown are M ± SD, statistically significant (p < 0.05) differences are indicated by asterisks

26, 39–43]. At the same time, there was no sufficient information about the mechanisms of immunoadjuvant action of agonists of TLR receptors. Effects of TLR agonists on the processes of presentation of target antigens of rAd in APCs and on the processes of activation of antigen-reactive T cells were poorly understood as well.

In this work we studied the mechanisms of adjuvant action of TLR3 and TLR4 agonists combined with rAd vaccine. We used Poly I:C and LPS as a classical well-studied agonists of TLR3 and TLR4 receptors with high immunostimulatory activity [44]. IMM (Immunomax®) is a pharmaceutical grade plant derived injectable TLR4 ligand. It is a large water-soluble polysaccharide which structure is solved [45]. In vitro IMM directly activates DCs and macrophages [29, 46, 47]. Activated DCs express co-activation receptors for T cells (CD86, CD80 and CD40), and secrete immunostimulatory cytokines (IL-12, IL-6, TNF-α, RANTES, MIP-1, MCP-1, IL-1), and antimicrobial substances (type I interferons, NO, peroxynitrite, CRAMP). After activation with IMM both types of APCs, DCs and macrophages, acquire antitumor properties, although their cancer-killing mechanisms are different [46]. The influence of IMM on DCs and macrophages is equivalent to LPS [29, 46, 47]. Using InvivoGen HEK-Blue™ TLR cell lines which express certain human TLRs, it has been shown that IMM activates only cells which express TLR4 but not those which express TLR2, TLR3, TLR5, TLR7, TLR8 or TLR9 [47]. IMM induces activation of MyD88 → NF-kB signaling axis. DCs' activation with IMM is abrogated with CLI-095, a specific inhibitor of TLR4 intracellular domain [29]. It also activates mouse and human NK cells and this activation is DC-mediated [47]. IMM does not activate DCs/macrophages obtained from the TLR4−/−knockout mice [46]. In vivo injections of IMM substantially changed cellular composition of spleen and lung of mice having 4 T1 breast cancer metastatic disease. It increased frequency of activated NK, CD4$^+$ and CD8$^+$ cells, and decreased frequency of myeloid-derived suppressor cells in spleens of mice [47]. In primary 4 T1 tumor-resected mice, repeated injections of IMM significantly prolonged overall survival and cured 30% of animals [47].

Administration of TLR3 and TLR4 agonists together with rAdTet-off H1 vaccine vector encoding haemagglutinin from the influenza virus (H1) significantly increased the intensity of responses of T-cells recognizing H1 epitopes (Fig. 1). Agonists of TLR3 (Poly-I:C) and TLR4 (LPS, IMM) doubled the amount of antigen-reactive CD4$^+$ T cells secreting IFN-γ in the spleen of mice immunized with rAdTet-off H1 (Fig. 1b). TLR4 agonists also increased the accumulation of antigen-reactive CD8$^+$ cells (Fig. 1a), while TLR3 agonist did not influence the responses of antigen-reactive CD8$^+$ T cells (Fig. 1a). Cytotoxic CD8$^+$ T-cells have a key role in the elimination of

intracellular infectious agents, at the same time, CD4$^+$ T helper cells are able to enhance the effector function of CD8$^+$ T cells [48, 49]. Thus, the ability of TLR4 agonists to improve both types of T-cell responses - CD4$^+$ and CD8$^+$ – is an important adjuvant property.

The adjuvant effect of TLR agonist is primarily associated with the activation of APCs [8–13]. TLR agonists up-regulate expression of co-stimulatory and MHC molecules, increasing antigen presentation properties, induce synthesis of cytokines and chemokines, facilitating the formation of a more intense immune response against foreign antigens [8]. We carried out detailed study of the effects of TLR3 and TLR4 agonists on the presentation of rAd antigens in DCs using in vitro models where DCs transduced with rAdTet-off H1 was stimulated with TLR3 or TLR4 agonists and co-cultured with H1-reactive T cells.

TLR3 and TLR4 agonists differently reactivated T cells specific to rAdTet-off H1 (Fig. 2, Additional file 1: Figure S2). TLR4 agonists increased the number of reactivated CD4$^+$ and CD8$^+$ T-cell at 4–10 times more. This allows a 10-fold decrease in the dose of the virus vector inducing a maximum response of T cells. TLR3 agonist Poly I:C doubled the amount of reactivated CD8$^+$ T cells co-cultured with DCs loaded with suboptimal doses of rAdTet-off H1. However, Poly I:C inhibited the responses of T cells reactivated with DCs loaded with maximum dose of rAd. Therefore, the adenovirus load of DC determines efficiency of antigen expression as well as reactivation of antigen-specific T cells. It can be proposed that studies demonstrating a positive effect of TLR3 agonist on rAd-immunisation was considered with non-maximal doses of rAd [7, 21, 22, 41, 42].

Activation of T cells following their interaction with complexes of antigens with MHCI/II depends on three key regulatory signals. The first signal occurs when the T cell receptor recognizes MHCI/II-antigen complex, which directly depends on the antigen binding affinity, and on the efficiency of target antigen expression in APCs in the case of adenoviral immunization. The second signal occurs, when T-cell receptors are linked to co-activation molecules (CD40, CD80, CD86) on the surface of APCs, which depends on it's the expression on the surface of the DCs. Finally, the third signal is determined by the T-cell's cytokine environment. In the absence of pro-inflammatory cytokines and type I interferons, activated T cells die before they have completed their function [31–36].

We investigated the influence of TLR3 and TLR4 agonists on each of three mentioned signals in antigen-presenting DCs. TLR4 agonists significantly increased expression of the target antigen encoded in rAd (Fig. 3a-d), stimulated expression of CD40, CD80 and CD86 molecules and enhanced secretion of pro-inflammatory cytokines TNFα, IL-12, IL-6, but not type I interferons (Fig. 4). TLR3 agonist suppressed expression of the target antigen encoded in rAd

(Fig. 3b-d), and strongly activated expression of CD40, but not CD80 and CD86 molecules, and did not substantially stimulated expression of TNF-α, IL-12, IL-6 genes (Fig. 4). Simultaneously, DCs stimulated with TLR3 agonist (Poly I:C) produced a large amount of *IFN-β* (Fig. 4e). It is known that type I interferons determine maturation of DCs and regulation of T cell responses in the presence of a TLR3 agonist. Blocking interferon signaling in IFNabR$^{-/-}$ mice resulted in a critical decrease of the CD40, CD86 proteins expression on the surface of DCs in the presence of Poly I:C and inhibition of antigen-specific T cell responses [50].

Cytokines and type I interferons produced by APCs in response to LPS, IMM and Poly I:C are able to determine the function of the third activation signal for T cells as well as the efficiency of production of the target rAd antigen in APCs. Both inhibition and enhancement of rAd expression could be regulated by cytokine signals. These signals are transmitted from the cells activated with TLR3 and TLR4 agonists to non-activated cells in a paracrine manner (Fig. 5). This is particularly shown for TNF-α and IFN-β, which are capable of enhancing and inhibiting the expression of the target antigen in APC transduced by rAd, respectively (Fig. 6). We demonstrated that intensive secretion of IFN-β promotes a decrease in expression level of rAdTet-off H1 in DCs stimulated with Poly I:C (Figs. 3b-d and 4e). In contrast, enhanced production of TNF-α following activation of APCs with LPS or IMM (Fig. 4d) promoted increased expression of rAd antigens in APCs (Fig. 3a-d). Previously, it was shown that the efficiency of rAd expression in vivo is determined by the interferon response of target cells [27, 28]. The expression of rAd in DCs and the induction of CD8$^+$ T cells responses were inversely correlated with the expression level of genes responsible for activation of interferon pathways in APCs [27]. Interferon-β has a mixed effect on the activation of T cells upon their contact with APCs [27, 28, 33, 34]. Particularly, IFN-β had an antiviral effect and inhibited production of target antigen encoded in rAd in APCs [27, 28]. Stimulation of APCs with Poly I:C (Fig. 3b-d) and IFN-β (Fig. 6a) caused a suppressed antigen expression of rAdTet-off H1 in macrophages and DC, which resulted in a decreased reactivation of H1-specific T cells (Fig. 2).

According to our data TLR3-activated DCs do express CD40 (Fig. 4a) but do not express CD86/80 (Fig. 4b and c). The expression of CD40 is a key co-stimulatory molecule for CD4$^+$ T cells, because the CD40L is expressed preferentially by CD4$^+$ T cells, but not CD8+ T cells [51]. Which means that TLR3-induced expression of CD40 on APCs should provide the co-stimulatory signal to CD4$^+$ T cells but not to CD8$^+$ T cells (Fig. 7). The latter are readily accepting the co-stimulatory signal generated via CD80/86-CD28 axis which is well induced by TLR4 but not TLR3 agonists.

Conclusions

We have identified the principal differences in the adjuvant action of TLR3 and TLR4 agonists used for rAd based immunization. TLR3 agonist stimulates accumulation of antigen-specific CD4$^+$ T cells, and TLR4 agonist increases accumulation of both CD4$^+$ and CD8$^+$ T cells in the spleen of rAd-immunized mice. The mechanisms of adjuvant action of TLR3 and TLR4 agonists were studied in the model of reactivation of antigen-specific T cells in vitro. Adjuvant action of TLR4 agonists accumulates from the stimulation of rAd target antigen expression, up-regulation of co-activation molecules and production of pro-inflammatory cytokines by antigen-presenting cells. These changes have a complex positive effect on the induction of T-cell responses to the target antigen. Poly I:C is not as strong as TLR4 agonists in stimulating the expression of co-activation molecules and cytokines. It even suppressed the rAd target antigen expression in APCs at high adenovirus load. The adjuvant effect of Poly I:C could be mediated by an elevated level of IFN-β and CD40 molecules.

Methods

Antibodies and reagents

Agonist of Toll-like receptor 4 lipopolysaccharide from *E. coli* serotype 055: B5 (LPS, Sigma, L-2880), agonist of Toll-like receptor 4 Immunomax® (IMM, Immapharma), agonist of Toll-like receptor 3, a synthetic analog of double-stranded RNA, Poly Inosine: Poly Cytidine acid (Poly I:C, Invivogen), recombinant tumor necrosis factor α (TNF-α, Sigma, T7539), recombinant interferon-β1 (IFN-β, BioLegend, 581,302), Influenza H1 (A/California/04/2009) Hemagglutinin/HA Antibodies (Sino biological, 11,055-RM10), recombinant hemagglutinin of influenza virus H1 (Sino biological, 11,085-V084), dihydrochloride DAPI (Sigma), CellTrace™ Violet (Invitrigen, C34557) were used in this study.

Animals

Female 8–10 weeks old BALB/c mice were obtained from the Stolbovaya Nursery of the Russian Academy of Medical Science and fed standard rodent food under standard animal house conditions in the vivarium of the National Research Center Institute of Immunology FMBA of Russia. All handling and experimental procedures with animals were carried out in strict accordance with the rules of research work with laboratory animals of the Institute of Immunology of FMBA Russia (Order of November 12, 2015), certified by the Local Ethics Committee (Resolution 4/17 of July 13, 2017).

Forimmunization animals were treated with low (10^7 PFU/mouse) and high (10^8 PFU/mouse) doses of rAdTet-off H1. The low vaccine dose was administered alone or in combination with 10 μg LPS or 10 μg IMM or 5 μg Poly I:C.

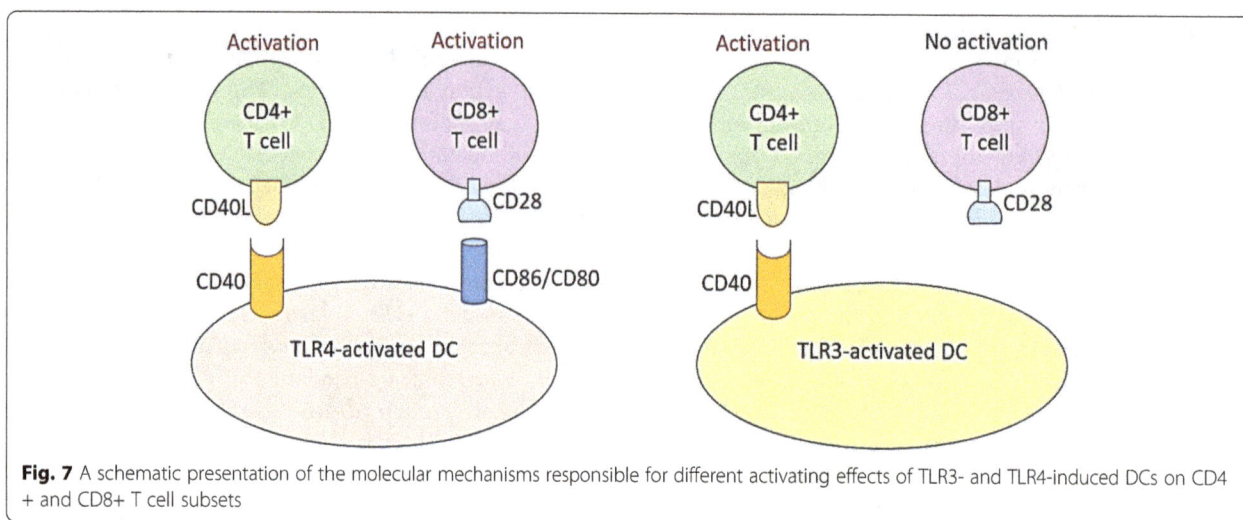

Fig. 7 A schematic presentation of the molecular mechanisms responsible for different activating effects of TLR3- and TLR4-induced DCs on CD4 + and CD8+ T cell subsets

Antigen-presenting cells

All cell cultures were incubated in a complete medium (CM) based on DMEM with 25 mM HEPES supplemented with a cocktail of nonessential amino acids, 10% fetal bovine serum (FBS, HyClone, Cat # SV30160.03 endotoxin level ≤ 10 EU/ml), 2 mM L- glutamine, 1 mM sodium pyruvate, and 10 μg/ml gentamycin at 37°C in a 5% CO_2 humidified atmosphere (all culture supplements were obtained from PanEco, Russia).

Bone marrow derived dendritic cells (DCs) were obtained in vitro by culturing bone marrow cells of BALB/c mice with a granulocyte-macrophage colony-stimulating factor (GM-CSF, BioLegend). Mice were euthanized in a CO2 chamber, and bone marrow was washed out from the femurs and the tibias, erythrocytes removed by osmotic shock, nuclear cells washed twice with PBS (Amresco, E404), followed by cultivation in a complete medium supplemented with 10 ng/ml GM-CSF (Sigma) for 7 days, media was changed at day 4. After 7 days of culture the non-adherent (dendritic cells) cells were gathered. Viability and purity were assayed with flow cytometry. Among viable cell (> 80% by DAPI staining) non-adherent population of cells were identified as 70% CD11b$^+$CD11c$^+$ dendritic cells (DCs).

Peritoneal macrophages were obtained by washing of the peritoneal cavity of euthanized BALB/c mice. The cells were pelleted by centrifugation, resuspended in CM, and cultured for 18–20 h at 37 °C in a humidified atmosphere of 5% CO2. Then non-adhesive cells were gently washed away with PBS. The remaining adherent cells comprised over 90% of macrophages assayed by flow cytometry analysis with F4/80 staining.

Constructing of the recombinant replication-defective adenovirus vector with a gene insert

In the study, we used GMP-grade rAds, which were produced in Federal Research Centre of Epidemiology and Microbiology named after N.F. Gamaleya.

Plasmid pShuttle-tet-off-tTA, carrying regulatory elements of the tet-off system, was obtained by cloning the required areas from plasmids pTet-off and pTRE-Tight (Tet-Off & Tet-On Gene Expression System, Clontech, USA) into plasmid pShuttle-CMV, using KpnI and EcoRV restriction endonucleases. Hemagglutinin H1 codon-optimized nucleotide sequence (synthesized by Evrogen JSC, Moscow, Russia) were cloned into the pShuttle-Tet-off-tTA plasmid. As a result, we got plasmid pShuttle-Tet-off-H1opt.

Nucleotide sequence of GFP gene was cloned into pShuttle CMV vector obtained from "The Ad-Easy Adenoviral Vector System (Stratagene, 240009)" according to manufacture's instruction. Also we used plasmid vectors pGreen (Carolina Biological Supply Company), p310D (pRcCMV-SEAP).

The Ad-Easy Adenoviral Vector System (Stratagene, 240,009) was used to construct rAd-GFP and rAd5-tet-H1opt, according to the manufacturer's instructions.

The GFP and H1 inserts in the corresponding constructs pShuttle-CMV-GFP, and pShuttle-Tet-off-H1 were verified by restriction analysis using EcoRI, NotI and EcoRV endonucleases and PCR. The presence of the genes *gfp* и *h1* in rAd was confirmed by PCR. rAds were grown in HEK-293 cells and chromatographically purified. The effective titer of the rAd-GFP and rAdTet-off H1 preparations was estimated using the plaque-forming assay in the HEK-293 cell culture.

The negative endotoxin content of rAds was demonstrated in LAL-test, InvivoGen HEK-Blue™ TLR4 reporter cell line assay and in the rabbit pyrogen test.

Transduction of cells with recombinant replication-defective adenovirus vectors

The cell cultures were transduced with rAd-GFP or rAdTet-off H1 at the dose of 3,5–350 PFU/cell in 150 μl of CM. The transduced cells were cultured in the presence or absence of LPS (0.1–10 µg/ml), Immunomax (1–10 µg/ml), Poly I:C (0.1–10 мкг/мл), TNF-α (1–30 ng/ml) or IFN-β (0.1–100 ng/ml).

CD4⁺ и CD8⁺ T-cell immune responses to H1 upon rAdTet-off H1immunization

Quantity and phenotype of hemagglutinin H1 specific T-cell were detected using the ELISPOT technique.

Immunised mice were euthanized in a CO2 chamber, suspension of cells from spleen of mice was separated at ficoll gradient (density 1.09 g/cm3) and mononuclear cells were gathered. Then mononuclear cells were treated with antibodies to CD4 (BioLegend, 100,412) and CD8 (BioLegend, 100,752). To obtain pure population of CD4+ and CD8+ T-cells we used flow cytometer FACSAria II. We excluded doubled events by FCS-A and FCS-H parameters. Dead cells were excluded by DAPI staining. Purity of sorted populations was approximately 90–95%. The purified populations of CD4⁺ and CD8⁺ T cells from the spleen ofimmunized mice were reactivated in vitro by culturing with antigen-presenting dendritic cells.

For restimulation of CD4+ T cells in vitro, we used dendritic cells that represent antigenic epitopes of the H1 in the context of MHC class II. For this purpose, dendritic cells were further activated with lipopolysaccharide from E. coli (1 µg/ml) and loaded with recombinant H1 protein (2 µg/ml). We also stimulated CD4⁺ T cells with dendritic cells transduced with rAdTet-off H1 (3.5–350 pfu per cell) to detect cross-presentation events. To restimulate CD8⁺ T cells in vitro, dendritic cells in which antigenic epitopes of the rAdTet-off H1 are present in the context of MHC class I were used. In this case, the dendritic cells were transduced with rAdTet-off H1 (3.5–350 PFU per cell).

ELISPOT

96-well plate for ELISPOT (mouse IFN-γ ELISPOT Kit, cat. 552,569, BD Biosciences) was loaded by 10,000 dendritic cells with 150 µl of complete culture medium per well. Antigen-presenting dendritic cells were transduced with rAdTet-off H1 (3.5–350 PFU per cell) or loaded with recombinant H1 protein (2 µg) and incubated overnight in the presence of 0.1–10 µg/ml of agonist of TLR3 or TLR4. On next day 50 µl of spleens cells suspension of interest – 100,000 CD4⁺ T-cells or 50,000 CD8⁺ T-cells, were added to each well. The plate was incubated for 23 h in CO₂-incubator strictly in the horizontal avoiding shaking. Then the plate was treated with accordance to manufacturer protocol (BD Biosciences). Wells of the plate were several times washed with distilled water and then 3 times with washer buffer (BD Biosciences). We added to each well 100 µl of detecting antibodies to IFN-γ and incubated them within 2 h at room temperature. Then we scoured them 4 times with washer buffer and added 100 µl/well streptavidin-peroxidase conjugate (BD

Biosciences), incubating within 1 h. After the incubation we elaborately scoured wells with washer buffer and then by PBS solution. Quickly added chromogenic substrate of 3-amino-9-ethylcarbazole (BD Biosciences), and incubated them within 15 min, after that elaborately washed them with distilled water, and left wells to dry at room temperature.

We took photo of each well using binocular microscope MBS-10 (magnification × 4) and digital camera Levenhuk DCM800 with 1280 × 960 pxls resolution. Quantification of spots with IFN-γ that had been formed by single cells in the wells of plate was done by using the software package ImageJ (National Institutes of Health, USA).

Measurement of production intensity of the GFP and H1 proteins encoded by rAd

Intracellular GFP accumulation was estimated by flow cytometry on FACS Aria II (BD Biosciences). Fluorescence was excited with the 488 nm laser, and emission intensity was measured between 515 and 545 nm.

Expression of membrane-bound H1 was examined by staining of cells with HA-specific primary and fluorochrome labeled secondary (Invitrogen, A-11034) antibodies, followed by flow cytometry by FACS Aria II.

Table 1 Nucleotide sequences of the primers used in the work

№	Gene Name	Primer name	5'-- > 3' sequence
1	gfp	EGFP-F	GACCACTACCAGCAGAACAC
		EGFP-R	CTTGTACAGCTCGTCCATGC
		EGFP-TP	FAM-AGCACCCAGTCCGCCCTGAGCA-RTQ
2	b-actin	β-actin-F	AGAGGGAAATCGTGCGTGAC
		β -actin-R	CAATAGTGATGACCTGGCCGT
		β -actin-TP	FAM-CACTGCCGCATCCTCTTCCTCCC-RTQ
3	gapdh	GAPDH-F	TTCACCACCATGGAGAAGGC
		GAPDH-R	GGCATGGACTGTGGTCATGA
		GAPDH-TP	FAM-TGCATCCTGCACCACCAACTGCTTAG-RTQ
4	tnfa	TNF-F	CATCTTCTCAAAATTCGAGTGACAA
		TNF-RV	TGGGAGTAGACAAGGTACAACCC
		TNF-TP	FAM-CACGTCGTAGCAAACCACCAAGTGGA-RTQ
5	H1	H1-F	CTGGATGGATTCTGGGCAAC
		H1-R	CAGGGTAGCATGTGCCGTTG
		H1-TP	FAM –TGTGAATCCCTGAGCACCGCCT-RTQ
6	ifnb	IFN-F	ACCACAGCCCTCTCCATC
		IFN-RV	GCATCTTCTCCGTCATCTCC
		IFN-TP	FAM-CAACCTCACCTACAGGGCGGAC-RTQ

Real-time PCR

Total RNA, DNA, and cDNA preparations were obtained using Sintol reagent kits (RNA-extran, S-sorb, RT reagent kit, respectively), following the manufacturer's instructions. The samples of purified total RNA were additionally treated with DNAse (Thermo Scientific, USA). RT-PCR was carried out by using primers which are shown in Table 1 following cycling on the DTprime-4 amplifier (DNA Technology Inc., Russia): 94 °C (5 min), 40 cycles at 94 °C (10 s) and 62 °C (20 s) and elongation at 72 °C for 5 s. The progress of cycling was monitored using FAM fluorescence. Expression of target mRNA was normalized to expression of β-actin or GAPDH mRNA using $2^{\wedge}\Delta\Delta Cp$ method.

Statistical analysis

Data are reported as means (M) ± standard deviation (SD). Statistical significance between groups was determined using the one-way ANOVA with Tukey post hoc comparison test or two-tailed unpaired t-test (p values < 0.05 were considered significant). All statistical parameters were calculated using GraphPad prism 5.0 Software.

Additional file

> **Additional file 1: Figure S1.** Effect of TLR agonists on the expression of rAd in DCs. DCs were transduced with rAdTet-off H1 (100 PFU per cell) in the presence of 10 μg/ml agonists of TLR3 (Poly I:C) or TLR4 (LPS, IMM); 24 h after transfection cells were stained with primary (H1-specific) and secondary fluorochrome labeled antibodies. The mean fluorescence (MFI) of H1-positive DCs in the test samples was detected by flow cytometry. Shown are M ± SD, statistically significant ($p < 0.05$) differences are indicated by asterisks. **Figure S2.** Effect of TLR3- and TLR4-activated APCs on the reactivation of CD4$^+$ and CD8$^+$ T-cells. Balb/c mice were immunized (i.m.) with 10^8 PFU rAdTet-off H1. Forty days after immunization, the pool of CD8$^+$ (**a, c**) and CD4$^+$ (**b, d**) T cells from the spleen of euthanized immune mice was re-activated in vitro. Sorted CD8$^+$ and CD4$^+$ T cells were co-cultured with bone marrow derived DCs (**c, d**) or macrophages (MF) (**a, b**) preloaded with 20 PFU/cell rAdTet-off H1 in the presence of 0–10 μg/ml agonists of TLR3 (Poly I:C) or TLR4 (LPS, IMM). The number of reactivated IFNγ-producing T-cells were detected by ELISPOT and calculated for 1 million spleen cells. Shown are M ± SD, statistically significant differences ($p < 0.05$) are indicated by asterisks. (PDF 123 kb)

Abbreviations

APCs: Antigen-presenting cells; BSA: Bovine serum albumin; DAPI: 4,6-diamidino-2-phenylindole; DCs: Dendritic cells; GAPDH: Glyceraldehyde 3-phosphate dehydrogenase; GFP: Green fluorescent protein; GM-CSF: Granulocyte-macrophage colony-stimulating factor; H1: Haemagglutinin of a human influenza virus H1 subtype; i.m.: Intramuscular injection; IMM: Immunomax; LPS: Lipopolysaccharide; M: Mean; MHC: Major histocompatibility complex; PBS: Phosphate-buffered saline; PFU: Plaque-forming unit; Poly I:C: Polyinosinic-polycytidylic acid; rAD: Recombinant adenovirus vector; SD: Standard deviation; TLR: Toll-like receptors

Funding

This work was supported by Russian Science Foundation Grant 15–15-00102.

Authors' contributions

EL: experimental work (design and optimization of each experimental stage), analysis and interpretation of data, drafting of the manuscript. AB: experimental work, interpretation of data, drafting of the manuscript. AP: experimental work (T cells sorting), interpretation of data. MC: primers design, RT-PCR results interpretation. AL + IT+MS + DL: experimental work (preparation of rAd constructs) and revising of the manuscript. BN: conception and design of rAd constructs, revising of the manuscript. RA: conception, design, revising of the manuscript. All authors read and approved the final manuscript.

Competing interests

The authors declare that they have no competing interests.

Author details

[1]National Research Center Institute of Immunology, Federal Medical-Biological Agency of Russia, Moscow, Russia. [2]Federal Research Centre of Epidemiology and Microbiology named after Honorary Academician N.F. Gamaleya, Ministry of Health, Moscow, Russia.

References

1. Coulie PG, Van den Eynde BJ, van der Bruggen P, Boon T. Tumour antigens recognized by T lymphocytes: at the core of cancer immunotherapy. Nat Rev Cancer. 2014;14:135–46.
2. Appay V, Douek DC, Price DA. CD8+ T cell efficacy in vaccination and disease. Nat Med. 2008;14:623–8.
3. Gilbert SC. T-cell-inducing vaccines - what's the future. Immunology. 2011;135:19–26.
4. Reed SG, Hsu FC, Carter D, Orr MT. The science of vaccine adjuvants: advances in TLR4 ligand adjuvants. Curr Opin Immunol. 2016;41:85–90.
5. Poteet E, Lewis P, Chen C, Ho SO, Do T, Chiang SM, et al. Toll-like receptor 3 adjuvant in combination with virus-like particles elicit a humoral response against HIV. Vaccine. 2016;34:5886–94.
6. Van Hoeven N, Joshi SW, Nana GI, Bosco-Lauth A, Fox C, Bowen RA, et al. A novel synthetic TLR-4 agonist adjuvant increases the protective response to a clinical-stage West Nile virus vaccine antigen in multiple formulations. PLoS One. 2016;11:e0149610.
7. Park H, Adamson L, Ha T, Mullen K, Hagen SI, Nogueron A, et al. Polyinosinic-polycytidylic acid is the most effective TLR adjuvant for SIV gag protein-induced T cell responses in nonhuman primates. J Immunol. 2013;190:4103–15.
8. Tsukasa S, Azuma M, Matsumoto M. Pattern recognition by dendritic cells and its application to vaccine adjuvant for antitumor immunotherapy. In: Immunother Cancer. Tokyo: Springer; 2016. p. 235–46.
9. Ngoi SM, Tovey MG, Vella AT. Targeting poly I:C to the TLR3-independent pathway boosts effector CD8 T cell differentiation through IFNα/β. J Immunol. 2009;181:7670–80.
10. Geurtsen J, Fransen F, Vandebriel RJ, Gremmer ER, de la Fonteyne-Blankestijn LJJ, Kuipers B, et al. Supplementation of whole-cell pertussis vaccines with lipopolysaccharide analogs: modification of vaccine-induced immune responses. Vaccine. 2008;26:899–906.
11. Quintilio W, Kubrusly FS, Iourtov D, Miyaki C, Sakauchi MA, Lúcio F, et al. Bordetella pertussis monophosphoryl lipid a as adjuvant for inactivated split virion influenza vaccine in mice. Vaccine. 2009;27:4219–24.
12. Salem ML, SA EL-N, Kadima A, Gillanders WE, Cole DJ. The adjuvant effects of the toll-like receptor 3 ligand polyinosinic-cytidylic acid poly (I:C) on antigen-specific CD8+ T cell responses are partially dependent on NK cells with the induction of a beneficial cytokine milieu. Vaccine. 2006;24:5119–32.
13. Zhu Q, Egelston C, Gagnon S, Sui Y, Belyakov IM, Klinman DM, et al. Using 3 TLR ligands as a combination adjuvant induces qualitative changes in T cell responses needed for antiviral protection in mice. J Clin Invest. 2010;120:607–16.
14. Afkhami S, Yao Y, Xing Z. Methods and clinical development of adenovirus-vectored vaccines against mucosal pathogens. Mol Ther Methods Clin Dev. 2016;3:16030.
15. Hollingdale MR, Sedegah M, Limbach K. Development of replication-deficient adenovirus malaria vaccines. Expert Rev Vaccines. 2016;16:261–71.

16. Shen CF, Jacob D, Zhu T, Bernier A, Shao Z, Yu X, et al. Optimization and scale-up of cell culture and purification processes for production of an adenovirus-vectored tuberculosis vaccine candidate. Vaccine. 2016;34:3381–7.

17. Hayes PJ, Cox JH, Coleman AR, Fernandez N, Bergin PJ, Kopycinski JT, et al. Adenovirus-based HIV-1 vaccine candidates tested in efficacy trials elicit CD8+ T cells with limited breadth of HIV-1 inhibition. AIDS. 2016;30:1703–12.

18. Li M, Jiang Y, Gong T, Zhang Z, Sun X. Intranasal vaccination against HIV-1 with adenoviral vector-based Nanocomplex using synthetic TLR-4 agonist peptide as adjuvant. Mol Pharm. 2016;13:885–94.

19. Appledorn DM, Aldhamen YA, DePas W, Seregin SS, Liu CJJ, Schuldt N, et al. A new adenovirus based vaccine vector expressing an Eimeria tenella derived TLR agonist improves cellular immune responses to an antigenic target. PLoS One. 2010;5:e9579.

20. Salucci V, Mennuni C, Calvaruso F, Cerino R, Neuner P, Ciliberto G, et al. CD8+ T-cell tolerance can be broken by an adenoviral vaccine while CD4+ T-cell tolerance is broken by additional co-administration of a toll-like receptor ligand. Scand J Immunol. 2006;63:35–41.

21. Peters W, Brandl JR, Lindbloom JD, Martinez CJ, Scallan CD, Trager GR, et al. Oral administration of an adenovirus vector encoding both an avian influenza a hemagglutinin and a TLR3 ligand induces antigen specific granzyme B and IFN-γ T cell responses in humans. Vaccine. 2013;31:1752–8.

22. Scallan CD, Tingley DW, Lindbloom JD, Toomey JS, Tucker SN. An adenovirus-based vaccine with a double-stranded RNA adjuvant protects mice and ferrets against H5N1 avian influenza in oral delivery models. Clin Vaccine Immunol. 2013;20:85–94.

23. Appledorn DM, Aldhamen YA, Godbehere S, Seregin SS, Amalfitano A. Sublingual administration of an adenovirus serotype 5 (Ad5)-based vaccine confirms toll-like receptor agonist activity in the oral cavity and elicits improved mucosal and systemic cell-mediated responses against HIV antigens despite preexisting Ad5 immuni. Clin Vaccine Immunol. 2011;18:150–60.

24. Hofmeyer KA, Duthie MS, Laurance JD, Favila MA, Van Hoeven N, Coler RN, et al. Optimizing immunization strategies for the induction of antigen-specific CD4 and CD8 T cell responses for protection against intracellular parasites. Clin Vaccine Immunol. 2016;23:785–94.

25. Rhee EG, Blattman JN, Kasturi SP, Kelley RP, Kaufman DR, Lynch DM, et al. Multiple innate immune pathways contribute to the immunogenicity of recombinant adenovirus vaccine vectors. J Virol. 2011;85:315–23.

26. Rhee EG, Kelley RP, Agarwal I, Lynch DM, La Porte A, Simmons NL, et al. TLR4 ligands augment antigen-specific CD8+ T lymphocyte responses elicited by a viral vaccine vector. J Virol. 2010;84:10413–9.

27. Quinn KM, Zak DE, Costa A, Yamamoto A, Kastenmuller K, Hill BJ, et al. Antigen expression determines adenoviral vaccine potency independent of IFN and STING signaling. J Clin Invest. 2015;125:1129–46.

28. Tsuzuki S, Tachibana M, Hemmi M, Yamaguchi T, Shoji M, Sakurai F, et al. TANK-binding kinase 1-dependent or -independent signaling elicits the cell-type-specific innate immune responses induced by the adenovirus vector. Int Immunol. 2016;28:105–15.

29. Bagaev AV, Pichugin AV, Lebedeva ES, Lysenko AA, Shmarov MM, Logunov DY, et al. Regulation of the target protein (transgene) expression in the adenovirus vector using agonists of toll-like receptors. Acta Nat. 2014;6:27–39.

30. Clarke SR. The critical role of CD40/CD40L in the CD4-dependent generation of CD8+ T cell immunity. J Leukoc Biol. 2000;67:607–14.

31. Curtsinger JM, Lins DC, Mescher MF. Signal 3 determines tolerance versus full activation of naive CD8 T cells: dissociating proliferation and development of effector function. J Exp Med. 2003;197:1141–51.

32. Curtsinger JM, Schmidt CS, Mondino A, Lins DC, Kedl RM, Jenkins MK, et al. Inflammatory cytokines provide a third signal for activation of naive CD4+ and CD8+ T cells. J Immunol. 1999;162:3256–62.

33. Huber JP, David FJ. Regulation of effector and memory T-cell functions by type I interferon. Immunology. 2011;132:466–74.

34. Welsh RM, Bahl K, Marshall HD, Urban SL. Type 1 interferons and antiviral CD8 T-cell responses. PLoS Pathog. 2012;8:e1002352.

35. Chowdhury FZ, Ramos HJ, Davis LS, Forman J, Farrar JD. IL-12 selectively programs effector pathways that are stably expressed in human CD8 + effector memory T cells in vivo. Blood. 2011;118:3890–900.

36. Mescher MF, Curtsinger JM, Agarwal P, Casey KA, Gerner M, Hammerbeck CD, et al. Signals required for programming effector and memory development by CD8+ T cells. Immunol Rev. 2006;211:81–92.

37. Hsu H, Xiong J, Goeddel DV. The TNF receptor 1-associated protein TRADD signals cell death and NF-κB activation. Cell. 1995;81:495–504.

38. Sadler AJ, Bryan RG. Williams. Interferon-inducible antiviral effectors. Nat Rev Immunol. 2009;8:559–68.

39. Karan D, Krieg AM, Lubaroff DM. Paradoxical enhancement of CD8 T cell-dependent anti-tumor protection despite reduced CD8 T cell responses with addition of a TLR9 agonist to a tumor vaccine. Int J Cancer. 2007;121:1520–8.

40. Brown THT, David J, Acosta-Ramirez E, Moore JM, Lee S, Zhong G, et al. Comparison of immune responses and protective efficacy of intranasal prime-boost immunization regimens using adenovirus-based and CpG/HH2 adjuvanted-subunit vaccines against genital chlamydia muridarum infection. Vaccine. 2012;30:350–60.

41. Diaz-San Segundo F, Dias CC, Moraes MP, Weiss M, Perez-Martin E, Salazar AM, et al. Poly ICLC increases the potency of a replication-defective human adenovirus vectored foot-and-mouth disease vaccine. Virology. 2014;468:283–92.

42. Chuai X, Chen H, Wang W, Deng Y, Wen B, Ruan L, et al. Poly(I:C)/alum mixed adjuvant priming enhances HBV subunit vaccine-induced immunity in mice when combined with recombinant adenoviral-based HBV vaccine boosting. PLoS One. 2013;8:e54126.

43. Wen Y-M, Wang Y-X. Biological features of hepatitis B virus isolates from patients based on full-length genomic analysis. Rev Med Virol. 2009;19:57–64.

44. Medzhitov R, Janeway C. The toll receptor family and microbial recognition. Trends Microbiol. 2000;8:452–6.

45. Ataullakhonov RI, Pichugin AV, Melnikova TM, Khaitov RM. Method of producing a substance with antimicrobial, antiviral, and immunostimulatory activities, a substance and a composition. In: Patents.com. 2015. http://patents.com/us-20160263175.html. Accessed 5 Jul 2018.

46. Bagaev A, Pichugin A, Nelson EL, Agadjanyan MG, Ghochikyan A, Ataullakhanov RI. Anticancer mechanisms in two murine bone marrow–derived dendritic cell subsets activated with TLR4 agonists. J Immunol. 2018;200:2656–69.

47. Ghochikyan A, Pichugin A, Bagaev A, Davtyan A, Hovakimyan A, Tukhvatulin A, et al. Targeting TLR-4 with a novel pharmaceutical grade plant derived agonist, Immunomax, as a therapeutic strategy for metastatic breast cancer. J Transl Med. 2014;12:1–12.

48. Provine NM, Larocca RA, Penaloza-MacMaster P, Borducchi EN, McNally A, Parenteau LR, et al. Longitudinal requirement for CD4+ T cell help for adenovirus vector-elicited CD8+ T cell responses. J Immunol. 2014;192:5214–25.

49. Provine NM, Badamchi-Zadeh A, Bricault CA, Penaloza-MacMaster P, Larocca RA, Borducchi EN, et al. Transient CD4 + T cell depletion results in the delayed development of functional vaccine-elicited antibody responses. J Virol. 2016;90:4278–88.

50. Hu W, Jain A, Gao Y, Dozmorov IM, Mandraju R, Wakeland EK, et al. Differential outcome of TRIF-mediated signaling in TLR4 and TLR3 induced DC maturation. Proc Natl Acad Sci. 2015;112:13994–9.

51. Elgueta R, Benso MJ, de Vries VS, Wasiuk A, Guo Y, Noelle RJ. Molecular mechanism and function of CD40/CD40L engagement in the immune system. Immunol Rev. 2013;229:152–72.

16

An optimized IFN-γ ELISpot assay for the sensitive and standardized monitoring of CMV protein-reactive effector cells of cell-mediated immunity

Sascha Barabas[1], Theresa Spindler[1], Richard Kiener[2], Charlotte Tonar[1], Tamara Lugner[1], Julia Batzilla[1], Hanna Bendfeldt[1], Anne Rascle[1], Benedikt Asbach[2], Ralf Wagner[2] and Ludwig Deml[1,2]*

Abstract

Background: In healthy individuals, Cytomegalovirus (CMV) infection is efficiently controlled by CMV-specific cell-mediated immunity (CMI). Functional impairment of CMI in immunocompromized individuals however can lead to uncontrolled CMV replication and severe clinical complications. Close monitoring of CMV-specific CMI is therefore clinically relevant and might allow a reliable prognosis of CMV disease as well as assist personalized therapeutic decisions.

Methods: Objective of this work was the optimization and technical validation of an IFN-γ ELISpot assay for a standardized, sensitive and reliable quantification of CMV-reactive effector cells. T-activated® immunodominant CMV IE-1 and pp65 proteins were used as stimulants. All basic assay parameters and reagents were tested and optimized to establish a user-friendly protocol and maximize the signal-to-noise ratio of the ELISpot assay.

Results: Optimized and standardized ELISpot revealed low intra-assay, inter-assay and inter-operator variability (coefficient of variation CV below 22%) and CV inter-site was lower than 40%. Good assay linearity was obtained between 6×10^4 and 2×10^5 PBMC per well upon stimulation with T-activated® IE-1 ($R^2 = 0.97$) and pp65 ($R^2 = 0.99$) antigens. Remarkably, stimulation of peripheral blood mononuclear cells (PBMC) with T-activated® IE-1 and pp65 proteins resulted in the activation of a broad range of CMV-reactive effector cells, including CD3+CD4+ (Th), CD3+CD8+ (CTL), CD3−CD56+ (NK) and CD3+CD56+ (NKT-like) cells. Accordingly, the optimized IFN-γ ELISpot assay revealed very high sensitivity (97%) in a cohort of 45 healthy donors, of which 32 were CMV IgG-seropositive.

Conclusion: The combined use of T-activated® IE-1 and pp65 proteins for the stimulation of PBMC with the optimized IFN-γ ELISpot assay represents a highly standardized, valuable tool to monitor the functionality of CMV-specific CMI with great sensitivity and reliability.

Keywords: Cytomegalovirus, CMV, IE-1, pp65, Cell-mediated immunity, ELISpot, CD4+, CD8+, T helper (Th), Cytotoxic T lymphocyte (CTL), Natural killer (NK), NKT-like

* Correspondence: Ludwig.Deml@lophius.com
[1]Lophius Biosciences GmbH, Am BioPark 13, 93053 Regensburg, Germany
[2]Institute of Medical Microbiology and Hygiene, University Regensburg,
Franz-Josef-Strauss-Allee 11, 93053 Regensburg, Germany

Background

Human cytomegalovirus (CMV) is endemic in all human populations, with a seroprevalence ranging from 36 to 100% depending on age, gender and location [1]. In healthy individuals, CMV replication is efficiently controlled by cell-mediated immunity (CMI). In immunocompromised individuals however, the reduced frequency and functionality of CMV-reactive effector cells is associated with severe clinical complications due to uncontrolled virus replication [1–3]. Quantitative assessment of functional CMV-reactive effector cells in immunocompromized individuals might help to identify patients at increased risk for CMV-mediated clinical complications and to adjust antiviral and immunosuppressive therapy [3, 4].

Reliable monitoring of CMV-specific CMI in immunocompromised individuals, such as solid-organ or allogeneic stem cell transplant recipients, requires a specific, standardized but also highly sensitive assay capable of detecting low numbers of CMV-reactive cells. Such sensitivity might be achieved by using highly immunogenic stimulants and via the reactivation of a broad spectrum of physiological effector cells involved in the protection against CMV replication in vivo, notably CD4$^+$ (T helper or Th), CD8$^+$ (cytotoxic T lymphocytes or CTL), but also natural killer (NK) and natural killer T (NKT) cells [5–12].

Current diagnostic methods to detect and monitor CMV-specific CMI are mostly based on the restimulation of CD4$^+$ and/or CD8$^+$ effector cells with pools of overlapping peptides, cocktails of preselected immunodominant CMV-peptides or lysates of CMV-infected cells and the subsequent measurement of induced cytokine production (e.g. IFN-γ) or cell proliferation, by flow cytometry, enzyme-linked immunosorbent assay (ELISA) or enzyme-linked immunospot assay (ELISpot). A different approach consists in the direct staining with CMV-peptide-loaded multimers and enumeration of CMV-specific CD8$^+$ T cells by flow cytometry. However, this method is lacking a functional readout and is restricted to certain HLA types, impeding its use in routine diagnostics.

ELISA-based assays, such as QuantiFERON®-CMV are advantageous in that they require low blood volumes and are easy to perform [13]. However, they are restricted to the detection of IFN-γ-producing CD8$^+$ T cells and do not allow single-cell-level measurement. Due to analyte dilution, ELISA-based assays usually result in reduced sensitivity [14, 15] and often yield indeterminate results, especially in immunocompromised patients [16–21]. Intracellular cytokine staining (ICS) and subsequent flow cytometric analysis is usually more sensitive than ELISA [15, 20] and allows the assessment of both the functionality and the phenotype of CMV-reactivated cytokine-producing cells. However, this method is difficult to standardize and only detects the intracellular analyte, not the biologically active cytokine secreted over the stimulation period.

ELISpot-based assays identify and enumerate biologically active, cytokine-secreting cells from isolated peripheral blood mononuclear cells (PBMC), at the single-cell level both qualitatively and quantitatively [22]. ELISpot represents the most sensitive read-out system and thus is most appropriate for the detection of low-level responses [23, 24]. In particular, ELISpot is more sensitive than ICS for the detection of antigen-specific cells, such as in vitro-reactivated memory T cells, which produce only low amounts of cytokines [15, 25]. ELISpot was recently successfully employed over ELISA in the detection of congenital CMV infection [26–28].

Conventional CMV-specific ELISpot assays are based on the detection of IFN-γ-producing CD4$^+$ and/or CD8$^+$ T cells, depending on the antigens used for PBMC stimulation [23, 24, 29, 30]. The careful selection and formulation of antigens is crucial to ensure specificity, sensitivity and thus a diagnostic value to the assay. We have previously shown that urea-formulated recombinant (T-activated®) proteins are processed by the exogenous and endogenous antigen processing machinery, resulting in the presentation of naturally generated peptides by MHC class II and class I molecules [31]. Stimulation of PBMC by T-activated® proteins thus mimics more closely a natural infection, resulting not only in the specific activation of memory T (CD4$^+$, CD8$^+$) and NK cells, but also possibly in the bystander activation of NK and NKT-like cells present in the PBMC population [31, 32].

We describe here the establishment, optimization and standardization of a highly sensitive ELISpot assay that takes advantage of both the IFN-γ ELISpot readout and the immunodominant and highly immunogenic T-activated® IE-1 and pp65 CMV proteins as stimulants. We also compared the performance of the optimized assay to that of intracellular staining and flow cytometry in healthy CMV-seropositive donors, and demonstrated the ability of T-activated® IE-1 and pp65 antigens to activate a broad spectrum of CMV-reactive cells, including CD3$^+$CD4$^+$ (Th), CD3$^+$CD8$^+$ (CTL), CD3$^-$CD56$^+$ (NK) and CD3$^+$CD56$^+$ (NKT-like) cells. Therefore, the combined use of T-activated® IE-1 and pp65 CMV proteins with our optimized IFN-γ ELISpot defines a highly sensitive assay meeting all conditions for a reliable and standardized immune monitoring diagnostic tool.

Methods

Proteins, ELISpot plate precoating and detection conjugate

Urea-formulated T-activated® proteins were prepared as previously described [31]. The T-activated® immunodominant region of CMV pp65 (amino acids 366 to 546, hCMV strain AD169 [33]) was provided by MIKROGEN (MIKROGEN GmbH, Neuried, Germany). Full length IE-1 (hCMV towne strain) was kindly provided by Christina Paulus and Michael Nevels (University of Regensburg, Germany). T-activation® of IE-1 was performed by Lophius Biosciences. Staphylococcal enterotoxin B (SEB; 11249738001, Roche Diagnostics GmbH, Mannheim, Germany) and phytohemagglutinin (PHA; S4881, Sigma-Aldrich Chemie GmbH, Munich, Germany) were used as positive controls for PBMC stimulation. 96-well ELISpot plates (MAIPS4510, Merck Millipore, Merck KGaA, Darmstadt, Germany) and 8-well ELISpot strips (M8IPS4510, Merck Millipore) each pre-coated with anti-human-IFN-γ mAb 1-D1K (MabTech, Nacka Strand, Sweden) as well as the detection conjugate mAb-AP (7-B6-1) (MabTech, Nacka Strand, Sweden) coupled with alkaline phosphatase (Roche, Basel, Switzerland) were obtained from Microcoat Biotechnologie GmbH.

Blood collection and PBMC preparation

Blood samples were collected in lithium heparin tubes (S-Monovette®, Sarstedt, SARSTEDT AG & Co., Nümbrecht, Germany) from healthy individuals with known CMV serostatus by venipuncture and stored for up to 8 hours at room temperature (18-25 °C) until further processing. Isolation of peripheral blood mononuclear cells (PBMC) was performed using standard Ficoll-Paque density centrifugation as specified by the manufacturer (Pancoll human, PAN-Biotech GmbH, Aidenbach, Germany). PBMC were finally suspended in serum-free AIM-V® medium (Life Technologies, Inc., Grand Island, NY) and counted either manually in a Neubauer's chamber or using the Hem-o-test 2000 cell-counting device (BGT BioGenTechnologies GmbH, Steinfurt, Germany). Automated cell counting was performed in the whole blood venous mode of the calibrated analyzer.

ELISpot assay

IFN-γ ELISpot assays were performed as previously described [31] unless specified otherwise in the Results section. Briefly, 2×10^5 freshly isolated PBMC were plated in four replicates into 96-well ELISpot plates or 8-well ELISpot strips precoated with anti-human-IFN-γ mAb 1-D1K (Microcoat Biotechnologie GmbH) and stimulated for 19 h at 37 °C under 5% CO_2 with either 3 μg/ml T-activated® pp65 antigen or 15 μg/ml T-activated® IE-1 protein. As unstimulated control (neg.), cells were incubated for 19 h in cell culture medium. After cell removal, plates were developed for 2 h at room temperature (18-25 °C) in the presence of 0.4 U/ml IFN-γ-specific alkaline phosphatase-coupled mAb 7-B6-1. Spot detection was performed following incubation for 6 min in the dark with a 1-step nitroblue

tetrazolium–5-bromo-4-chloro-3-indolylphosphate substrate (Thermo Fischer Scientific, Waltham, USA). IFN-γ-specific spot-forming cells (SFC) were counted using a Bioreader® 5000 Eα (BIO-SYS GmbH, Karben, Germany). Of note, comparable results were obtained on two other readers (AID Elispot Robotic System ELROB05i and CTL ImmunoSpot® S6).

Intracellular cytokine staining

Intracellular cytokine staining was performed as previously described [31], with the following modifications. PBMC from six healthy CMV-seropositive donors were isolated and four replicates each were stimulated for 6 h at 37 °C and 5% CO_2 with 3 μg/ml T-activated® pp65 antigen or with 15 μg/ml T-activated® IE-1 protein in the presence of co-stimulatory anti-CD28 and anti-CD49d monoclonal antibodies (BD, Heidelberg, Germany). The unstimulated PBMC control cells were incubated with co-stimulatory anti-CD28 and anti-CD49d molecules only. Stimulation with SEB and anti-CD28 + anti-CD49d served as positive control. After the first two hours of incubation, 1 μg/ml brefeldin A (BFA, Sigma-Aldrich Chemie GmbH, Steinheim, Germany) was added to prevent cytokine secretion from activated cells. Surface markers (CD3, CD4, CD8, CD56) were stained for 30 min at 4 °C using the following conjugated antibodies (all from Biolegend, London, UK): anti-CD3 APC-Cy7, anti-CD4 Brilliant Violet 421, anti-CD8 FITC, anti-CD56 PerCP. Cells were fixed and permeabilized for 30 min at 4 °C in BD Cytofix/Cytoperm (BD, Heidelberg, Germany). Intracellular staining of IFN-γ was performed using anti-IFN-γ APC (Biolegend, London, UK) in BD Perm/Wash Buffer (BD, Heidelberg, Germany) for 45 min at 4 °C. Samples were analyzed on a BD FACS-Canto™ II flow cytometer (Becton Dickinson, USA). Live-gating of cells was performed during acquisition. Mean (SD) number of event acquisition was 172,904 (108,298). Results were reported as percentage of the gated population producing IFN-γ (dot plots) and as the number of IFN-γ⁺ cells/200,000 lymphocytes (bar graphs).

Serology

The CMV serological testing of blood donors was performed using the fully automated CMV immunoglobulin M (IgM) and IgG tests on the Architect instrument (Abbott Laboratories, Abbott Park, IL) or the BEP® III system (Siemens Healthcare) by the diagnostics department of the Institute for Medical Microbiology and Hygiene (University of Regensburg, Germany). CMV IgG-serology was used as primary reference measurement procedure (gold standard method).

Statistics

Statistics applied to assay development was performed using SigmaPlot Version 11.0 and GraphPad Prism 5.04. At the start of this study, a positive ELISpot test result was defined by a statistically significant difference between quadruplicate SFC values of non-stimulated and specifically stimulated approaches of at least one of the two antigens used, calculated using the Mann–Whitney U-Test (MWU) (SigmaPlot). Two-sided exact P values are reported. P values < 0.05 were considered statistically significant. Statistical analyses to assess variations between two or more settings were performed by generating arithmetic means for all replicates of each given setting. Those means were grouped to generate an overall arithmetic mean and standard deviation. The coefficient of variation in % (ratio of the standard deviation to the mean multiplied by 100) was calculated in Microsoft Excel. The curve fitting for sigmoidal curves of the titration experiment (Fig. 1) was performed using the four parameter logistic function of GraphPad Prism 5.04. For the assessment of the ELISpot assay sensitivity in seropositive healthy blood donor collectives, the non-parametric Mann–Whitney U-Test (MWU test) was performed to determine if a significant difference exists between the groups of negative control and stimulation quadruplicates. Multiple-group comparisons were performed using a non-parametric One-way ANOVA (Kruskal-Wallis test) with Dunn's multiple comparison post test. SFC values were depicted using GraphPad Prism 5.04 either as Tukey box plots showing median values (horizontal line), interquartile ranges (IQR: Q3-Q1), lower and upper whiskers (Q1-1.5xIQR and Q3 + 1.5xIQR

respectively) and outliers (below Q1-1.5xIQR and above Q3 + 1.5xIQR; black dots), or as histograms. For assay validation of optimized ELISpot, positivity cut-off was calculated on IFN-γ ELISpot results obtained from a collective of 45 healthy donors using SAS 9.2 Software and VFP (Variance Function Program; option "Simple variance function estimate") version 12.0.

Results

IFN-γ ELISpot assay optimization following PBMC stimulation with T-activated® IE-1 and pp65 CMV antigens

Freshly isolated PBMC were used for the ELISpot assay. To prevent loss in T cell functionality, for instance due to activated granulocytes [34], heparinized blood samples were processed with no further additives within 8 h. A total number of 2×10^5 PBMC per well was chosen for the development of the ELISpot assay protocol as this cell count is below confluency and can usually be obtained from samples of less than 15 ml whole blood. The CMV immediate-early protein IE-1 and the late tegument protein pp65 represent well-characterized immunodominant T cell antigens [1, 24, 35]. Full-length IE-1 and a 181 amino-acid C-terminal fragment of pp65 were produced and formulated in the presence of urea (T-activation®) to increase their stimulatory capacity for different types of CMV-reactive effector cells of cell-mediated immunity [31]. Optimal T-activated® antigen concentration was first determined by performing dose–response experiments. Freshly isolated PBMC of one healthy CMV-seropositive donor were stimulated with 31.6 fg/ml to 31.6 µg/ml T-activated® pp65 or with 0.01 to 31.6 µg/ml T-activated® IE-1, and the number of IFN-γ secreting cells was determined by IFN-γ ELISpot. T-activated® pp65 revealed a much stronger capacity to stimulate IFN-γ secreting effector cells than T-activated® IE-1, reaching a plateau of responsiveness between 0.316 and 3.16 ng/ml pp65 vs. approximately 31.6 µg/ml for IE-1 (Fig. 1). Accordingly, T-activated® antigen concentrations of 3 µg/ml pp65 and 15 µg/ml IE-1 were selected for further PBMC stimulations and ELISpot assays.

Assay sensitivity and specificity were determined by stimulating PBMC isolated from 10 each CMV-seropositive and CMV-seronegative healthy donors with the defined pp65 and IE-1 T-activated® antigen concentrations. The number of reactive effector cells was quantified by IFN-γ ELISpot. Significant stimulation was defined using a Mann–Whitney U-Test as a statistically significant difference between SFC values of non-stimulated and CMV antigen-stimulated conditions (each in quadruplicate). T-activated® pp65 and IE-1 induced a significant activation of responsive effector cells in 10 out of 10 and 9 out of 10 PBMC preparations from individual CMV-seropositive donors, respectively (Fig. 2).

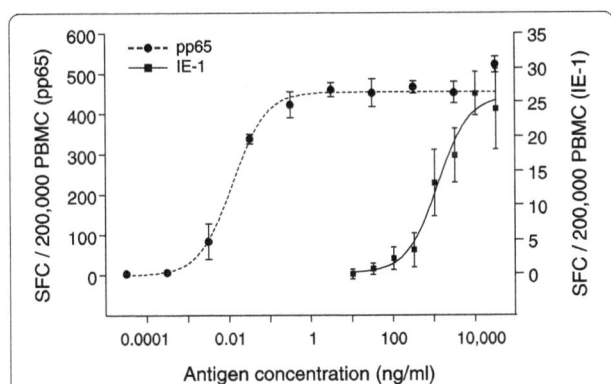

Fig. 1 Determination of optimal concentrations of T-activated® pp65 and IE-1 for the stimulation of PBMC. PBMC were isolated from one CMV-seropositive healthy donor blood sample and stimulated for 19 h with increasing concentrations of T-activated® pp65 (31.6 fg/ml-31.6 µg/ml; black circles) or IE-1 (0.01-31.6 µg/ml; black squares). IFN-γ ELISpot results of four replicates are expressed as mean SFC/200,000 PBMC. Error bars represent standard deviations. The Y-axis scale was adjusted to pp65- (left) and IE-1- (right) specific values to optimize data resolution. Curve fitting was made using the four parameter logistic function of GraphPad Prism 5.04

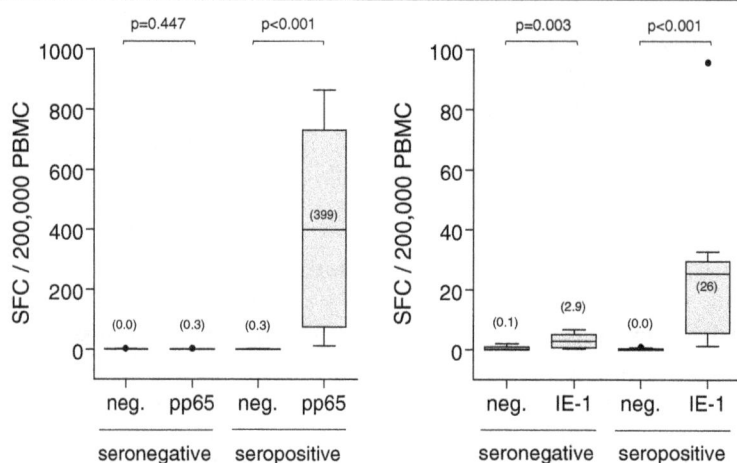

Fig. 2 Determination of assay sensitivity and specificity. PBMC from 10 each CMV-seropositive and CMV-negative healthy blood donors were left unstimulated (neg.) or were stimulated with T-activated® pp65 or IE-1 and IFN-γ ELISpot assays were conducted as before. Mean SFC values per 200,000 PBMC of 4 replicates are shown as box plots. Median values (horizontal black lines) are indicated in brackets. Y-axis scales were adjusted in each graph for better resolution of SFC counts. Median age and range of CMV-seronegative and CMV-seropositive subjects was 28 (24–53) and 31 (23–56) years. Gender distribution in CMV-seronegative (30% male and 70% female) and CMV-seropositive (25% male and 75% female) groups was comparable. Differences between unstimulated and stimulated conditions were tested using the non-parametric two-sided Mann–Whitney U (MWU) test. P-values < 0.05 were considered statistically significant

In this collective, T-activated® pp65 showed an overall greater capacity to activate responsive cells with a median of 399 SFC/200,000 PBMC (range 12–864 SFC/200,000 PBMC), compared to T-activated® IE-1 with a median of 26 SFC/200,000 PBMC (range 1.3-96 SFC/200,000 PBMC). Nevertheless, substantial response of up to 96 SFC/200,000 PBMC was detected in response to T-activated® IE-1 in individual samples of CMV-seropositive donors (Fig. 2). All 10 PBMC samples (100%) from different CMV-seronegative donors showed negative test results after stimulation with pp65 (median 0.3 SFC/200,000 PBMC; range 0–2.8), while 9 out of 10 (90%) PBMC samples from CMV-seronegative individuals were negative after stimulation with IE-1 (median 2.9 SFC/200,000 PBMC; range 0.3-6.8). Spot count within CMV-seronegative IE-1-stimulated PBMC was higher than in CMV-seronegative pp65-stimulated PBMC but did not exceed 7 SFC/200,000 PBMC (Fig. 2).

IFN-γ has been shown to be secreted continuously during antigen stimulation. Thus, signal intensity in IFN-γ ELISpot is dependent on the duration of stimulation [14, 36]. The duration of antigen stimulation in IFN-γ ELISpot reported in the literature usually ranges from 16 to 24 h [37–42]. To address the influence of the incubation time on the test results, IFN-γ ELISpot were performed on PBMC from 3 independent CMV-seropositive healthy donors following stimulation with T-activated® pp65 and IE-1 antigens for 17, 19 and 21 h. No statistically significant differences in SFC numbers were detected between the 3 conditions (Fig. 3), demonstrating signal stability in this time range. Thus, an

incubation time of 19 h was chosen for the optimized ELISpot assay.

Numerous protocol variables can affect ELISpot test results. For instance, the medium used for primary cell culture often includes serum which contains various batch-dependent non-characterized bioactive molecules in different concentrations [43]. In order to define standardized cell culture conditions, the impact on the assay performance of different serum-containing media (RPMI 1640 supplemented with 5% of either FCS, human AB, synthetic NTA or synthetic NTS) and of serum-free media (AIM-V®, UltraCulture) was investigated. Serum-free media yielded the best effector cell responses, comparable to that of RPMI 1640 supplemented with 5% FCS (Fig. 4a). In addition, AIM-V® exhibited lowest background signals in unstimulated conditions (Fig. 4b), thus maximizing signal-to-noise ratio. Consequently, the ELISpot protocol was further established using AIM-V® serum-free medium.

ELISpot assays can be performed with various membrane materials, including nitrocellulose (NC), mixed cellulose ester (MCE) and polyvinylidene fluoride (PVDF). We compared IFN-γ ELISpot results from PBMC samples of six healthy individuals (four replicates each, two preparations per donor) employing the most commonly used MCE plates, PVDF plates and PVDF strips from Millipore (Merck Millipore, Merck KGaA, Darmstadt, Germany). PVDF membranes require an activation step with ethanol prior to binding of the capture antibody. In addition, more stringent washing steps prior to spot development were needed using PVDF-based

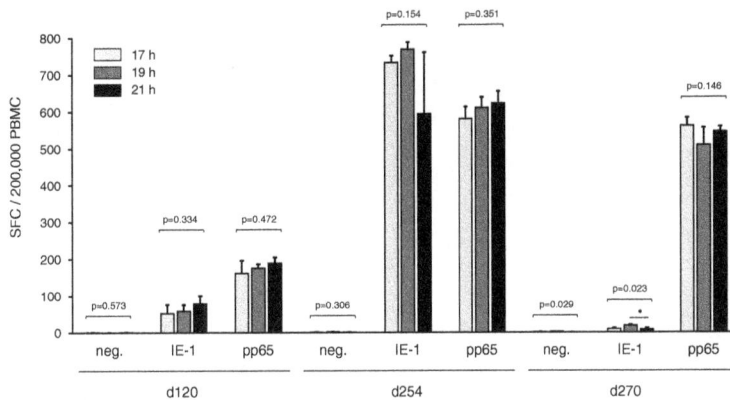

Fig. 3 Effect of duration of antigen stimulation on IFN-γ ELISpot test results. SFC counts (means of four replicates) in IFN-γ ELISpot following stimulation of PBMC samples from three CMV-seropositive healthy donors (d120, 32-year-old male; d254, 62-year-old female; d270, 22-year-old female) with T-activated® IE-1 or pp65 for 17, 19 and 21 h. Unstimulated PBMC (neg.) were used as a negative control. Differences between stimulation durations were tested using the non-parametric two-sided One-way ANOVA Kruskal-Wallis test (*$P < 0.05$). P-values < 0.05 were considered statistically significant

plates compared to MCE plates, to avoid undesirable background staining of membranes. Nevertheless, the resolution of the detected spots in terms of sharpness and homogeneity was improved on PVDF membranes (not shown), resulting in higher spot counts compared to MCE membranes (up to 10-times more in the case of IE-1 stimulations, with a median SFC of 155 vs. 13/ 200,000 PBMC, respectively; Fig. 5). Since PVDF 8-well strips were more performant and because their use might allow reduced costs, in particular when single patient samples are tested in clinical routine, the PVDF 8-well-strip format was chosen for the optimized assay development.

Optimal coating of microtiter plates with capture antibody is crucial for a robust assay performance. The density of IFN-γ capture antibody bound to the PVDF membrane should not be limiting and, in particular, should allow the reliable detection of high spot counts. PVDF strips were coated with increasing concentrations (2.5 to 7.5 µg/ml) of anti-IFN-γ antibody. PBMC from five CMV-seropositive donors were seeded into the coated wells and either left unstimulated or stimulated with T-activated® IE-1 or pp65. In the range of 2.5 to 7.5 µg/ml, increasing antibody concentrations had no effect on background staining in unstimulated PBMC (median SFC of 0 to 0.5/200,000 PBMC regardless of IFN-γ capture antibody concentration; Figs. 6a-b). Similarly, IE-1-specific low-to-moderate SFC levels (medians of 19 to 26 SFC/200,000 PBMC) were comparable in all coating-antibody conditions (Fig. 6a). The same was true for pp65-specific responses up to ~300 SFC/ 200,000 PBMC (donors d032, d120 and d241; Fig. 6c).

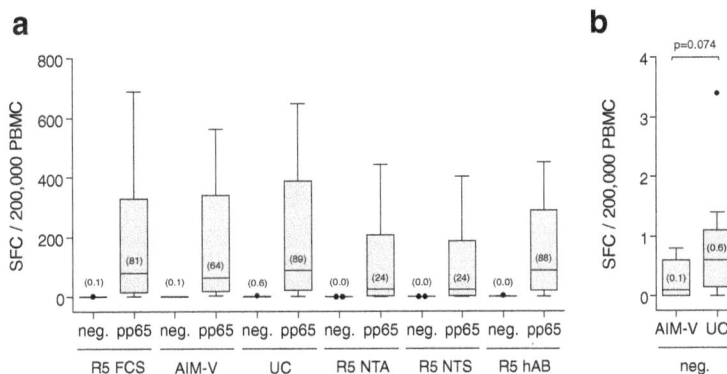

Fig. 4 Evaluation of different cell culture media on the performance of IFN-γ ELISpot. **a** Boxplot diagram showing ELISpot results upon stimulation of PBMC of 10 CMV-seropositive healthy blood donors (median age and range of 31 (26–54) years; 40% male and 60% female) with T-activated® pp65 in various cell culture media. Median values (horizontal black lines) are indicated in brackets. Differences between medium conditions among stimulated conditions were tested using the non-parametric two-sided One-way ANOVA Kruskal-Wallis test (p = 0.613). **b** ELISpot results of the non-stimulated cells incubated in AIM-V or in UltraCulture (UC) serum-free media are shown separately with an expanded Y-axis scale. Differences between both conditions were tested using the non-parametric two-sided MWU test (p = 0.074). P-values < 0.05 were considered statistically significant. Serum-containing media were composed of RPMI 1640 supplemented with 5% serum (R5): FCS, NTA, NTS or human AB (hAB)

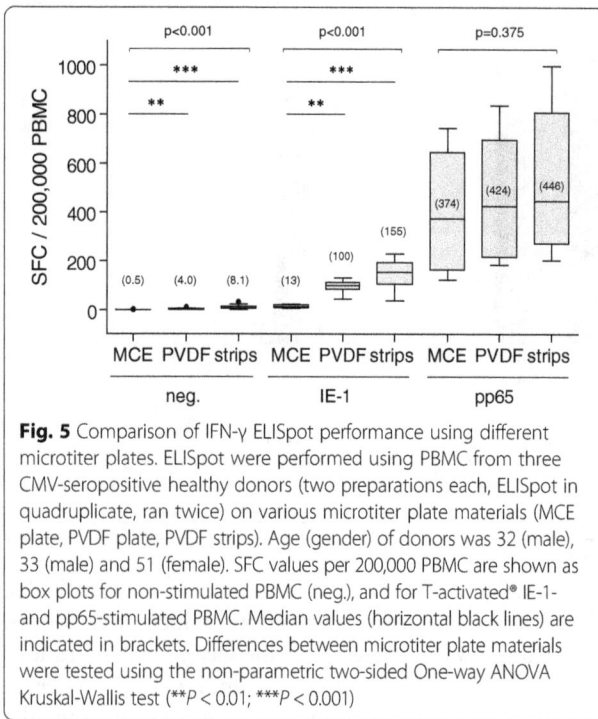

Fig. 5 Comparison of IFN-γ ELISpot performance using different microtiter plates. ELISpot were performed using PBMC from three CMV-seropositive healthy donors (two preparations each, ELISpot in quadruplicate, ran twice) on various microtiter plate materials (MCE plate, PVDF plate, PVDF strips). Age (gender) of donors was 32 (male), 33 (male) and 51 (female). SFC values per 200,000 PBMC are shown as box plots for non-stimulated PBMC (neg.), and for T-activated® IE-1- and pp65-stimulated PBMC. Median values (horizontal black lines) are indicated in brackets. Differences between microtiter plate materials were tested using the non-parametric two-sided One-way ANOVA Kruskal-Wallis test (**P < 0.01; ***P < 0.001)

In contrast, in individual donors with higher spot counts (e.g., d172, d202; Fig. 6c), detection of pp65-reactive cells increased in a dose-dependent manner with the concentration of IFN-γ capture antibody used for coating, especially between 2.5 and 5 µg/ml antibody. At antibody concentrations of 5 µg/ml and beyond, spot counts remained stable (Figs. 6b-c). Based on these results, a concentration of 5 µg/ml IFN-γ capture antibody was chosen for coating in the optimized ELISpot protocol.

ELISpot assays rely on the detection of captured cytokine by cytokine-specific antibodies, which can be either directly coupled to a reporter enzyme (one-step assay development), like alkaline phosphatase (AP), or a combination of a biotinylated secondary antibody and a streptavidin-conjugated reporter enzyme (two-step assay development). A one-step assay development saves handling time and prevents operator errors. AP-conjugated mAb (7-B6-1) (MicroCoat Biotechnologie GmbH, Bernried, Germany) was used as detection conjugate for the standardized ELISpot protocol. Different incubation parameters (e.g., 0.5 – 3 h at 37 °C, 2 h at room temperature [RT, 18-25 °C]) were tested. Spot counts were comparable in all conditions. However, spot

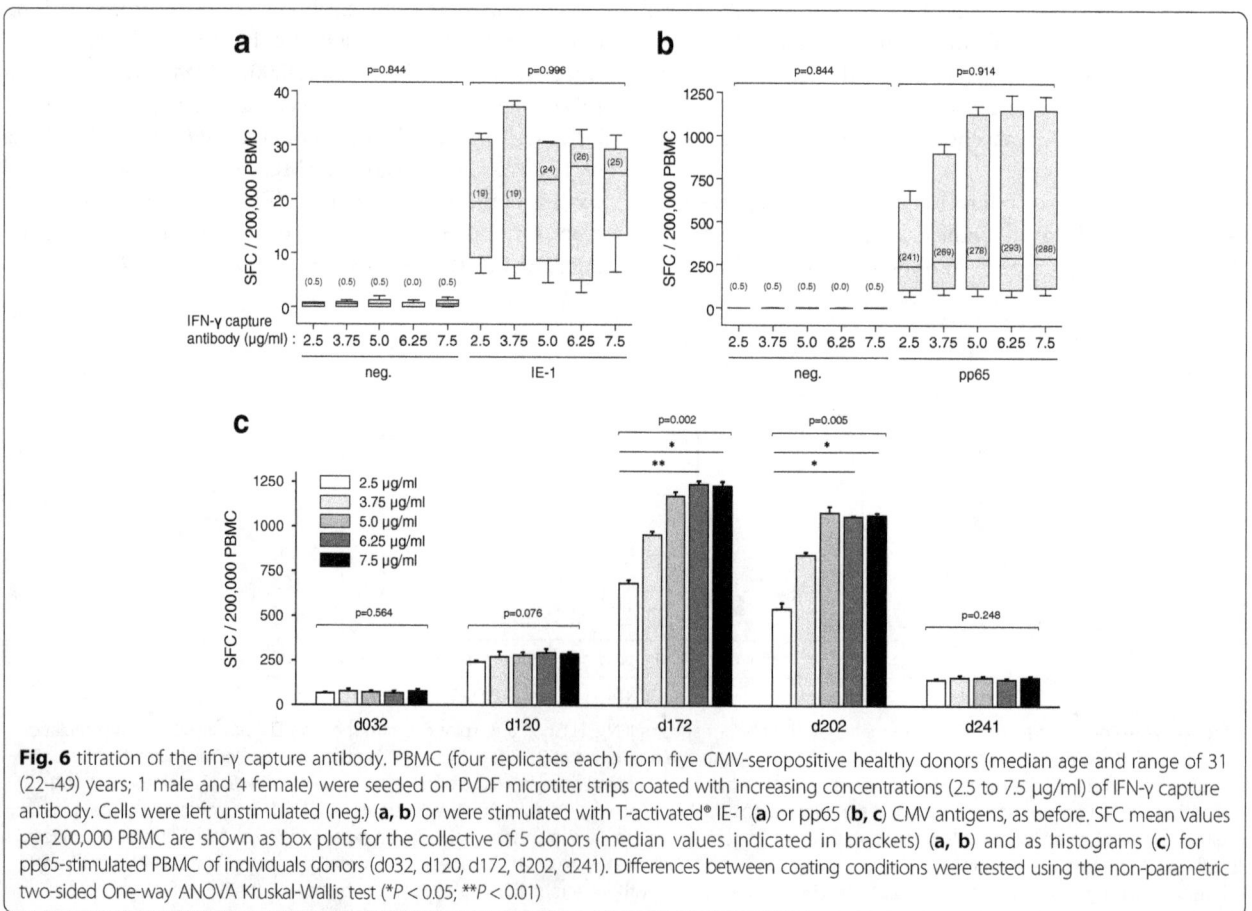

Fig. 6 titration of the ifn-γ capture antibody. PBMC (four replicates each) from five CMV-seropositive healthy donors (median age and range of 31 (22–49) years; 1 male and 4 female) were seeded on PVDF microtiter strips coated with increasing concentrations (2.5 to 7.5 µg/ml) of IFN-γ capture antibody. Cells were left unstimulated (neg.) (**a, b**) or were stimulated with T-activated® IE-1 (**a**) or pp65 (**b, c**) CMV antigens, as before. SFC mean values per 200,000 PBMC are shown as box plots for the collective of 5 donors (median values indicated in brackets) (**a, b**) and as histograms (**c**) for pp65-stimulated PBMC of individuals donors (d032, d120, d172, d202, d241). Differences between coating conditions were tested using the non-parametric two-sided One-way ANOVA Kruskal-Wallis test (*P < 0.05; **P < 0.01)

morphology and thus proper detection was best upon incubation with AP-conjugate for 2 h at RT, compared to other conditions (not shown). Increase in the concentration of the detection conjugate from 0.025 to 0.4 U/ml resulted in slightly elevated SFC median values for pp65, and the maximum spot counts exceeded those generated by the two-step assay development (not shown). Therefore, a one-step assay development for 2 h at RT with 0.4 U/ml detection conjugate was chosen.

Finally, standardization of the SFC staining reaction was addressed to complete assay optimization. Duration of incubation with the AP substrate affects spot size and/or background level, and is thus critical for reliable spot enumeration. A one-step chromogenic alkaline phosphatase substrate NBT/BCIP (Thermo Fischer Scientific, Waltham, USA) was used as staining solution, and incubation times ranging from 2 to 13 min in the dark were evaluated. SFC counts were comparable in all conditions. However, shorter incubation times resulted in smaller spot diameter, while longer incubation times yielded enhanced background levels (data not shown). Therefore, a staining duration of six minutes in the dark was defined for the optimized ELISpot protocol.

Linearity and precision of the optimized CMV ELISpot assay

The optimized ELISpot protocol was used to determine the working range of PBMC that ensure assay linearity. PBMC from one healthy CMV-seropositive donor were seeded at a density ranging from 2×10^4 to 2.5×10^5 PBMC per well. For cell numbers between 6×10^4 and 2×10^5 PBMC per well, ELISpot counts were directly proportional to the number of PBMC seeded, following stimulation with either IE-1 (linear regression analysis; $R^2 = 0.97$) or pp65 ($R^2 = 0.99$) (Fig. 7a). Because of the usually lower spot count resulting

from IE-1 stimulation, the use of 2×10^5 PBMC per well was chosen for the standardized ELISpot assay, to ensure sufficient SFC values.

To further verify the linearity between the number of CMV-reactive effector cells and enumerated SFC, increasing numbers of PBMC from one CMV-seropositive healthy donor were seeded and the total number of PBMC was adjusted to 2×10^5 per well using PBMC from one CMV-seronegative donor. Two donor pairs (d034 + d219, d204 + d067) that showed no allo-reactivity in a 19-h co-culture were chosen for these experiments. Due to low SFC numbers (below 20 SFC/200,000 PBMC), IE-1 stimulation results showed increased variability compared to pp65 and did not allow a reliable linearity calculation (R^2 values below 0.96; data not shown). ELISpot assay results following pp65 stimulation showed a good linear correlation for both donor pairs, with R^2 values of 0.99 (d034 + d219) and 0.98 (d204 + d067) in the linear regression analysis (Fig. 7b).

Precision and repeatability of the optimized assay were evaluated by calculating the intra-assay, inter-assay, inter-operator and inter-site variability. In each case, PBMC from three CMV-seropositive healthy donors were tested in quadruplicate, and variability was assessed by calculating the coefficient of variation (CV), defined as the ratio of the standard deviation to the mean. CV for ELISpot values < 10 SFC/200,000 PBMC were not calculated (see positivity cut-off calculation below). CV intra-assay reached 14% for IE-1 stimulation and 6% for pp65 stimulation (Additional File 1: Table S1). CV inter-assay did not exceed 17% for IE-1 and 22% for pp65 (Additional File 1: Table S2). CV inter-operator was below 13% and 18% for IE-1 and pp65 respectively (Additional File 1: Table S3). Finally, inter-site variation, which is essential for assay validation for diagnostics

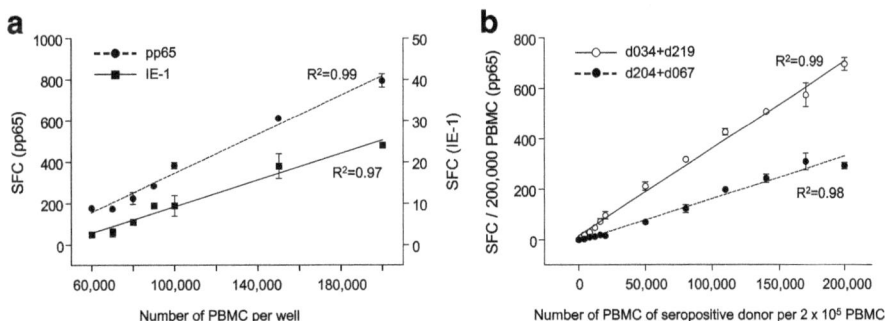

Fig. 7 IFN-γ ELISpot assay linearity. **a** Working range of PBMC per ELISpot assay. Increasing number of PBMC from one CMV-seropositive healthy donor were seeded per well and ELISpot assays were performed as described, following stimulation with T-activated® IE-1 or pp65. Mean SFC values and standard deviation obtained for 60,000-200,000 PBMC per well are depicted. Scale of the Y-axes was adjusted for pp65 (left) and IE-1 (right) for a better data resolution. **b** Linearity between the number of CMV-reactive PBMC and enumerated SFC. The indicated numbers of PBMC from one CMV-seropositive healthy donor were mixed with PBMC from one CMV-seronegative donor (up to 200,000 total PBMC) and stimulated with T-activated® pp65 antigen according to the optimized protocol. Mean SFC values and standard deviation of quadruplicate measurements are shown for two donor pairs (d034 + d219, d204 + d067). In both panels, regression lines and corresponding coefficient of determination R^2 were generated using the regression line tool of GraphPad Prism 5.04

purposes, was evaluated. Whole blood samples were simultaneously collected from three CMV-seropositive healthy donors and shipped (under constant condition at RT) to four different laboratories in Germany. PBMC were freshly isolated and ELISpot assays performed according to the optimized protocol by a total of 7 operators. CV inter-site reached a maximum of 39% for IE-1 and of 28% for pp65 (Additional File 1: Table S4).

Evaluation of at least four independent measurements has been recommended to achieve statistically significant ELISpot results [44–46]. To address the influence of intra-replicate variations on the assay outcome, we compared ELISpot results of quintuplicate and quadruplicate measurements of each control and antigen stimulations. No significant variation of test results was found (data not shown). Therefore, quadruplicate measurements of unstimulated and T-activated® IE-1- and pp65-stimulated conditions allow assay reliability, as well as practicability in combination with the use of 8-well strips.

Staphylococcal enterotoxin B (SEB) is a powerful superantigen, and phytohemagglutinin (PHA) a potent mitogen, both inducing massive IFN-γ secretion by T cells [47, 48]. Thus SEB and PHA are suitable positive controls for cell viability, successful stimulation of cytokine secretion and overall T cell functionality. This is particularly important for result interpretation when low T cell frequency is expected, for instance in recipients of allogeneic stem cell transplantation. In the optimized ELISpot assay, stimulations of test samples with either SEB or PHA are performed in duplicate.

In addition, an effector cell-independent operator control was established to validate proper assay performance. This operator control is based on the detection of recombinant IFN-γ upon direct incubation with the immobilized anti-human-IFN-γ mAb (1-D1K) capture antibody. This control, also performed in duplicate, should yield a homogeneous dark staining of the PVDF membrane.

Technical assay validation: definition of a positivity cut-off

To ease result interpretation of the IFN-γ ELISpot assay and to maximize specificity (i.e. avoid false positives within unstimulated conditions and within stimulated conditions in CMV-seronegative individuals), a technical cut-off was defined. IFN-γ ELISpot assays were performed according to the optimized protocol on PBMC from 45 healthy donors, of which 32 were CMV IgG-seropositive (Table 1).

Median and range of SFC values from unstimulated PBMC of CMV-seronegative and CMV-seropositive individuals were comparable [median SFC (range) of 0.7 (0.5-8.6) and 0.7 (0.5-2.5)/200,000 PBMC, respectively; Fig. 8]. Spot counts in IE-1- and pp65-stimulated PBMC of CMV-seronegative subjects were low [median SFC

Table 1 Technical validation cohort of healthy donors

Median age (range) in years	33 (21; 64)
Gender, N (%)	
Male	11 (24.4%)
Female	34 (75.6%)
CMV serostatus, N (%)	
Positive	32 (71.1%)
Negative	13 (28.9%)

(range) of 4.0 (2.0-52) and 1.4 (0.6-7.6)/200,000 PBMC, respectively; Fig. 8]. In CMV-seropositive individuals, SFC levels in IE-1- and pp65-stimulated PBMC reached 1114 and 954 spot counts/200,000 PBMC (median of 22 and 265 respectively; Fig. 8). For the determination of a technical cut-off, spot counts in the unstimulated control as well as in T-activated® pp65- and IE-1-stimulated conditions of CMV-seronegative and CMV-seropositive individuals were taken into consideration. Positivity threshold was determined using z-statistics (α-level = 0.05) on log10-transformed geometric mean

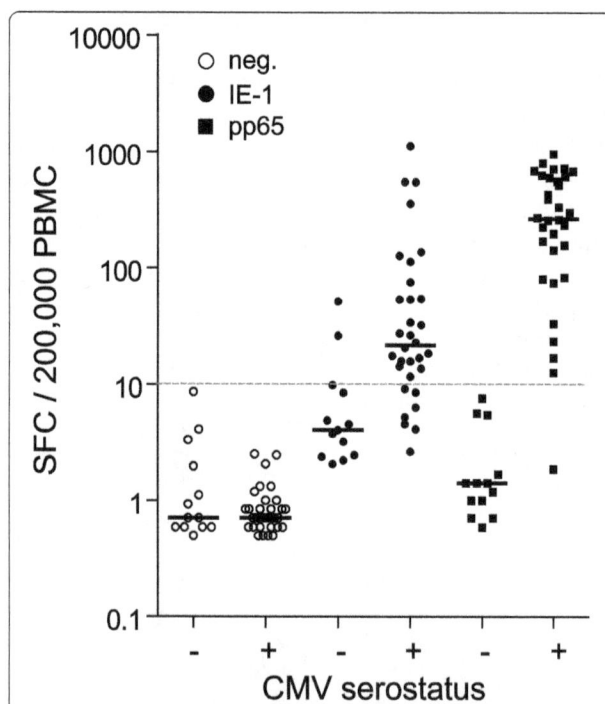

Fig. 8 Assay validation in immunocompetent donors. PBMC isolated from whole blood of 45 healthy donors (Table 1) were assayed using the optimized IFN-γ ELISpot. A positivity cut-off of 10 SFC/200,000 PBMC (grey horizontal dashed line) was defined (see text and Additional File 2). Considering a test result as positive when the geometric mean for at least one of the IE-1 or pp65 stimulated approach is ≥ 10 SFC/200,000 PBMC and when the ratio of geometric means of stimulated to unstimulated conditions is ≥ 2.5, positive agreement (sensitivity) and negative agreement (specificity) of the optimized IFN-γ ELISpot test results with CMV serology within this collective of healthy donors was 97% and 85% respectively

values. Values = 0 were replaced by values near detection limit, which was assumed to be 0.5. Standard deviation (SD) of ELISpot measurements for the unstimulated control, IE-1 stimulation and pp65 stimulation was respectively 0.234, 0.192 and 0.136. Considering a SD of 0.2 and assuming that 4 replicates are measured for each negative control and test samples, a criterion that the ratio of geometric means of stimulated to unstimulated values is at least 2.5 was calculated. On the other hand, precision profiles were generated from both IE-1- and pp65-specific test results, whereby a coefficient of variation (CV) no higher than 40% was used as a limit of acceptance of assay validity to determine the respective limit of quantitation (LoQ). Precision profiles for IE-1- and pp65-specific ELISpot results from the 45 healthy donors yielded LoQ values of 8.6 and 7.1 respectively (Additional File 2). Of note, a similar analysis performed on a cohort of 124 hemodialysis patients provided comparable SD values within unstimulated and antigen-stimulated conditions (range 0.199-0.240) and yielded LoQ values of 7.8 (IE-1) and 8.3 (pp65) [49]. Based on these analyses, a cut-off of 10 SFC/200,000 PBMC was chosen to define positive test results.

Altogether, using T-activated® pp65 and IE-1 antigens and the optimized IFN-γ ELISpot assay, test results are considered positive if the geometric mean of the spots resulting from pp65 or IE1 stimulations are ≥ 10 SFC/200,000 PBMC and if the ratio of the geometric means of stimulated to non-stimulated conditions is ≥ 2.5. According to these definitions, the collective of 45 healthy donors (32 CMV IgG-seropositive, 13 CMV IgG-seronegative) revealed a sensitivity (defined as the positive agreement with CMV IgG-serology, used as primary reference measurement procedure) of 97% and a specificity (negative agreement with CMV IgG-serology) of 85% (Fig. 8).

Functional assay validation: T-activated antigens stimulate a broad spectrum of clinically relevant CMV-reactive effector cells

Urea-formulated recombinant (T-activated®) proteins are processed by both the exogenous (MHC class II) and endogenous (MHC class I) antigen processing and presentation pathways [31]. Stimulation of PBMC by T-activated® proteins thus reproduces more closely a natural infection, potentially resulting in the activation of a broad spectrum of clinically relevant CMV-reactive cells (e.g., Th, CTL, NK, NKT cells; [5–12]), which might contribute to the high sensitivity of the IFN-γ ELISpot assay. To further characterize the cells targeted by T-activated® IE-1 and pp65 antigens and to investigate the possible inter-individual variability in the effector cells response, intracellular IFN-γ staining and flow

cytometry analyses were performed in parallel to IFN-γ ELISpot assays. Freshly isolated PBMC from six CMV-seropositive healthy donors were stimulated with T-activated® IE-1 and pp65 proteins for 19 h and IFN-γ-producing cells enumerated according to the optimized ELISpot assay. The same PBMC preparations (4 replicates each) were stimulated for 6 h with the same batch of T-activated® IE-1 and pp65 proteins in the presence of co-stimulatory anti-CD28 and anti-CD49d antibodies. Surface markers (CD3, CD4, CD8, CD56) and intracellular IFN-γ staining were analysed by flow cytometry, as described in the Methods section. IFN-γ$^+$ subpopulations of CD3$^+$CD4$^+$ (Th), CD3$^+$CD8$^+$ (CTL), CD3$^+$CD56$^+$ (NKT-like) and CD3$^-$CD56$^+$ (NK) lymphocytes were enumerated following the gating strategy illustrated in Additional File 3. All six donors differed in their capacity to elicit an IE-1- and/or pp65-dependent response in the IFN-γ ELISpot assay. The intensity of the response was also heterogeneous among the six donors, with values ranging from 7 to 1,054 SFC (IE-1 stimulation) and from 28 to 780 SFC (pp65 stimulation) per 200,000 PBMC (Fig. 9a). Similarly, individual donors differed in the frequency and ratio of the various cell subpopulations investigated by flow cytometry (Fig. 9b). Interestingly, healthy CMV-seropositive individuals with lower spot counts (d120, d300, d343; Fig. 9a) also showed lower frequencies of IFN-γ$^+$ lymphocytes by flow cytometry (Fig. 9b), highlighting the ability of the ELISpot assay to distinguish low from high responders. Activation of each lymphocyte subpopulation investigated was detected in some but not all donors. For instance, weak to strong CD4$^+$ T cell activation was detected in 4 out of 6 donors (d120, d172, d300, d343) in response to either IE-1, pp65, or both. Similarly, 5 out of 6 donors (d172, d290, d300, d343, d361) showed CD8$^+$ T cell activation in one or both stimulation conditions. CD3-CD56$^+$ (NK cells) were apparent in one donor (d120) in response to both antigens. CD3$^+$CD56$^+$ (NKT-like) cells were weakly activated in 4 out of 6 individuals (d120, d172 d300, d361) in response to both IE-1 and pp65 (Fig. 9b). Remarkably, a strong pp65-specific CD4$^+$ activation in d172 correlated with a strong pp65-specific response in ELISpot, and a strong pp65-specific (d290) and IE-1-specific (d361) CD8$^+$ activation was associated with a high spot count in the corresponding ELISpot (Figs. 9a-b), suggesting that these CMV-reactive effector cells significantly contribute to the detected ELISpot signals. Altogether, these data demonstrate the ability of T-activated® IE-1 and pp65 proteins to stimulate a broad range of CMV-specific effector cells. These experiments also revealed the high heterogeneity of responses among healthy CMV-seropositive individuals. Notably, the observation that some individuals respond to either IE-1 or pp65 emphasizes the importance of assessing the response to both antigens. Monitoring both IE-1- and pp65-specific

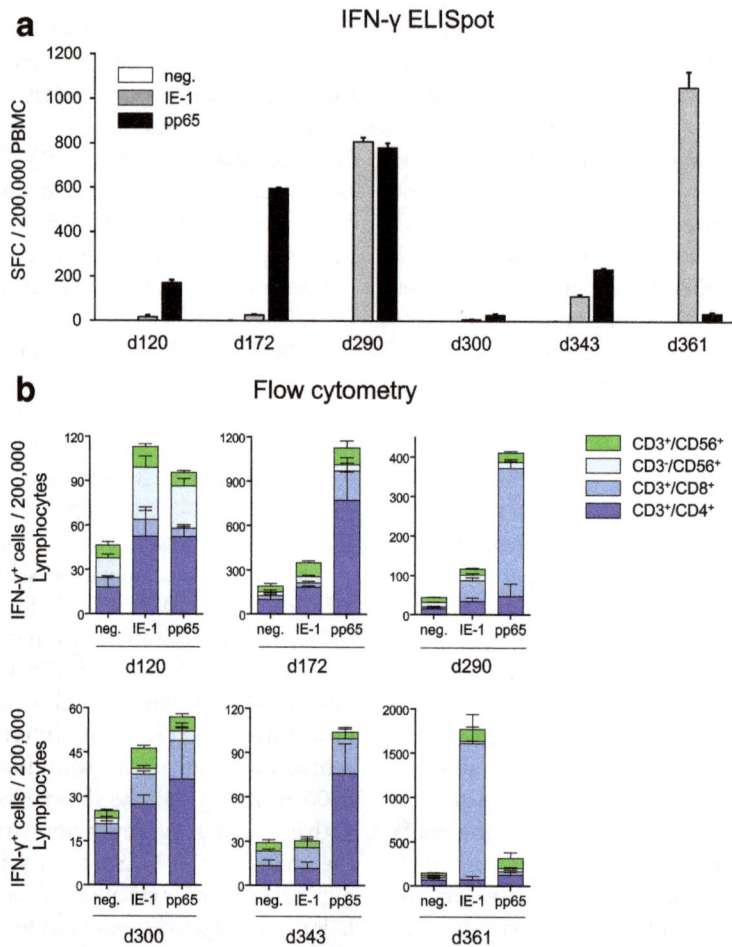

Fig. 9 T-activated® pp65 and IE-1 CMV antigens stimulate a broad range of CMV-reactive effector cells. Comparative analysis of IFN-γ secreting cells by ELISpot (**a**) and flow cytometry (**b**) following stimulation of PBMC with T-activated® pp65 and IE-1 antigens. PBMC (4 replicates each) from six CMV-seropositive healthy donors (median age and range of 39 (22–55) years; 2 male and 4 female) were stimulated with T-activated® pp65 and IE-1 antigens according to the optimized IFN-γ ELISpot (**a**) and to the protocol of intracellular and surface marker staining and flow cytometry described in the Methods section (**b**). Bar graphs in (**a**) depict IFN-γ-dependent SFC per 200,000 PBMC, as before. Bar graphs in (**b**) represent the number of IFN-γ-expressing $CD3^+CD4^+$ (Th), $CD3^+CD8^+$ (CTL), $CD3^-CD56^+$ (NK) and $CD3^+CD56^+$ (NKT-like) cells per 200,000 lymphocytes. Note that the Y-axis scales in (**b**) were adjusted for a better resolution of the respective data. Individual age and gender of donors were as follows: d120, 37-year-old male; d172, 55-year-old female; d290, 46-year-old female; d300, 41-year-old female; d343, 24-year-old female; d361, 22-year-old male

responses in the optimized IFN-γ ELISpot assay might improve the overall sensitivity of the test.

Discussion

We describe here the development and technical validation of an optimized and standardized IFN-γ ELISpot protocol for the monitoring of CMV-reactive effector cells of cell-mediated immunity (CMI).

The particularity of the assay is the use of T-activated® proteins [31] as stimulant of CMV-reactive effector cells. We now demonstrate that urea-formulated IE-1 and pp65 proteins are capable of activating not only CMV-reactive CD4+ (Th) and CD8+ (CTL) lymphocytes, but also innate lymphocytes (CD3−CD56+ NK and CD3+CD56+ NKT-like cells), likely

by bystander activation as well as by activation of CMV-specific memory NK cells [5, 7, 8, 32, 50, 51]. This finding is important given the acknowledged role played by these effector cells in the protection against CMV reactivation in vivo [5–12]. Inter-individual variability in the response of lymphocyte subpopulations was high among CMV-seropositive healthy donors, therefore further emphasizing the importance of an antigen formulation capable of activating a broad spectrum of CMV-reactive effector cells. In this, the optimized IFN-γ ELISpot assays outperforms existing ELISpot- and ELISA-based CMV-specific CMI monitoring tools. In addition, the characteristics and high sensitivity of our assay predict a performance independent of the HLA-type of the donor.

The second particularity of the described assay is the combined use of two T-activated® proteins, IE-1 and pp65, as antigens. We show here that both antigens can elicit the activation of distinct CMV-specific effector cells and that while some CMV-seropositive healthy individuals are reactive to both antigens, some are only reactive to one (either IE-1 or pp65), as previously reported [52]. Therefore, consideration of both test results is expected to improve the sensitivity of the assay, notably in cohort studies. This is particularly relevant for the monitoring of CMV-specific CMI in immunocompromised patients. Accordingly, we recently demonstrated the benefit of measuring the response to both T-activated® IE-1 and pp65 antigens in terms of assay sensitivity, in clinical studies assessing CMV-specific CMI during pregnancy [53], in hemodialysis patients [49] and in renal transplant recipients (submitted).

The assessment of the response to both IE-1 and pp65 antigens is further justified by the respective relevance and differential contribution of IE-1- and pp65-reactive effector cells to the protection against CMV reactivation and related clinical complications, both in healthy CMV-seropositive individuals and in transplant recipients [1, 6, 54–59]. The differential contribution of IE-1- and pp65-specific effector cells likely reflect the dynamic of the cell-mediated immune response [10, 60–64]. Mechanisms of immune evasion inhibiting MHC-I-dependent IE-1 antigen processing and presentation might also explain the lower frequency of IE-1-specific IFN-γ-producing cells detected in our ELISpot assay [65]. In addition, reduced processing and presentation efficiency due to protein stability, size and nuclear localization might play a role in the reduced reactivity to IE-1, as opposed to pp65 [64, 66, 67]. This proposition is supported by the observation that higher concentrations of IE-1 were required in our ELISpot assay, in comparison to pp65, to trigger a significant response.

Another particularity of our IFN-γ ELISpot assay was its ability to elicit positive test results in CMV-seronegative individuals, notably following stimulation with IE-1. In the cohort of 45 healthy donors, out of the 13 CMV-seronegative individuals 2 showed IE-1-specific values ≥ 10 SFC/200,000 PBMC (Additional File 2), corresponding to a negative agreement with CMV IgG-serology of 85%. Similar results were obtained in a cohort of 124 hemodialysis patients [49]. Numerous studies reported discordant results between cellular and humoral immunity against CMV [68–71]. Given the high sensitivity of our ELISpot assay and its ability to detect a broad range of CMV-reactive cells, it is possible that cellular reactivity in CMV-seronegative individuals reflects a previous exposure to CMV that failed to mount a humoral immune response, rather than a false-positive ELISpot result. Further experiments will

be necessary to address this possibility. Nonetheless, this observation raises the question of the accuracy of CMV serology to identify immunocompromised patients at increased risk of CMV reactivation [3, 70, 72].

The optimized and standardized IFN-γ ELISpot assay exhibited robust performance in terms of assay variability, precision and linearity. Intra-assay, inter-assay and inter-operator coefficients of variations (CV) did not exceed 22%, which is below the range of recommended precision (% of relative standard deviation or %RSD) for cell-based assays [73]. As predicted, inter-site variability involving different operators was higher, but remained acceptable with a CV of no more than 39%. This is an important criterion for the reliable longitudinal monitoring of CMV-specific immune responses in patients. Linearity of the assay is also a critical parameter, in particular for the monitoring of immunocompromised patients with reduced and/or functionally impaired T cells, such as children or recipients of allogeneic stem cell transplantation. Good linearity and high signal-to-noise ratio were obtained for both IE-1 ($R^2 = 0.97$) and pp65 ($R^2 = 0.99$) in the range of 60,000 to 200,000 PBMC per well. Two multi-center clinical studies are currently being conducted, in renal transplant recipients under immunosuppressive therapy and in allogeneic stem cell transplantation patients, to assess the sensitivity of the optimized CMV-specific IFN-γ ELISpot assay in this clinical context and to correlate results of the assay to clinical outcome.

Conclusions

Altogether, this optimized, standardized and user-friendly CMV-specific IFN-γ ELISpot assay meet all the conditions of a sensitive and reliable diagnostic test for the monitoring of the functionality of CMV-specific CMI. Beside its validation in healthy individuals (this study), its suitability to assess CMV-specific cell-mediated immunity in a cohort of hemodialysis patients representative of patients prior to transplantation has been demonstrated [49]. Further validation of the assay in immunocompromised patients, such as transplant recipients is necessary to determine its suitability in assisting clinicians to evaluate the risk of CMV reactivation and disease, and possibly individualize the therapeutic management of patients.

Abbreviations
CMI: Cell-mediated immunity; CMV: Cytomegalovirus; CTL: Cytotoxic T lymphocyte; CV: Coefficient of variation; ELISA: Enzyme-linked immunosorbent assay; ELISpot: Enzyme-linked immunospot; HLA: Human leukocyte antigen; ICS: Intracellular cytokine staining; IE-1: Immediate early-1 protein; IFN-γ: Interferon gamma; LoQ: Limit of quantitation; NK: Natural killer cell; NKT: Natural killer T cell; PBMC: Peripheral blood mononuclear cell; pp65: 65 kDa lower matrix phosphoprotein; RSD: Relative standard deviation; SD: Standard deviation; SFC: Spot-forming cell; Th: T helper cell

Acknowledgements

We thank Christina Paulus and Michael Nevels (University of Regensburg) for their support in IE-1 production and purification, and Thomas Keller (ACOMED Statistik) for statistical evaluation.

Funding

This project was funded by the Bayerische Forschungsstiftung Grants AZ 924–10 and AZ 1070–13 (ForBiMed project D5). The funding body had no role in the design of the study and in collection, analysis and interpretation of data and in writing the manuscript.

Authors' contributions

SB and LD designed and supervised assay development. TS, CT, TL and SB performed experiments for assay development and analysed data. BA, RW and RK designed and supervised the flow cytometry experiment. RK performed the intracellular cytokine staining and flow cytometry experiment, and analysed data. AR, JB and HB drafted the manuscript and figures. All authors edited, read and/or approved the final version.

Competing interests

SB, JB, HB, LD, AR, TS, CT and TL are or were employees of Lophius Biosciences GmbH. LD is co-founder and Chief Scientific Officer of Lophius Biosciences GmbH. RW is Chairman of the Board of Lophius Biosciences GmbH. RW, SB and LD are shareholders of Lophius Biosciences GmbH.

Additional files

Additional File 1: Assay variability. Intra-assay (**Table S1.**), inter-assay (**Table S2.**), inter-operator (**Table S3.**) and inter-site (**Table S4.**) variability was assessed as described in the respective legends. (PDF 128 kb)**Additional File 2:** Positivity cut-off definition. Results obtained using the optimized IFN-γ ELISpot assay on PBMC isolated from whole blood of 45 healthy donors (Table 1 and Fig. 8) were used to generate precision profiles for each IE-1 and pp65 stimulation. Limits of quantitation (LoQ) for IE-1 and pp65 were 8.6 and 7.1 SFC/200,000 PBMC respectively. LoQ calculated on a cohort of 124 hemodialysis patients [49] were in a similar range (7.8 and 8.3 for IE-1 and pp65 respectively). Therefore, a positivity cut-off of 10 SFC/200,000 PBMC was chosen for the standardized assay. In addition, intra-assay standard deviation (SD) within both cohorts of healthy donors (n = 45) and hemodialysis patients (n = 124) for stimulated and unstimulated measurements was the basis for the calculation of a criterion that the ratio of geometric means of stimulated to unstimulated values is at least 2.5. Finally, considering a test result as positive when geometric mean for at least one of the IE-1 or pp65 stimulated approach is ≥

10 SFC/200,000 PBMC, positive agreement (sensitivity) and negative agreement (specificity) of the optimized IFN-γ ELISpot test results with CMV serology within the collective of 45 healthy donors was 97% and 85% respectively (Fig. 8). (PDF 73 kb)**Additional File 3:** Gating strategy of flow cytometry analyses following surface marker (CD3, CD4, CD8, CD56) and intracellular IFN-γ staining. PBMC (4 replicates each) from six CMV-seropositive healthy donors were stimulated with T-activated® pp65 and IE-1 antigens for 6 h, as indicated in the legend to Fig. 9. (**A**) Cells were first gated on single events in a Forward Scatter-Area (FSC-A) x FSC-Height (FSC-H) dot plot (Gating #1). Based on FSC-A x Side Scatter-Area (SSC-A) properties, a gate was next set around lymphocytes (Gating #2). By plotting CD3 against CD56, CD56 single positive cells (Gating #3), CD3/CD56 double positive cells (Gating #4) and CD3 single positive cells (Gating #5) were separated. CD3 single positive cells (Gating #5) were further subdivided into CD3/CD4 double positive (Gating #6) and CD3/CD8 double positive cells (Gating #7). (**B**) Representative dot plots (1 out of 4 replicates) of stained PBMC of donor d290. In each plot, percentage value in gated area is the mean frequency (from 4 replicates) of IFN-γ-expressing CD3$^+$CD4$^+$ (Th), CD3$^+$CD8$^+$ (CTL), CD3$^-$CD56$^+$ (NK) and CD3$^+$CD56$^+$ (NKT-like) cells. (PDF 351 kb)

References

1. Crough T, Khanna R. Immunobiology of human cytomegalovirus: from bench to bedside. Clin Microbiol Rev. 2009;22:76–98.
2. Fisher RA. Cytomegalovirus infection and disease in the new era of immunosuppression following solid organ transplantation. Transpl Infect Dis Off J Transplant Soc. 2009;11:195–202.
3. Kotton CN, Kumar D, Caliendo AM, Asberg A, Chou S, Danziger-Isakov L, et al. Updated international consensus guidelines on the management of cytomegalovirus in solid-organ transplantation. Transplantation. 2013;96:333–60.
4. Lisboa LF, Kumar D, Wilson LE, Humar A. Clinical utility of cytomegalovirus cell-mediated immunity in transplant recipients with cytomegalovirus viremia. Transplantation. 2012;93:195–200.
5. van Dommelen SLH, Tabarias HA, Smyth MJ, Degli-Esposti MA. Activation of natural killer (NK) T cells during murine cytomegalovirus infection enhances the antiviral response mediated by NK cells. J Virol. 2003;77:1877–84.
6. Sylwester AW, Mitchell BL, Edgar JB, Taormina C, Pelte C, Ruchti F, et al. Broadly targeted human cytomegalovirus-specific CD4+ and CD8+ T cells dominate the memory compartments of exposed subjects. J Exp Med. 2005;202:673–85.
7. Kamath AT, Sheasby CE, Tough DF. Dendritic cells and NK cells stimulate bystander T cell activation in response to TLR agonists through secretion of IFN-alpha beta and IFN-gamma. J Immunol. 2005;174:767–76.
8. Min-Oo G, Lanier LL. Cytomegalovirus generates long-lived antigen-specific NK cells with diminished bystander activation to heterologous infection. J Exp Med. 2014;211:2669–80.
9. Sester M, Sester U, Gärtner B, Heine G, Girndt M, Mueller-Lantzsch N, et al. Levels of virus-specific CD4 T cells correlate with cytomegalovirus control and predict virus-induced disease after renal transplantation. Transplantation. 2001;71:1287–94.
10. Sester M, Sester U, Gärtner BC, Girndt M, Meyerhans A, Köhler H. Dominance of virus-specific CD8 T cells in human primary cytomegalovirus infection. J Am Soc Nephrol JASN. 2002;13:2577–84.
11. Gamadia LE, Remmerswaal EBM, Weel JF, Bemelman F, van Lier RAW, Ten Berge IJM. Primary immune responses to human CMV: a critical role for IFN-

gamma-producing CD4+ T cells in protection against CMV disease. Blood. 2003;101:2686–92.

12. Hanley PJ, Bollard CM. Controlling cytomegalovirus: helping the immune system take the lead. Viruses. 2014;6:2242–58.

13. Walker S, Fazou C, Crough T, Holdsworth R, Kiely P, Veale M, et al. Ex vivo monitoring of human cytomegalovirus-specific CD8+ T-cell responses using QuantiFERON-CMV. Transpl Infect Dis Off J Transplant Soc. 2007;9:165–70.

14. Lehmann PV, Zhang W. Unique strengths of ELISPOT for T cell diagnostics. Methods Mol Biol Clifton NJ. 2012;792:3–23.

15. Tassignon J, Burny W, Dahmani S, Zhou L, Stordeur P, Byl B, et al. Monitoring of cellular responses after vaccination against tetanus toxoid: comparison of the measurement of IFN-gamma production by ELISA, ELISPOT, flow cytometry and real-time PCR. J Immunol Methods. 2005;305:188–98.

16. Abate D, Saldan A, Mengoli C, Fiscon M, Silvestre C, Fallico L, et al. Comparison of cytomegalovirus (CMV) enzyme-linked immunosorbent spot and CMV quantiferon gamma interferon-releasing assays in assessing risk of CMV infection in kidney transplant recipients. J Clin Microbiol. 2013;51:2501–7.

17. Abate D, Saldan A, Forner G, Tinto D, Bianchin A, Palù G. Optimization of interferon gamma ELISPOT assay to detect human cytomegalovirus specific T-cell responses in solid organ transplants. J Virol Methods. 2014;196:157–62.

18. Abate D, Cesaro S, Cofano S, Fiscon M, Saldan A, Varotto S, et al. Diagnostic utility of human cytomegalovirus-specific T-cell response monitoring in predicting viremia in pediatric allogeneic stem-cell transplant patients. Transplantation. 2012;93:536–42.

19. Manuel O, Husain S, Kumar D, Zayas C, Mawhorter S, Levi ME, et al. Assessment of cytomegalovirus-specific cell-mediated immunity for the prediction of cytomegalovirus disease in high-risk solid-organ transplant recipients: a multicenter cohort study. Clin Infect Dis Off Publ Infect Dis Soc Am. 2013;56:817–24.

20. Clari MÁ, Muñoz-Cobo B, Solano C, Benet I, Costa E, Remigia MJ, et al. Performance of the QuantiFERON-cytomegalovirus (CMV) assay for detection and estimation of the magnitude and functionality of the CMV-specific gamma interferon-producing CD8(+) T-cell response in allogeneic stem cell transplant recipients. Clin Vaccine Immunol CVI. 2012;19:791–6.

21. Fleming T, Dunne J, Crowley B. Ex vivo monitoring of human cytomegalovirus-specific CD8(+) T-Cell responses using the QuantiFERON-CMV assay in allogeneic hematopoietic stem cell transplant recipients attending an Irish hospital. J Med Virol. 2010;82:433–40.

22. Cox JH, Ferrari G, Janetzki S. Measurement of cytokine release at the single cell level using the ELISPOT assay. Methods San Diego Calif. 2006;38:274–82.

23. Karlsson AC, Martin JN, Younger SR, Bredt BM, Epling L, Ronquillo R, et al. Comparison of the ELISPOT and cytokine flow cytometry assays for the enumeration of antigen-specific T cells. J Immunol Methods. 2003;283:141–53.

24. Tischer S, Dieks D, Sukdolak C, Bunse C, Figueiredo C, Immenschuh S, et al. Evaluation of suitable target antigens and immunoassays for high-accuracy immune monitoring of cytomegalovirus and Epstein-Barr virus-specific T cells as targets of interest in immunotherapeutic approaches. J Immunol Methods. 2014;408:101–13.

25. Meierhoff G, Ott PA, Lehmann PV, Schloot NC. Cytokine detection by ELISPOT: relevance for immunological studies in type 1 diabetes. Diabetes Metab Res Rev. 2002;18:367–80.

26. Forner G, Saldan A, Mengoli C, Gussetti N, Palù G, Abate D. CMV-ELISPOT but not CMV-QuantiFERON assay is a novel biomarker to determine the risk of congenital CMV infection in pregnant women. J Clin Microbiol. 2016;54:2149–54.

27. Saldan A, Forner G, Mengoli C, Tinto D, Fallico L, Peracchi M, et al. Comparison of the Cytomegalovirus (CMV) Enzyme-Linked Immunosorbent Spot and CMV QuantiFERON Cell-Mediated Immune Assays in CMV-Seropositive and -Seronegative Pregnant and Nonpregnant Women. J Clin Microbiol. 2016;54:1352–6.

28. Saldan A, Forner G, Mengoli C, Gussetti N, Palù G, Abate D. Strong cell-mediated immune response to human cytomegalovirus is associated with increased risk of fetal infection in primarily infected pregnant women. Clin Infect Dis Off Publ Infect Dis Soc Am. 2015;61:1228–34.

29. Godard B, Gazagne A, Gey A, Baptiste M, Vingert B, Pegaz-Fiornet B, et al. Optimization of an elispot assay to detect cytomegalovirus-specific CD8+ T lymphocytes. Hum Immunol. 2004;65:1307–16.

30. Schmittel A, Keilholz U, Scheibenbogen C. Evaluation of the interferon-gamma ELISPOT-assay for quantification of peptide specific T lymphocytes from peripheral blood. J Immunol Methods. 1997;210:167–74.

31. Barabas S, Gary R, Bauer T, Lindner J, Lindner P, Weinberger B, et al. Urea-mediated cross-presentation of soluble Epstein-Barr virus BZLF1 protein. PLoS Pathog. 2008;4:e1000198.

32. Cerwenka A, Lanier LL. Natural killer cell memory in infection, inflammation and cancer. Nat Rev Immunol. 2016;16:112–23.

33. Rowe WP, Hartley JW, Waterman S, Turner HC, Huebner RJ. Cytopathogenic agent resembling human salivary gland virus recovered from tissue cultures of human adenoids. Proc Soc Exp Biol Med Soc Exp Biol Med N Y N. 1956; 92:418–24.

34. McKenna KC, Beatty KM, Vicetti Miguel R, Bilonick RA. Delayed processing of blood increases the frequency of activated CD11b + CD15+ granulocytes which inhibit T cell function. J Immunol Methods. 2009;341:68–75.

35. Xu J, Wu R, Xiang F, Kong Q, Hong J, Kang X. Diversified phenotype of antigen specific CD8+ T cells responding to the immunodominant epitopes of IE and pp 65 antigens of human cytomegalovirus. Cell Immunol. 2015; 295:105–11.

36. Hesse MD, Karulin AY, Boehm BO, Lehmann PV, Tary-Lehmann M. A T cell clone's avidity is a function of its activation state. J Immunol. 2001;167: 1353–61.

37. Elkington R, Walker S, Crough T, Menzies M, Tellam J, Bharadwaj M, et al. Ex vivo profiling of CD8 + –T-cell responses to human cytomegalovirus reveals broad and multispecific reactivities in healthy virus carriers. J Virol. 2003;77:5226–40.

38. Avetisyan G, Aschan J, Hägglund H, Ringdén O, Ljungman P. Evaluation of intervention strategy based on CMV-specific immune responses after allogeneic SCT. Bone Marrow Transplant. 2007;40:865–9.

39. Mattes FM, Vargas A, Kopycinski J, Hainsworth EG, Sweny P, Nebbia G, et al. Functional impairment of cytomegalovirus specific CD8 T cells predicts high-level replication after renal transplantation. Am J Transplant Off J Am Soc Transplant Am Soc Transpl Surg. 2008;8:990–9.

40. Costa C, Balloco C, Sidoti F, Mantovani S, Rittà M, Piceghello A, et al. Evaluation of CMV-specific cellular immune response by EliSPOT assay in kidney transplant patients. J Clin Virol Off Publ Pan Am Soc Clin Virol. 2014; 61:523–8.

41. Costa C, Astegiano S, Terlizzi ME, Sidoti F, Curtoni A, Solidoro P, et al. Evaluation and significance of cytomegalovirus-specific cellular immune response in lung transplant recipients. Transplant Proc. 2011;43:1159–61.

42. Bestard O, Lucia M, Crespo E, Van Liempt B, Palacio D, Melilli E, et al. Pretransplant immediately early-1-specific T cell responses provide protection for CMV infection after kidney transplantation. Am J Transplant Off J Am Soc Transplant Am Soc Transpl Surg. 2013;13:1793–805.

43. Smith SG, Joosten SA, Verscheure V, Pathan AA, McShane H, Ottenhoff THM, et al. Identification of major factors influencing ELISpot-based monitoring of cellular responses to antigens from Mycobacterium tuberculosis. PLoS One. 2009;4:e7972.

44. Moodie Z, Price L, Janetzki S, Britten CM. Response determination criteria for ELISPOT: toward a standard that can be applied across laboratories. Methods Mol Biol Clifton NJ. 2012;792:185–96.

45. Moodie Z, Price L, Gouttefangeas C, Mander A, Janetzki S, Löwer M, et al. Response definition criteria for ELISPOT assays revisited. Cancer Immunol Immunother CII. 2010;59:1489–501.

46. Dittrich M, Lehmann PV. Statistical analysis of ELISPOT assays. Methods Mol Biol Clifton NJ. 2012;792:173–83.

47. Krakauer T. Immune response to staphylococcal superantigens. Immunol Res. 1999;20:163–73.

48. Hao XS, Le JM, Vilcek J, Chang TW. Determination of human T cell activity in response to allogeneic cells and mitogens. An immunochemical assay for gamma-interferon is more sensitive and specific than a proliferation assay. J Immunol Methods. 1986;92:59–63.

49. Banas B, Böger CA, Lückhoff G, Krüger B, Barabas S, Batzilla J, Schemmerer M, Köstler J, Bendfeldt H, Rascle A, Wagner R, Deml L, Leicht J, Krämer BK. Validation of T-Track® CMV to assess the functionality of cytomegalovirus-reactive cell-mediated immunity in hemodialysis patients. BMC Immunology. 2017. doi:10.1186/s12865-017-0194-z.

50. Reschner A, Hubert P, Delvenne P, Boniver J, Jacobs N. Innate lymphocyte and dendritic cell cross-talk: a key factor in the regulation of the immune response. Clin Exp Immunol. 2008;152:219–26.

51. Ferlazzo G, Morandi B. Cross-talks between natural killer cells and distinct subsets of dendritic cells. Front Immunol. 2014;5:159.

52. Kern F, Surel IP, Faulhaber N, Frömmel C, Schneider-Mergener J, Schönemann C, et al. Target structures of the CD8(+)-T-cell response to human cytomegalovirus: the 72-kDa major immediate-early protein revisited. J Virol. 1999;73:8179–84.

53. Reuschel E, Barabas S, Zeman F, Bendfeldt H, Rascle A, Deml L, et al. Functional impairment of CMV-reactive cellular immunity during pregnancy. J Med Virol. 2017;89:324–31.

54. Nickel P, Bold G, Presber F, Biti D, Babel N, Kreutzer S, et al. High levels of CMV-IE-1-specific memory T cells are associated with less alloimmunity and improved renal allograft function. Transpl Immunol. 2009;20:238–42.

55. Egli A, Binet I, Binggeli S, Jäger C, Dumoulin A, Schaub S, et al. Cytomegalovirus-specific T-cell responses and viral replication in kidney transplant recipients. J Transl Med. 2008;6:29.

56. Bunde T, Kirchner A, Hoffmeister B, Habedank D, Hetzer R, Cherepnev G, et al. Protection from cytomegalovirus after transplantation is correlated with immediate early 1-specific CD8 T cells. J Exp Med. 2005; 201:1031–6.

57. Tormo N, Solano C, Benet I, Nieto J, de la Cámara R, Garcia-Noblejas A, et al. Kinetics of cytomegalovirus (CMV) pp 65 and IE-1-specific IFNgamma CD8+ and CD4+ T cells during episodes of viral DNAemia in allogeneic stem cell transplant recipients: potential implications for the management of active CMV infection. J Med Virol. 2010;82:1208–15.

58. Meij P, Jedema I, Zandvliet ML, van der Heiden PLJ, van de Meent M, van Egmond HME, et al. Effective treatment of refractory CMV reactivation after allogeneic stem cell transplantation with in vitro-generated CMV pp 65-specific CD8+ T-cell lines. J Immunother. 2012;35:621–8.

59. Feuchtinger T, Opherk K, Bethge WA, Topp MS, Schuster FR, Weissinger EM, et al. Adoptive transfer of pp 65-specific T cells for the treatment of chemorefractory cytomegalovirus disease or reactivation after haploidentical and matched unrelated stem cell transplantation. Blood. 2010;116:4360–7.

60. Widmann T, Sester U, Gärtner BC, Schubert J, Pfreundschuh M, Köhler H, et al. Levels of CMV specific CD4 T cells are dynamic and correlate with CMV viremia after allogeneic stem cell transplantation. PLoS One. 2008;3:e3634.

61. Sacre K, Carcelain G, Cassoux N, Fillet A-M, Costagliola D, Vittecoq D, et al. Repertoire, diversity, and differentiation of specific CD8 T cells are associated with immune protection against human cytomegalovirus disease. J Exp Med. 2005;201:1999–2010.

62. Gerna G, Lilleri D, Fornara C, Comolli G, Lozza L, Campana C, et al. Monitoring of human cytomegalovirus-specific CD4 and CD8 T-cell immunity in patients receiving solid organ transplantation. Am J Transplant Off J Am Soc Transplant Am Soc Transpl Surg. 2006;6:2356–64.

63. Sester M, Sester U, Gärtner B, Kubuschok B, Girndt M, Meyerhans A, et al. Sustained high frequencies of specific CD4 T cells restricted to a single persistent virus. J Virol. 2002;76:3748–55.

64. Tabi Z, Moutaftsi M, Borysiewicz LK. Human cytomegalovirus pp 65- and immediate early 1 antigen-specific HLA class I-restricted cytotoxic T cell responses induced by cross-presentation of viral antigens. J Immunol. 2001;166:5695–703.

65. Gilbert MJ, Riddell SR, Li CR, Greenberg PD. Selective interference with class I major histocompatibility complex presentation of the major immediate-early protein following infection with human cytomegalovirus. J Virol. 1993;67:3461–9.

66. Scheller N, Furtwängler R, Sester U, Maier R, Breinig T, Meyerhans A. Human cytomegalovirus protein pp 65: an efficient protein carrier system into human dendritic cells. Gene Ther. 2008;15:318–25.

67. Delmas S, Martin L, Baron M, Nelson JA, Streblow DN, Davignon J-L. Optimization of CD4+ T lymphocyte response to human cytomegalovirus nuclear IE1 protein through modifications of both size and cellular localization. J Immunol. 2005;175: 6812–9.

68. Loeth N, Assing K, Madsen HO, Vindeløv L, Buus S, Stryhn A. Humoral and cellular CMV responses in healthy donors; identification of a frequent population of CMV-specific, CD4+ T cells in seronegative donors. PLoS One. 2012;7:e31420.

69. Lúcia M, Crespo E, Melilli E, Cruzado JM, Luque S, Llaudó I, et al. Preformed frequencies of cytomegalovirus (CMV)-specific memory T and B cells identify protected CMV-sensitized individuals among seronegative kidney transplant recipients. Clin Infect Dis Off Publ Infect Dis Soc Am. 2014;59: 1537–45.

70. Sester M, Gärtner BC, Sester U, Girndt M, Mueller-Lantzsch N, Köhler H. Is the cytomegalovirus serologic status always accurate? A comparative analysis of humoral and cellular immunity. Transplantation. 2003;76:1229–30.

71. Zhu J, Shearer GM, Marincola FM, Norman JE, Rott D, Zou JP, et al. Discordant cellular and humoral immune responses to cytomegalovirus infection in healthy blood donors: existence of a Th1-type dominant response. Int Immunol. 2001;13: 785–90.

72. Schmidt T, Ritter M, Dirks J, Gärtner BC, Sester U, Sester M. Cytomegalovirus-specific T-cell immunity to assign the infection status in individuals with passive immunity: a proof of principle. J Clin Virol Off Publ Pan Am Soc Clin Virol. 2012;54:272–5.

73. Tuomela M, Stanescu I, Krohn K. Validation overview of bio-analytical methods. Gene Ther. 2005;12 Suppl 1:S131–138.

17

5-Aminolevulinic acid regulates the immune response in LPS-stimulated RAW 264.7 macrophages

Yuta Sugiyama[1], Yukari Hiraiwa[1], Yuichiro Hagiya[1], Motowo Nakajima[2], Tohru Tanaka[2] and Shun-ichiro Ogura[1*] ⓘ

Abstract

Background: Macrophages are crucial players in a variety of inflammatory responses to environmental cues. However, it has been widely reported that macrophages cause chronic inflammation and are involved in a variety of diseases, such as obesity, diabetes, metabolic syndrome, and cancer. In this study, we report the suppressive effect of 5-aminolevulinic acid (ALA), via the HO-1-related system, on the immune response of the LPS-stimulated mouse macrophage cell line RAW264.7.

Results: RAW264.7 cells were treated with LPS with or without ALA, and proinflammatory mediator expression levels and phagocytic ability were assessed. ALA treatment resulted in the attenuation of iNOS and NO expression and the downregulation of proinflammatory cytokines (TNF-α, cyclooxygenase2, IL-1β, IL-6). In addition, ALA treatment did not affect the phagocytic ability of macrophages. To our knowledge, this study is the first to investigate the effect of ALA on macrophage function. Our findings suggest that ALA may have high potential as a novel anti-inflammatory agent.

Conclusions: In the present study, we showed that exogenous addition of ALA induces HO-1 and leads to the downregulation of NO and some proinflammatory cytokines. These findings support ALA as a promising anti-inflammatory agent.

Keywords: 5-Aminolevulinic acid, Macrophage, Heme oxygenase-1, LPS, Anti inflammation

Background

Recent research has revealed a variety of macrophage roles and functions, and macrophages have a very important role in maintaining homeostasis and a normal physiological condition by adjusting various biological activities. When the elaborate balance of macrophage activity collapses, macrophages can cause various diseases [1]. For example, a number of recent investigations have indicated the important relationship between the particular steps of colorectal cancer development and inflammation due to obesity, which is mediated by proinflammatory cytokines (e.g., interleukin-6 (IL-6)) and tumor necrosis factor-α (TNF-α) secreted by macrophages [2, 3]. Therefore, to avoid lifestyle-related diseases caused by macrophages, it is important to prevent abnormal activation and to keep macrophages within their proper range of activity. Lipopolysaccharide (LPS) is a component of the outer membrane of Gram-negative bacteria. Since LPS is widely used in studies of inflammation and chronic inflammation can be modeled by administration of LPS in vivo [4, 5], we used LPS to study inflammation in an in vitro model.

Heme oxygenase-1 (HO-1) is a well-known antioxidant that catalyzes the degradation of heme [6]. Heme digestion implemented by HO-1 leads to the production of biliverdin, ferrous iron, and carbon monoxide. Biliverdin is reduced promptly to bilirubin by biliverdin reductase. It is generally assumed that these heme-related catabolites have antioxidant activity [7]. For example, carbon monoxide mediates potent anti-inflammatory

* Correspondence: sogura@bio.titech.ac.jp
[1]School of Life Science and Technology, Tokyo Institute of Technology, Yokohama, Kanagawa, Japan
Full list of author information is available at the end of the article

effects. Otterbein et al. (2000) revealed that carbon monoxide at low concentrations inhibited the expression of the lipopolysaccharide (LPS)-induced proinflammatory cytokines TNF-α, interleukin-1β (IL-1β), and others [8].

5-Aminolevulinic acid (ALA) is a natural amino acid and a precursor in the porphyrin synthesis pathway leading to heme [9]. The first and normally rate-limiting step of heme synthesis is the mitochondrial enzyme 5-aminolevulinic acid synthase (ALAS). Thus, exogenous ALA addition leads to the upregulation of heme synthesis and heme-related enzymes. In addition, it is well known that ALA exposure results in HO-1 induction. In particular, Nishio (2014) reported that the addition of ALA to a macrophage cell line (RAW 264 cells) increases heme, which inactivates Bach1, and that HO-1 expression is induced via activation of MAPK [10]. However, the functions of macrophage cells under HO-1 induction by ALA are not well understood.

In this study, we investigated the effect of ALA on macrophage function. To this end, we utilized the LPS-stimulated mouse macrophage cell line RAW264.7, and evaluated the effect of ALA on inflammatory cytokine expression levels and macrophage phagocytic ability.

Results

HO-1 protein expression analysis of ALA-treated RAW264.7 macrophages

We first examined the effect of ALA on the RAW264.7 macrophage cell line by western blot analysis of HO-1 and MTT viability assays (Fig. 1). Cells were seeded and incubated with medium containing 1 mM ALA. After 24 h of incubation, cells were used for each assessment. HO-1 protein expression levels of the 1 mM ALA-added group were significantly upregulated compared with those of the control group in a time-dependent manner (Fig. 1a). These results are consistent with previous studies [10]. No decrease in cell viability was observed in 1 mM ALA (Fig. 1b). These results suggest that ALA addition induces HO-1 protein expression without noticeable cell damage in RAW264.7 cells.

iNOS and NO expression analysis of RAW264.7 macrophages under LPS stimulation with ALA

Since we evaluated the effect of ALA alone on HO-1, we investigated the effect of ALA on the activity of the macrophage cell RAW264.7. Nitric oxide (NO), a free radical produced by nitric oxide synthase (NOS), has been shown to have a number of important biological functions, including tumor cell killing and host defense against intracellular pathogens. iNOS is generally not present in inactive cells but is induced by various stimuli such as LPS [11]. Therefore, iNOS and NO expression analysis of RAW264.7 macrophages under LPS stimulation with ALA was performed to assess the effect of ALA on the immune response.

RAW264.7 cells were cultured in 1 μg/mL of LPS with or without 1 mM ALA for 24 h. After culture, mRNA and protein expression levels of iNOS were assessed by quantitative real-time PCR and western blot analysis, respectively (Fig. 2). iNOS mRNA expression levels were clearly upregulated under LPS treatment;

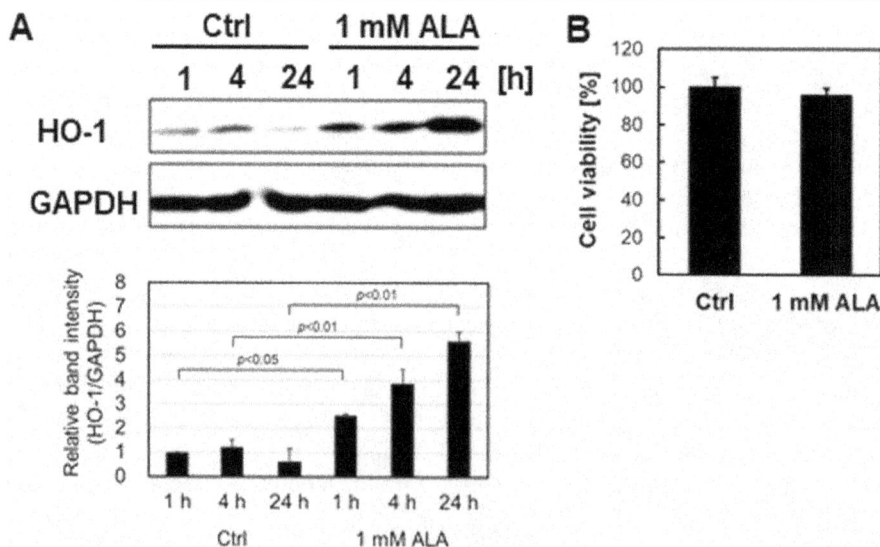

Fig. 1 ALA induced HO-1 protein expression level without reducing cell viability in RAW264.7 macrophage. **a** RAW264.7 cells were incubated with or without 1 mM of ALA for 24 h. After treatment, HO-1 protein expression level was analyzed by the Western blotting method. Upper panel, representative Western blot bands. Lower panel, summarized bar graph shows band intensity presented as ratio of HO-1 over GAPDH. Values are means ± SD, n = 2. **b** The viability of RAW264.7 cells were tested by MTT assay after 24-h incubation in medium containing 1 mM of ALA. Values are means ± SD, n = 3, p values are shown in figures

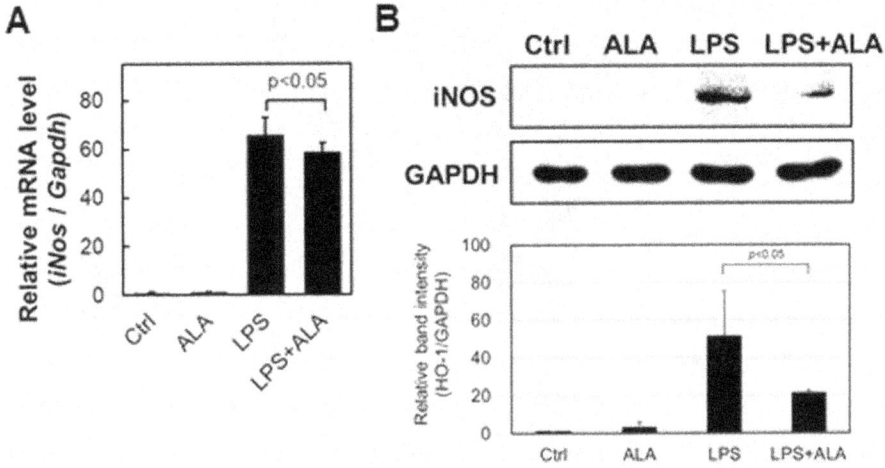

Fig. 2 ALA significantly reduced LPS-induced iNOS mRNA and protein expression. RAW264.7 was incubated in 1 μg/mL LPS condition with or without 1 mM ALA. After incubation, **a** iNOS mRNA levels were analyzed by Real-time PCR (Values are means ± SD, n = 3) and **b** iNOS protein levels were analyzed by Western blotting (Upper panel, representative Western blot bands. Lower panel, summarized bar graph shows band intensity presented as ratio of iNOS over GAPDH. Values are means ± SD, n = 2, p values are shown in figures)

there was no significant effect on iNOS expression by ALA. However, LPS-stimulated iNOS mRNA expression with ALA was significantly lower than that without ALA ($p < 0.05$). Similarly, iNOS protein expression levels were increased by LPS stimulation and were decreased by ALA treatment. These results therefore confirmed that iNOS was induced by LPS stimulation, which is similar to other reports suggesting that ALA reduced iNOS induction by LPS [12].

Next, NO expression levels of RAW264.7 cells cultured 24 h with each concentration of LPS and ALA were measured by the Griess assay (Fig. 3). First, NO expression levels were tested under the LPS-alone condition. NO was increased in an LPS dose-dependent manner (Fig. 3a). Second, the fluctuation of NO levels with ALA under 1000 ng/mL LPS was measured. A significant reduction of NO was observed in an ALA dose-dependent manner (Fig. 3b). These data indicated

that ALA has the ability to downregulate mRNA and protein expression of iNOS, which followed NO synthesis in RAW264.7 cells stimulated by LPS. Since several reports have suggested the relationship of HO-1 and iNOS to NO production, it was suggested that ALA-induced HO-1 may cause the downregulation of iNOS and NO expression [13, 14].

Proinflammatory cytokine expression analysis of RAW264.7 macrophages under LPS stimulation with ALA

Since ALA showed a decreasing effect on iNOS and NO, we investigated other proinflammatory cytokines known to be induced by LPS stimulation. After LPS stimulation in 24-h culture with or without ALA, the mRNA expression levels of TNF-α, cyclooxygenase2 (COX2), IL-1β, and IL-6 were assessed by real-time PCR analysis (Fig. 4). The mRNA levels of each of the proinflammatory cytokines were upregulated by LPS

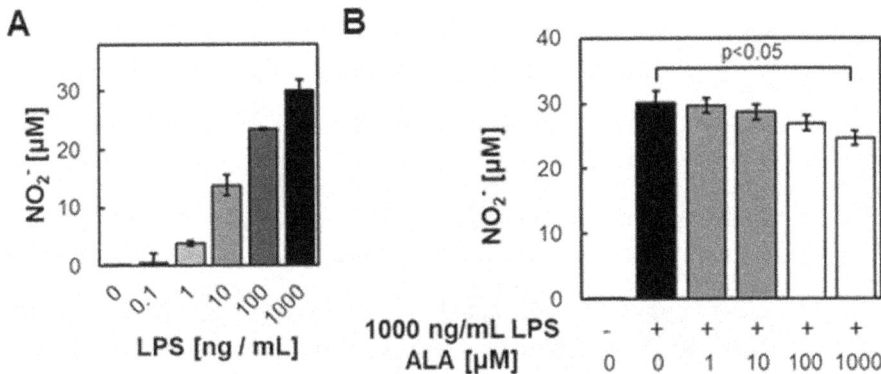

Fig. 3 ALA-treatment significantly reduced NO$_2^-$ expression in RAW264.7 macrophages stimulated by LPS. NO$_2^-$ expression levels of RAW264.7 were tested after incubation with several conditions of (**a**) LPS or (**b**) ALA with 1000 ng/mL LPS. Values are means ± SD, n = 3, p values are shown in figures

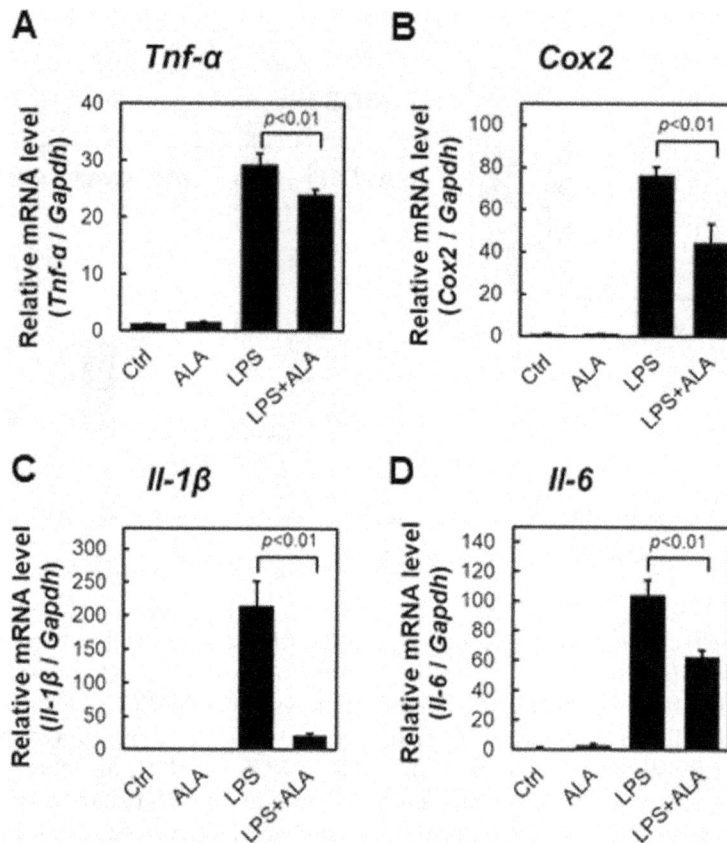

Fig. 4 ALA-treatment shown significant inhibitory effect on proinflammatory cytokines. **a** TNF-α, **b** COX2, **c** IL-1β and **d** IL-6 mRNA expression levels of RAW264.7 were analyzed after 1 mL ALA treatment and/or 1 μg/mL LPS. Values are means ± SD, $n = 3$, p values are shown in figures

treatment. In contrast, all of the LPS-inducible cytokines were significantly reduced with ALA addition compared with the LPS-alone condition. These results are consistent with Otterbein et al. (2000) and they suggested that carbon monoxide, which is the by-product of heme degradation by HO-1, inhibits the expression of LPS-induced proinflammatory cytokines. Thus, our data indicated that the addition of ALA leads to HO-1 expression and a downregulative effect on proinflammatory mediators.

Phagocytic ability assays of RAW264.7 macrophages under LPS stimulation with ALA

In general, phagocytosis is a characteristic feature of macrophages. We tested the effect of ALA on the phagocytic ability of macrophages because it was revealed that ALA has a downregulative effect on proinflammatory cytokines. To examine the phagocytic ability of RAW264.7 cells, we used fluorescence beads. After pretreatment with 1 μg/mL LPS with or without 1 mM ALA for 24 h, RAW264.7 cells were cultured in a medium containing 1×10^8 particles of fluorescence beads for 5 h. Cells were then observed by fluorescence microscopy, and digital images were obtained. Figure 5a

shows the intracellular beads in red fluorescence. Figure 5b shows the relative particle intake normalized by cellular protein as phagocytic ability. LPS stimuli induced the upregulation of phagocytic ability ($p < 0.05$). Moreover, the co-incubation of LPS and ALA resulted in significantly higher particle intakes ($p < 0.01$ compared with the LPS-alone condition). These data show that ALA alone has no influence on phagocytic ability. Although our finding show that ALA exhibits a downregulative effect on proinflammatory cytokines, they also show that ALA significantly upregulated phagocytic ability with LPS stimulation.

Discussion

In this study, we evaluated the functions of ALA-induced expression of HO-1 by macrophage cells by ALA under LPS treatment. First, we showed that ALA addition induces HO-1 protein expression without noticeable cell damage. Second, we revealed that ALA causes changes in several proinflammatory factors induced by LPS stimulation. In particular, ALA treatment induced the attenuation of iNOS and NO expression and the downregulation of proinflammatory cytokines (TNF-α, COX2, IL-1β, and IL-6), with no reductive

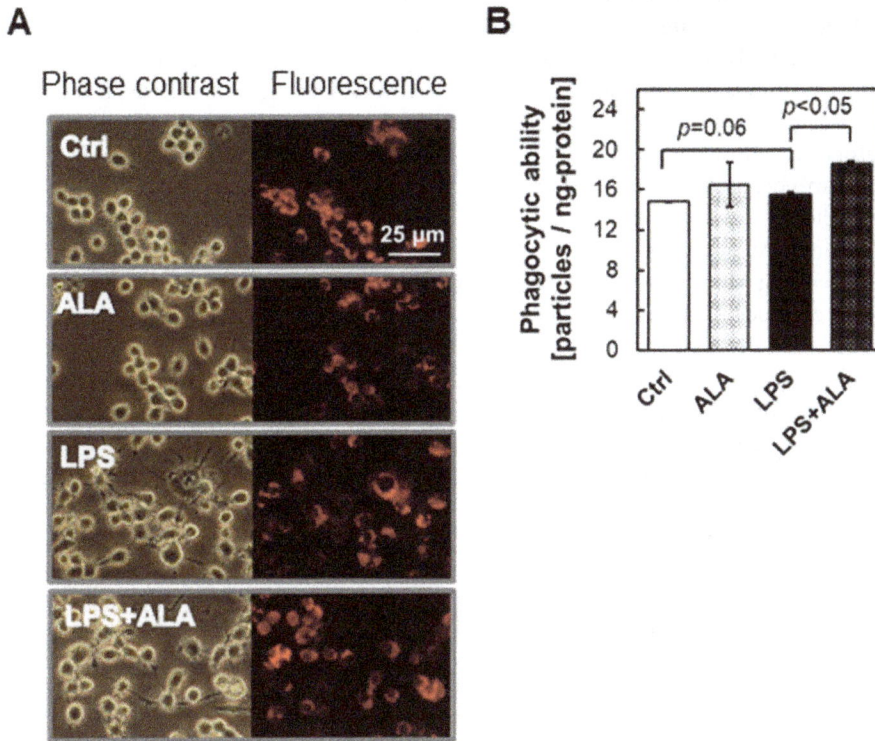

Fig. 5 Phagocytotic ability was more strongly increased by co-administration of LPS and ALA than by LPS alone. Phagocytotic ability was estimated using fluorescence beads. RAW264.7 was treated with 1 µg/mL LPS and/or 1 mM ALA for 24 h and incubated for 5 h in culture medium containing 1×10^8 particles of fluorescence beads. **a** Fluorescence microscopy observation was performed (left, phase contrast; right, fluorescence). **b** Fluorescence beads uptake was assessed as phagocytotic ability by using fluorescence spectrophotometer (Ex. 535 nm, Em. 570 nm). Values are means ± SD, $n = 3$, p values are shown in figure

effect of phagocytic ability, were shown. These data indicate that ALA, as a HO-1 inducer, has promise as a novel anti-inflammatory agent.

HO-1 is the first and rate-limiting enzyme in the action of degrade of heme into carbon monoxide, ferritin, and biliverdin. Accumulating evidence suggests that carbon monoxide and bilirubin, produced from biliverdin by the enzyme biliverdin reductase, are potent anti-inflammatory mediators [6]. It is generally assumed that this HO-1 and a bi-product-related system may act as a crucial regulator in inflammatory processes, and regulates the balance between proinflammatory and anti-inflammatory mediators.

As an immune response to LPS stimulation, macrophages upregulate their production of various inflammatory cytokines. Indeed, there are several reports on the relationship between HO-1 and the LPS-inducible reaction in macrophages. For example, it has been suggested that HO-1 expression is induced via depletion of intracellular glutathione by LPS-induced ROS [15]. Otterbein et al. (2000) have shown that carbon monoxide produced by HO-1 inhibits the expression of LPS-induced proinflammatory cytokines such as TNF-α and IL-1β [8]. They suggest that the effect of HO-1 is based on the mechanism of p38 MAPK inhibition. In addition, carbon monoxide can bind to the iron atom of heme in heme proteins, such as NOS, and modulate their function [16]. Thus, carbon monoxide may weaken the activity of iNOS by combining with heme. On the other hand, bilirubin is generally well known as a potent reducer that can scavenge radical compounds. Since NO produced by iNOS in the immune response is a radical, bilirubin reduces NO, thus suppressing a series of NO reactions [17]. As a broad reaction by several kinds of radicals or immune-responsible factors may occur against immune stimulation, it can be said that bilirubin has an important role in arresting these reactions [18, 19]. To our knowledge, Fe^{2+} does not have an anti-inflammatory role. Rather, Fe^{2+} has a cytotoxic effect via the Fenton reaction [20]. Thus, we consider that Fe^{2+} did not have a key function as an anti-inflammatory agent of ALA in our study. Berberat et al. reported that the ferritin heavy chain induced by Fe^{2+} protects endothelial cells from apoptosis induced by a variety of stimuli, such as ischemia-reperfusion injury in vitro and in vivo [21]. This finding may offer an anti-oxidative role of Fe^{2+} as the downstream molecule of HO-1. From the above consideration, we hypothesize the following mechanism of the anti-inflammatory effect of ALA. ALA may upregulate heme synthesis, which in turn increases HO-1, which then acts to degrade heme. At the same time, the catabolites of heme increase and show a suppressive effect on iNOS and other proinflammatory cytokines.

Macrophage cells have been shown to contribute to inflammation-related diseases through the secretion of proinflammatory cytokines. As many researchers have reported, the HO-1-related system of macrophages may be a therapeutic target for chronic inflammation [22–24]. For example, Hualin (2012) revealed that hemin upregulated HO-1 expression in rat alveolar macrophages, and that pretreatment with hemin inhibited LPS-induced NO production, developed arginase activity, and enhanced phagocytotic ability via the p38 MAPK pathway in these cells [25]. In addition, Oh et al. showed that HO-1 is induced by the addition of H_2S [26]. They found that H_2S suppressed the activation of NF-κB by LPS, which in turn then suppressed iNOS expression and NO production. They also showed that knock down of HO-1 with siRNA cancels the effect of suppression of iNOS expression and NO production. More interestingly, they suggested that CO is a particularly important factor since the same effect as that by adding H_2S is also obtained by adding CO alone, which is a product of HO-1. We observed HO-1 upregulation (Fig. 1) and attenuation of iNOS and NO expression by ALA exposure (Figs. 2 and 3); therefore, we suggest that a similar mechanism is involved.

In the classical classification, there are two types of macrophages: M1 and M2. The features of M1 macrophages are glycolysis and the secretion of proinflammatory cytokines. On the other hand, M2 macrophages show higher oxidative metabolism and anti-inflammatory cytokine production, such as IL-10. Vats (2006) revealed that the metabolic shift by overexpression of PGC1β attenuates macrophage-mediated inflammation (e.g., suppression of IL-6 expression) [27]. On the other hand, our previous study demonstrated that ALA has an upregulative effect on aerobic respiration based on the induction of the mitochondrial respiratory chain complex IV, a heme protein enzyme named as cytochrome c oxidase [28, 29]. We consider that the mechanism of this phenomenon is that ALA administration upregulates heme synthesis. This leads to the induction of hemoprotein synthesis, which is followed by the induction of heme protein assembling, as we have previously shown in cytochrome P450, a heme protein that catalyzes the oxidation of lipophilic substrates [30]. The ALA-effect of NO attenuation and the downregulation of proinflammatory cytokines may be caused by not only the HO-1-related system but also a metabolic shift caused by ALA.

ALA is the natural biochemical precursor of porphyrin synthesis and broadly exists in animals and plants. In animal cells, the synthesized porphyrin is converted to heme with iron by ferrochelatase. The rate-limiting enzyme in porphyrin synthesis is ALA synthetase, the role of which is ALA synthesis from glycine and succinyl CoA in mitochondria. Therefore, exogeneous ALA addition causes the upregulation of porphyrin synthesis. Moreover, in cancer cells, ALA administration induces the accumulation of fluorescent porphyrins [9]. Thus, ALA is a widely used compound for tumor photodynamic diagnosis. For example, the W. Stummer group reported that there are no concerns regarding the toxicological safety of fluorescence-guided surgery with 5-aminolevulinic acid in phase III clinical trials [31].

Conclusions

In this study, we showed that exogenous addition of ALA, the precursor of heme, induces HO-1 and leads to the downregulation of NO and some proinflammatory cytokines. To our knowledge, this study is the first to investigate the effects of ALA on macrophage function. These findings support ALA as a promising anti-inflammatory agent. Further studies are needed to comprehensively examine the effect of ALA on macrophages.

Methods
Biochemicals

The substrate ALA hydrochloride was purchased from Cosmo Oil Co., Ltd. (Tokyo, Japan). RPMI-1640 medium and Antibiotic-Antimycotic solution (ABAM, Penicillin-Streptomycin-Amphotericin B mixture) were obtained from Nacalai Tesque (Kyoto, Japan). Fetal bovine serum (FBS) was purchased from Invitrogen (Carlsbad, CA, USA). The MTT reagent was purchased from Sigma-Aldrich (St. Louis, MO, USA). All other chemicals used were of analytical grade.

Cell culture and viability assays

The mouse macrophage cell line RAW264.7 was purchased from RIKEN Cell Bank (Ibaraki, Japan). The cells were grown in DMEM, supplemented with 10% FBS and ABAM, and incubated at 37 °C in an incubator with a controlled humidified atmosphere containing 5% CO_2. Cell viability was measured by the MTT assay as described previously [32].

Western blot analysis

Western blot analysis was performed as previously described with some modifications [33]. For immunoblot analysis, samples were first treated with the SDS-PAGE sample buffer solution containing 10% (v/v) 2-mercaptoethanol. Thereafter, sample proteins were electrophoretically separated by 15% polyacrylamide gels and then electroblotted onto a polyvinylidene fluoride membrane (Millipore, Bedford, MA). The membrane was incubated in blocking solution containing 5% (*w/v*) skim milk in TTBS [20 mM Tris-HCl (pH 7.4), 150 mM NaCl, 0.05% (v/v) Tween 20] at 4 °C overnight. We used an antibody specific to HO-1-1 (1:200, mouse monoclonal, ab13248, Abcam, Cambridge, UK) [34], iNOS (1:500, inducible nitric oxide synthase, mouse monoclonal, sc-7271, Santa Cruz Biotechnology, Inc., TX, USA) [35] or GAPDH (1:1000, mouse monoclonal, 05–50,118, American Research Products, Inc., Belmont, MA, USA) [36] as the primary antibody. For the secondary antibody, we used anti-mouse IgG horseradish peroxidase (HRP)-conjugated antibody (Cell Signaling Technology, Inc., Beverly, MA, USA) at 1:3000 dilution. HRP-dependent luminescence was developed with Western Lightning Chemiluminescent Reagent Plus (PerkinElmer Life and Analytical Sciences, Inc., Waltham, MA, USA) and detected with a Lumino Imaging Analyzer ImageQuant LAS 4000 mini (GE Healthcare UK, Amersham Place, England). The intensity of chemiluminescence was determined with an ImageQuantTM TL Analysis Toolbox (GE Healthcare UK, Amersham Place, England).

Quantitative real-time PCR analysis using SYBR green assays

Total RNA was isolated using a NucleoSpin® RNA II (Macherey-Nagel, Düren, Mannheim, Germany) kit according to the manufacturer's instructions. The concentration and quality of RNA were analyzed using a UV-Vis spectrophotometer (Shimadzu). Subsequently, cDNA was synthesized from total RNA using a Prime-Script RT reagent kit with a gDNA Eraser (TaKaRa Bio, Otsu, Japan) according to the manufacturer's instructions. The expressions of iNOS, COX2 (cyclooxygenase2), TNF-α, IL-1β, IL-6, and GAPDH mRNAs were determined using a Thermal Cycler Dice® Real-Time System Single (TaKaRa Bio, Shiga, Japan) with a SYBR Premix Ex Taq (TaKaRa Bio). Primers are shown in Table 1.

The amplification conditions included 30 s at 95 °C; 50 cycles at 95 °C for 5 s and 60 °C for 60 s each; dissociation for 15 s at 95 °C and 30 s at 60 °C; and then 15 s at 95 °C on a Thermal Cycler Dice Real-Time System. Thermal Cycler Dice Real-Time System analysis software (TaKaRa, Shiga, Japan) was used for data analysis. The Ct values (cycle threshold) were calculated using the crossing-point method, and the genes expression levels were measured by comparison with a standard curve. The expression levels of target genes were normalized to those of GAPDH.

Measurement of nitric oxide (NO)

Nitrite, a stable metabolite of NO, was measured with a Griess Reagent System (Promega, Madison, WI, USA) according to the manufacturer's instructions.

Phagocytic ability assays

Phagocytosis assays were performed using Fluoresbrite™ Yellow Orange (YO) Carboxylate Microspheres (18720–10,

Table 1 Sequences of primers used in real-time PCR

iNOS	forward	5'-CCTCCTCCACCCTACCAAGT-3'
	reverse	5'-CACCCAAAGTGCTTCAGTCA-3'
COX2	forward	5'-AGGAGACATCCTGATCCTGGT-3'
	reverse	5'-GTTCAGCCTGGCAAGTCTTT-3'
TNF-α	forward	5'-GTGGAACTGGCAGAAGAGGC-3'
	reverse	5'-AGACAGAAGAGCGTGGTGGC-3'
IL-1β	forward	5'-CCTCGTGCTGTCGGACCCAT-3'
	reverse	5'-CAGGCTTGTGCTCTGCTTGTGA-3'
IL-6	forward	5'-CCGGAGAGGAGACTTCACAG-3'
	reverse	5'-CAGAATTGCCATTGCACAAC-3'
GAPDH	forward	5'-TGTGTCCGTCGTGGATCTGA-3'
	reverse	5'-TTGCTGTTGAAGTCGCAGGAG-3'

Polysciences, Inc., Warrington, PA, USA) according to the manufacturer's instructions. Briefly, 5×10^6 cells were inoculated in a 3 cm dish and incubated with LPS and ALA for 24 h following medium change. After the incubation, medium was changed to 2 mL of fresh medium without FBS and 20 μL of 1×10^8 particles/mL of Fluoresbrite® Microparticles solution was added. After 5 h of incubation, cells were washed three times with PBS. Cells were then observed with a fluorescence microscope (CKX41, Olympus, Japan) equipped with a digital camera (E620, Olympus), and digital images were obtained. Fluoresbrite® Microparticle fluorescence was measured at excitation and emission wavelengths of 535 nm and 570 nm, respectively. To determine the intracellular particle number, the macrophages were collected by a cell scraper and resuspended in PBS. The Fluorescence intensity was measured (excitation and emission wavelengths of 465 nm and 550 nm, respectively) and compared to a standard curve obtained from fluorescence particles alone in PBS. After measurement, cells were lysed by 0.1 M NaOH and protein concentration was measured by Bradford protein assay.

Statistical analysis

Data are expressed as means ± standard deviation in two or three independent experiments. Statistical significances were analyzed using the Tukey-Kramer's test with an α level of 0.05. Statistical analyses were performed using a software, JMP® 13 (SAS Institute Inc., Cary, NC, USA).

Abbreviations
ABAM: Antibiotic-Antimycotic solution; ALA: 5-Aminolevulinic acid; ALAS: 5-Aminolevulinic acid synthase; COX2: Cyclooxygenase2; FBS: Fetal bovine serum; HO-1: Heme oxygenase-1; IL-1β: Interleukin-1β; iNOS: Inducible nitric oxide synthase; LPS: Lipopolysaccharide; NO: Nitric oxide; TNF-α: Tumor necrosis factor-α

Acknowledgements
Not applicable

Funding

SBI Pharmaceuticals CO., LTD., provided support in the form of salaries for authors [MN, TT] but did not have any additional role in the study design, data collection and analysis, decision to publish, or preparation of the manuscript. The specific roles of these authors are articulated in the 'author contributions' section.

Authors' contributions

YS designed the study and a major contributor in writing the manuscript. All other authors have contributed to data collection and interpretation, and critically reviewed the manuscript. All authors approved the final version of the manuscript and agree to be accountable for all aspects of the work in ensuring that questions related to the accuracy or integrity of any part of the work are appropriately investigated and resolved.

Competing interests

We have the following interests: Motowo Nakajima and Tohru Tanaka are employed by SBI Pharmaceuticals CO., LTD. There are no patents, products in development or marketed products to declare in relation to the contents of the manuscript. This does not alter our adherence to all the BMC policies on sharing data and materials, as detailed online in the guide for authors.

Author details

[1]School of Life Science and Technology, Tokyo Institute of Technology, Yokohama, Kanagawa, Japan. [2]SBI Pharma CO., LTD., Roppongi, Tokyo 106-6020, Japan.

References

1. Wynn TA, Chawla A, Pollard JW. Macrophage biology in development, homeostasis and disease. Nature. 2013;496:445–55.
2. Pietrzyk L, Torres A, Maciejewski R, Torres K. Obesity and obese-related chronic low-grade inflammation in promotion of colorectal Cancer development. Asian Pac J Cancer Prev. 2015;16:4161–8.
3. Zeyda M, Stulnig TM. Adipose tissue macrophages. Immunol Lett. 2007;112:61–7.
4. Ostos MA, Recalde D, Zakin MM, Scott-Algara D. Implication of natural killer T cells in atherosclerosis development during a LPS-induced chronic inflammation. FEBS Lett. 2002;519:23–9.
5. Noailles A, Maneu V, Campello L, Lax P, Cuenca N. Systemic inflammation induced by lipopolysaccharide aggravates inherited retinal dystrophy. Cell Death Dis. 2018;9:350.
6. Kirkby KA, Adin CA. Products of heme oxygenase and their potential therapeutic applications. Am J Physiol Physiol. 2006;290:F563–71.
7. Schumacher A, Zenclussen AC. Effects of heme oxygenase-1 on innate and adaptive immune responses promoting pregnancy success and allograft tolerance. Front Pharmacol. 2015;5:288.
8. Choi AMK, Otterbein LE, Bach FH, Alam J, Soares M, Tao Lu H, et al. Carbon monoxide has anti-inflammatory effects involving the mitogen-activated protein kinase pathway. Nat Med. 2000;6:422–8.
9. Ishizuka M, Abe F, Sano Y, Takahashi K, Inoue K, Nakajima M, et al. Novel development of 5-aminolevurinic acid (ALA) in cancer diagnoses and therapy. Int Immunopharmacol. 2011;11:358–65.
10. Nishio Y, Fujino M, Zhao M, Ishii T, Ishizuka M, Ito H, et al. 5-Aminolevulinic acid combined with ferrous iron enhances the expression of heme oxygenase-1. Int Immunopharmacol. 2014;19:300–7.
11. Chan ED, Riches DWH, Altmeyer M, Barthel M, Eberhard M, Rehrauer H, et al. IFN-γ + LPS induction of iNOS is modulated by ERK , JNK / SAPK , and p38 mapk in a mouse macrophage cell line; 2012;
12. Jacobs AT, Ignarro LJ. Lipopolysaccharide-induced expression of interferon-beta mediates the timing of inducible nitric-oxide synthase induction in RAW 264.7 macrophages. J Biol Chem. 2001;276:47950–7.
13. Kim Y-S, Pi S-H, Lee Y-M, Lee S-I, Kim E-C. The anti-inflammatory role of Heme Oxygenase-1 in lipopolysaccharide and cytokine-stimulated inducible nitric oxide synthase and nitric oxide production in human periodontal ligament cells. J Periodontol. 2009;80:2045–55.
14. Ashino T, Yamanaka R, Yamamoto M, Shimokawa H, Sekikawa K, Iwakura Y, et al. Negative feedback regulation of lipopolysaccharide-induced inducible nitric oxide synthase gene expression by heme oxygenase-1 induction in macrophages. Mol Immunol. 2008;45:2106–15.
15. Srisook K, Cha Y-N. Super-induction of HO-1 in macrophages stimulated with lipopolysaccharide by prior depletion of glutathione decreases iNOS expression and NO production. Nitric Oxide. 2005;12:70–9.
16. Kachalova GS, Popov AN, Bartunik HD. A Steric Mechanism for Inhibition of CO Binding to Heme Proteins. Science. 1999;284:473–6.
17. Wang WW, Smith DLH, Zucker SD. Bilirubin inhibits iNOS expression and NO production in response to endotoxin in rats. Hepatology. 2004;40:424–33.
18. Baranano DE, Rao M, Ferris CD, Snyder SH. Biliverdin reductase: a major physiologic cytoprotectant. Proc Natl Acad Sci U S A. 2002;99:16093–8.
19. McDonagh AF. The biliverdin–bilirubin antioxidant cycle of cellular protection: missing a wheel? Free Radic Biol Med. 2010;49:814–20.
20. Winterbourn CC. Toxicity of iron and hydrogen peroxide: the Fenton reaction. Toxicol Lett. 1995;82–83:969–74.
21. Berberat PO, Katori M, Kaczmarek E, Anselmo D, Lassman C, Ke B, et al. Heavy chain ferritin acts as an anti-apoptotic gene that protects livers from ischemia-reperfusion injury. FASEB J. 2003;17:1724–6.
22. Vijayan V, Mueller S, Baumgart-Vogt E, Immenschuh S. Heme oxygenase-1 as a therapeutic target in inflammatory disorders of the gastrointestinal tract. World J Gastroenterol. 2010;16:3112–9.
23. Poss KD, Tonegawa S. Heme oxygenase 1 is required for mammalian iron reutilization. Proc Natl Acad Sci U S A. 1997;94:10919–24.
24. Yachie A, Niida Y, Wada T, Igarashi N, Kaneda H, Toma T, et al. Oxidative stress causes enhanced endothelial cell injury in human heme oxygenase-1 deficiency. J Clin Invest. 1999;103:129–35.
25. Hualin C, Wenli X, Dapeng L, Xijing L, Xiuhua P, Qingfeng P. The anti-inflammatory mechanism of Heme Oxygenase-1 induced by hemin in primary rat alveolar macrophages. Inflammation. 2012;35:1087–93.
26. Oh GS, Pae HO, Lee BS, Kim BN, Kim JM, Kim HR, et al. Hydrogen sulfide inhibits nitric oxide production and nuclear factor-κB via heme oxygenase-1 expression in RAW264.7 macrophages stimulated with lipopolysaccharide. Free Radic Biol Med. 2006;41:106–19.
27. Vats D, Mukundan L, Odegaard JI, Zhang L, Smith KL, Morel CR, et al. Oxidative metabolism and PGC-1β attenuate macrophage-mediated inflammation. Cell Metab. 2006;4:13–24.
28. Ogura S-I, Maruyama K, Hagiya Y, Sugiyama Y, Tsuchiya K, Takahashi K, et al. The effect of 5-aminolevulinic acid on cytochrome c oxidase activity in mouse liver. BMC Res Notes. 2011;4:66.
29. Sugiyama Y, Hagiya Y, Nakajima M, Ishizuka M, Tanaka T, Ogura S-I. The heme precursor 5-aminolevulinic acid disrupts the Warburg effect in tumor cells and induces caspase-dependent apoptosis. Oncol Rep. 2013;31:1282–6.
30. Miura M, Ito K, Hayashi M, Nakajima M, Tanaka T, Ogura S. The Effect of 5-Aminolevulinic Acid on Cytochrome P450-Mediated Prodrug Activation. PLoS One. 2015;10:e0131793.
31. Stummer W, Pichlmeier U, Meinel T, Wiestler OD, Zanella F, Reulen H-J, et al. Fluorescence-guided surgery with 5-aminolevulinic acid for resection of malignant glioma: a randomised controlled multicentre phase III trial. Lancet Oncol. 2006;7:392–401.
32. Tamura A, Onishi Y, An R, Koshiba S, Wakabayashi K, Hoshijima K, et al. In vitro evaluation of photosensitivity risk related to genetic polymorphisms of human ABC transporter ABCG2 and inhibition by drugs. Drug Metab Pharmacokinet. 2007;22:428–40.
33. Adachi T, Nakagawa H, Chung I, Hagiya Y, Hoshijima K, Noguchi N, et al. Nrf2-dependent and -independent induction of ABC transporters ABCC1, ABCC2, and ABCG2 in HepG2 cells under oxidative stress. J Exp Ther Oncol. 2007;6:335–48.

34. Sun Y, Zhang Y, Zhao D, Ding G, Huang S, Zhang A, et al. Rotenone remarkably attenuates oxidative stress, inflammation, and fibrosis in chronic obstructive Uropathy. Mediat Inflamm. 2014;2014:1–9.

35. Huang SC-C, Everts B, Ivanova Y, O'Sullivan D, Nascimento M, Smith AM, et al. Cell-intrinsic lysosomal lipolysis is essential for alternative activation of macrophages. Nat Immunol. 2014;15:846–55.

36. Hashimoto M, Murata K, Ishida J, Kanou A, Kasuya Y, Fukamizu A. Severe Hypomyelination and developmental defects are caused in mice lacking protein arginine methyltransferase 1 (PRMT1) in the central nervous system. J Biol Chem. 2016;291:2237–45.

18

Variation in IL-21-secreting circulating follicular helper T cells in Kawasaki disease

Meng Xu[1†], Yanfang Jiang[2,3,4†], Jian Zhang[5], Yan Zheng[5], Deying Liu[6], Lishuang Guo[1] and Sirui Yang[1*] 🔟

Abstract

Objective: Circulating follicular helper T (cTfh) cells are a specialized subset of CD4[+] T cells that express the CXC-chemokine receptor 5 (CXCR5). These cells exhibit immune activities by inducing B cell differentiation and proliferation via the secretion of interleukin (IL)-21. Multiple studies have demonstrated that cTfh cells are associated with the progression and severity of numerous diseases. To investigate the role of cTfh cells in the development of Kawasaki disease (KD), we analyzed the distinct subpopulations of cTfh cells and serum IL-21 levels in different phases of KD.

Methods: According to the differential expression of inducible co-stimulator (ICOS) and programmed cell death protein 1 (PD-1), cTfh cells were divided into distinct subsets. We used flow cytometry and flow cytometric bead arrays (CBA) to analyze subsets of CD4[+]CXCR5[+] T cells and serum IL-21 levels. The samples were collected from control subjects and Kawasaki disease patients in the acute and remission phases.

Results: In the acute phase (AP), the percentages of ICOS^{high}PD-1^{high}, ICOS[+]PD-1[+], ICOS[−]PD-1[+], CD45RA[−]IL-21[+] cTfh cells and serum IL-21 levels significantly increased. Furthermore, the percentages of ICOS^{high}PD-1^{high} and ICOS[+]PD-1[+] cTfh cells positively correlated with erythrocyte sedimentation rate (ESR) and C-reactive protein (CRP) values, whereas the percentage of ICOS[−]PD-1[+] cTfh cells indicated negative correlations. The percentages of ICOS[+]PD-1[+], ICOS^{high}PD-1^{high} and CD45RA[−]IL-21[+] cTfh cells correlated positively with serum IL-21 levels. In the remission phase (RP), the percentages of ICOS[−]PD-1[+], CD45RA[−]IL-21[+] cTfh cells and serum IL-21 levels were significantly decreased. In contrast, the percentages of ICOS[+]PD-1[+], ICOS^{high}PD-1^{high}, and ICOS[+]PD-1[−] cTfh cells were further increased. Among these subsets, only CD45RA[−]IL-21[+] cTfh cells correlated positively with serum IL-21 levels.

Conclusions: The present study is the first investigation that examined the distribution of circulating cTfh cell subsets in Kawasaki disease. Both cTfh cells and serum IL-21 are essential to the pathogenesis of KD. Our study provides further understanding of the immune response involved in KD and offers novel insights in the pathogenetic mechanism of this disease.

Keywords: Circulating follicular helper T cells, Kawasaki disease, Interleukin-21, Immune response

Background

Kawasaki disease (KD) is an acute febrile vasculitis that was first reported in 1967 [1]. KD most commonly occurs in infants and children under five years of age and is characterized initially by high fever, mucocutaneous inflammation, edema of the extremities, polymorphous rash, and cervical lymphadenopathy (≥1.5 cm diameter) [2]. The exact pathogenesis of Kawasaki disease remains unknown. Generally, it is believed that KD is secondary to infectious agents, triggering an aberrant immune response in genetically susceptible individuals [3, 4]. The treatment efficacy of intravenous immunoglobulin (IVIG) administered during the acute phase of the disease further confirms the fundamental involvement of immune response dysregulation in the pathogenesis of KD. Therefore, the understanding of the factors that regulate the abnormal immune response in KD is important for developing strategies for the management of KD patients.

Both innate and adaptive immune systems are involved in the pathogenesis of KD. The innate immune system presents high numbers of activated circulating

* Correspondence: sryang@jlu.edu.cn
†Meng Xu and Yanfang Jiang contributed equally to this work.
[1]Department of Pediatric Rheumatology and Allergy, The First Hospital of Jilin University, Changchun 130021, China
Full list of author information is available at the end of the article

neutrophils and elevated levels of serum cytokines, such as interleukin (IL)-1, IL-6, and tumor necrosis factor alpha (TNFα) [5]. The reduction in the numbers of neutrophils and cytokines levels following IVIG administration [6] is regarded as a consequence of the downregulation of the nuclear factor kappa B (NF-κB) signaling pathway in monocytes/macrophages [7]. Although T cells have traditionally been considered to play essential roles in adaptive immune responses, the alterations in the percentage of T cells in KD are a subject of controversy and different investigators have reported conflicting results [8–10]. It has been concluded that the variation in T cells could be further investigated based on of their subpopulations and cytokine levels [5]. Current studies that examined the variation of T-cell subpopulations with regard to KD have generally investigated T helper cells [11, 12], regulatory T cells [13], and cytotoxic T cells [14]; however, the role of follicular helper T (Tfh) cells in KD remains to be elucidated. B cells are also important participants in the adaptive immune responses. In acute phase of KD, studies about B cells found increased CD19$^+$ cells [15] and elevated levels of serum immunoglobulins (IgA, IgG, IgM and IgE) [16]. Accordingly, it can be speculated that Tfh cells may be involved in the pathogenesis of KD due to their ability in homing B cell to the germinal centers (GC), regulating GC positive selection, and inducing B cell differentiation to plasma cells and memory B cells via the secretion of IL-21 [17–19]. However, suppressed plasmablast responses [20] and reduced IgA-expressing B cells [21] in KD were also reported. Hence, the studies conducted on Tfh cells are important in clarifying the role of B cells in KD, since Tfh cells can aid the function of B cells.

Tfh cells were initially identified in the GC of secondary lymphoid tissues and have been shown to express the CXC-chemokine receptor 5 (CXCR5). The percentage of Tfh cells can be detected by the expression of inducible co-stimulator (ICOS) and programmed cell death protein 1 (PD-1), two CD28 superfamily molecules [22, 23]. ICOS delivers positive signals to CD4$^+$ T cells by interacting with dendritic cells and B cells that express an ICOS ligand, which is involved in Tfh cell differentiation [24, 25]. In contrast to ICOS, the inhibitory signals [26, 27] that block the interactions between PD-1 and the ligands PD-L1 and/or PD-L2 have been shown to increase the differentiation of Tfh cells [28, 29]. The assessment of GC Tfh cells in patients, particularly in children, is subject to huge limitations, due to poor access to lymphoid organ samples. Despite these disadvantages, the establishment of circulating Tfh (cTfh) cells [26] from blood samples offers a surrogate strategy to analyze Tfh responses. Circulating Tfh cells are believed to represent a memory compartment

of GC Tfh cells that express B-cell lymphoma 6 protein (Bcl-6), which is downregulated when the cells enter the circulation [30]. Circulating Tfh cells share the phenotype and functional properties of GC Tfh cells [31, 32]. Current understanding of cTfh cells suggests that they can be classified into distinct subsets according to the differential expression of ICOS and PD-1. Typically, they were divided into one activated subset (ICOS$^+$PD1^{++}) and two quiescent subsets (ICOS$^-$PD1$^-$ and ICOS$^-$PD1$^+$) [33]. The majority of ICOS$^+$PD1^{++} cTfh cells express Ki67, which is a cellular marker for proliferation. On the contrary, the two quiescent subsets lack the expression of Ki67 [34]. Furthermore, in comparison, ICOS$^+$PD1^{++} cTfh cells display the most efficient capacity in helping naïve or memory B cells. Thus, investigation on the variation in cTfh-cell subsets would be beneficial for better understanding the level of their activation. IL-21 is recognized as a hallmark for cTfh cells [33] and belongs to the type I cytokine family. This cytokine is a highly potent stimulator of plasma cell proliferation and differentiation [35]. IL-21 is also believed to be an autocrine growth factor for Tfh cells [36]. However, the role of IL-21 in cTfh cells remains to be fully elucidated.

T cells comprise a heterogeneous population; therefore, in the present study, we aimed to analyze the distinct subsets of circulating Tfh cells that were defined by characteristic Tfh markers and serum IL-21 levels. The examination of their expression levels and the correlation among the subgroups can be used to further clarify the immunopathogenesis of KD.

Materials and methods
Patients

A total of 24 hospitalized pediatric patients with KD ranging from six months to five years in age and 20 age-matched control subjects were enrolled from May 2015 to November 2016 (14 cases in the Department of Pediatrics, The First Hospital of Jilin University, China and another 10 cases in the Department of Pediatrics, Children's Hospital, Changchun, China). Among the KD patients, only one was diagnosed with coronary artery lesions by echocardiography. All KD patients underwent detailed physical and laboratory examinations, and were diagnosed according to the criteria of the 2004 American Heart Association (AHA) statement [37]. Patients with other autoimmune diseases were excluded. All individuals were treated with IVIG at a cumulative dose of 2 g/kg within two days and 30–100 mg/kg/d of aspirin in divided doses from the time at which the diagnosis was established until defervescence. Disease remission was achieved following treatment without recurrence in all patients. None of these children had received other medical therapy for at least one month. The samples were collected from patients in both the acute and remission phases of KD. Acute phase (AP) refers to the period from diagnosis establishment to IVIG administration. Remission phase (RP) is defined as the time from which patients are afebrile for at least 48 h before discharge. The control group comprised eight children with hexadactyly, four children with wryneck, and eight children with hernias and without any other autoimmune diseases or infections in the previous month. The samples were obtained before surgery. The study protocol was approved by the ethics committee of The First Hospital of Jilin University. Written informed consent was obtained from the parents of each child.

The following laboratory parameters were recorded: white blood cell count, absolute neutrophil and lymphocyte counts, serum immunoglobulins (Ig) G, A and M, C-reactive protein (CRP) and erythrocyte sedimentation rate (ESR).

Flow cytometric analysis

Blood samples were collected separately from controls and KD patients in different phases. Peripheral blood mononuclear cells (PBMCs) were isolated from individual KD patients and control subjects by density-gradient centrifugation at $800 \times g$ for 30 min at 25 °C using Ficoll-Paque Plus (Amersham Biosciences, Little Chalfont, UK). Freshly isolated PBMCs (4×10^6/mL) were cultured in 10% fetal calf serum RPMI-1640 (Hyclone, Logan, UT, USA) in U-bottom 24-well tissue culture plates (Costar, Lowell, MA, USA) and stimulated for 1 h with or without 50 ng/mL of phorbol myristate acetate (PMA) in the presence of 2 µg/mL of ionomycin (Sigma, St. Louis, MO, USA). The cells were then treated with Brefeldin A (10 µg/mL, GolgiStop™, BD Biosciences, San Jose, CA, USA) for an additional 5 h. For flow cytometric analysis, PBMCs were stained in duplicate with BV510-anti-CD3, APC-H7-anti-CD4, BB515-anti-CXCR5, PE-Cy5-anti-CD45RA, PE-CF594-anti-CD279 and BV421-anti-CD278 (Becton Dickinson, San Jose, CA, USA) at room temperature for 30 min. Subsequently, the cells were fixed, permeabilized, and stained with PE-anti-IL-21 (Becton Dickinson). Multicolor flow cytometry (FACSAria™ II, BD Biosciences) was used to determine the percentages of distinct cTfh cells, and the data were analyzed with FlowJo software (v5.7.2; FlowJo, Ashland, OR, USA).

Measurement of serum IL-21 levels by cytometric bead array (CBA)

Serum IL-21 concentrations were detected using a CBA human soluble protein master buffer kit (BD Biosciences) according to the manufacturer's instructions. The samples were further analyzed with a flow cytometer (FACSAria™ II, BD Biosciences), and

quantified using the CellQuest Pro and CBA softwares (Becton Dickinson).

Statistical analysis

Statistical data were performed with SPSS version 22.0 software. A P value lower than 0.05 ($P < 0.05$) was considered to indicate statistical significance. All data were expressed as the median and range values. The differences between groups were analyzed using the Kruskal–Wallis test. The Wilcoxon matched pairs test was applied to assess the differences between the AP and RP data. The relationship between different variables was evaluated using the Spearman's rank correlation test.

Results

Patient characteristics

A total of 24 patients with KD and 20 control subjects were recruited in the present study. Five samples of KD patients in RP were unavailable due to advanced discharge. The demographic and clinical characteristics of patients and control subjects are shown in Table 1. No significant differences were detected with regard to the paremeters age and sex between the KD and the control groups. Although white blood cell count and the number of absolute neutrophils were significantly higher in the KD group, no significant differences were noted in absolute lymphocyte counts between the two groups. The CRP and ESR values were significantly elevated in the KD group compared with that noted in the control group. In addition, serum IgG levels were significantly lower in the KD group than those in the control group. However, no significant differences were

Table 1 The demographic and clinical characteristics of the study participants

Parameters	Kawasaki disease		Controls ($n = 20$)
	Acute phase ($n = 24$)	Remission phase ($n = 19$)	
Age, year	2.75 (0.6–5)	NA	2.38 (0.9–4.5)
Sex, Female/Male	11/14	NA	8/12
CRP, mg/L	76.25 (20–151)[#, *]	2.76 (0.8–5.28)	2.35 (0.7–3.28)
ESR, mm/h	51.37 (11–98)[#]	53.67 (9–76)[#]	7 (3–11)
IgG, g/L	6.295 (1.82–16.1)[#]	NA	10.22 (6.08–14.37)
IgA, g/L	1.715 (0.91–2.92)	NA	1.91 (0.71–3.1)
IgM, g/L	0.99 (0.19–1.77)	NA	1.035 (0.69–1.93)
WBC, 10^9/L	14.31 (5.89–35)[#, *]	8.729 (4.82–13.79)	7.735 (5.31–10.03)
Neutrophils, 10^9/L	10.14 (2.52–33.69)[#, *]	2.98 (1.98–5.09)	2.58 (2.06–4.69)
Lymphocytes, 10^9/L	2.915 (0.88–8.82)	3.736 (1.92–6.75)	4.085 (1.01–5.28)

Data shown are median (range) or number of cases. *CRP* C-reactive protein, *ESR* erythrocyte sedimentation rate, *Ig* immunoglobulin, *WBC* white blood cell counts, *NA* not available. [#]$P < 0.05$ vs. the controls. [*]$P < 0.05$ vs. remission phase noted in the serum IgM and IgA levels between the two groups. In the RP, the white blood cell count, absolute neutrophil count and CRP values were dramatically decreased compared with those in the AP.

Circulating CD4$^+$CXCR5$^+$ T cells subsets and serum IL-21 levels in the different phases of KD

To investigate the role of circulating Tfh cells in KD, PBMCs from control subjects and patients in different phases of KD were immunostained for CD3, CD4, CXCR5, CD278, CD279, CD45RA and IL-21 expression, and further analyzed by flow cytometry. Initially, five subsets of cTfh cells were described by flow cytometry that were based on the differential expression of ICOS and PD-1, namely CD4$^+$CXCR5$^+$ICOS^{high}PD-1^{high}, CD4$^+$CXCR5$^+$I-COS$^+$PD-1$^+$, CD4$^+$CXCR5$^+$ICOS$^-$PD-1$^+$, CD4$^+$CXCR5$^+$I-COS$^-$PD-1$^-$ and CD4$^+$CXCR5$^+$ICOS$^+$PD-1$^-$. To ensure proper gating strategy, isotype controls were used to determine the gating parameters (Additional file 1: Figure S1). These cell populations were measured by gating initially live lymphocytes, subsequently CD3$^+$CD4$^+$ T cells, and finally CD4$^+$CXCR5$^+$ T cells (Fig. 1A). CD4$^+$CXCR5$^+$ T cells were considered circulating Tfh cells. No significant differences were noted in the percentages of total cTfh cells in the AP and RP KD groups compared with the control group ($P = 0.2964$ and $P = 0.7369$, respectively; Fig. 1Ba). The percentages of ICOS^{high}PD-1^{high} cells were significantly higher in both the AP and RP groups than those noted in the control groups ($P = 0.0001$ and $P < 0.0001$,

respectively; Fig. 1Bb) and a similar pattern was observed in the percentages of ICOS$^+$PD-1$^+$ cells ($P = 0.0003$ and $P < 0.0001$, respectively; Fig. 1Bc). However, the percentage of ICOS$^-$PD-1$^+$ cells was significantly increased in the AP, but not in the RP groups ($P = 0.0007$ and $P > 0.9999$, respectively; Fig. 1Bd). In contrast, the percentages of ICOS$^-$PD-1$^-$ cTfh cells in both the AP and RP were significantly lower than those in the control group ($P < 0.0001$ and $P = 0.0002$, respectively; Fig. 1Be). Moreover, a significant elevation in the percentage of ICOS$^+$PD-1 cTfh cells was noted only in the RP of KD and not in the AP ($P = 0.0251$ and $P = 0.5349$, respectively; Fig. 1Bf). Subsequenlty, we analyzed the serum IL-21 levels and the percentage of the T cell subpopulation, namely CD4$^+$CXCR5$^+$CD45RA$^-$IL-21$^+$ T cells, by gating initially live lymphocytes, subsequently CD3$^+$CD4$^+$ T cells, and finally CXCR5$^+$CD45RA$^-$ T cells (Fig. 2a). A significant increase in the percentage of CD45RA$^-$IL-21$^+$ cTfh cells was observed in both AP and RP KD patients ($P < 0.0001$ and $P = 0.0002$, respectively; Fig. 2b). Similarly, serum IL-21 levels were significantly elevated in both the AP and RP ($P < 0.0001$ and $P = 0.0011$, respectively; Fig. 2c). The data indicated that although the overall percentage of cTfh cells remained stable, significant variations were noted among the cTfh cell subpopulations and serum IL-21 levels. This further suggested that the RP represents a transitional period from the AP to recovery, in which clinical symptoms and characteristics improve, despite the continuation of the immune response.

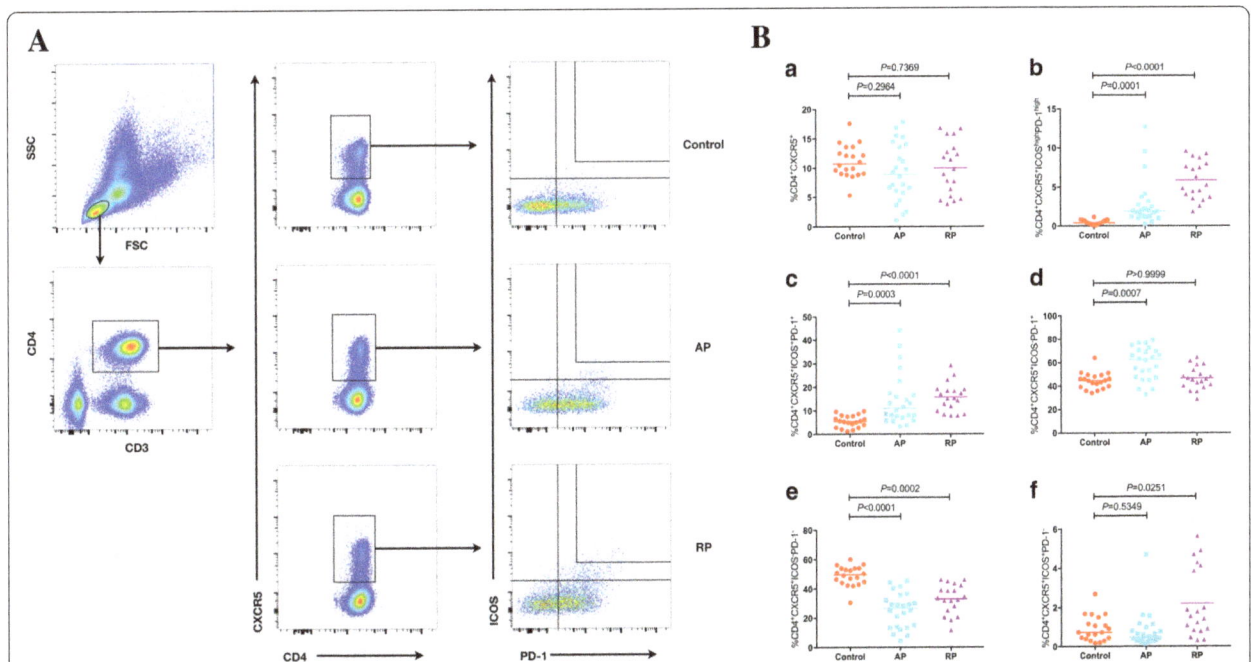

Fig. 1 Flow cytometry analysis of the frequency of circulating Tfh cells in KD patients. **A** Flow cytometry analysis. **B** Quantitative analysis. The data shown are representative dot plots or are expressed as the mean percentage of T cells of individual subjects. The horizontal lines represent the median values. PBMC, peripheral blood mononuclear cell. AP, Acute phase. RP, Remission phase

Correlation of the percentages of distinct cTfh-cells subsets with clinical characteristics and IL-21 levels in the AP of KD

To understand the importance of cTfh cells in the pathogenesis of KD, the associations of the percentages of distinct cTfh-cells subsets with the levels of the biomarkers CRP and ESR and of the IL-21 in the AP were analyzed. We demonstrated that both serum CRP and ESR levels positively correlated with the percentage of ICOS^{high}PD-1^{high} cTfh cells ($r = 0.5961$, $P = 0.0021$, Fig. 3a; $r = 0.4373$, $P = 0.0326$, respectively; Fig. 3b). A similar pattern was observed for the percentage of ICOS^{+}PD-1^{+} cTfh cells ($r = 0.5442$, $P = 0.0060$, Fig. 3c; $r = 0.5262$, $P = 0.0083$, respectively; Fig. 3d). In contrast to this finding, serum CRP levels and serum ESR negatively correlated with the percentage of ICOS^{-}PD-1^{+} cTfh cells ($r = 0.4287$, $P = 0.0366$, Fig. 3e; $r = 0.4173$, $P = 0.0425$, respectively; Fig. 3f). Furthermore, serum IL-21 levels positively correlated with the percentage of ICOS^{high}PD-1^{high} ($r = 0.5416$, $P = 0.0063$, Fig. 3g), ICOS^{+}PD-1^{+} ($r = 0.7498$, $P < 0.0001$, Fig. 3h) and CD45RA^{-}IL-21^{+} ($r = 0.6314$, $P = 0.0009$, Fig. 3i) cTfh cells. No additional significant correlations were noted among these parameters (data not shown). The data

indicated that different cTfh-cell subsets play distinct roles in acute KD.

Variation of cTfh-cells subsets and serum IL-21 levels after treatment

To further investigate the role of cTfh cells in KD patients, we explored the percentages of distinct cTfh-cells subsets in the RP. As shown in Fig. 4, heterogeneous variations were noted in the cTfh-cell subsets, although this effect was not statistically significant in the CD4^{+}CXCR5^{+} T cells ($P = 0.9563$, Fig. 4a). However, the percentages of ICOS^{high}PD-1^{high} and ICOS^{+}PD-1^{+} cTfh cells further increased in the RP ($P < 0.0001$, Fig. 4b; $P = 0.0003$, Fig. 4c). Furthermore, the percentages of ICOS^{+}PD-1^{-} and ICOS^{-}PD-1^{-} cTfh cells were also significantly increased ($P < 0.0001$, Fig. 4d; $P = 0.0017$, Fig. 4e). In contrast to these observations, the percentages of ICOS^{-}PD-1^{+} cTfh cells and CD45RA^{-}IL21^{+} cTfh cells, as well as the serum IL-21 levels were significantly decreased ($P < 0.0001$, Fig. 4f; $P = 0.0008$, Fig. 4g; $P < 0.0001$, Fig. 4h). The data of the present study demonstrated that certain cTfh cell subsets further increased following drug administration and clinical improvement. It was notable that in the RP, only the

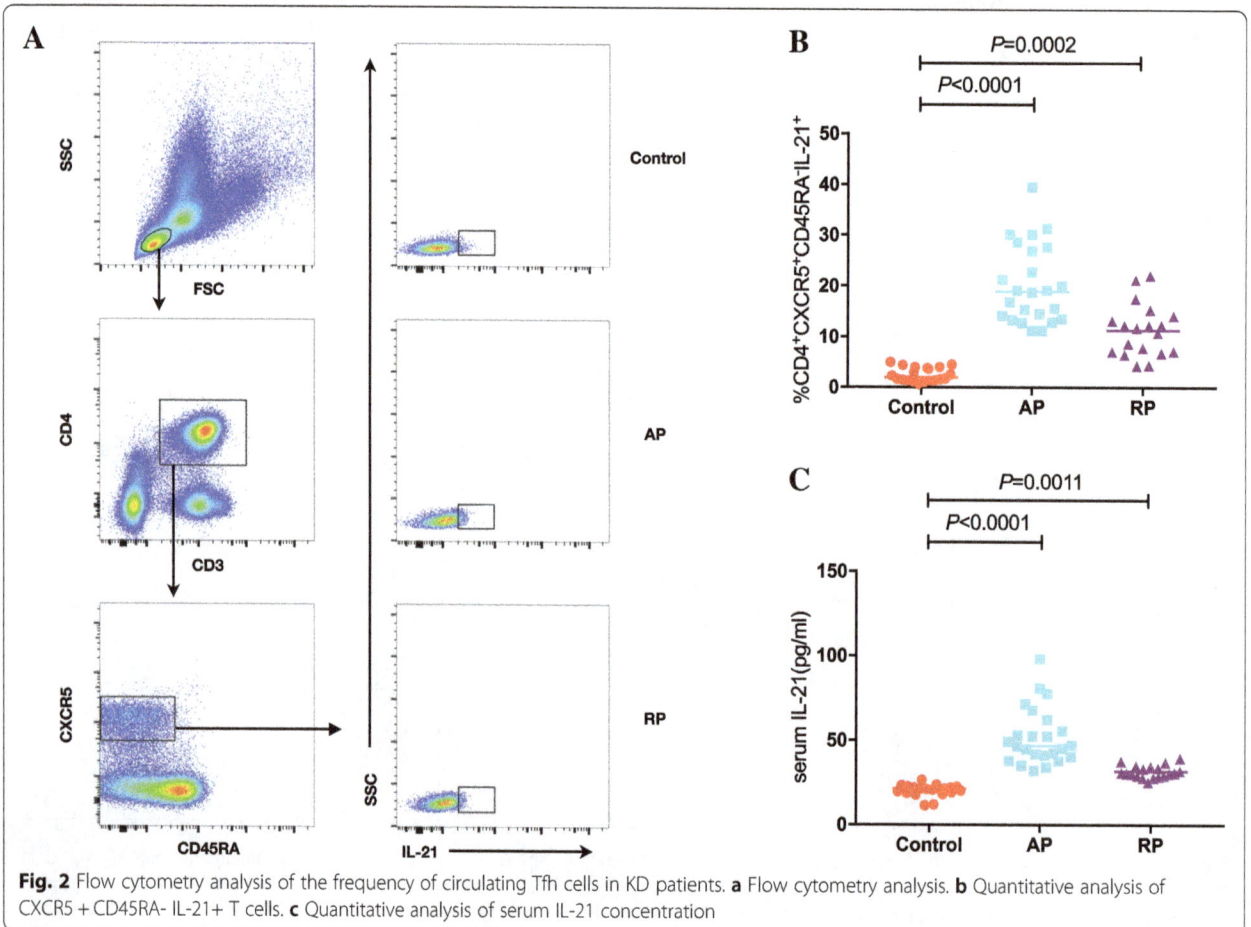

Fig. 2 Flow cytometry analysis of the frequency of circulating Tfh cells in KD patients. **a** Flow cytometry analysis. **b** Quantitative analysis of CXCR5 + CD45RA- IL-21+ T cells. **c** Quantitative analysis of serum IL-21 concentration

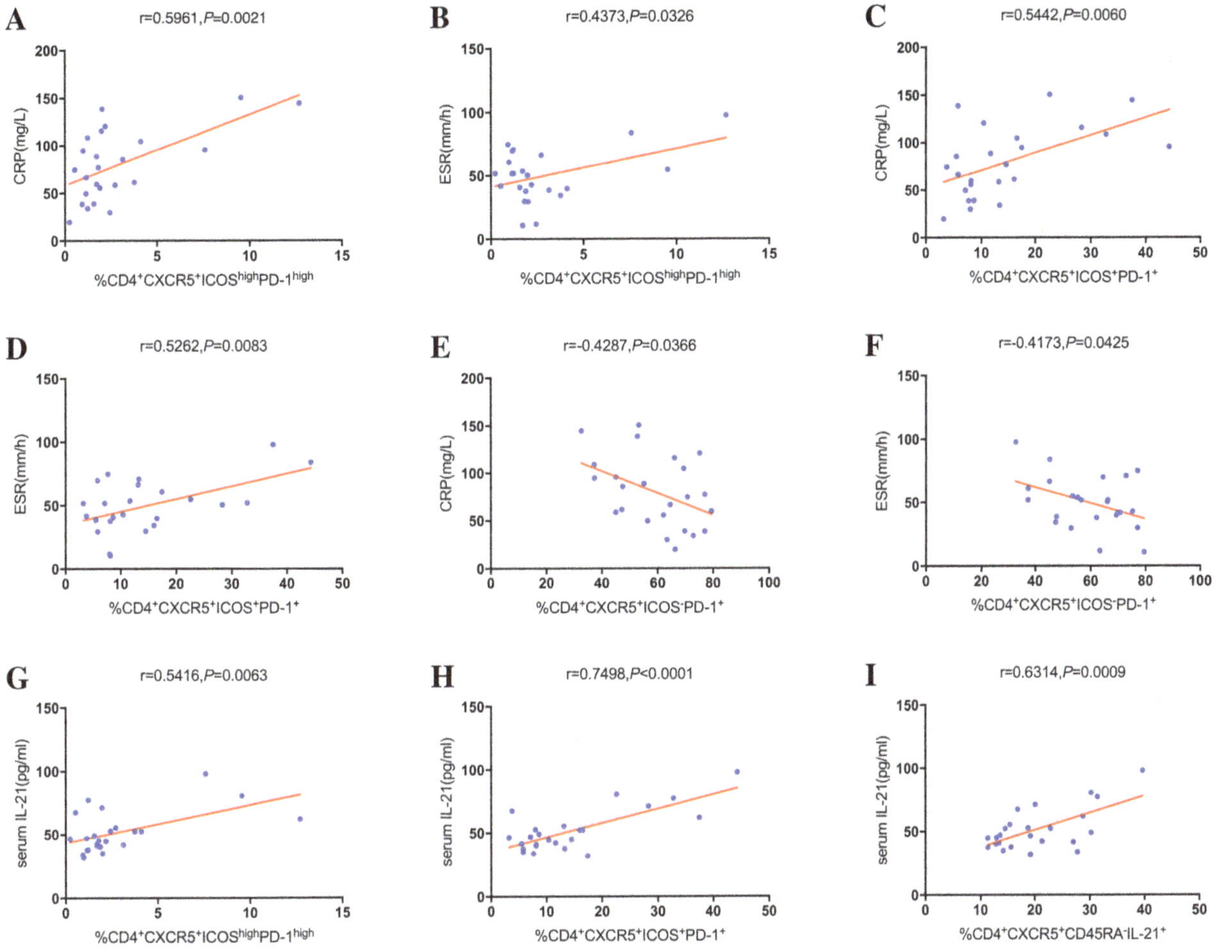

Fig. 3 Correlation analysis during the acute phase of KD. **a–h** The correlation between the subsets of cTfh cells and the serum CRP and IL-21 levels and/or ESR

CD45RA⁻IL21⁺ cTfh cells correlated with serum IL-21 levels ($r = 0.5141$, $P = 0.0243$, Fig. 4i).

Discussion

The roles of circulating Tfh cells in different disease models have already been widely investigated. A previous study conducted on systemic lupus erythematosus indicated that PD-1 expression on cTfh cells contributed to the regulation of germinal center B-cell function and humoral response [38]. Szabo et al. reported that ICOS⁺PD-1⁺ cTfh cells and IL-21-producing CD4⁺CXCR5⁺PD-1⁺ T cells were significantly increased in Sjögren's syndrome subjects [39]. Our previous study in children indicated that the percentage of cTfh cells correlated with the pathogenesis and progression of Henoch–Schönlein purpura [40]. In the present study, we found that although the overall percentage of cTfh cells remained stable, marked variations were noted in the percentages of cTfh-cell subsets and the levels of cytokines. In the AP, the percentages of $ICOS^{high}PD\text{-}1^{high}$, ICOS⁺PD-1⁺, ICOS⁻PD-1⁺, and CD45RA⁻IL-21⁺ cTfh cells and serum IL-21 levels were significantly elevated. It is apparent that aberrant distribution of cTfh cells is ubiquitous in rheumatic diseases, although the precise mechanism remains unclear. Based on our data, $ICOS^{high}PD\text{-}1^{high}$, ICOS⁺PD-1⁺, ICOS⁻PD-1⁺ cTfh cells correlated positively with CRP and ESR, which suggested that these three subsets contribute to innate immune responses. Correlation analysis with IL-21 levels implied that $ICOS^{high}PD\text{-}1^{high}$, ICOS⁺PD-1⁺ and CD45RA⁻IL-21⁺ cTfh cells affected KD development via IL-21 secretion. It seems difficult to explain that although the clinical symptoms had been improved in the RP, the percentages of the $ICOS^{high}PD\text{-}1^{high}$ and ICOS⁺PD-1⁺, and ICOS⁺PD-1⁻ cTfh cells were further increased. However, among these subsets, $ICOS^{high}PD\text{-}1^{high}$ population may be a representative subset of cTfh cells. Not only because $ICOS^{high}PD\text{-}1^{high}$ population can be regarded as a subpopulation of $ICOS^{+}PD1^{++}$ cTfh cells, which is an activated subset, but also because this phenotype is similar to that of GC Tfh cells, which are ICOS⁺

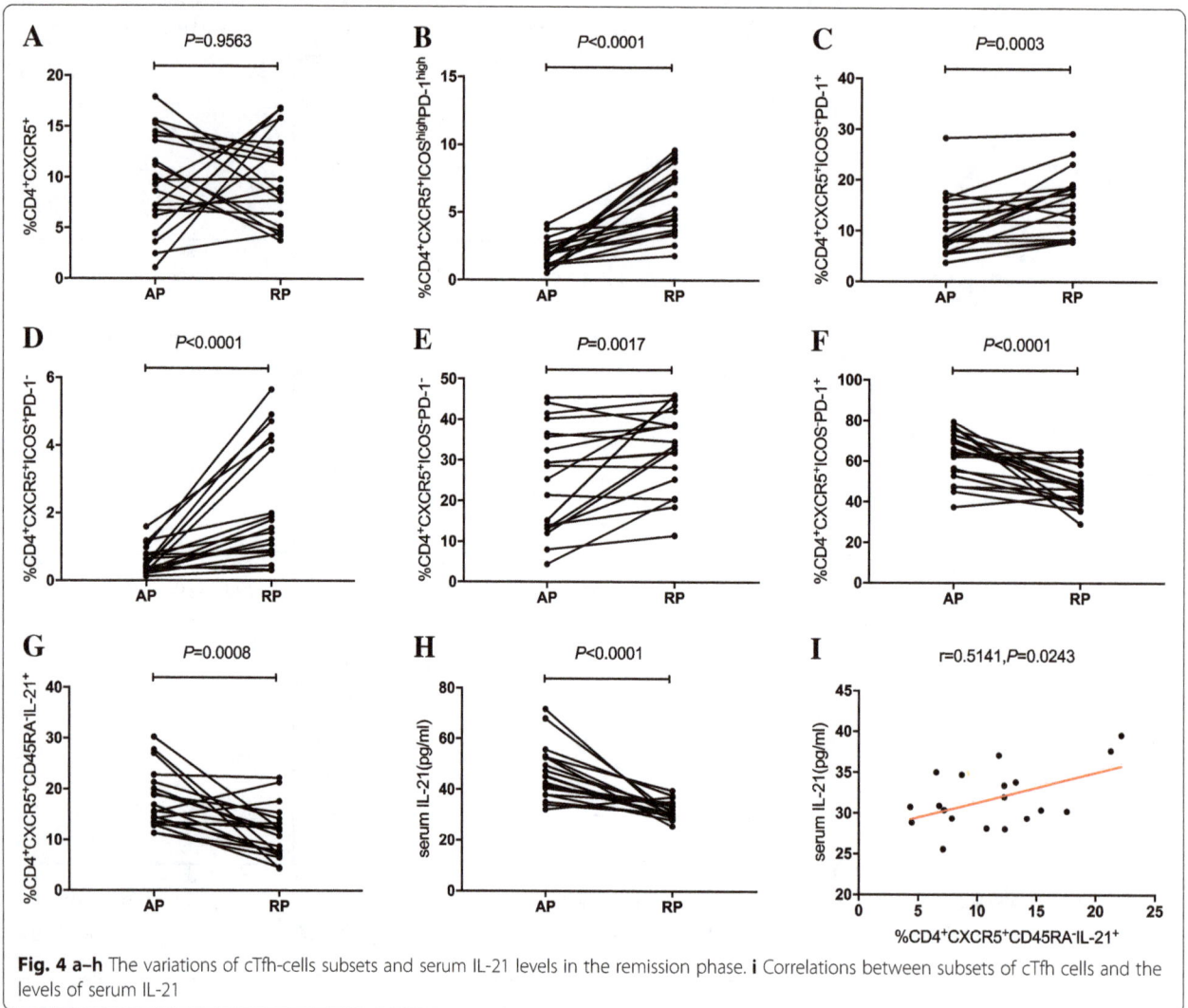

Fig. 4 a–h The variations of cTfh-cells subsets and serum IL-21 levels in the remission phase. **i** Correlations between subsets of cTfh cells and the levels of serum IL-21

+PD-1++ [35]. In other words, the increase of ICOS[high]PD-1[high] cTfh cells likely represents the activation of cTfh cells. Hence, our results suggested that cTfh cells were activated in the AP, and they were persistently activated in the RP. Although the function of these subsets cannot be clarified in the present analysis, the absence of a correlation with IL-21 levels despite the increased percentages of these subsets, indicates that these cells may not secrete IL-21 efficiently in RP [34, 41, 42]. Furthermore, Franco et al. [43] indicated that the expansion of circulating central memory T cells but not effector memory T cells could be detected even at 1 to 3 months following the onset of the disease. This expansion aims to protect patients against future exposure to the stimuli of KD. Whether these further increased subsets in RP are circulating central memory cells remains to be clarified.

Since its discovery in 2000, IL-21 has been shown to perform antitumor and antiviral functions and to participate in the development of autoimmune diseases via

the Janus kinase (JAK)-signal transducer, the activator of transcription (STAT), the mitogen-activated protein kinase (MAPK) and the phosphoinositide 3-kinase (PI3K)-AKT signaling pathways [44]; however, the mechanism underlying the role in KD is unknown. Several studies have been conducted on the role of IL-21 in KD. One study in a Korean cohort demonstrated that IL-21 represents a sensitive and specific biomarker of KD [45]. In accordance with this report, we found elevated serum IL-21 levels in the AP, while the corresponding levels were reduced in the RP. However, Engelberg et al. reported that IL-21 levels were also elevated in febrile controls [46]. Therefore, serum IL-21 levels appear to be a sensitive, but not specific, indicator of active KD. Additionally, serum IL-21 levels may be regulated by IgG levels [45]. In the present study, we observed lower levels of serum IgG and higher expression levels of IL-21 in the AP, while in the RP the IgG levels were shown to increase [47] and IL-21 levels decreased. Nevertheless, further analysis indicated no correlation between serum levels of IL-21 and IgG in the AP. It can be speculated that this finding may have been produced by the increase in the normal range of IgG with age. Furthermore, IL-21 is not exclusively expressed in cTfh cells, but also in Th17 and NKT cells [48, 49]. IL-21 was further found to be suppressed by activated plasma cells [50]. Thus, in addition to cTfh cells, multiple factors, such as Th17, NKT and plasma cells, might affect serum IL-21 levels.

The relationship between IL-21 expression and Tfh cell differentiation remains controversial. It has been postulated that IL-21 contributes to the efficient development of Tfh cells by upregulating BCL-6 and MAF [51, 52], while other studies have indicated that Tfh cells can be generated without IL-21 expression [53]. Alternatively, it has been shown that IL-21 alone is insufficient to enhance the expression of CXCR5 [54]. Thus, it can be hypothesized that IL-21 acts as a cooperator, rather than a conductor of Tfh cell differentiation, which is a complex process regulated by IL-21, IL-12, IL-6, BCL-6, and ICOS [35, 54]. In the present study, we investigated the percentage of total cTfh cells and the serum IL-21 levels in KD patients during different phases of the disease progression. It is interesting to note, that no significant variation was noted in the percentage of CXCR5 cells regardless of the levels of IL-21, indicating that no definite correlation between IL-21 levels and cTfh cell differentiation in KD.

Unfortunately, the correlations between coronary artery lesions and cTfh cells were not analyzed in the present study. However, a recent study revealed associations of coronary artery lesions with a number of clinical characteristic, particularly CRP and ESR [55]. It was noted that KD patients with CRP levels higher than 30 mg/L and ESR higher than 40 mm/h exhibited a higher incidence of coronary artery lesion. Moreover, the percentage of ICOS⁻PD-1⁺ cTfh cells correlated negatively with ESR and CRP, indicating the possibility of an increased percentage of ICOS⁻PD-1⁺cTfh cells to act as a protective barrier against coronary artery lesions. This hypothesis may provide a new therapeutic approach in preventing coronary artery lesions. According to our clinical observations, coronary artery lesions were present in the patients without significant elevation of CRP and ESR. In addition, not all of the patients with high CRP and ESR possessed coronary artery lesions. It can be speculated that the pathogenesis of coronary artery lesions in KD is diverse, possibly due to epigenetic effects [56] and genetic polymorphisms [57]. Therefore, investigation of the association between cTfh cells and the development of coronary lesions are required. Besides, another limitation of the present study shoud be mentioned. The

exact function and mechanism underlying the further increase in the cTfh cell population during the RP remain to be elucidated. Focus will be given on these issues in the subsequent studies.

Conclusions

In summary, significant variations were identified in the percentages of cTfh-cell subsets and the level of serum IL-21 in Kawasaki disease. Our results indicated that IL-21-secreting cTfh cells were essential for both the acute and remission phase of KD. It also can be concluded that cTfh cells were activated in the acute phase and persistently activated in remission phase. To the best of our knowledge, this is the first investigation of serum IL-21 levels in terms of the distribution of circulating cTfh cell subsets in KD. Our data provide further understanding of the immune responses of KD and novel insights in the pathogenesis of this disease.

Abbreviations
AP: Acute phase; CBA: Cytometric bead array; cTfh cells: Circulating follicular helper T cells; CXCR5: CXC-chemokine receptor 5; GC: Germinal center; ICOS: Inducible co-stimulator; IL: Interleukin; KD: Kawasaki disease; NF-κB: Nuclear factor kappa B; PBMC: Peripheral blood mononuclear cells; PD-1: Programmed cell death protein 1; RP: Remission phase

Acknowledgements
The authors thank the patients for their participation in this study. This work was supported by the Key Laboratory of Zoonoses Research of The First Hospital of Jilin University.

Funding
This work was supported by Natural Science Foundation of Jilin provincial science and Technology Department (20180101116JC). The funders had no role in study design, data collection and analysis, decision to publish, or preparation of the manuscript.

Authors' contributions
MX and YJ carried out the experiments, and analyzed, and interpreted the data. JZ, YZ, DL and LG interpreted the data and discussed the results, which are vital for formation of conception. SY contributed to the conception and design of the study, the analysis and interpretation of the data, and drafting and revising the manuscript. All authors read and approved the final manuscript.

Competing interests
The authors declare that they have no competing interests.

Author details
[1]Department of Pediatric Rheumatology and Allergy, The First Hospital of Jilin University, Changchun 130021, China. [2]Genetic Diagnosis Center, The First Hospital of Jilin University, Changchun 130021, China. [3]Key Laboratory of Zoonoses Research, Ministry of Education, The First Hospital of Jilin University, Changchun 130021, China. [4]Jiangsu Co-innovation Center for Prevention and Control of Important Animal Infectious Diseases and Zoonoses, Yangzhou 225009, China. [5]Department of Pediatric, Children's Hospital, Changchun 130021, China. [6]Department of Pediatric Rheumatology and Immunology, Wuhan Children's Hospital, Tongji Medical College, Huazhong University of Science & Technology, Wuhan 430000, China.

References

1. Kawasaki T. Acute febrile mucocutaneous syndrome with lymphoid involvement with specific desquamation of the fingers and toes in children. Arerugi. 1967;16(3):178–222.
2. McCrindle B, et al. Diagnosis, treatment, and long-term Management of Kawasaki Disease: a scientific statement for health professionals from the American Heart Association. Circulation. 2017;135(17):e927–99.
3. Shulman ST, Rowley AH. Kawasaki disease: insights into pathogenesis and approaches to treatment. Nat Rev Rheumatol. 2015;11(8):475–82.
4. Onouchi Y, et al. A genome-wide association study identifies three new risk loci for Kawasaki disease. Nat Genet. 2012;44(5):517–21.
5. Matsubara T, Ichiyama T, Furukawa S. Immunological profile of peripheral blood lymphocytes and monocytes/macrophages in Kawasaki disease. Clin Exp Immunol. 2005;141(3):381–7.
6. Furukawa S, et al. Reduction of peripheral blood macrophages/monocytes in Kawasaki disease by intravenous gammaglobulin. Eur J Pediatr. 1990; 150(1):43–7.
7. Ichiyama T, et al. NF-kappaB activation in peripheral blood monocytes/ macrophages and T cells during acute Kawasaki disease. Clin Immunol. 2001;99(3):373–7.
8. Abe J, et al. Selective expansion of T cells expressing T-cell receptor variable regions V beta 2 and V beta 8 in Kawasaki disease. Proc Natl Acad Sci U S A. 1992;89(9):4066–70.
9. Brogan P, et al. T cell Vbeta repertoires in childhood vasculitides. Clin Exp Immunol. 2003;131(3):517–27.
10. Nomura Y, et al. Twenty-five types of T-cell receptor Vbeta family repertoire in patients with Kawasaki syndrome. Eur J Pediatr. 1998;157(12):981–6.
11. Kimura J, et al. Th1 and Th2 cytokine production is suppressed at the level of transcriptional regulation in Kawasaki disease. Clin Exp Immunol. 2004; 137(2):444–9.
12. Guo MM, et al. Th17- and Treg-related cytokine and mRNA expression are associated with acute and resolving Kawasaki disease. Allergy. 2015;70(3):310–8.
13. Ni F, et al. Regulatory T cell microRNA expression changes in children with acute Kawasaki disease. Clin Exp Immunol. 2014;178(2):384–93.
14. Ye Q, et al. Intravenous immunoglobulin treatment responsiveness depends on the degree of CD8+ T cell activation in Kawasaki disease. Clin Immunol. 2016;171:25–31.
15. Ding Y, et al. Profiles of responses of immunological factors to different subtypes of Kawasaki disease. BMC Musculoskelet Disord. 2015;16:315.
16. Lin CY, Hwang B. Serial immunologic studies in patients with mucocutaneous lymph node syndrome (Kawasaki disease). Ann Allergy. 1987;59(4):291–7.
17. Breitfeld D, et al. Follicular B helper T cells express CXC chemokine receptor 5, localize to B cell follicles, and support immunoglobulin production. J Exp Med. 2000;192(11):1545–52.
18. Schaerli P, et al. CXC chemokine receptor 5 expression defines follicular homing T cells with B cell helper function. J Exp Med. 2000;192(11):1553–62.
19. Shulman Z, et al. T follicular helper cell dynamics in germinal centers. Science. 2013;341(6146):673–7.
20. Martin M, Wrotniak BH, Hicar M. Suppressed plasmablast responses in febrile infants, including children with Kawasaki disease. PLoS One. 2018;13(3): e0193539.
21. Shingadia D, et al. Surface and cytoplasmic immunoglobulin expression in circulating B-lymphocytes in acute Kawasaki disease. Pediatr Res. 2001;50(4):538–43.
22. Hutloff A, et al. ICOS is an inducible T-cell co-stimulator structurally and functionally related to CD28. Nature. 1999;397(6716):263–6.
23. Sharpe A, Freeman G. The B7-CD28 superfamily. Nat Rev Immunol. 2002; 2(2):116–26.
24. Bossaller L, et al. ICOS deficiency is associated with a severe reduction of CXCR5+CD4 germinal center Th cells. J Immunol. 2006;177(7):4927–32.
25. Nurieva R, et al. Generation of T follicular helper cells is mediated by interleukin-21 but independent of T helper 1, 2, or 17 cell lineages. Immunity. 2008;29(1):138–49.
26. Crotty S. T follicular helper cell differentiation, function, and roles in disease. Immunity. 2014;41(4):529–42.
27. Ueno H, Banchereau J, Vinuesa CG. Pathophysiology of T follicular helper cells in humans and mice. Nat Immunol. 2015;16(2):142–52.
28. Good-Jacobson KL, et al. PD-1 regulates germinal center B cell survival and the formation and affinity of long-lived plasma cells. Nat Immunol. 2010; 11(6):535–42.
29. Hamel KM, et al. B7-H1 expression on non-B and non-T cells promotes distinct effects on T- and B-cell responses in autoimmune arthritis. Eur J Immunol. 2010;40(11):3117–27.
30. Schmitt N, Bentebibel S, Ueno H. Phenotype and functions of memory Tfh cells in human blood. Trends Immunol. 2014;35(9):436–42.
31. Morita R, et al. Human blood CXCR5(+)CD4(+) T cells are counterparts of T follicular cells and contain specific subsets that differentially support antibody secretion. Immunity. 2011;34(1):108–21.
32. Ueno H. T follicular helper cells in human autoimmunity. Curr Opin Immunol. 2016;43:24–31.
33. Ueno H, Human Circulating T. Follicular helper cell subsets in health and disease. J Clin Immunol. 2016;36(Suppl 1):34–9.
34. Locci M, et al. Human circulating PD-1+CXCR3-CXCR5+ memory Tfh cells are highly functional and correlate with broadly neutralizing HIV antibody responses. Immunity. 2013;39(4):758–69.
35. Crotty S. Follicular helper CD4 T cells (TFH). Annu Rev Immunol. 2011;29:621–63.
36. King C, Tangye SG, Mackay CR. T follicular helper (TFH) cells in normal and dysregulated immune responses. Annu Rev Immunol. 2008;26:741–66.
37. Newburger JW, et al. Diagnosis, treatment, and long-term management of Kawasaki disease: a statement for health professionals from the committee on rheumatic fever, endocarditis and Kawasaki disease, council on cardiovascular disease in the young, American Heart Association. Circulation. 2004;110(17):2747–71.
38. Choi JY, et al. Circulating follicular helper-like T cells in systemic lupus erythematosus: association with disease activity. Arthritis Rheumatol. 2015; 67(4):988–99.
39. Szabo K, et al. A comprehensive investigation on the distribution of circulating follicular T helper cells and B cell subsets in primary Sjogren's syndrome and systemic lupus erythematosus. Clin Exp Immunol. 2016; 183(1):76–89.
40. Liu D, et al. Distinct phenotypic subpopulations of circulating CD4+CXCR5+ follicular helper T cells in children with active IgA vasculitis. BMC Immunol. 2016;17(1):40.
41. Bentebibel S, et al. Induction of ICOS+CXCR3+CXCR5+ TH cells correlates with antibody responses to influenza vaccination. Sci Transl Med. 2013; 5(176):176ra32.
42. Boswell K, et al. Loss of circulating CD4 T cells with B cell helper function during chronic HIV infection. PLoS Pathog. 2014;10(1):e1003853.
43. Franco A, et al. Memory T-cells and characterization of peripheral T-cell clones in acute Kawasaki disease. Autoimmunity. 2010;43(4):317–24.
44. Spolski R, Leonard W. Interleukin-21: a double-edged sword with therapeutic potential. Nat Rev Drug Discov. 2014;13(5):379–95.
45. Bae Y, et al. Elevated serum levels of IL-21 in Kawasaki disease. Allergy Asthma Immunol Res. 2012;4(6):351–6.
46. Engelberg R, et al. Observational study of Interleukin-21 (IL-21) does not distinguish Kawasaki disease from other causes of fever in children. Pediatr Rheumatol Online J. 2017;15(1):32.
47. Han J, et al. Correlation between elevated platelet count and immunoglobulin levels in the early convalescent stage of Kawasaki disease. Medicine (Baltimore). 2017;96(29):e7583.
48. Coquet J, et al. IL-21 modulates activation of NKT cells in patients with stage IV malignant melanoma. Clin Transl Immunology. 2013;2(10):e6.

49. Korn T, et al. IL-21 initiates an alternative pathway to induce proinflammatory T(H)17 cells. Nature. 2007;448(7152):484–7.
50. Pelletier N, et al. Plasma cells negatively regulate the follicular helper T cell program. Nat Immunol. 2010;11(12):1110–8.
51. Bauquet AT, et al. The costimulatory molecule ICOS regulates the expression of c-Maf and IL-21 in the development of follicular T helper cells and TH-17 cells. Nat Immunol. 2009;10(2):167–75.
52. Ozaki K, et al. Regulation of B cell differentiation and plasma cell generation by IL-21, a novel inducer of Blimp-1 and Bcl-6. J Immunol. 2004;173(9):5361–71.
53. Tangye S, et al. The good, the bad and the ugly - TFH cells in human health and disease. Nat Rev Immunol. 2013;13(6):412–26.
54. Eto D, et al. IL-21 and IL-6 are critical for different aspects of B cell immunity and redundantly induce optimal follicular helper CD4 T cell (Tfh) differentiation. PLoS One. 2011;6(3):e17739.
55. Bai L, et al. Retrospective analysis of risk factors associated with Kawasaki disease in China. Oncotarget. 2017;8(33):54357–63.
56. Kuo H, et al. Epigenetic hypomethylation and upregulation of matrix metalloproteinase 9 in Kawasaki disease. Oncotarget. 2017;8(37):60875–91.
57. Kuo H, et al. Genome-wide association study identifies novel susceptibility genes associated with coronary artery aneurysm formation in Kawasaki disease. PLoS One. 2016;11(5):e0154943.

19

Oncolytic herpes simplex virus and immunotherapy

Wenqing Ma, Hongbin He[*] and Hongmei Wang[*]

Abstract

Background: Oncolytic viruses have been proposed to be employed as a potential treatment of cancer. Well targeted, they will serve the purpose of cracking tumor cells without causing damage to normal cells. In this category of oncolytic viral drugs human pathogens herpes simplex virus (HSV) is especially suitable for the cause. Although most viral infection causes antiviral reaction in the host, HSV has multiple mechanisms to evade those responses. Powerful anti-tumor effect can thus be achieved via genetic manipulation of the HSV genes involved in this evading mechanism, namely deletions or mutations that adapt its function towards a tumor microenvironment. Currently, oncolytic HSV (oHSV) is widely use in clinical; moreover, there's hope that its curative effect will be further enhanced through the combination of oHSV with both traditional and emerging therapeutics.

Results: In this review, we provide a summary of the HSV host antiviral response evasion mechanism, HSV expresses immune evasion genes such as ICP34.5, ICP0, Us3, which are involved in inducing and activating host responses, so that the virus can evade the immune system and establish effective long-term latent infection; we outlined details of the oHSV strains generated by removing genes critical to viral replication such as ICP34.5, ICP0, and inserting therapeutic genes such as *LacZ*, granulocyte macrophage colony-stimulating factor (GM-CSF); security and limitation of some oHSV such G207, 1716, OncoVEX, NV1020, HF10, G47 in clinical application; and the achievements of oHSV combined with immunotherapy and chemotherapy.

Conclusion: We reviewed the immunotherapy mechanism of the oHSV and provided a series of cases. We also pointed out that an in-depth study of the application of oHSV in cancer treatment will potentially benefits cancer patients more.

Keywords: Oncolytic herpes simplex virus, Cancer, Immune escape, Genetically engineered, Oncolytic viral therapy

Introduction

For the past few years,despite constant new attempts finding phenomenal cancer treatments, chemotherapy, radiation and targeted drugs therapy are still the main therapeutic method in clinical practice. However, many problems remain in these methods, such as incompleteness, severe side effects, easy development of drug resistance, and lack of control in tumor recurrence and metastasis, etc., all of which lead to unsatisfactory result in treating tumor. The shortcomings of these major therapies call for new strategies in the field of cancer [1].

The Oncolytic virus is a subtype of a lytic virus that selectively replicates and kills cancer cells and spreads within the tumor without damaging normal tissue. The activities of oncolytic virus reflect the basic biological principles of the virus and the interaction of host-virus in the fight between pathogenesis and the immune system [2].

HSV, a member of the alpha-herpesviruses subfamily, shares many similarities with pseudorabies virus, varicella-zoster virus and infectious bovine rhinotracheitis virus [3]. The virus contains double stranded DNA genomes of at least 120 kb, encoding for 70 or more genes. At present, lysotype HSV is the first virus to be developed into a recombinant oncolytic viral therapeutic vector, and the first oncolytic virus to fight cancer. As a cytolytic virus HSV possesses the following advantages: (1) HSV replicate quickly in cells and has capability to

* Correspondence: hongbinhe@sdnu.edu.cn; hongmeiwang@sdnu.edu.cn
Ruminant Diseases Research Center, Shandong Provincial Key Laboratory of Animal Resistance Biology, College of Life Sciences, Shandong Normal University, Jinan 250014, China

infect multiple types of cancer cells; (2) HSV has a large genome, which can be easily modified and be inserted with multiple additional transgenes [4, 5]; (3) HSV can be prevented with antiviral drugs when the dose start to impose threat to the patients' lives [6–8]; (4) Modifying the glycoprotein of HSV can improve the targeting of tumor cells [9].

As efficient OVs, HSV has some ability to escape the host's immune response including: To complement and incapacitate immunoglobulins via viral glycoproteins; to inhibit the production of cytokine/chemokine from infected cells [10]; to block the antigen presenting cells' (APCs) maturation [11]; to evade host immunological surveillance via negative-regulation of the expression of MHC class I [12] and to inhibit the apoptosis and cell death induced by cytotoxic T lymphocyte(TL) [13]. For deletion or mutation of those genes that were involved

in HSV's escape through its host' immune defense will prohibit its replication in normal cells. Tumor microenvironment is often in an immunosuppressive state, which may allow the virus' entry and replication, which in turns eventually leads to the dissolution and death of tumor cells (Fig. 1). oHSV can also reverse the immune suppression of tumor microenvironment, enhance tumor immunogenicity, promote the infiltration of inflammatory cells, and play an effective anti-tumor effect.

This review elaborates on how the HSV surmounts the anti-viral defense mechanism of the host; the oHSVs' involvements in deletion or modification of viral gene and the clinical development of oHSV. A better understanding of the complex pattern of the interaction between HSV and host, and combination with current clinical oHSV is essential to the refinements the strategy of oHSV, thus to improve the

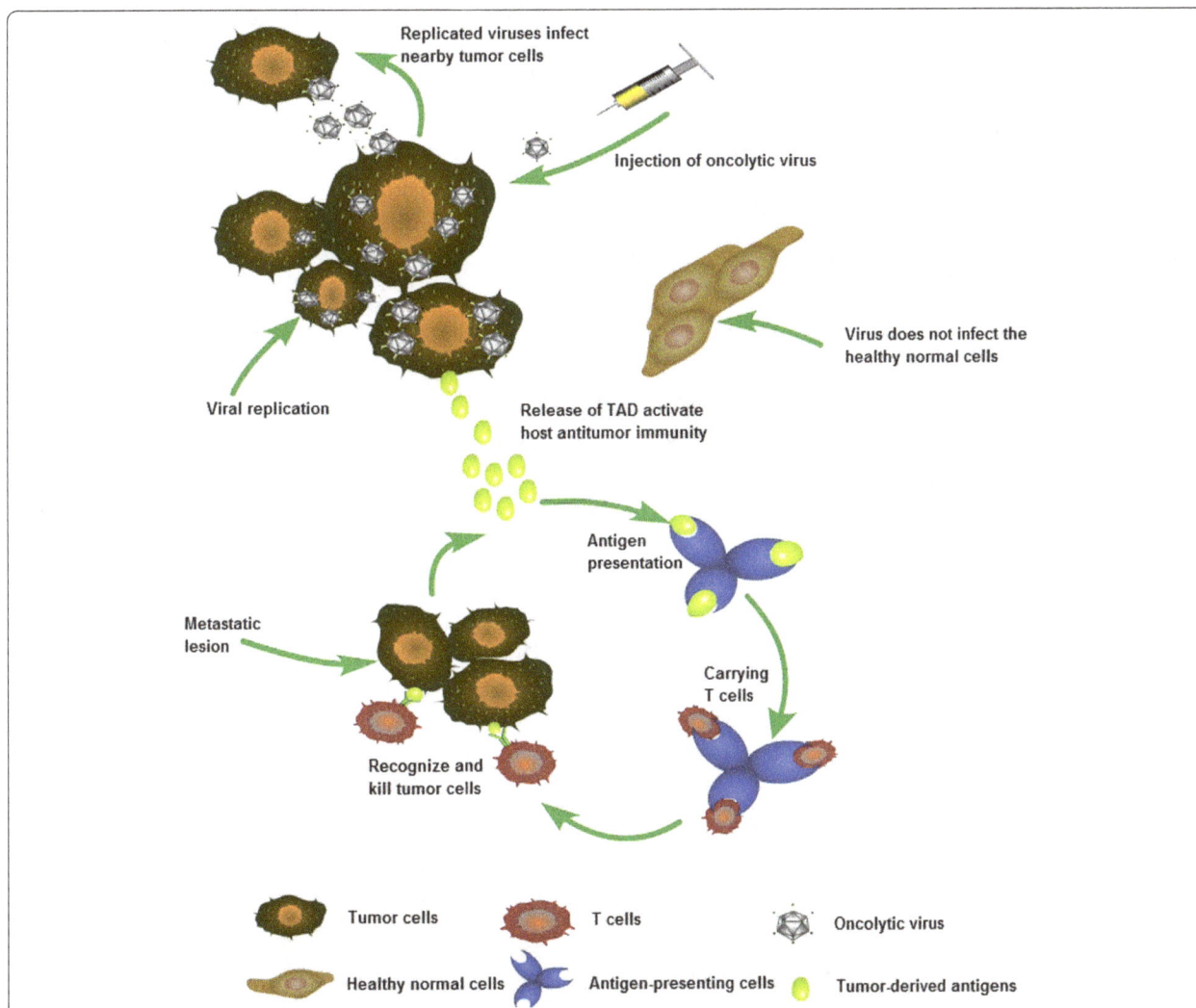

Fig. 1 Mechanisms of oncolytic virus selective killing tumor cells. Local replication of oncolytic virus induces lysis of tumor cells results in release of tumor-derived antigens which promote the activity of the cancer-immunity cycle, resulting in the specific antitumor immunity in the course of its oncolytic activities that act on remote lesions, ultimately killing the tumor cells selectively

therapeutic effects and to comprehend the oHSV immune imperfection.

The mechanism of HSV confronted the host immune response

The infection of HSV causes to a cascade reaction of host anti-viral immunity responses. As a successful pathogen, HSV expresses proteins which are involved in inducing and activating host responses, so that the virus can escape from the immune system and set up effective long-term latent infection. HSV has various mechanisms to escape the host reactions (Fig. 2):

Envelope glycoprotein

The envelope glycoproteins of HSV can escape humoral immunity mechanisms, such as Glycoprotein C binding and inactivating properdin and complement protein C3b, C5 to protect the virus from virus neutralization mediated by complement induced via natural IgM and antibody-independent complement neutralization [14, 15]. gE and gI encode Fc receptors, which can attach to

IgG [16]. This binding inactivation of complement mediated via antibody and cytotoxicity of antibody dependence conduce pathogenicity [17]. gD inhibit the expression of CD112, which binds to the natural killer (NK) cells excitating receptors DNAX accessory molecule 1 (DNAM1), leading to a noneffective binding and lysis to HSV-infected or gD-transfected cells via NK [18]. HSV inhibits the expression of CD1d, surface molecules of APCs, and thus reduces NKT cells stimulate [19].

Immune evasion genes

A series of genes encoded via HSV escape the host antiviral immune monitoring mechanism [10, 20]. In cancer cells, some of these pathways are flawed [21]. Interferon (IFN) 1 signaling pathway, crucial for antiviral innate immunity [22], relates to genes that are involved in pathways such as the TLR signaling pathway: Us3 inhibit the signal transmission of TLR3 and TLR2 to TRAF6 [23], deubiquitinase for UL36 down-regulate the expression of TRAF3 [20], ICP0 inhibit the expression of P50 and

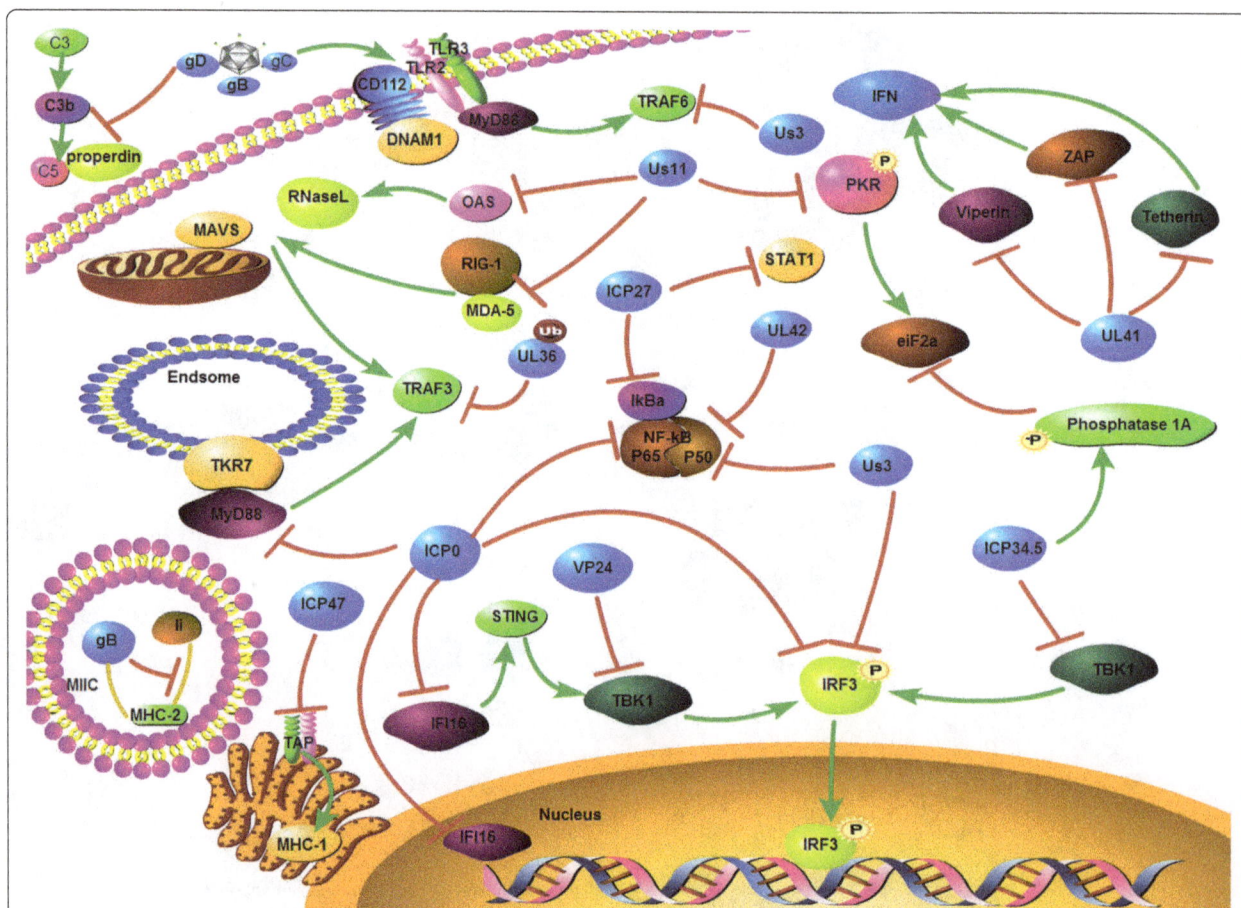

Fig. 2 Mechanism of HSV evades host immune responses. HSV expresses genes which evade host immune surveillance via inactive immune regulation factor involved in the antiviral inmate immunity pathway, such the TLR signaling pathway, RLR signaling pathway and the DNA sensor signaling pathway

P65, the subunits of MyD88 and NF-κB [24], UL42 and Us3 inhibit the process of nuclear translocation via NF-κB [25, 26], and ICP27 bind to IκBa inhibits NF-κB [27]. In the RLR signaling pathway: the Us11 can combine with RIG-I and MDA-5, thus inhibits the integration with MAVS [28, 29]. ICP34.5 inhibit the phosphorylation of IRF3 by binding TBK1 [30], US3 inhibit production of IFN-β via hyperphosphorylation of IFN regulatory factor 3 (IRF3) [31], ICP0 prevents IRF3 sustained activation, thus inhibiting translocation from the nucleus to cytoplasm [32]. Influence of the DNA sensor signaling pathway is also present: IFI16, involved in sensing pathogen DNA and initiating signaling pathways, inhibits via ICP0 in the nucleus [33]. In addition, IFN-stimulated genes, UL41 the virion host shutoff protein (Vhs), inhibits viperin, ZAP, and tetherin via degraded mRNA [20, 34], Us11 inhibits OAS [35] and protein kinase R (PKR) [36]. Eukaryotic Initiation Factor 2 (eIF2a) phosphorylated via PKR, shuts down the synthesis of protein. ICP27 blocks the phosphorylation and activation of STAT-1 [37]. Due to the defection of cancer cells in IFN signaling [38], deletion or mutation in these immune evasion genes such as ICP34.5, ICP0, Us3 in oHSV will avail ourselves of a cancer therapy [21].

Block dendritic cells function

Dendritic cells (DCs) are polymorphisms and heterogeneous antigen presenting cells, it has vital function for the recognition of pathogens at the site of infection and the initiation of protective HSV-specific T cells [39]. HSV has numerous mechanisms to inhibit DCs function [11]. ICP34.5 binds to TBK1 and IKKα/β, impeding the maturation of DCs and inhibits autophagy by interfering with antigen presentation [40, 41]. ICP0 induces CD83 degradation as a DCs maturation marker, leading to a decrease in T cell stimulation [42] ICP47 blocks transporter associated with antigen presentation (TAP), inhibits MHC I-peptide presentation, and thus leads to a mediated by MHC I to CD8+ T-cells to escapes immunological surveillance in host cells without antigen presentation. Pourchet A et al. showed that oHSV express UL49.5 from BHV-1 has a high efficacy treating cancer models, which is rely on CD8+ T cells [43]. gB binds to HLA-DM and HLA-DR, which yields a negtive-regulation of MHC II pathway in CD4+ T cells [44]. ICP34.5 and UL41 interfere with antigen presentation of CD4+ T cells via down-regulated MHC II accumulation on the surface of glioblastoma cells [45].

T cells are also influenced via HSV infection. Firstly Us3 inhibits LAT, which is the linker activating T cells, and in turns blocks TCR signaling [24]. Secondly oHSV infection has an impact on the pathway in T cells, such as inhibiting NF-κB, activating STAT3, JNK and MAPK p38 pathways, and suppressing the pro-inflammatory cytokines synthesis, such as IL-2, TNF-a and increasing IL-10 synthesis [46].

Inhibition of autophagy

Autophagy is an important cellular degradative pathway [47], which exerts on cellular pathogens like oHSV with a process similar to the MHC I and II presented in APCs [48]. ICP34.5 targets Beclin1 and interacts with PPP1CA, blocking the formation of autophagosome [49–51]. HSV induced EIF2AK2 activation down-regulates the Beclin1-mediated autophagy [49, 51]. In additional, ICP34.5 directly inhibits TBK1, which can regulated the phosphorylation of autophagic receptors SQSTM1/p62 and optineurin (OPTN) to mediate substances recruitment into phagophores for degradation [52]. Us11 interacts with EIF2AK2, inhibiting the phosphorylation of EIF2S1, mediated via EIF2AK2, to block autophagy [53].

Inhibition of apoptosis

Apoptosis, the programmed cell death, can clear up the infected cells. HSV encoding anti-apoptotic virulence factors to suppress apoptosis then gives the virus enough time to replicate after infection [13, 54]. After HSV infection, some genes like ICP6, Us3, gD and Us5 (gJ) play role in the suppression of cells apoptosis. Us3 suppresses the expression of cytochrome c and the activation of caspase-3 [54], Us3 protein kinase activates the proapoptotic proteins Bad and Bid [55]. Us5 (gJ) antagonizes Fas/UV-induced apoptosis and weakens the granzyme B-mediated pathways of CTL-induced apoptosis [56]. Compared to gJ, Us6 (gD) blocks apoptosis at different stages of the viral life cycle. Necroptosis, another programmed cell death, which absence of caspases. ICP6 suppress apoptosis by blocking caspase 8 mediated via TNF-α and Fas ligand [57], also blocking necroptosis induced by TNF via inhibits the binding of RIP1 and RIP3 [58]. However, ICP6 had the reverse effect, in mice [13, 59].

The interactions of these host viruses are crucial to harmonize the OV activity, regulate the OVs anti-viral immune responses, and inducing anti-tumor immunity.

Genetically engineered oHSV

The key to eradicate tumors in this new therapy is to improve the precision when targeting oHSV for tumors, and enhance the suppression. Genetic engineering can affect many aspects of how viruses' work. To enhance tumor selectivity by removing key genes in healthy cells that replicate with the virus. Table 1 summarizes the modified viral genes in oHSV and the functions of viral proteins encoded by these genes.

Dlsptk, the first type 1 herpes simplex virus mutants, includes a mutation within the UL23 gene that encodes the thymidine kinase (TK) gene. Dlsptk can inhibit the growth of glioma in nude rat brain [60, 61]. Nevertheless, high

Table 1 Immune evasion genes of HSV

Gene	Protein	Function	oHSV name
UL27	gB	Part of initial attachment of the virus to the cell by binding to heparan sulfate. With gH/gL, enables fusion of the envelope with the cell membrane. Down-regulation of MHC II processing pathway in CD4+ cells.	R5141; KNE
UL44	gC	Forms the initial attachment of the virus to the cell by binding to heparan sulfate. Inactivates serum complement proteins.	R5141
US6	gD	Binds to HVeM and/or nectin-1, leading to a conformation change that initiates fusion. Down-regulates NK receptor ligand and NK-mediated lysis; inhibition of apoptosis.	R5141; R-LM249; HSV1716EGFR; KNE
RL1	ICP34.5	Major neurovirulence gene. Suppression of PKR/eIF-2a signaling pathway and IFN-induced anti-viral mechanisms; Inhibits DC maturation and antigen. Presentation; Blocks MHC class II accumulation on the cell surface; Binds to Beclin-1, inhibiting autophagy.	HSV1716; R3616; OncoVex^{GMCSF}; G47; ΔG207; DM33;
RL2	ICP0	Blocks NF-κB-mediated transcription of immunomodulatory cytokines, and IRF3-induced and IRF7-induced anti-viral signaling pathways; inhibits IRF3 translocation to the nucleus; inhibits IFI16; degradation of mature DC marker (CD83). Involved in transcription of viral genes. Has ubiquitin ligase activity. Inhibits interferon response. Alters the cellular environment to promote viral replication.	R7020 (NV1020);
UL39	ICP6	Major subunit of ribonucleotide reductase. Blocks TNF-a-mediated and Fas ligand-mediated apoptosis through interacting with caspase 8 and necroptosis.	hrR3; G47Δ
UL54	ICP27	Inhibits cellular mRNA splicing. Recruits necessary proteins involved in viral transcription and translation. Activates cellular pathways to promote viral replication. Blocks NF-κB and IRF3 signaling pathways; blocks STAT1 activation and its translocation to the nucleus.	HF10
US12	ICP47	Down-regulates MHC class I by inhibiting TAP.	G47Δ; OncoVex^{GMCSF}
US11	US11	Binds to and is phosphorylated by PKR, preventing cellular inhibition of protein synthesis and autophagy; blocks OAS.	G47Δ
US3	US3	Inhibits NF-κB activation and reduces cytokine expression, such as IL-8; inhibits induction of apoptosis; hyperphosphorylates IRF3 to block activation of RLR signaling pathway.	R7041
UL48	VP16	Initiates transcription of immediate early genes. Inhibits NF-κB activation and blocks IRF3 pathway and IFN-β production.	KM100

doses of Dlsptk can cause fatal encephalitis. For this reason, it is necessary to look for other engineered herpes mutants with low toxicity [62].

HrR3, the recombinant HSV-1, insert a *LacZ* in HSV-1 UL39 (encode ICP6), alternatively replicates in cancer cells, which has remarkable anticancer activity [63, 64].

HSV1716 was isolated from HSV-1 (17+) strain, deletes two copies of the main neurotoxic determinant generepeat RL1, which encodes neurotoxic determinant ICP34.5). PKR phosphorylates eIF2a, thus inhibits protein translation and induces cell apoptosis and kills the virus. ICP34.5 mediated dephosphorylation of eIF2a prevent cell apoptosis and protect the survival and reproduction of virus [65]. 1716 targets cancer cells that uncontrollable protein synthesis [66].

R3616, isolated from HSV-1 (F) strain, deletes the two replicas of ICP34.5 genes. R3616 can effectively induce host anti-tumor immune response by inducing a series of immune cells [67]. Kanzaki et al. showed that R3616 infects tumor antigen-specific lymphocytes; this not only effect on primary tumors, but also regulates multiple metastases [68].

NV1020 is an attenuated HSV that contains a diploid gene (RL1, RL2 and s1), with UL56 in the genome

deleted [69]. Moreover, NV1020 attenuated via delete the TK gene and the UL24 genes promoter, and then inserts an exogenous copy of TK gene. These changes allow NV1020 highly attenuated and only proliferates in tumor cells.

G207, the first oHSV to be tested in clinical trials, deletes the ICP34.5 and inserted the *LacZ* gene, so the virus can selectively spread in tumor cells [70]. The deletion mutants ICP34.5 induced the down-regulate of late viral genes including US11 via PKR [9]. G207 can induce systemic anti-tumor immunity, which is related to the activation of cytotoxic T lymphocytes [8].

G47Δ derived from G207, contain two of the mutations in the RL1 and ICP47 genes, and insert the *LacZ* in ICP6 gene (coding ribonucleic acid reductase large subunit) area cause its inactivation. Inactivation of ICP6 then induces the oHSV's only replicate in proliferating cells. Furthermore, the ICP47 mutation can effectively activate the host's anti-tumor immune response via enhanced MHC-I expression [71]. Due to the three remoulds in the genome, G47Δ may be less toxic and more secure than G207 and T-Vec.

DM33 includes deletions of ICP34.5 and LAT gene. Unlike Dlsptk, DM33 was isolated from the McKrae strain, which promotes viral growth and kills cancer cells [72, 73].

HF10, remove the 3.9 kb connection point between the right end of UL and UL/IRL, which caused the loss expression of UL56, and reproduction of UL53 (gK), UL54 (ICP27) and UL55 [9]. HF10 enhances angiogenesis and induces acytotoxic T lymphocytes anti-tumor response [62].

Oncovex^{GM-CSF}, ICP34.5 and ICP47 genes in HSV-1 were strike out, and the integration of human GM-CSF was step in the ICP34.5 site. A series of cytokines such as IL12, GM-CSF, IFN-α and tumor necrosis factor (TNF-α) used with oHSV can modify and enhance the anti-tumor immunity. The GM-CSF shows the most effective results. TNF-α, IL-12 and IFN-α preclinical cancer studies have also show promising contributions [74, 75]. Oncovex^{GM-CSF} enhanced antigen-specific T cell response and decreased inhibitory CD4+ regulation of T cell expression, with a specific antitumor effects achieved in CD8+ T cells [76].

Clinical development and limitations of oHSV

Oncolytic viruses have assessment for treatment of a series of mlignation tumors. The first clinical trials of engineered virus was conducted in the 1990s [77]. Several different oHSV have been or will be tested worldwide for various cancers; some have been developed to phase II/III trials, such as G207, 1716, OncoVEX, NV1020, HF10, G47Δ (Table 2) [78].

Initially, oHSVs lay emphasis on security vectors, which included the deletes ICP34.5 gene, such as HSV1716. HSV1716 was first demonstrated to be safe and toxic in patients with pleomorphic glioblastoma and

intersex astrocytoma [79]. The results showed that HSV1716 had good tolerance and no adverse reactions occurred after high dose of 1×10^5 PFU treatment. HSV1716 has been used in the treatment of glioma and oral squamous cell carcinoma [80–82].

Then strains with additional multiple deletions or mutations in case of the reversion of wild type virus, like the G207 [83], became the first oHSVs used in clinical trial. G207 has been used for recurrent malignant glioma in phase I studies, untoward effect have been moderated to slight fever and local erythema/inflammation reactions at the sites of injection [84].

G47Δ enhances the anti-tumor efficacy while retaining the safety characteristics of G207 [85–87]. G47Δ showed efficacy in all solid tumor models tested in vivo, such as hepatocellular carcinoma [88], schwannoma [89], prostate cancer [87, 90, 91], nasopharyngeal carcinoma [71], glioma, thyroid carcinoma [92], colorectal cancer, breast cancer [93] and malignant peripheral nerve sheath tumor. G47Δ has the ability to killing cancer stem cells [94]. At present, G47 Δ is the only third generation oHSVs tested on humans [85].

NV1020 safety and efficacy have been demonstrated in some cancer diseases, such as colon carcinoma, pleural cancer, bladder cancer and pancreatic cancer [95–98]. Kemeny N et.al investigated the safety and tolerance of NV1020 in liver metastasis of colorectal cancer in a phase I clinical trial [99]. NV1020 was also tested for liver metastasis from colorectal cancer in phase II trials. The results show that NV1020 is safe and effective in anti-tumor therapy [100]. In phase III trials, NV1020 was used in combination with cytotoxic and targeted drugs [62].

Table 2 oHSVs of genetic engineering and its clinical application

oHSV name	Genetic modification	Descrption	Clinical application
DIsptk	TK⁻(UL23)	Internal deletion within UL23	Malignant human gliomas
hrR3	UL39	Insertion of *LacZ* (encodes β-galactosidase) in UL39	Pancreatic cancer; colon carcinoma; liver cancers
HSV1716	ICP34.5	Deletion in both copies of ICP34.5	Glioblastoma multiforme; anaplastic astrocytoma; oral squamous cell carcinoma
R3616	ICP34.5	Deletion of two copies of ICP34.5	Pancreatic cancer; colon carcinoma
G207	ICP34.5	Deletions of two copies of the ICP34.5; insertion of an *Escherichia coli LacZ*	Prostate adenocarcinoma; glioblastoma; hepatocellular carcinoma; colorectal cancer
R7020 (NV1020)	UL23, UL55, UL56, RL1, RL2, RS1	Deletion of UL23, as well as the region encoding UL55, UL56, and one copy of RL1, RL2, and RS1 (though not the RS1 promoter)	Pancreatic cancer; colon carcinoma; bladder cancer; pleural cancer
G47Δ	RL1, UL39, US11, US12	Deletion of the overlapping US11 promoter/US12 region, putting expression of the normally late US11 gene under the immediate early US12 promoter	Prostate adenocarcinoma; glioblastoma; rectal cancer; nasopharyngeal carcinoma; breast cancer
OncoVex^{GM-CSF}	ICP34.5 and ICP47	Deletion of two copies of ICP34.5 gene and the viral ICP47 genes; insertion of GM-CSF	Breast cancer; head and neck cancer; gastrointestinal cancers; malignant melanoma
HF10	UL53, UL54, UL55, UL56	Spontaneous deletion of UL56 as well as duplication of UL53, UL54, and UL55	Breast cancer; malignant melanoma; pancreatic cancer
DM33	ICP34.5	Deletions of γ-34.5 and LAT gene	Human gliomas and glioma cell line

Oncovex^{GM-CSF} is the first type of oncolytic virus. After genetic engineering, oncogm-csf can selectively replicate in tumor cells, directly inject into the lesion, express GM-CSF, and enhance systemic anti-tumor immune response [68, 101]. GM-CSF insertion can promote complementary anti-tumor immune response by recruiting APCs [102]. After intratumoral injection of oncovex^{GM-CSF}, the lesions of 8/50 patients with metastatic malignant melanoma disappeared completely [103]. The safety of an oncovex^{GM-CSF} has been determined in phase I studies [104]. Direct injection of oncovex^{GM-CSF} into melanoma lesions yielded an objective response rate of 28% in phase II clinical trials. Phase III clinical trials are ongoing [62].

However, oncolytic viruses all have the peculiarity of parental viruses and have some defects. Although HSV-1 is transmitted between cells and does not cause viremia, the most effective method for oncolytic HSV-1 is intracellular administration, which may not be suitable for intravenous infusion [105]. Because there are some drawbacks in intravenous administration, circulating antibodies may reduce the efficacy [106]. Viremia naturally causes viruses to be easily neutralized by antibodies; so the antineoplastic effect of intravenous administration of such viruses is limited in patients who have been treated or vaccinated. Clinical trials using oncolytic measles virus in the treatment of multiple myeloma fully demonstrated the adverse effects of circulating antibodies [107]. In dose-increasing studies, intravenous measles virus injection showed efficacy only when the dose reached a high dose of 10^{11} TCID50. In mice with transplanted tumors, intravenous injection of reovirus (REV) for 3 weeks after initial inhibition of tumor growth resulted in tumor regeneration, while the serum titer of anti- REVs antibodies increased [108]. Phase I study showed that 12 of 33 patients (36%) reached the maximum neutralizing REV antibody titer on the 7th day and 20 patients (61%) reached the maximum neutralizing REV antibody titer on the 14th day [109]. Hence, in the first week of treatment, speediness, repetitive, high-dose administration should be given before serum neutralizing antibodies rise, and should be combined with other anticancer therapies [106].

Increase the efficacy of oHSV deliver to tumor cells

At present, in the application of ohsv, there are some problems that limit its therapeutic effect, whether intratumoral or intravenous injection, there are some defects. Intratumoral injection can ensure that virus particles reach the lesion directly, but it is difficult to spread to the lesion area outside the injection area. Intravenous injection provides an opportunity for the virus to infect all cancer cells, and is particularly effective in the treatment of metastatic lesions [110]. Nevertheless, viral particles

injected into veins are bound to suffer innate immune responses from the host [111], which may result in the virus particles being neutralized by antibodies before reaching the target cells.

The receptors that bind oHSV to cells are repositioned to ensure that the virus is more readily accessible to cancer cells. The co-injection of oHSV and collagenase can degrade the extracellular matrix of tumors by collagenase, and make the region outside the injection site of virus particles diffuse. The method for delivery of the oHSV can be enhanced or reduced by pretreatment with antiangiogenesis molecules. When oHSV was administered by direct injection, prior injection of cyclic RGD peptide, an antiangiogenic agent, reduced tumor vascular permeability and infiltration of leukocytes [112]. When oHSV is injected intravenously, the blood-brain barrier will increase the difficulty of injection. In order to solve this problem, it has been proved that destruction of the blood-brain barrier through hypertonic solution of mannitol can increase the number of viruses reaching tumors [110]. Ultrasound technique is also used to enhance the permeability of cell membrane and the efficacy of chemotherapeutic drugs anti-cancer [113]. Shintani et al. showed that effective use of ultrasound technology to help oHSV-1 enter squamous cell carcinomas [114]. Combination with key immunoregulatory inhibitors can improve the efficacy of oncolytic virus. For example, a study showed that intravenous injection of anti-PD-1 antibodies combined with Reolysin was significantly more effective in treating subcutaneous melanoma in mice than intravenous injection of Reolysin or anti-PD-1 alone [115]. Combination of anti-PD-1 antibody therapy can improve NK cells' effective lysis of REV infected malignant cells by reducing the activity of regulatory T cells. Phase I study of combined therapy of oncolytic virus T-Vec and pembrolizumab (anti-PD-1) for head and neck cancer has been completed [105].

Besides, the oHSV combination with chemotherapy is also an effective strategy for tumor treatment. Toyoizumi et al. showed that combining the HSV1716 with chemotherapeutic drug MMC to treat the human non-small cell lung cancer yielded profound efficacy [116]. This study showed that chemotherapy and oHSV can work together treat cancer, and this synergistic effect will strengthen anti-tumor ability. Co-administrated with cyclophosphamide, the anticancer activity of HrR3 improved effectively [117]. Cyclophosphamide can enhance the replication of oncolytic virus by inhibiting the immune response of the system and has better anti-cancer effect [118]. However, in all oncolytic theatmets, the long range of side effects of inducing via body anti-tumor immunity, such as the emergence of AIDs, requires close study.

Conclusion

Oncolytic therapy, successes or failure hangs on the interaction of antiviral and antitumor immune responses between virus and host. HSV has been shown to be a site virus gets for oncolytic treatment because it is susceptible to genetic changes, deletions or mutations in genes with immunoregulatory function like ICP0, ICP 34.5, ICP 27, Us3 and UL39. This genetic alteration may result in an enhanced innate immune response, weakening viral replication and spreading in tumors.

At present, oHSV applied in clinical trials have not experienced serious adverse result and has achieved some effectiveness. For example, HSV1716 has been used for the treatment of oral squamous cell carcinoma and gloma [85–87]; G47Δ showed efficacy in glioma, breast cancer [93], malignant peripheral nerve sheath tumor [92], schwannoma [89], nasopharyngeal carcinoma [71], hepatocellular carcinoma [88], prostate cancer [87, 90, 91], colorectal cancer and thyroid carcinoma; NV1020 can effectively control liver metastasis and prolong survival via re-sensitizing to chemotherapy [100].

Although the deleted or mutated genes confer safety and selectivity to oHSV in the treatments of tumor cells, efficacy has been attenuated. Direct injection of oHSVs is usually preferred during treatment, but this procedure limits the delivery to the sites where the tumor actually occurs. Physical factors like the extracellular matrix can limit the initial distribution and external diffusion of oHSV in the tumors [119]. The inborn and acquired anti-virus immunity can limit the replication and spread of oHSV [120]. In oncolytic virotherapy, these are only some examples of the many hurdles to be overcome. This made it necessary to combine oHSV with other therapies. The expectations are to develop a combination therapy regimen that produces synergic action against tumor cells without overlapping side effects. For examples, the combinations of oHSV with collagenase can degrade the extracellular matrix of tumors by collagenase, and make the region outside the injection site of virus particles diffuse; Injection of circulating RGD peptide before oHSV infection can reduce the permeability of blood vessels and infiltration of leukocytes in tumors [112]; and many published combination joint research tested the efficacy of oHSV combined with immunotherapies and chemotherapies in vitro. These identified combinations have achieved some good results.

With the development of preclinical research into clinical application, it is more likely to achieve greater success in understanding the combination of oHSV and other treatments. In a word, there are many areas to be researched in development of oHSV combined with other therapies. But hopefully all would join hand to cure cancer patients.

Abbreviations

APC: antigen presenting cell; DC: Dendritic cell; DNAM1: DNAX accessory molecule 1; EIF2a: eukaryotic Initiation Factor 2; GM-CSF: granulocyte macrophage colony-stimulating factor; IFN: interferon; oHSV: oncolytic herpes simplex virus; OPTN: optineurin; PKR: protein kinase R; RR: ribonucleotide reductase; TAP: transporter associated with antigen presentation; TK: thymidine kinase; TL: T lymphocyte; TNF-α: tumor necrosis factor; Vhs: virion host shutoff protein

Acknowledgements

Not applicable.

Funding

This work was partially supported by National Key Research and Development Program of China (2018YFD0501600), Shandong province Key Research and Development program Fund (2018GNC113011), National Natural Science Fund of China (31872490, 31672556, 31502064), Taishan Scholar and Distinguished Experts (H. H.).

Authors' contributions

WQM, HMW and HBH participated in conception, data collection and data analysis and writing the manuscript; WQM prepared Figs. 1, 2; HMW and HBH critical review and making revisions. All authors read and approved the manuscript.

Competing interests

The authors declare that they have no competing interests.

References

1. Sanchala DS, Bhatt LK, Prabhavalkar KS. Oncolytic Herpes Simplex viral therapy: a stride toward selective targeting of Cancer cells. Front Pharmacol. 2017;8:270.
2. Hamid O, Hoffner B, Gasal E, Hong J, Carvajal RD. Oncolytic immunotherapy: unlocking the potential of viruses to help target cancer. Cancer Immunol Immunother. 2017;66(10):1249–64.
3. Hou P, Wang H, Zhao G, He C, He H. Rapid detection of infectious bovine Rhinotracheitis virus using recombinase polymerase amplification assays. BMC Vet Res. 2017;13(1):386.
4. Dai MH, Zamarin D, Gao SP, Chou TC, Gonzalez L, Lin SF, Fong Y. Synergistic action of oncolytic herpes simplex virus and radiotherapy in pancreatic cancer cell lines. Br J Surg. 2010;97(9):1385–94.
5. Eisenberg DP, Adusumilli PS, Hendershott KJ, Yu Z, Mullerad M, Chan MK, Chou TC, Fong Y. 5-fluorouracil and gemcitabine potentiate the efficacy of oncolytic herpes viral gene therapy in the treatment of pancreatic cancer. J Gastrointest Surg. 2005;9(8):1068–77 discussion 1077-1069.
6. Hartkopf AD, Fehm T, Wallwiener D, Lauer U. Oncolytic virotherapy of gynecologic malignancies. Gynecol Oncol. 2011;120(2):302–10.
7. De Clercq E. Antiviral drugs in current clinical use. J Clin Virol. 2004;30(2): 115–33.
8. Todo T. "Armed" oncolytic herpes simplex viruses for brain tumor therapy. Cell Adhes Migr. 2008;2(3):208–13.
9. Sokolowski NA, Rizos H, Diefenbach RJ. Oncolytic virotherapy using herpes simplex virus: how far have we come? Oncolytic Virother. 2015;4:207–19.

10. Suazo PA, Ibanez FJ, Retamal-Diaz AR, Paz-Fiblas MV, Bueno SM, Kalergis AM, Gonzalez PA. Evasion of early antiviral responses by herpes simplex viruses. Mediat Inflamm. 2015;2015:593757.

11. Bedoui S, Greyer M. The role of dendritic cells in immunity against primary herpes simplex virus infections. Front Microbiol. 2014;5:533.

12. Rombout JH, Yang G, Kiron V. Adaptive immune responses at mucosal surfaces of teleost fish. Fish Shellfish Immunol. 2014;40(2):634–43.

13. Yu X, He S. The interplay between human herpes simplex virus infection and the apoptosis and necroptosis cell death pathways. Virol J. 2016;13:77.

14. Hook LM, Lubinski JM, Jiang M, Pangburn MK, Friedman HM. Herpes simplex virus type 1 and 2 glycoprotein C prevents complement-mediated neutralization induced by natural immunoglobulin M antibody. J Virol. 2006; 80(8):4038–46.

15. Wang X, Ju Z, Huang J, Hou M, Zhou L, Qi C, Zhang Y, Gao Q, Pan Q, Li G, Zhong J, Wang C. The relationship between the variants of the bovine MBL2 gene and milk production traits, mastitis, serum MBL-C levels and complement activity. Vet Immunol Immunopathol. 2012;148(3–4):311–9.

16. Dubin G, Frank I, Friedman HM. Herpes simplex virus type 1 encodes two fc receptors which have different binding characteristics for monomeric immunoglobulin G (IgG) and IgG complexes. J Virol. 1990;64(6):2725–31.

17. Lubinski JM, Lazear HM, Awasthi S, Wang F, Friedman HM. The herpes simplex virus 1 IgG fc receptor blocks antibody-mediated complement activation and antibody-dependent cellular cytotoxicity in vivo. J Virol. 2011; 85(7):3239–49.

18. Grauwet K, Cantoni C, Parodi M, De Maria A, Devriendt B, Pende D, Moretta L, Vitale M, Favoreel HW. Modulation of CD112 by the alphaherpesvirus gD protein suppresses DNAM-1-dependent NK cell-mediated lysis of infected cells. Proc Natl Acad Sci U S A. 2014;111(45):16118–23.

19. Yuan W, Dasgupta A, Cresswell P. Herpes simplex virus evades natural killer T cell recognition by suppressing CD1d recycling. Nat Immunol. 2006;7(8):835–42.

20. Su C, Zhan G, Zheng C. Evasion of host antiviral innate immunity by HSV-1, an update. Virol J. 2016;13:38.

21. Peters C, Rabkin SD. Designing Herpes viruses as Oncolytics. Mol Ther Oncolytics. 2015;2:15010.

22. Shan S, Qi C, Zhu Y, Li H, An L, Yang G. Expression profile of carp IFN correlate with the up-regulation of interferon regulatory factor-1 (IRF-1) in vivo and in vitro: the pivotal molecules in antiviral defense. Fish Shellfish Immunol. 2016;52:94–102.

23. Yang Y, Wu S, Wang Y, Pan S, Lan B, Liu Y, Zhang L, Leng Q, Chen D, Zhang C, He B, Cao Y. The Us3 protein of Herpes Simplex virus 1 inhibits T cell signaling by confining linker for activation of T cells (LAT) activation via TRAF6 protein. J Biol Chem. 2015;290(25):15670–8.

24. van Lint AL, Murawski MR, Goodbody RE, Severa M, Fitzgerald KA, Finberg RW, Knipe DM, Kurt-Jones EA. Herpes simplex virus immediate-early ICP0 protein inhibits toll-like receptor 2-dependent inflammatory responses and NF-kappaB signaling. J Virol. 2010;84(20):10802–11.

25. Zhang J, Wang S, Wang K, Zheng C. Herpes simplex virus 1 DNA polymerase processivity factor UL42 inhibits TNF-alpha-induced NF-kappaB activation by interacting with p65/RelA and p50/NF-kappaB1. Med Microbiol Immunol. 2013;202(4):313–25.

26. Wang K, Ni L, Wang S, Zheng C. Herpes simplex virus 1 protein kinase US3 hyperphosphorylates p65/RelA and dampens NF-kappaB activation. J Virol. 2014;88(14):7941–51.

27. Kim JC, Lee SY, Kim SY, Kim JK, Kim HJ, Lee HM, Choi MS, Min JS, Kim MJ, Choi HS, Ahn JK. HSV-1 ICP27 suppresses NF-kappaB activity by stabilizing IkappaBalpha. FEBS Lett. 2008;582(16):2371–6.

28. Xing J, Wang S, Lin R, Mossman KL, Zheng C. Herpes simplex virus 1 tegument protein US11 downmodulates the RLR signaling pathway via direct interaction with RIG-I and MDA-5. J Virol. 2012;86(7):3528–40.

29. Zhu YY, Xing WX, Shan SJ, Zhang SQ, Li YQ, Li T, An L, Yang GW. Characterization and immune response expression of the rig-I-like receptor mda5 in common carp Cyprinus carpio. J Fish Biol. 2016;88(6):2188–202.

30. Ma Y, Jin H, Valyi-Nagy T, Cao Y, Yan Z, He B. Inhibition of TANK binding kinase 1 by herpes simplex virus 1 facilitates productive infection. J Virol. 2012;86(4):2188–96.

31. Wang S, Wang K, Lin R, Zheng C. Herpes simplex virus 1 serine/threonine kinase US3 hyperphosphorylates IRF3 and inhibits beta interferon production. J Virol. 2013;87(23):12814–27.

32. Paladino P, Collins SE, Mossman KL. Cellular localization of the herpes simplex virus ICP0 protein dictates its ability to block IRF3-mediated innate immune responses. PLoS One. 2010;5(4):e10428.

33. Everett RD. Dynamic response of IFI16 and Promyelocytic leukemia nuclear body components to Herpes Simplex virus 1 infection. J Virol. 2015;90(1): 167–79.

34. Zenner HL, Mauricio R, Banting G, Crump CM. Herpes simplex virus 1 counteracts tetherin restriction via its virion host shutoff activity. J Virol. 2013;87(24):13115–23.

35. Sanchez R, Mohr I. Inhibition of cellular 2'-5' oligoadenylate synthetase by the herpes simplex virus type 1 Us11 protein. J Virol. 2007;81(7):3455–64.

36. Poppers J, Mulvey M, Khoo D, Mohr I. Inhibition of PKR activation by the proline-rich RNA binding domain of the herpes simplex virus type 1 Us11 protein. J Virol. 2000;74(23):11215–21.

37. Johnson KE, Song B, Knipe DM. Role for herpes simplex virus 1 ICP27 in the inhibition of type I interferon signaling. Virology. 2008;374(2):487–94.

38. Kaufman HL, Kohlhapp FJ, Zloza A. Oncolytic viruses: a new class of immunotherapy drugs. Nat Rev Drug Discov. 2015;14(9):642–62.

39. Saha D, Wakimoto H, Rabkin SD. Oncolytic herpes simplex virus interactions with the host immune system. Curr Opin Virol. 2016;21:26–34.

40. Ma Y, He B. Recognition of herpes simplex viruses: toll-like receptors and beyond. J Mol Biol. 2014;426(6):1133–47.

41. Gobeil PA, Leib DA. Herpes simplex virus gamma34.5 interferes with autophagosome maturation and antigen presentation in dendritic cells. MBio. 2012;3(5):e00267–12.

42. Heilingloh CS, Muhl-Zurbes P, Steinkasserer A, Kummer M. Herpes simplex virus type 1 ICP0 induces CD83 degradation in mature dendritic cells independent of its E3 ubiquitin ligase function. J Gen Virol. 2014;95(Pt 6): 1366–75.

43. Pourchet A, Fuhrmann SR, Pilones KA, Demaria S, Frey AB, Mulvey M, Mohr I. CD8(+) T-cell immune evasion enables oncolytic virus immunotherapy. EBioMed. 2016;5:59–67.

44. Neumann J, Eis-Hubinger AM, Koch N. Herpes simplex virus type 1 targets the MHC class II processing pathway for immune evasion. J Immunol. 2003; 171(6):3075–83.

45. Trgovcich J, Johnson D, Roizman B. Cell surface major histocompatibility complex class II proteins are regulated by the products of the gamma(1)34. 5 and U(L)41 genes of herpes simplex virus 1. J Virol. 2002;76(14):6974–86.

46. Sloan DD, Jerome KR. Herpes simplex virus remodels T-cell receptor signaling, resulting in p38-dependent selective synthesis of interleukin-10. J Virol. 2007;81(22):12504–14.

47. Xie W, Zhou J. Aberrant regulation of autophagy in mammalian diseases. Biol Lett. 2018;14(1):20170540.

48. O'Connell D, Liang C. Autophagy interaction with herpes simplex virus type-1 infection. Autophagy. 2016;12(3):451–9.

49. Orvedahl A, Alexander D, Talloczy Z, Sun Q, Wei Y, Zhang W, Burns D, Leib DA, Levine B. HSV-1 ICP34.5 confers neurovirulence by targeting the Beclin 1 autophagy protein. Cell Host Microbe. 2007;1(1):23–35.

50. Orvedahl A, Levine B. Autophagy and viral neurovirulence. Cell Microbiol. 2008;10(9):1747–56.

51. Kanai R, Zaupa C, Sgubin D, Antoszczyk SJ, Martuza RL, Wakimoto H, Rabkin SD. Effect of gamma34.5 deletions on oncolytic herpes simplex virus activity in brain tumors. J Virol. 2012;86(8):4420–31.

52. Pilli M, Arko-Mensah J, Ponpuak M, Roberts E, Master S, Mandell MA, Dupont N, Ornatowski W, Jiang S, Bradfute SB, Bruun JA, Hansen TE, Johansen T, Deretic V. TBK-1 promotes autophagy-mediated antimicrobial defense by controlling autophagosome maturation. Immunity. 2012;37(2): 223–34.

53. Lussignol M, Queval C, Bernet-Camard MF, Cotte-Laffitte J, Beau I, Codogno P, Esclatine A. The herpes simplex virus 1 Us11 protein inhibits autophagy through its interaction with the protein kinase PKR. J Virol. 2013;87(2):859–71.

54. You Y, Cheng AC, Wang MS, Jia RY, Sun KF, Yang Q, Wu Y, Zhu D, Chen S, Liu MF, Zhao XX, Chen XY. The suppression of apoptosis by alpha-herpesvirus. Cell Death Dis. 2017;8(4):e2749.

55. Cartier A, Broberg E, Komai T, Henriksson M, Masucci MG. The herpes simplex virus-1 Us3 protein kinase blocks CD8T cell lysis by preventing the cleavage of bid by granzyme B. Cell Death Differ. 2003;10(12):1320–8.

56. Jerome KR, Chen Z, Lang R, Torres MR, Hofmeister J, Smith S, Fox R, Froelich CJ, Corey L. HSV and glycoprotein J inhibit caspase activation and apoptosis induced by granzyme B or Fas. J Immunol. 2001;167(7):3928–35.

57. Dufour F, Sasseville AM, Chabaud S, Massie B, Siegel RM, Langelier Y. The ribonucleotide reductase R1 subunits of herpes simplex virus types 1 and 2 protect cells against TNFalpha- and FasL-induced apoptosis by interacting with caspase-8. Apoptosis. 2011;16(3):256–71.

58. Guo H, Omoto S, Harris PA, Finger JN, Bertin J, Gough PJ, Kaiser WJ, Mocarski ES. Herpes simplex virus suppresses necroptosis in human cells. Cell Host Microbe. 2015;17(2):243–51.

59. Wang X, Li Y, Liu S, Yu X, Li L, Shi C, He W, Li J, Xu L, Hu Z, Yu L, Yang Z, Chen Q, Ge L, Zhang Z, Zhou B, et al. Direct activation of RIP3/MLKL-dependent necrosis by herpes simplex virus 1 (HSV-1) protein ICP6 triggers host antiviral defense. Proc Natl Acad Sci U S A. 2014;111(43):15438–43.

60. Martuza RL, Malick A, Markert JM, Ruffner KL, Coen DM. Experimental therapy of human glioma by means of a genetically engineered virus mutant. Science. 1991;252(5007):854–6.

61. Markert JM, Coen DM, Malick A, Mineta T, Martuza RL. Expanded spectrum of viral therapy in the treatment of nervous system tumors. J Neurosurg. 1992;77(4):590–4.

62. Liu S, Dai M, You L, Zhao Y. Advance in herpes simplex viruses for cancer therapy. Sci China Life Sci. 2013;56(4):298–305.

63. D J. GOLDSTEIN. And WELLER. SK. Herpes Simplex virus type 1-induced ribonucleotide reductase activity is dispensable for virus growth and DNA synthesis: isolation and characterization of an ICP6 lacZ insertion mutant. J Virol. 1988;62(1):196–205.

64. Preston GV, Palfreyman WJ, Dutia MB. Identification of a Herpes Simplex virus type 1 polypeptide which is a component of the virus-induced ribonucleotide reductase. J Gen Virol. 1984;65(9):1457 1466.

65. He B, Gross M, Roizman B. The gamma(1)34.5 protein of herpes simplex virus 1 complexes with protein phosphatase 1alpha to dephosphorylate the alpha subunit of the eukaryotic translation initiation factor 2 and preclude the shutoff of protein synthesis by double-stranded RNA-activated protein kinase. Proc Natl Acad Sci U S A. 1997;94(3):843–8.

66. Chou J, Roizman B. The gamma 1(34.5) gene of herpes simplex virus 1 precludes neuroblastoma cells from triggering total shutoff of protein synthesis characteristic of programed cell death in neuronal cells. Proc Natl Acad Sci U S A. 1992;89(8):3266–70.

67. Shirota T, Kasuya H, Kodera Y, Nishikawa Y, Shikano T, Sahin TT, Gewen T, Yamamura K, Fukuda S, Kanzaki A, Yamada S, Fujii T, Sugimoto H, Nomoto S, Takeda S, Nakao A. Oncolytic herpes virus induces effective anti-cancer immunity against murine colon cancer. Hepato-Gastroenterology. 2011; 58(110–111):1482–9.

68. Kanzaki A, Kasuya H, Yamamura K, Sahin TT, Nomura N, Shikano T, Shirota T, Tan G, Fukuda S, Misawa M, Nishikawa Y, Yamada S, Fujii T, Sugimoto H, Nomoto S, Takeda S, et al. Antitumor efficacy of oncolytic herpes simplex virus adsorbed onto antigen-specific lymphocytes. Cancer Gene Ther. 2012;19(4):292–8.

69. Koshizuka T, Kawaguchi Y, Nishiyama Y. Herpes simplex virus type 2 membrane protein UL56 associates with the kinesin motor protein KIF1A. J Gen Virol. 2005;86(Pt 3):527–33.

70. Kramm CM, Chase M, Herrlinger U, Jacobs A, Pechan PA, Rainov NG, Sena-Esteves M, Aghi M, Barnett FH, Chiocca EA, Breakefield XO. Therapeutic efficiency and safety of a second-generation replication-conditional HSV1 vector for brain tumor gene therapy. Hum Gene Ther. 1997;8(17):2057–68.

71. Wang JN, Hu P, Zeng MS, Liu RB. Anti-tumor effect of oncolytic herpes simplex virus G47delta on human nasopharyngeal carcinoma. Chinese J Cancer. 2011;30(12):831–41.

72. Samoto K, Ehtesham M, Perng GC, Hashizume K, Wechsler SL, Nesburn AB, Black KL, Yu JS. A herpes simplex virus type 1 mutant with gamma 34.5 and LAT deletions effectively oncolyses human U87 glioblastomas in nude mice. Neurosurgery. 2002;50(3):599–605 discussion 605-596.

73. Samoto K, Perng GC, Ehtesham M, Liu Y, Wechsler SL, Nesburn AB, Black KL, Yu JS. A herpes simplex virus type 1 mutant deleted for gamma34.5 and LAT kills glioma cells in vitro and is inhibited for in vivo reactivation. Cancer Gene Ther. 2001;8(4):269–77.

74. Liu BL, Robinson M, Han ZQ, Branston RH, English C, Reay P, McGrath Y, Thomas SK, Thornton M, Bullock P, Love CA, Coffin RS. ICP34.5 deleted herpes simplex virus with enhanced oncolytic, immune stimulating, and anti-tumour properties. Gene Ther. 2003;10(4):292–303.

75. Cui LL, Yang G, Pan J, Zhang C. Tumor necrosis factor alpha knockout increases fertility of mice. Theriogenology. 2011;75(5):867–76.

76. Kaufman HL, Kim DW, DeRaffele G, Mitcham J, Coffin RS, Kim-Schulze S. Local and distant immunity induced by intralesional vaccination with an oncolytic herpes virus encoding GM-CSF in patients with stage IIIc and IV melanoma. Ann Surg Oncol. 2010;17(3):718–30.

77. Kirn D, Martuza RL, Zwiebel J. Replication-selective virotherapy for cancer: biological principles, risk management and future directions. Nat Med. 2001; 7(7):781–7.

78. Kanai R, Wakimoto H, Cheema T, Rabkin SD. Oncolytic herpes simplex virus vectors and chemotherapy: are combinatorial strategies more effective for cancer? Future Oncol. 2010;6(4):619–34.

79. Rampling R, Cruickshank G, Papanastassiou V, Nicoll J, Hadley D, Brennan D, Petty R, MacLean A, Harland J, McKie E, Mabbs R, Brown M. Toxicity evaluation of replication-competent herpes simplex virus (ICP 34.5 null mutant 1716) in patients with recurrent malignant glioma. Gene Ther. 2000; 7(10):859–66.

80. Mace AT, Ganly I, Soutar DS, Brown SM. Potential for efficacy of the oncolytic Herpes simplex virus 1716 in patients with oral squamous cell carcinoma. Head Neck. 2008;30(8):1045–51.

81. Papanastassiou V, Rampling R, Fraser M, Petty R, Hadley D, Nicoll J, Harland J, Mabbs R, Brown M. The potential for efficacy of the modified (ICP 34.5(-)) herpes simplex virus HSV1716 following intratumoural injection into human malignant glioma: a proof of principle study. Gene Ther. 2002;9(6):398–406.

82. Harrow S, Papanastassiou V, Harland J, Mabbs R, Petty R, Fraser M, Hadley D, Patterson J, Brown SM, Rampling R. HSV1716 injection into the brain adjacent to tumour following surgical resection of high-grade glioma: safety data and long-term survival. Gene Ther. 2004;11(22):1648–58.

83. Moore AE. Viruses with oncolytic properties and their adaptation to tumors. Ann N Y Acad Sci. 1952;54(6):945–52.

84. Markert JM, Medlock MD, Rabkin SD, Gillespie GY, Todo T, Hunter WD, Palmer CA, Feigenbaum F, Tornatore C, Tufaro F, Martuza RL. Conditionally replicating herpes simplex virus mutant, G207 for the treatment of malignant glioma: results of a phase I trial. Gene Ther. 2000;7(10):867–74.

85. Todo T, Martuza RL, Rabkin SD, Johnson PA. Oncolytic herpes simplex virus vector with enhanced MHC class I presentation and tumor cell killing. Proc Natl Acad Sci U S A. 2001;98(11):6396–401.

86. Passer BJ, Wu CL, Wu S, Rabkin SD, Martuza RL. Analysis of genetically engineered oncolytic herpes simplex viruses in human prostate cancer organotypic cultures. Gene Ther. 2009;16(12):1477–82.

87. Fukuhara H, Martuza RL, Rabkin SD, Ito Y, Todo T. Oncolytic herpes simplex virus vector g47delta in combination with androgen ablation for the treatment of human prostate adenocarcinoma. Clin Cancer Res. 2005;11(21): 7886–90.

88. Wang J, Xu L, Zeng W, Hu P, Zeng M, Rabkin SD, Liu R. Treatment of human hepatocellular carcinoma by the oncolytic herpes simplex virus G47delta. Cancer Cell Int. 2014;14(1):83.

89. Prabhakar S, Messerli SM, Stemmer-Rachamimov AO, Liu TC, Rabkin S, Martuza R, Breakefield XO. Treatment of implantable NF2 schwannoma tumor models with oncolytic herpes simplex virus G47Delta. Cancer Gene Ther. 2007;14(5):460–7.

90. Varghese S, Rabkin SD, Liu R, Nielsen PG, Ipe T, Martuza RL. Enhanced therapeutic efficacy of IL-12, but not GM-CSF, expressing oncolytic herpes simplex virus for transgenic mouse derived prostate cancers. Cancer Gene Ther. 2006;13(3):253–65.

91. Fukuhara H, Ino Y, Kuroda T, Martuza RL, Todo T. Triple gene-deleted oncolytic herpes simplex virus vector double-armed with interleukin 18 and soluble B7-1 constructed by bacterial artificial chromosome-mediated system. Cancer Res. 2005;65(23):10663–8.

92. Antoszczyk S, Spyra M, Mautner VF, Kurtz A, Stemmer-Rachamimov AO, Martuza RL, Rabkin SD. Treatment of orthotopic malignant peripheral nerve sheath tumors with oncolytic herpes simplex virus. Neuro-Oncology. 2014; 16(8):1057–66.

93. Liu R, Martuza RL, Rabkin SD. Intracarotid delivery of oncolytic HSV vector G47Delta to metastatic breast cancer in the brain. Gene Ther. 2005;12(8): 647–54.

94. Cheema TA, Wakimoto H, Fecci PE, Ning J, Kuroda T, Jeyaretna DS, Martuza RL, Rabkin SD. Multifaceted oncolytic virus therapy for glioblastoma in an immunocompetent cancer stem cell model. Proc Natl Acad Sci U S A. 2013; 110(29):12006–11.

95. McAuliffe PF, Jarnagin WR, Johnson P, Delman KA, Federoff H, Fong Y. Effective treatment of pancreatic tumors with two multimutated herpes simplex oncolytic viruses. J Gastroint Surg. 2000;4(6):580–8.

96. Gutermann A, Mayer E, von Dehn-Rothfelser K, Breidenstein C, Weber M, Muench M, Gungor D, Suehnel J, Moebius U, Lechmann M. Efficacy of oncolytic herpesvirus NV1020 can be enhanced by combination with chemotherapeutics in colon carcinoma cells. Hum Gene Ther. 2006;17(12): 1241–53.

97. Cozzi PJ, Malhotra S, McAuliffe P, Kooby DA, Federoff HJ, Huryk B, Johnson P, Scardino PT, Heston WD, Fong Y. Intravesical oncolytic viral therapy using

attenuated, replication-competent herpes simplex viruses G207 and Nv1020 is effective in the treatment of bladder cancer in an orthotopic syngeneic model. FASEB J. 2001;15(7):1306–8.

98. Ebright MI, Zager JS, Malhotra S, Delman KA, Weigel TL, Rusch VW, Fong Y. Replication-competent herpes virus NV1020 as direct treatment of pleural cancer in a rat model. J Thorac Cardiovasc Surg. 2002;124(1):123–9.

99. Kemeny N, Brown K, Covey A, Kim T, Bhargava A, Brody L, Guilfoyle B, Haag NP, Karrasch M, Glasschroeder B, Knoll A, Getrajdman G, Kowal KJ, Jarnagin WR, Fong Y. Phase I, open-label, dose-escalating study of a genetically engineered herpes simplex virus, NV1020, in subjects with metastatic colorectal carcinoma to the liver. Hum Gene Ther. 2006;17(12):1214–24.

100. Geevarghese SK, Geller DA, de Haan HA, Horer M, Knoll AE, Mescheder A, Nemunaitis J, Reid TR, Sze DY, Tanabe KK, Tawfik H. Phase I/II study of oncolytic herpes simplex virus NV1020 in patients with extensively pretreated refractory colorectal cancer metastatic to the liver. Hum Gene Ther. 2010;21(9):1119–28.

101. McGeoch DJ, Dalrymple MA, Davison AJ, Dolan A, Frame MC, McNab D, Perry LJ, Scott JE, Taylor P. The complete DNA sequence of the long unique region in the genome of herpes simplex virus type 1. J Gen Virol. 1988;69(Pt 7):1531–74.

102. van de Laar L, Coffer PJ, Woltman AM. Regulation of dendritic cell development by GM-CSF: molecular control and implications for immune homeostasis and therapy. Blood. 2012;119(15):3383–93.

103. Senzer NN, Kaufman HL, Amatruda T, Nemunaitis M, Reid T, Daniels G, Gonzalez R, Glaspy J, Whitman E, Harrington K, Goldsweig H, Marshall T, Love C, Coffin R, Nemunaitis JJ. Phase II clinical trial of a granulocyte-macrophage colony-stimulating factor-encoding, second-generation oncolytic herpesvirus in patients with unresectable metastatic melanoma. J Clin Oncol. 2009;27(34):5763–71.

104. Hu JC, Coffin RS, Davis CJ, Graham NJ, Groves N, Guest PJ, Harrington KJ, James ND, Love CA, McNeish I, Medley LC, Michael A, Nutting CM, Pandha HS, Shorrock CA, Simpson J, et al. A phase I study of OncoVEXGM-CSF, a second-generation oncolytic herpes simplex virus expressing granulocyte macrophage colony-stimulating factor. Clin Cancer Res. 2006;12(22):6737–47.

105. Fukuhara H, Ino Y, Todo T. Oncolytic virus therapy: a new era of cancer treatment at dawn. Cancer Sci. 2016;107(10):1373–9.

106. Gong J, Sachdev E, Mita AC, Mita MM. Clinical development of reovirus for cancer therapy: An oncolytic virus with immune-mediated antitumor activity. World J Methodol. 2016;6(1):25–42.

107. Russell SJ, Federspiel MJ, Peng KW, Tong C, Dingli D, Morice WG, Lowe V, O'Connor MK, Kyle RA, Leung N, Buadi FK, Rajkumar SV, Gertz MA, Lacy MQ, Dispenzieri A. Remission of disseminated cancer after systemic oncolytic virotherapy. Mayo Clin Proc. 2014;89(7):926–33.

108. Hirasawa K, Nishikawa SG, Norman KL, Coffey MC, Thompson BG, Yoon CS, Waisman DM, Lee PW. Systemic reovirus therapy of metastatic cancer in immune-competent mice. Cancer Res. 2003;63(2):348–53.

109. White CL, Twigger KR, Vidal L, De Bono JS, Coffey M, Heinemann L, Morgan R, Merrick A, Errington F, Vile RG, Melcher AA, Pandha HS, Harrington KJ. Characterization of the adaptive and innate immune response to intravenous oncolytic reovirus (Dearing type 3) during a phase I clinical trial. Gene Ther. 2008;15(12):911–20.

110. Simpson GR, Han Z, Liu B, Wang Y, Campbell G, Coffin RS. Combination of a fusogenic glycoprotein, prodrug activation, and oncolytic herpes simplex virus for enhanced local tumor control. Cancer Res. 2006;66(9):4835–42.

111. Yang HT, Zou SS, Zhai LJ, Wang Y, Zhang FM, An LG, Yang GW. Pathogen invasion changes the intestinal microbiota composition and induces innate immune responses in the zebrafish intestine. Fish Shellfish Immunol. 2017; 71:35–42.

112. Mullerad M, Bochner BH, Adusumilli PS, Bhargava A, Kikuchi E, Hui-Ni C, Kattan MW, Chou TC, Fong Y. Herpes simplex virus based gene therapy enhances the efficacy of mitomycin C for the treatment of human bladder transitional cell carcinoma. J Urol. 2005;174(2):741–6.

113. Fechheimer M, Boylan JF, Parker S, Sisken JE, Patel GL, Zimmer SG. Transfection of mammalian cells with plasmid DNA by scrape loading and sonication loading. Proc Natl Acad Sci U S A. 1987;84(23):8463–7.

114. Shintani M, Takahashi G, Hamada M, Okunaga S, Iwai S, Yura Y. Effect of ultrasound on herpes simplex virus infection in cell culture. Virol J. 2011;8:446.

115. Rajani K, Parrish C, Kottke T, Thompson J, Zaidi S, Ilett L, Shim KG, Diaz RM, Pandha H, Harrington K, Coffey M, Melcher A, Vile R. Combination therapy with Reovirus and anti-PD-1 blockade controls tumor growth through innate and adaptive immune responses. Mol Ther. 2016;24(1):166–74.

116. Toyoizumi T, Mick R, Abbas AE, Kang EH, Kaiser LR, Molnar-Kimber KL. Combined therapy with chemotherapeutic agents and herpes simplex virus type 1 ICP34.5 mutant (HSV-1716) in human non-small cell lung cancer. Hum Gene Ther. 1999;10(18):3013–29.

117. Wakimoto H, Fulci G, Tyminski E, Chiocca EA. Altered expression of antiviral cytokine mRNAs associated with cyclophosphamide's enhancement of viral oncolysis. Gene Ther. 2004;11(2):214–23.

118. Ikeda K, Ichikawa T, Wakimoto H, Silver JS, Deisboeck TS, Finkelstein D, GRt H, Louis DN, Bartus RT, Hochberg FH, Chiocca EA. Oncolytic virus therapy of multiple tumors in the brain requires suppression of innate and elicited antiviral responses. Nat Med. 1999;5(8):881–7.

119. Yun CO. Overcoming the extracellular matrix barrier to improve intratumoral spread and therapeutic potential of oncolytic virotherapy. Curr Opin Mol Ther. 2008;10(4):356–61.

120. Fukuhara H, Todo T. Oncolytic herpes simplex virus type 1 and host immune responses. Curr Cancer Drug Targets. 2007;7(2):149–55.

Permissions

All chapters in this book were first published in IMMUNOLOGY, by BioMed Central; hereby published with permission under the Creative Commons Attribution License or equivalent. Every chapter published in this book has been scrutinized by our experts. Their significance has been extensively debated. The topics covered herein carry significant findings which will fuel the growth of the discipline. They may even be implemented as practical applications or may be referred to as a beginning point for another development.

The contributors of this book come from diverse backgrounds, making this book a truly international effort. This book will bring forth new frontiers with its revolutionizing research information and detailed analysis of the nascent developments around the world.

We would like to thank all the contributing authors for lending their expertise to make the book truly unique. They have played a crucial role in the development of this book. Without their invaluable contributions this book wouldn't have been possible. They have made vital efforts to compile up to date information on the varied aspects of this subject to make this book a valuable addition to the collection of many professionals and students.

This book was conceptualized with the vision of imparting up-to-date information and advanced data in this field. To ensure the same, a matchless editorial board was set up. Every individual on the board went through rigorous rounds of assessment to prove their worth. After which they invested a large part of their time researching and compiling the most relevant data for our readers.

The editorial board has been involved in producing this book since its inception. They have spent rigorous hours researching and exploring the diverse topics which have resulted in the successful publishing of this book. They have passed on their knowledge of decades through this book. To expedite this challenging task, the publisher supported the team at every step. A small team of assistant editors was also appointed to further simplify the editing procedure and attain best results for the readers.

Apart from the editorial board, the designing team has also invested a significant amount of their time in understanding the subject and creating the most relevant covers. They scrutinized every image to scout for the most suitable representation of the subject and create an appropriate cover for the book.

The publishing team has been an ardent support to the editorial, designing and production team. Their endless efforts to recruit the best for this project, has resulted in the accomplishment of this book. They are a veteran in the field of academics and their pool of knowledge is as vast as their experience in printing. Their expertise and guidance has proved useful at every step. Their uncompromising quality standards have made this book an exceptional effort. Their encouragement from time to time has been an inspiration for everyone.

The publisher and the editorial board hope that this book will prove to be a valuable piece of knowledge for researchers, students, practitioners and scholars across the globe.

List of Contributors

Ying-Ying Hey
Research School of Biology, Australian National University, Canberra, ACT, Australia
Clem Jones Research Centre for Regenerative Medicine, Bond University, Gold Coast, Queensland, Australia

Helen C. O'Neill
Clem Jones Research Centre for Regenerative Medicine, Bond University, Gold Coast, Queensland, Australia

Benjamin Quah
John Curtin School of Medical Research, Australian National University, Canberra, Australia

Ana Moreno, Ashanty M. Melo and Derek G. Doherty
Paediatrics, Trinity College, the University of Dublin, Dublin, Ireland
Trinity Translational Medicine Institute (TTMI), Trinity College Dublin, Dublin, Ireland

Eleanor J. Molloy
Paediatrics, Trinity College, the University of Dublin, Dublin, Ireland
Trinity Translational Medicine Institute (TTMI), Trinity College Dublin, Dublin, Ireland
Paediatrics, Tallaght Hospital, Dublin, Ireland
Coombe Women and Infants University Hospital, Dublin, Ireland
Neonatology, Our Lady's Children's Hospital, Crumlin, Dublin, Ireland
National Children's Research Centre, Our Lady's Children's Hospital, Crumlin, Dublin, Ireland

Dean Huggard
Paediatrics, Trinity College, the University of Dublin, Dublin, Ireland
Trinity Translational Medicine Institute (TTMI), Trinity College Dublin, Dublin, Ireland
Paediatrics, Tallaght Hospital, Dublin, Ireland
National Children's Research Centre, Our Lady's Children's Hospital, Crumlin, Dublin, Ireland
Department of Paediatrics, Trinity Centre for Health Sciences, Tallaght Hospital, Dublin 24, Ireland

Fiona McGrane, Niamh Lagan, Edna Roche and Joanne Balfe
Paediatrics, Trinity College, the University of Dublin, Dublin, Ireland
Paediatrics, Tallaght Hospital, Dublin, Ireland

Timothy Ronan Leahy
Paediatrics, Trinity College, the University of Dublin, Dublin, Ireland
Immunology, Our Lady's Children's Hospital, Crumlin, Dublin, Ireland

Orla Franklin
Paediatrics, Trinity College, the University of Dublin, Dublin, Ireland
Cardiology, Our Lady's Children's Hospital, Crumlin, Dublin, Ireland

Xi-Yao Huang, Hai-Bo Huang, Xing Zhao, Ning-Ya Li, Zhi-Jian Sun, Ke-Mei Peng and Hua-Zhen Liu
Department of Basic Veterinary Medicine, College of Animal Science and Veterinary Medicine, Huazhong Agricultural University, Wuhan, Hubei 430070, China

Abdur Rahman Ansari
Department of Basic Veterinary Medicine, College of Animal Science and Veterinary Medicine, Huazhong Agricultural University, Wuhan, Hubei 430070, China
Section of Anatomy and Histology, Department of Basic Sciences, College of Veterinary and Animal Sciences (CVAS) Jhang, University of Veterinary and Animal Sciences (UVAS), Lahore, Pakistan

Juming Zhong
Department of Basic Veterinary Medicine, College of Animal Science and Veterinary Medicine, Huazhong Agricultural University, Wuhan, Hubei 430070, China
Department of Anatomy, Physiology and Pharmacology, College of Veterinary Medicine, Auburn University, Auburn, USA

Zhengzhong Xu, Aihong Xia, Xin Li, Zhaocheng Zhu, Chuang Meng and Lin Sun
Jiangsu Key Laboratory of Zoonosis, Yangzhou University, No. 48 Wenhui East Road, Yangzhou 225009, Jiangsu, China

Xiang Chen
Jiangsu Key Laboratory of Zoonosis, Yangzhou University, No. 48 Wenhui East Road, Yangzhou 225009, Jiangsu, China
Jiangsu Co-Innovation Center for Prevention and Control of Important Animal Infectious Diseases and Zoonoses, Yangzhou University, Yangzhou, China

Yechi Shen, Shanshan Jin, Tian Lan, Yuqing Xie, Han Wu and Yuelan Yin
Key Laboratory of Prevention and Control of Biological Hazard Factors (Animal Origin) for Agrifood Safety and Quality, MOA of China, Yangzhou University, Yangzhou, China

Xinan Jiao
Key Laboratory of Prevention and Control of Biological Hazard Factors (Animal Origin) for Agrifood Safety and Quality, MOA of China, Yangzhou University, Yangzhou, China
Jiangsu Co-Innovation Center for Prevention and Control of Important Animal Infectious Diseases and Zoonoses, Yangzhou University, Yangzhou, China

Xiaojia Xu, Yaping Liang, Mingjuan Yin, Yan Zhang, Lingfeng Huang and Jindong Ni
Department of Environmental and Occupational Health, Dongguan Key Laboratory of Environmental Medicine, School of Public Health, Guangdong Medical University, Dongguan 523808, China

Yulian Li and Zuwei Yu
Dalang Community Health Service Centers, Dongguan 523770, China

María Morales, Mayte Gallego, Victor Iraola, Raquel Moya and Jerónimo Carnés
Research & Development, Laboratorios LETI, S.L., Calle del Sol n° 5, 28760 Madrid, Tres Cantos, Spain

Marta Taulés
Centres Científics i Tecnològics, Universitat de Barcelona, Barcelona, Spain

Eliandre de Oliveira
Plataforma de Proteòmica, Parc Científic de Barcelona, Barcelona, Spain

L. E. Amoah, H. B. Abagna, K. Akyea-Mensah, K. A. Kusi and B. A. Gyan
Noguchi Memorial Institute for Medical Research, University of Ghana, Accra, Ghana

A. C. Lo
Noguchi Memorial Institute for Medical Research, University of Ghana, Accra, Ghana
Present address: University Cheikh Anta DIOP, Dakar, Senegal

Masayuki Shiozawa and Satoru Takeda
Department of Obstetrics and Gynecology, Juntendo University Hospital, 3-1-3 Hongo, Bunkyo-ku, Tokyo, Japan

Chuan-Hsin Chang and Yi-Ching Chen
Department of Radiation Therapy and Oncology, Shin Kong Wu Ho-Su Memorial Hospital, No.95, Wenchang Road, Shilin District, Taipei, Taiwan
Department of Research and Development, Johnpro Biotech Inc., 2F., No. 118, Hougang St., Shilin Dist., Taipei City, Taiwan

Yu-Shan Wang
Department of Radiation Therapy and Oncology, Shin Kong Wu Ho-Su Memorial Hospital, No.95, Wenchang Road, Shilin District, Taipei, Taiwan
Department of Research and Development, Johnpro Biotech Inc., 2F., No.118, Hougang St., Shilin Dist.,Taipei City, Taiwan
Institute of Molecular Medicine and Bioengineering, National Chiao Tung University, Room 117 Lab Building 1, 75 Bo-Ai Street, Hsinchu, Taiwan

Mau-Shin Chi
Department of Radiation Therapy and Oncology, Shin Kong Wu Ho-Su Memorial Hospital, No.95, Wenchang Road, Shilin District, Taipei, Taiwan
Institute of Molecular Medicine and Bioengineering, National Chiao Tung University, Room 117 Lab Building 1, 75 Bo-Ai Street, Hsinchu, Taiwan

Kwan-Hwa Chi
Department of Radiation Therapy and Oncology, Shin Kong Wu Ho-Su Memorial Hospital, No.95, Wenchang Road, Shilin District, Taipei, Taiwan

Institute of Veterinary Clinical Science,School of Veterinary Medicine, National Taiwan University, Taipei, Taiwan
Department of Biomedical Imaging and Radiological Sciences, National Yang-Ming University, Taipei, Taiwan

Yi-Chun Huang
Department of Research and Development, Johnpro Biotech Inc., 2F., No.118, Hougang St., Shilin Dist., Taipei City, Taiwan

Hsu-Chao Hao
Department of Biotechnology, Hungkuang University, No. 1018, Sec. 6, Taiwan Boulevard, Shalu District, Taichung City, Taiwan

Yue-Cune Chang
Department of Mathematics, Tamkang University, No.151, Yingzhuan Rd.,Tamsui Dist., New Taipei City, Taiwan

Minna Hietikko, Outi Koskinen, Kaija Laurila and Katri Lindfors
Celiac Disease Research Center, Faculty of Medicine and Life Sciences, University of Tampere, Tampere, Finland

Teea Salmi
Celiac Disease Research Center, Faculty of Medicine and Life Sciences, University of Tampere, Tampere, Finland
Department of Dermatology, Tampere University Hospital, Tampere, Finland

Tuire Ilus
Celiac Disease Research Center, Faculty of Medicine and Life Sciences, University of Tampere, Tampere, Finland
Department of Gastroenterology and Alimentary Tract Surgery, Tampere University Hospital, Tampere, Finland

Katri Kaukinen
Celiac Disease Research Center, Faculty of Medicine and Life Sciences, University of Tampere, Tampere, Finland
Department of Internal Medicine, Tampere University Hospital, Tampere, Finland

Kalle Kurppa
Tampere Center for Child Health Research, University of Tampere, Tampere, Finland

Department of Paediatrics, Tampere University Hospital, Tampere, Finland

Päivi Saavalainen
Department of Medical and Clinical Genetics and the Research Programs Unit, Immunobiology, University of Helsinki, Helsinki, Finland

Heini Huhtala
Faculty of Social Sciences, University of Tampere, Tampere, Finland

Yusuf Omosun, Tankya Simoneaux, Camilla C. Mills, Francis O. Eko and Qing He
Department of Microbiology, Biochemistry, and Immunology, Morehouse School of Medicine, 720 Westview Drive S.W., Atlanta, GA 30310, USA

Khamia Ryans and Danielle N. McKeithen
Department of Microbiology, Biochemistry, and Immunology, Morehouse School of Medicine, 720 Westview Drive S.W., Atlanta, GA 30310, USA
Department of Biology, Clark Atlanta University, Atlanta, GA 30314, USA

Joseph U. Igietseme
Department of Microbiology, Biochemistry, and Immunology, Morehouse School of Medicine, 720 Westview Drive S.W., Atlanta, GA 30310, USA
Centers for Disease Control & Prevention (CDC), Atlanta, GA 30333, USA

Nathan Bowen
Department of Biology, Clark Atlanta University, Atlanta, GA 30314, USA

Carolyn M. Black
Centers for Disease Control & Prevention (CDC), Atlanta, GA 30333, USA

Kristin Paulsen Rye, Steinar Sørnes and Øystein Bruserud
Department of Clinical Science, Lab-building 8.floor, University of Bergen, N-5021 Bergen, Norway

Kurt Hanevik, Kristine Mørch and Nina Langeland
Department of Clinical Science, Lab-building 8.floor, University of Bergen, N-5021 Bergen, Norway
Center for Tropical Infectious Diseases, Haukeland University Hospital, Bergen, Norway

Einar Kristoffersen
Department of Clinical Science, Lab-building 8.floor, University of Bergen, N-5021 Bergen, Norway

Department of immunology and transfusion medicine, Haukeland University Hospital, Bergen, Norway

Staffan Svärd
Department of Cell and Molecular biology, Uppsala University, Uppsala, Sweden

Lothar Marischen, Anne Englert, Anna-Lena Schmitt, Hermann Einsele and Juergen Loeffler
Department of Internal Medicine II, WÜ4i, University Hospital Wuerzburg, Wuerzburg, Germany

Irini A. Doytchinova
Faculty of Pharmacy, Medical University of Sofia, 2 Dunav st, 1000 Sofia, Bulgaria

Darren R. Flower
School of Life and Health Sciences, Aston University, Aston Triangle, Birmingham B4 7ET, UK

Bernhard Banas and Carsten A. Böger
Department of Nephrology, University Medical Center Regensburg, Regensburg, Germany

Gerhard Lückhoff
Dialysis Center Landshut, Landshut, Germany

Bernd Krüger and Bernhard K. Krämer
5th Department of Medicine, University Medical Center Mannheim, Medical Faculty Mannheim of the University Heidelberg, Mannheim, Germany

Sascha Barabas, Julia Batzilla, Hanna Bendfeldt, Anne Rascle and Ludwig Deml
Lophius Biosciences GmbH, Regensburg, Germany

Mathias Schemmerer
Lophius Biosciences GmbH, Regensburg, Germany
Institute of Clinical Microbiology and Hygiene, University of Regensburg, Regensburg, Germany

Josef Köstler and Ralf Wagner
Institute of Clinical Microbiology and Hygiene, University of Regensburg, Regensburg, Germany

Joachim Leicht
Dialysis Center Schwandorf, Schwandorf, Germany

Ekaterina Lebedeva, Alexander Bagaev, Alexey Pichugin, Marina Chulkina and Ravshan Ataullakhanov
National Research Center Institute of Immunology, Federal Medical-Biological Agency of Russia, Moscow, Russia

Andrei Lysenko, Irina Tutykhina, Maxim Shmarov, Denis Logunov and Boris Naroditsky
Federal Research Centre of Epidemiology and Microbiology named after Honorary Academician N.F. Gamaleya, Ministry of Health, Moscow, Russia

Sascha Barabas, Theresa Spindler, Charlotte Tonar, Tamara Lugner, Julia Batzilla, Hanna Bendfeldt and Anne Rascle
Lophius Biosciences GmbH, Am BioPark 13, 93053 Regensburg, Germany

Ludwig Deml
Lophius Biosciences GmbH, Am BioPark 13, 93053 Regensburg, Germany
Institute of Medical Microbiology and Hygiene, University Regensburg, Franz-Josef-Strauss-Allee 11, 93053 Regensburg, Germany

Richard Kiener, Benedikt Asbach and Ralf Wagner
Institute of Medical Microbiology and Hygiene, University Regensburg, Franz-Josef-Strauss-Allee 11, 93053 Regensburg, Germany

Yuta Sugiyama, Yukari Hiraiwa, Yuichiro Hagiya, and Shun-ichiro Ogura
School of Life Science and Technology, Tokyo Institute of Technology, Yokohama, Kanagawa, Japan.

Motowo Nakajima and Tohru Tanaka
SBI Pharma CO., LTD., Roppongi, Tokyo 106-6020, Japan

Meng Xu, Lishuang Guo and Sirui Yang
Department of Pediatric Rheumatology and Allergy, The First Hospital of Jilin University, Changchun 130021, China

Yanfang Jiang
Genetic Diagnosis Center, The First Hospital of Jilin University, Changchun 130021, China

Key Laboratory of Zoonoses Research, Ministry of Education, The First Hospital of Jilin University, Changchun 130021, China
Jiangsu Co-innovation Center for Prevention and Control of Important Animal Infectious Diseases and Zoonoses, Yangzhou 225009, China

Jian Zhang and Yan Zheng
Department of Pediatric, Children's Hospital, Changchun 130021, China

Deying Liu
Department of Pediatric Rheumatology and Immunology, Wuhan Children's Hospital, Tongji Medical College, Huazhong University of Science & Technology, Wuhan 430000, China

Wenqing Ma, Hongbin He and Hongmei Wang
Ruminant Diseases Research Center, Shandong Provincial Key Laboratory of Animal Resistance Biology, College of Life Sciences, Shandong Normal University, Jinan 250014, China

Index

www.ingramcontent.com/pod-product-compliance
Lightning Source LLC
Chambersburg PA
CBHW082033190326
41458CB00010B/3349